ID0819985

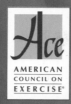

AMERICAN
COUNCIL ON
EXERCISE®

Aerobics Instructor Manual

Manual

The Resource for Group Fitness Instructors

Richard T. Cotton
Managing Editor

Robert L. Goldstein
Editor

American Council on Exercise
San Diego, California

Library of Congress Cataloging-in-Publication Data

Aerobics Instructor Manual: the resource for fitness professionals /
    Richard T. Cotton, managing editor: Robert L. Goldstein, editor—
    2nd ed.
        p. cm.
    Rev. ed. of: Aerobic dance-exercise instructor manual. c1987.
    Includes bibliographical references and index.
    ISBN 0-9618161-3-9: $39.95
        1. Aerobic dancing—Study and teaching—Handbooks, manuals, etc.
        2. Aerobic exercises—Study and teaching—Handbooks, manuals, etc.
I. Cotton, Richard T. (Richard Thomas), 1951-   . II. Goldstein,
Robert l. (Robert Louis), 1946-   . III. Aerobic dance-exercise instructor manual.
RA781.15.A35   1993
613.7'1—dc20   93-28250
                                                                        CIP

ISBN 0-9618161-3-9

EFG

Distributed by:
American Council on Exercise
P.O. Box 910449
San Diego, CA 92191-0449
(619) 535-8227
(619) 535-1778 (FAX)
http://www.acefitness.org

Design: Mires Design, John Ball
Production: Mires Design, Gale Spitzley
Photographer: John Johnson
Anatomical Illustrations: James Staunton
Variations Chapter Coordinator: Karen Kelly Duncanson
Technical Consultants: Karen Kelly Duncanson,
Deborah Ellison, Barbara Gauthier
Glossary: Holli K. Spicer
Index: Theresa Schaffer
Copy Editors: Michelle V. Stoia, Barbara Gauthier
Proofreaders: Michelle V. Stoia, Holli K. Spicer
Chapter Models: Karen Kelly Duncanson, Peter Bissell,
Holli K. Spicer, Ann Buck
Cover Models: Melissa Mayer, Denise Lee-Yohn, Mike
Johnson, Barbara Gauthier, Karen Kelly Duncanson,
Holli K. Spicer
Chapter Lead Models: Richard Cotton, Linda Dillard,
Dee Dorsey, Troy Freeman, Alesia Garcia, Barbara
Gauthier, Mike Johnson, Karen Kelly Duncanson,
Denise Lee-Yohn, Melissa Mayer, Mary Reeves,
Tiffany Rombold, Russ Russell, Mitch Sudy, Karen Spicer

Acknowledgements: To the entire American Council on Exercise
staff for their support and guidance through this process.

Reviewers

Anthony, Jeff, D.O. Physician, general practice, sports medicine; team physician for San Diego State University, the U.S. Men's Olympic Volleyball and the San Diego Sockers; clinical instructor at University of California at San Diego; member of IDEA's board of advisors.

Beasley Bob, Ph.D. Associate professor of exercise physiology, University of South Florida, Tampa; researcher in water exercise and designer of water-specific exercise equipment; water exercise instructor; author of numerous articles on the subject of water exercise.

Bissell, Peter, B.S. Aerobics program director at Premier Athletic and Squash Club, San Diego, California; ACE-certified Aerobics Instructor with 14 years experience teaching a variety of group exercise classes.

Blahnik, Jay, B.S. Owner of Body Dynamics Fitness Instructor Training in Southern California; health education consultant for the American Heart Association; international workshop and master class presenter; featured instructor for the Sports Club Company; ACE-certified Aerobics Instructor and Personal Trainer; ACE Continuing Education Committee and Role Delineation Committee member.

Boyer, John L., M.D., F.A.C.P., F.A.C.C. Author of over 40 professional publications on exercise physiology, sports medicine, heart disease prevention and rehabilitation, early detection of heart disease in children, the treatment of hypertension and cardiovascular adaptations to altitude; consultant, symposium director and participant in health maintenance programs for business and industry; past president of the American College of Sports Medicine.

Buono, Michael J., Ph.D. Professor of human physiology and exercise physiology, San Diego State University; researcher in the area of thermal regulation and sweat gland function during exercise.

Caparosa, Susan, M.A. Coordinator of Project HELPS, Hypertension, Exercise and Lifestyle Program for Seniors, a NIA/NIH-funded research program; designer of fitness programs for women of all ages; certified exercise specialist by the American College of Sports Medicine.

Carter, Lindsay, Ph.D. Professor, San Diego State University, department of physical education; kinesiologist and kinanthropometry consultant.

Chu, Donald A., R.P.T., Ph.D. Founder and director of the Ather Sports Injury Clinic; author of Jumping into Plyometrics and Plyometric Exercises with the Medicine Ball; co-author of *Everybody's Aerobic Book*; chairman of the Executive Council of the Certified Strength & Conditioning Specialist Agency.

Davis, Steven C., Ph.D. Associate professor of exercise science, physical education department, California Polytechnic State University, San Luis Obispo; certified exercise specialist and program director of the American College of Sports Medicine.

Dressendorfer, Rudy, Ph.D., F.A.C.S.M. Professor of human performance and sport and director of the exercise science laboratory, New Mexico Highlands University, Las Vegas, New Mexico; certified preventive and rehabilitative exercise program director by the American College of Sports Medicine.

Ellison, Deborah, R.P.T. Private practitioner in San Diego, California specializing in ergonomics and women's health care issues; video consultant; author of *Advanced Exercise Design*; founder of Movement that Matters™; member of NIKE's national training team, Body Elite.

Herbert, David L., J.D. Attorney at law; president of Professional Reports Corporation & PRC Publishing, Inc.; co-editor, *The Exercise Standards and Malpractice*

Reporter and *The Sports Medicine Standards and Malpractice Reporter*, author of *Legal Aspects of Preventive & Rehabilitative Exercise Programs* and *Legal Aspects of Sports Medicine*; medical/legal editor for *The Physician and Sportsmedicine*.

Horwitz, Louis, M.D., F.A.C.E.P. Director, Community Hospital of Bedford, Emergency Department; board certified in emergency medicine; fellow of the American College of Emergency Physicians; teaching appointment at University Hospitals of Cleveland.

Koeberle, Brian E., J.D. Sports/entertainment attorney; director of operations for the Major League Baseball Players Alumni Association; author of *The Legal Aspects of Personal Fitness Training* and various sports/fitness law articles; lecturer on various sports/fitness law topics.

Meshkov, Sasha, M.S. Founder and director of Sasha & Company—The Workout Studio, Denver, Colorado and Professional Fitness Instructor Training, one of the first instructor training schools accredited by the American Council on Exercise; United States head judge, National Aerobic Championships; World Aerobic Championships judge; ACE Aerobics Certification Examination Committee member.

Midtlyng, Joanna, Ph.D. Professor of physical education and researcher in water exercise at Ball State University, Muncie, Indiana; author of several professional aquatic books; director of the Aquatic Council Instruction & Credentialing Advisory Committee for AAHPERD; recipient of the Honor Award by the Association for Research, Administration, Professional Councils & Societies (ARAPCS).

Minear, Alisa, M.S., R.D. Director of nutrition services and health education at Scripps Clinic and Research Foundations; clinical dietitian specializing in weight control at Scripps Clinic; adjunct clinical instructor for Loma Linda University; writer and lecturer; member of the American Dietetic Association.

Sallis, James F., Ph.D. Professor of psychology, San Diego State University, assistant adjunct professor of pediatrics, University of California at San Diego; co-author of *Health and Human Behavior*.

Wiswell, Robert, A., Ph.D. Associate professor of exercise sciences and department chair, University of Southern California, Los Angeles, California; research associate, Andrus Gerontology Center; author of numerous papers, research abstracts and books on exercise and aging, exercise and pregnancy and cardiopulmonary and metabolic responses to physical activity.

Contents

⑤ Endurance
Body Comp.

Foreword

The benefits of regular physical activity on the body and mind have been intuitively known for hundreds of years. With each decade we have learned more about the importance and value of exercise, pushing our knowledge past intuition to lay a scientific foundation. The U.S. Department of Health and Human Services has identified physical activity and fitness as a critical activity in our nation's health promotion and disease prevention plan. And recently, in 1996, the Surgeon General's Report on Physical Activity and Health found that regular physical activity reduces the risk of developing or dying from some of the leading causes of illness and death in the United States. Backed by this kind of reinforcement, it is unlikely that the value of, and support for, physical fitness will decline.

Despite this new support, the known benefits and the ongoing coordinated efforts of institutions and the organizations, a mere 20 percent of the population in America exercise regularly. The task of motivating millions of people to exercise regularly is not and likely will not be an easy one. We know that exercisers tend to be young, educated and affluent. In order to reach older, less educated and less affluent groups, we will need to readdress our approach and capitalize on known techniques to motivate and maintain exercise compliance.

Of all the variables that can affect exercise compliance, perhaps the most important is the quality of the exercise instructor. Research has verified that qualified, enthusiastic instructors can improve exercise compliance among their participants more than any other factor influencing compliance. Lending credence to this belief are the many effective exercise practices incorporated by qualified instructors such as prescribing progressive exercise to minimize injury, ensuring variety and fun in the routine, establishing realistic goals, providing periodic evaluations, keeping adequate records and recognizing accomplishments through rewards and recognition.

Perhaps this is why each day, the American Council on Exercise hears more about clubs looking for quality instructors and requiring degrees in health and physical education or certification by credible organizations for employment. As the demand for quality exercise increases, the exercising public and the fitness employer will demand better qualified instructors. Fitness professionals will be expected to be conversant with the information provided in this publication, experienced in the techniques and skills required to implement programs and current on emerging technologies and programs.

The fitness industry will continue to grow. By the year 2005, the U.S. Department of Labor predicts a 14 to 24 percent increase in the number of people employed as fitness instructors. With this growth will come innumerable opportunities for those who believe in fitness to become a part of this profession that dedicates itself to the health and well being of others. If you are or desire to be a part of this growing force of change, I hope that this publication can assist your efforts. The task is formidable. The cause is great.

Sheryl Marks Brown
Executive Director
American Council on Exercise

Introduction

This second edition of the *ACE Aerobics Instructor Manual* began nearly 12 months ago with a comprehensive review of the skills and knowledge needed by group fitness instructors to perform their job with a basic level of competency. The outcome of this review, referred to as a role delineation, was used as the basis for developing the content of this manual.

This new manual presents the most current, complete picture of the knowledge, instructional techniques and professional responsibilities group fitness instructors need to teach safe and effective exercise. It is designed to serve as a study aid for exam candidates preparing for the ACE certification exam and as a comprehensive fitness resource for new and veteran group fitness instructors.

It is important to note, however, that the scope of information presented in this manual will not exactly match the scope of information tested in the ACE certification exam. Exam candidates should refer to the Exam Content Outline in Appendix B for a detailed syllabus of information covered in the certification exam. In addition, ACE acknowledges various experience and skill levels among group fitness exam candidates. As such, we encourage candidates lacking the practical skills and experience related to teaching aerobics to take advantage of supervised training programs, such as the training programs accredited by ACE, to prepare for the ACE examinations.

Four completely new chapters have been added to the manual to reflect new areas of emphasis and changes in focus in the fitness industry. They address: biomechanics and kinesiology; adherence and motivation; special populations and health concerns; and new variations to the traditional aerobics class. The remaining 11 chapters have been completely revised and updated to bring you the latest insights and applications of current fitness research. Throughout the chapters, reference tools are provided to help readers locate subjects quickly and easily. Each chapter opens with "In this Chapter," a bulleted list of the primary topics addressed. These topics appear throughout the chapter in the right margin for easy referencing.

In Part I of the manual, Scientific Foundations, readers learn the basics of cardiorespiratory, metabolic, neuromuscular and environmental exercise physiology and get a detailed review of the cardiorespiratory and nervous systems and musculoskeletal anatomy. Chapter 3, Biomechanics and Applied Kinesiology, examines the critical relationship between biomechanics and kinesiology with regard to safe and effective exercise. Excellent detail of the function of every major muscle in the body is presented along with strength and flexibility exercises. To follow up, a very thorough overview of basic nutrition as it applies to both health maintenance and weight control is presented in Chapter 4.

If Part I is the foundation from which to acquire a solid knowledge base, Part II offers the "nuts and bolts" of the group fitness instructor profession. Assessment, Programming and Instruction reviews the application of the exercise science principles presented in Part I to the assessment, design and leading of an aerobics class. Chapter 5, Health Screening, presents the most up-to-date information related to the preexercise screening of fitness clients. Chapter 6, Fitness Testing and Aerobic Programming, demonstrates a battery of fitness tests that are easy to administer and concludes with the basics of aerobic exercise programming including type, intensity, frequency and progression of activity.

In Chapters 7 and 8, teaching strategies, choreography and music selection are discussed and then implemented in a detailed review of the critical components of designing and leading a group fitness class. Variations: From Step to Strength Training, Chapter 9, presents the basics of programming for six of the newest and hottest variations to the traditional group fitness class: step, water fitness, flexibility, strength, circuit and funk.

Catering to individual needs of exercisers is and will continue to be a challenging task for group fitness instructors. Part III, Individual Needs, examines a wide range of issues related to the varied needs of exercisers. Early on, you'll read about techniques to motivate your clients and keep them on track with their exercise programs. Then you'll learn how to personally tailor programs for exercisers with common health challenges such as cardiovascular disease, diabetes and arthritis, and how to create programs for specific groups of people such as older adults, children and individuals with hearing impairments. To close the section, we've devoted an entire chapter to exercise and pregnancy. This chapter offers a nice application of exercise science and obstetrics to group exercise programming.

Part IV, Instructor Responsibilities, the fourth and final section of the manual, provides information on the prevention, detection and treatment of musculoskeletal injuries, basic emergency procedures and the legal and professional responsibilities of group fitness instructors. While group fitness instructors may not need to draw upon this information on a daily basis, sound knowledge, judgment and application of these principles are essential to your future success in this dynamic field.

Richard T. Cotton, MA
Vice President, Publications
American Council on Exercise

Aerobics Instructor Manual

The Resource for Group Fitness Instructors

Part 1
Scientific Foundations

Chapter 1

Exercise Physiology

By Christine L. Wells

Bioenergetics of exercise

- Adenosine triphospate (ATP)
- The phosphagen system
- Aerobic and anaerobic production of ATP
- Muscles and metabolism

The neuromuscular system

- Types of muscular contractions
- Muscular response to training

The cardiovascular respiratory systems

- Carrying, delivering and extracting oxygen
- Responses to and benefits of aerobic exercise

Environmental considerations

- Exercising in the heat
- Exercising in the cold
- Exercising at high altitudes

The versatility of human movement is staggering to consider. The structure and function of the body allows an extraordinarily wide range of possible movements requiring complex mechanisms of neuromuscular coordination and metabolism. For example the human body is capable of movements requiring large bursts of energy over very brief periods of time and movements requiring low levels of energy over prolonged periods of time. Knowledge of exercise physiology, the focus of this chapter, is essential to understand these functions.

Christine L. Wells, Ph.D., professor of exercise science and physical education at Arizona State University, is a widely recognized authority on women and sports. She has been president of the Research Consortium of the American Alliance for Health, Physical Education, Recreation and Dance (AAHPERD), vice president of education of the American College of Sports Medicine (ACSM), and a member of the IDEA board of advisors. Dr. Wells is the author of Women, Sport, and Performance: A Physiological Perspective.

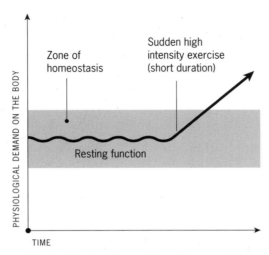

a. High physiological demand disrupts homeostasis.

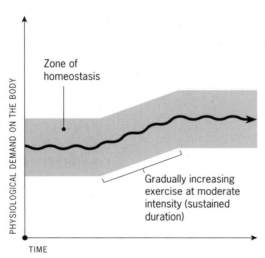

b. Low to moderate physiological demand allows re-establishment of homeostasis at a higher state.

Figure 1.1

The concept of homeostasis.

Exercise physiology is the study of how the body functions during exercise. Such knowledge provides the basis for understanding how the body functions at rest, how these functions change during exercise, and how the body adapts to physical training. When the body is at rest, physiological functions are basically in a state of equilibrium or balance. This state of stability is known as **homeostasis**. An easy way to envision homeostasis is to consider the concept of supply and demand: When at rest, the normal, healthy body is functioning comfortably and physiological demands are easily met. The body is experiencing little or no stress and one feels comfortable. Although defined as a stable state, homeostasis is not a static or unchanging state; rather, homeostasis is a dynamic state of being that requires the continuous production of energy and the removal of metabolic waste products even though metabolic processes are proceeding at a low rate of function when the body is at rest.

Fig. 1.1 illustrates that commencement of exercise disrupts the body's resting state of homeostasis. Movement patterns requiring a sudden burst of energy for relatively short periods are extremely stressful, placing such high metabolic demands on the body that the re-establishment of homeostasis at a higher level of function is impossible (Fig. 1.1a). Such forms of exercise can only be carried out for brief periods of time. Less demanding movement patterns that are begun gradually and require only a moderate amount of energy production over a sustained period, may allow the person to re-establish a new level of homeostasis (Fig. 1.1b). When exercise is terminated, physiological responses gradually return to their original resting level of homeostasis. A person's level of physical fitness largely determines the level of exercise intensity at which homeostasis can be re-established. A physically fit person can re-establish relative homeostasis over a wider range of exercise intensity levels than a less fit person.

PHYSICAL FITNESS

Physical fitness is a complex concept that has different meanings to different people. In this manual, **physical fitness** refers to the capacity of the heart, blood vessels, lungs and muscles to function at a high level of efficiency. One who is physically fit has an enhanced functional capacity that allows for a high **quality of life**.

Although a somewhat vague phrase, quality of life generally implies an overall positive feeling and enthusiasm for life, and the ability to do enriching and enjoyable activities without fatigue or exhaustion. A high level of physical fitness enables people to perform required daily tasks without fatigue, thus enabling participation in additional pleasurable activities for personal enjoyment. As physiological or functional capacity increases, one's capacity for physical activity or exercise increases. In other words, a person can lift heavier weights or run farther or faster—in short, participate in more strenuous activities. Being physically fit makes possible a lifestyle that the unfit cannot enjoy. Increased physical fitness is often reflected by physiological adaptations, such as a lowered heart rate during a standardized exercise test or an improved ability to mobilize and use body fuels. A high level of physical fitness suggests optimal physical performance and good health.

There are five major components of physical fitness. (Note, components are health-related as opposed to skill-related.) The development of a high degree of **motor skill** is sometimes confused with physical fitness, but these two attributes are not necessarily related to each other. A highly skilled person may have a low level of physical fitness, and the reverse may also be true. Motor skill (sometimes referred to as motor performance or motor fitness) is thought to be related to such attributes as agility, balance and coordination—terms that defy precise definition.

The five components of physical fitness are:

1. **Muscular strength**. The maximal force a muscle or muscle group can exert during contraction.

2. **Muscular endurance**. The ability of a muscle or muscle group to exert force against a resistance over a sustained period of time. Muscular endurance is assessed by measuring the length of time (duration) a muscle can exert force without fatigue, or by measuring the number of times (repetitions) that a given task can be performed without fatigue.

3. **Cardiovascular** or **cardiorespiratory endurance** (sometimes referred to as aerobic power or **aerobic fitness**). The capacity of the heart, blood vessels and lungs to deliver nutrients and oxygen to the working muscles and tissues during sustained exercise and to remove the metabolic waste products that would result in fatigue. Efficient functioning of the cardiorespiratory system is essential for optimal enjoyment of vigorous physical activities, such as running, swimming and cycling. This component is also important to good health. The performance of regular, moderately intense aerobic exercise is the key to developing and maintaining an efficient cardiorespiratory system.

4. **Flexibility**. The ability to move joints through their normal full range of motion (ROM). An adequate degree of flexibility is important to prevent injury and to maintain body mobility.

5. **Body composition**. Body composition refers to the makeup of the body using the concept of a two-component model: lean body mass and body fat. The **lean body mass** consists of the muscles, bones, nervous tissue, skin, blood and organs. These tissues have a high metabolic rate and make a direct, positive contribution to energy production during exercise. **Body fat** or adipose tissue represents that component of the body whose primary role is to store energy for later use. Body fat does not contribute in a direct sense to exercise performance. Body fat is further classified into essential body fat and storage body fat.

Chapter 1

Essential body fat is that amount of fat thought to be necessary for maintenance of life and reproductive function; 3 percent to 5 percent body fat is generally thought to be essential for men, and 8 percent to 12 percent for women. (Percent body fat refers to its portion of total body weight.) Storage fat is contained in the fatty deposits or fat pads found under the skin **(subcutaneous fat)** and deep inside the body **(internal fat)**. A large amount of storage fat is considered excess fat and is referred to as obesity.

BIOENERGETICS OF EXERCISE

he body's cells require a continuous supply of energy in order to function. Ultimately, the food eaten supplies this energy. However, cells do not directly use the energy contained in the food eaten, rather they need a chemical compound called **adenosine triphosphate (ATP)**.

ATP is the immediately usable form of chemical energy needed for cellular function, including muscular contraction.

The foods people eat are made up of carbohydrates, fats and proteins. The process of digestion breaks these nutrients down to their simplest components (**glucose**, **fatty acids** and **amino acids**, respectively), which are absorbed into the blood and transported to metabolically active cells, such as muscle, nerve or liver cells. These components either enter a metabolic pathway to produce ATP, or are stored in body tissues for later use (Fig. 1.2).

Some of the ATP formed is used immediately to carry on cellular function, and some is stored in the cells for future use. However, the body's storage capacity for ATP is quite limited, and therefore, most excess food energy is stored in another form. For example, excess glucose will be stored as **glycogen** in muscle or liver cells.

Figure 1.2

Foods consumed ultimately produce the chemical energy required for cellular function.

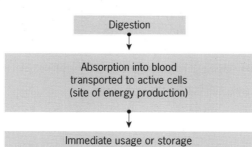

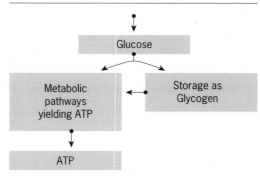

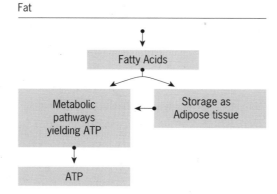

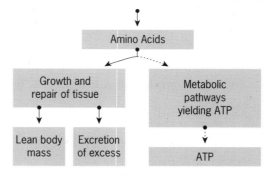

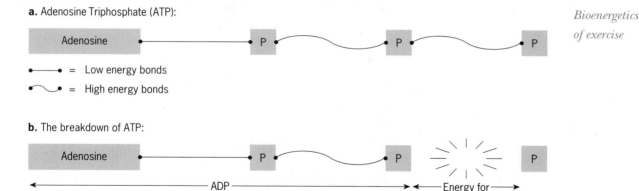

a. Adenosine Triphosphate (ATP):

•—————• = Low energy bonds

•⌇⌇⌇⌇• = High energy bonds

b. The breakdown of ATP:

ATP → ADP + energy for biological work + P

(ADP = Adenosine Diphosphate)

Figure 1.3

The ATP molecule.

Fatty acids that are not immediately used for ATP production will be stored as **adipose tissue** (body fat). In contrast, relatively little of the protein (amino acids) one eats is used for energy production. Instead, it is used for the growth or repair of cellular structures, or is excreted in waste products.

ATP—The Immediate Energy Source

ATP is a complicated chemical structure made up of a substance called adenosine and three simpler groups of atoms called phosphate groups (P). Special high-energy bonds (~) exist between two of the phosphate groups (Fig. 1.3a). Breaking the terminal phosphate bond, a high-energy bond, releases energy (E) that the cell uses directly to perform its cellular function. The specific cellular function performed depends on the cell type. In a muscle cell, the breakdown of ATP results in mechanical work known as muscular contraction. All "biological work" requires the breakdown of ATP (Fig. 1.3b).

ATP can be stored in the cells. The largest stores are found in cells with the highest metabolic activity—in the cells that need ATP most. Even so, the immediately available energy for muscle contraction is extremely limited—sufficient for only a few seconds of muscular work. Therefore, ATP must be continuously resynthesized to sus-tain muscular contraction for more than a few seconds. ATP can be resynthesized in several ways—immediately with the phosphagen system, somewhat more slowly with the anaerobic production of ATP from carbohydrate, or still more slowly with the aerobic production of ATP from either carbohydrate or fat.

The Phosphagen System. **Creatine phosphate (CP)** is another high-energy phosphate compound found in close association with ATP. Together, these compounds are referred to as the **phosphagens**. When the high-energy phosphate bond in CP is broken down, the released energy is immediately used to resynthesize ATP from the available products of ATP breakdown. Consequently, as rapidly as ATP is broken down for muscular contraction, it is reformed from **ADP (adenosine diphosphate)** and P (the phosphate group broken off from ATP) by the energy released from the breakdown of CP. This process is shown in Fig. 1.4.

The total amount of ATP and CP stored in the muscle is very small, and thus the amount of energy available for muscular contraction is extremely limited. In fact, there is probably enough energy available from the phosphagens for only about 10 seconds of all-out exertion. However, this energy is instantaneously available for muscular contraction, and

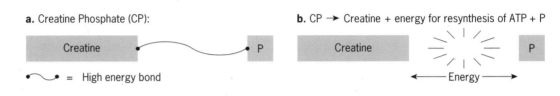

Figure 1.4

The immediate resynthesis of ATP by CP.

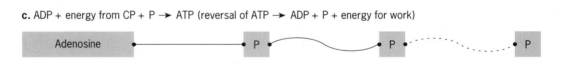

therefore is essential at the onset of physical activity, and during short-term, high-intensity activities such as sprinting 50 yards, performing a weight-lifting movement, or leaping across a stage.

In summary, the following **coupled reactions** allow for the release of energy from ATP for biological work, and the instantaneous resynthesis of ATP using the energy available from the breakdown of CP:

1. ATP → ADP + P + E *(energy for work)*

2. CP → C + P + E

(energy for ATP resynthesis in 3)

3. ADP + P + E → ATP

The ATP-CP system is referred to as the **phosphagen system**. Because oxygen is not required in the above process, the phosphagen system is an anaerobic pathway.

Anaerobic Production of ATP From Carbohydrates. The anaerobic production of ATP from carbohydrate sources is known as **anaerobic glycolysis. Anaerobic** means without the presence of oxygen, and **glycolysis** refers to the breakdown of glucose, or its storage form, glycogen. Thus, anaerobic glycolysis is a metabolic pathway that does not require oxygen and whose purpose is to transfer the bond energy contained in glucose (or glycogen) to the formation of ATP.

Anaerobic glycolysis is capable of producing ATP quite rapidly, and thus is required when energy (ATP) is needed to perform activities requiring large bursts of energy over somewhat longer periods of time than the phosphagen system will al-

low. This metabolic pathway occurs within the main body of the cell and involves the incomplete breakdown of glucose (or glycogen) to a simpler substance called **lactic acid (LA)**. In this process, bond energy is made available to form 2 units of ATP:

4a. Glucose → 2 ATP + 2 LA + heat

4b. Glycogen → 3 ATP + 2 LA + heat

Equation 4a indicates that 1 unit of glucose—the digested component of carbohydrate foods—breaks down without the presence of oxygen to yield 2 units of ATP and 2 units of LA. When glycogen (the storage form of glucose) is broken down, 3 units of ATP are formed. This is one reason why glycogen is the preferred fuel during high-intensity exercise.

Some energy is always lost in metabolic processes. This energy represents lost or "uncoupled energy" and is represented in the above formulas as heat. Because lactic acid is a simpler form of glucose that still contains significant bond energy, anaerobic glycolysis is considered an "incomplete" or partial combustion of glucose.

The formation of LA poses a significant problem because when it accumulates in large amounts, it is associated with muscle fatigue. If the removal of lactic acid by the circulatory system cannot keep pace with its production in the active muscles, temporary muscle fatigue occurs with painful symptoms usually referred to as "the burn." Thus, anaerobic glycolysis can only be used to a limited extent during sustained activity.

Aerobic Production of ATP From Carbohydrates or Fats. The aerobic production of ATP is used for activities requiring sustained energy production. Since **aerobic** means in the presence of oxygen, aerobic metabolic pathways require a continuous supply of oxygen delivered by the circulatory system. Without oxygen, these pathways fail to produce ATP. In the aerobic metabolism of carbohydrates, glucose (or glycogen) is broken down in the presence of oxygen (O_2) to yield approximately 36 units of ATP, carbon dioxide (CO_2), water (H_2O), and heat (lost energy):

5. Glucose + O_2 → 36 ATP + CO_2 + H_2O + heat

Aerobic glycolysis is considered the complete oxidation of glucose (or glycogen) because CO_2 and H_2O (unlike LA) do not contain additional bond energy. This metabolic pathway, called **aerobic glycolysis** or **oxidative glycolysis**, occurs within highly specialized cell structures called the **mitochondria**. Mitochondria, often called the powerhouses of the cell, contain specific enzymes (**oxidative enzymes**) needed by the cell to utilize oxygen. This highly efficient metabolic process—note the large amount of ATP produced for each unit of glucose oxidized—is limited mainly by the capacity of the cardiorespiratory system to deliver oxygen to the active cells.

Aerobic pathways are also available to break down fatty acids (the digested component of dietary fat) for the production of ATP:

6. Fatty Acid + O_2 → 129 ATP + CO_2 + H_2O + heat

This metabolic pathway, called **fatty acid oxidation**, also occurs within the mitochondria and requires a continuous supply of oxygen (as does aerobic glycolysis). The aerobic metabolism of fat yields a very large amount of ATP; therefore, fat is said to have a high caloric density. A **calorie** is a unit of energy. Fat yields 9 **kilocalories** per gram compared to 4 kilocalories per gram

of glucose. That is why body fat is such an excellent source of stored energy. (Note: 1,000 calories equals 1 kilocalorie [kcal]).

During rest, the body uses both glucose and fatty acid for energy production via aerobic pathways. The cardiorespiratory system can easily supply the oxygen necessary for this low rate of energy metabolism. With exercise, however, supplying the required amount of oxygen rapidly enough becomes more difficult. Because glucose metabolism requires less oxygen than fatty acid metabolism, the body will use more glucose for energy production and less fat as exercise intensity increases. Significant amounts of fatty acid will be used to produce energy only when relatively low-intensity exercise is sustained over a long period (20 minutes or more), because the sympathetic nervous system must stimulate the release of fatty acids into the blood from fat storage sites (adipose tissue) before fatty acid oxidation can occur. In summary, with low-intensity, long-duration exercise, aerobic metabolism uses fatty acids as the primary fuel source. With higher intensity-shorter duration exercise, the primary fuel source for aerobic metabolism is glucose (or glycogen).

ATP and the Continuum of Human Movement

The human body is capable of explosive, powerful movements as well as sustained, less powerful movements. Sprinting, jumping and throwing are examples of brief, high-intensity movement. Walking and jogging are characteristic of sustained, low-intensity movement. Of course, many movements are somewhere between these extremes.

Often sports and dance combine movements requiring powerful jumps or sprints with slower, less intense movements. This continuum of human movement is almost ideally matched with the continuum of energy production. Extremely intense, powerful muscular contractions (for example, an all-out sprint for 100 yards) require a metabolic system that provides energy instantaneously, (i.e., the rate of energy production must be extremely high). Unfortunately, an extremely high rate of energy production cannot be maintained very long; therefore, the total amount of energy produced is relatively low. (The total amount of energy produced is referred to as **capacity**.) The phosphagen system is characterized by a very rapid rate of ATP production, but its total capacity for ATP production is very limited.

Slightly less intense exercise can be sustained somewhat longer. For example, running a quarter-mile would require a metabolic system capable of supplying energy rapidly—not as fast as the phosphagen system, but more rapidly than required for slower, sustained activities. Such a metabolic system is provided by anaerobic glycolysis, which can supply energy at a high rate and has a higher capacity than the phosphagen system.

The aerobic forms of ATP production—aerobic glycolysis and fatty acid oxidation—are appropriate for slower, more sustained activities, such as walking, jogging and other forms of aerobic exercise performed over a much longer time. Aerobic metabolism has an almost unlimited capacity for total energy production given certain conditions, but at a lower rate because it cannot supply energy very rapidly.

Metabolic pathways are not mutually exclusive. At any moment in time, these pathways are working simultaneously to produce the ATP the body requires. The physiological demands of the activities one performs determine which metabolic system predominates. In other words, the relative proportion of energy derived

from each system varies with the type of movements one performs. In general, slow, low-intensity physical activities are performed using primarily aerobic processes, and fast, high-intensity physical activities are performed using primarily anaerobic processes.

Comparison of Anaerobic and Aerobic Production of ATP

The metabolic pathways described above also differ in several other ways. As explained above, although the phosphagens are available for immediate use, total energy production is extremely limited. This system of ATP production is limited mainly by the supply of CP available in the muscles.

The primary advantage of anaerobic glycolysis is that it can be mobilized almost instantaneously because oxygen is not required. However, compared with aerobic pathways, relatively little ATP is formed per unit of glucose substrate utilized (i.e., 2 units of ATP are formed for each unit of glucose used). Therefore, this is not a very efficient use of the glycogen stored in the muscles or liver. In addition, lactic acid (LA), a substance highly associated with muscle fatigue, occurs as a by-product of anaerobic ATP production. The primary limiting factor of anaerobic glycolysis is the amount of LA that can be tolerated before exhaustion occurs. Finally, since only glucose (or glycogen) can be used as a **substrate,** a secondary limiting factor is substrate depletion.

Aerobic metabolism produces ATP much more slowly than the above pathways because it requires a continuous supply of oxygen to the metabolically active cells. This is its major limitation. Another possible limitation of aerobic glycolysis is substrate (glycogen) depletion, which probably will not occur until 2 or more hours of continuous exercise have occurred. The aerobic production of ATP is more efficient than the other metabolic pathways because it yields a considerably higher amount of ATP per unit of substrate (glucose or fat) used. The only disadvantage of aerobic glycolysis or fatty acid oxidation is that the rate of ATP production is limited by the rate of oxygen delivery to the mitochondria and by the capacity of the cardiorespiratory and vascular systems. Table 1.1 presents a comparison of the aerobic and anaerobic systems of ATP production.

Muscles and Metabolism

Muscles are composed of several kinds of fibers that differ in their ability to utilize the metabolic pathways outlined above. **Fast twitch (FT) fibers** are rather poorly equipped in terms of the oxygen delivery system, but have an outstanding capacity for the phosphagen system and a very high capacity for anaerobic glycolysis. Therefore, FT fibers are specialized for anaerobic metabolism. They are recruited by the nervous system predominantly for rapid, powerful movements, such as jumping, throwing and sprinting.

Slow twitch (ST) fibers, on the other hand, are exceptionally well-equipped for oxygen delivery and have a high quantity of aerobic or oxidative enzymes. Although they do not have a highly developed mechanism for use of the phosphagens or anaerobic glycolysis, ST fibers have a large number of mitochondria, and consequently, are particularly well-designed for use of aerobic glycolysis and fatty acid oxidation. Thus, ST fibers are recruited primarily for low-intensity, longer duration activities, such

Bioenergetics of exercise

Table 1.1

COMPARISON OF ANAEROBIC AND AEROBIC SYSTEMS OF ATP PRODUCTION

Anaerobic Systems	Rate of ATP Production	Substrate	Capacity of System	Major Limitation	Major Use
Phosphagens (stored ATP & CP)	Very rapid rate	Creatine phosphate (CP)	Very limited ATP production	Very limited supply of CP	Very high-intensity, short-duration sprint activities. Predominates during activities of 1–10 seconds.
Anaerobic glycolysis (GLU → ATP + LA)	Rapid metabolic rate	Blood glucose Glycogen	Limited ATP production	Lactic acid by-product causes rapid fatigue	High-intensity, short duration activities. Predominates during activities of 1–3 minutes.

Aerobic Systems	Rate of ATP Production	Substrate	Capacity of System	Major Limitation	Major Use
Aerobic glycolysis	Slow metabolic rate	Blood glucose Glycogen	Unlimited ATP production	Relatively slow rate of oxygen delivery to cells Glycogen Storage	Lower intensity, longer duration, endurance activities. Predominates during activities longer than 3 minutes.
Fatty acid oxidation	Slow metabolic rate	Fatty acids	Unlimited ATP production	Relatively slow rate of oxygen delivery to cells Large amount of O_2 needed	Lower intensity, longer duration, endurance activities. Fatty acid oxidation predominates after about 20 minutes of continuous activity.

A motor neuron

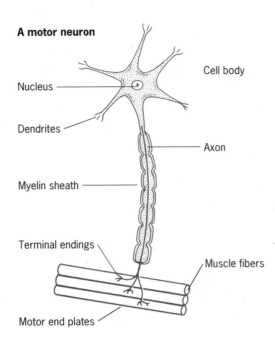

Figure 1.5

Basic anatomical structure of a neuron (or nerve cell) and motor end plate.

as walking, jogging and swimming.

Persons who excel in activities characterized by sudden bursts of energy, but who tire relatively rapidly, probably have a high percentage of FT fibers. Persons who are best at lower intensity, endurance activities probably have a large percentage of ST fibers. Most people have roughly equal percentages of both fiber types. There are also a number of "intermediate" muscle fibers that have a fairly high capacity for both fast anaerobic and slow aerobic movements.

Muscle fiber distribution (fast twitch, intermediate, or slow twitch) is determined by genetic makeup. This is not to say, however, that metabolic capacity is unresponsive to activity lifestyle. All three types of muscle fibers are highly trainable; that is, they are capable of adapting to the specific metabolic demands placed on them. If a person regularly engages in low-intensity endurance activities, improvement is seen in aerobic capacity. Although all three types of muscle fibers will show some improvement in aerobic ability, the ST fibers will be most responsive to this kind of training and will show the largest improvement

in aerobic capacity. If, on the other hand, short-duration, high-intensity exercise like interval training is pursued, other metabolic pathways will be emphasized, enhancing the capabilities of the FT fibers to perform anaerobically. ST fibers will be less responsive to this kind of training.

It is important for physical fitness professionals to have a thorough understanding of the different metabolic systems in order to prescribe specific exercise programs that will enable participants to achieve desired results. As discussed, exercise intensity and duration is directly related to the continuum of metabolic pathways and movement patterns. For example, prescribing quick, explosive movements specific to the use of the phosphagens and anaerobic glycolysis will be ineffective if the goal of the exercise program is to develop cardiorespiratory endurance. This concept, known as **exercise specificity**, is probably the single most important principle of exercise physiology to understand.

THE NEUROMUSCULAR SYSTEM

Exercise instructors need to understand how a motor skill is executed. To do so requires a basic appreciation of the neuromuscular system, which includes both the nervous system and the skeletal muscle system. The nervous system is responsible for coordinating movement. It is possible for a person to have well-developed muscles and still have poor coordination.

Basic Organization of the Nervous System

The basic anatomical unit of the nervous system is the **neuron**, or **nerve cell**. There are two kinds of neurons, sensory and motor. **Sensory neurons** convey electrical impulses from sensory organs in the periphery (such as the skin) to the spinal cord and brain (called the **central nervous** system). **Motor neurons** conduct impulses from the central nervous system (CNS) to the periphery. Because the motor neurons carry electrical impulses from the CNS to the muscle cells, they signal the muscles to contract or to relax and, therefore, regulate muscular movement. The endings of the motor neuron connect, or synapse, with muscle cells in the periphery of the body. This motor neuron—muscle cell synapse is called the neuromuscular junction or **motor end plate**. (Fig. 1.5 shows a motor neuron and motor end plate.) The basic functional unit of the neuromuscular system is the **motor unit**, which consists of one motor neuron and the muscle cells that it innervates. Motor units are arranged according to muscle fiber type. A neuron capable of conducting nervous impulses very rapidly will synapse with the cells of FT muscle fibers. The cells of ST muscle fibers will be controlled by somewhat slower conducting neurons.

Basic Organization of the Muscular System

The skeletal muscle cell is a complicated organ and is described only briefly

here. Basically, the muscle is entirely surrounded by connective tissue that extends from the tendon, which connects the muscle to the bone. Various sublayers of connective tissue divide each muscle into bundles of individual muscle cells. The connective tissues provide an important element of strength and structural integrity to the muscular system and are thought to be involved with delayed onset muscle soreness (DOMS).

An individual muscle cell is composed of many thread-like protein strands called **myofibrils** (Fig. 1.6), which contain the contractile proteins. The basic functional unit of the myofibril is the **sarcomere**. Within the sarcomere are two protein myofilaments: the thick myofilament is **myosin** and the thinner myofilament is **actin**. The myosin and actin myofilaments are arranged to interdigitate in a prescribed, regular way, revealing a pattern of alternating light and dark bands or striations within the sarcomere. Tiny projections called **cross-bridges** extend from the myosin myofilaments toward the actin myofilaments.

According to the **sliding filament theory**,

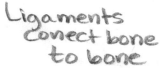

Figure 1.6

Muscle organization.

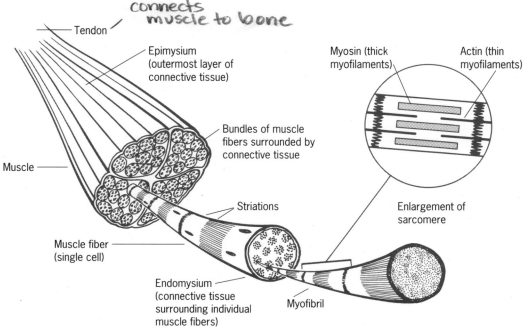

muscular contraction occurs when the cross-bridges extending from the myosin myofilaments attach (or couple) to the actin myofilaments and pull them over the myosin myofilaments. As the cross-bridges produce tension, the muscle shortens. The actual muscle shortening occurs as the actin myofilaments are pulled toward the center of the sarcomere, and the sarcomere shortens. The coupling of myosin and actin and the shortening process depend on the breakdown of ATP for energy.

Types of Muscular Contraction

What has been described above is a form of **isotonic muscular contraction**. The actin myofilaments slide over the myosin myofilaments toward the center of the sarcomere. Thus, each sarcomere in a stimulated myofibril is reduced in length (Fig. 1.7). The muscle visibly shortens, and

joint movement occurs. Tension (or force) develops throughout the muscle as it contracts, but the tension changes with the total length of the muscle and the angle of the joint. The greatest force is generated at the muscle's optimal length—the position of greatest strength—where the actin and myosin myofilaments are aligned so that the largest number of cross-bridges between the myofilaments are activated simultaneously. At all other lengths, fewer cross-bridges are simultaneously coupled to actin myofilaments and therefore, less force can be developed. The relationship of muscle tension (force) to muscle length is illustrated in Fig. 1.8a. This form of isotonic muscle contraction is also called **concentric contraction**, which means shortening muscle contraction.

Eccentric contraction is the opposite of concentric contraction in that the muscle

Figure 1.7

The sliding filament theory.

a. Myofibril at rest.

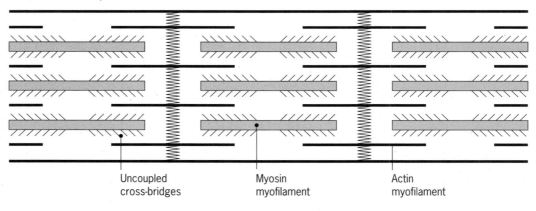

Uncoupled cross-bridges   Myosin myofilament   Actin myofilament

b. Contracted myofibril.

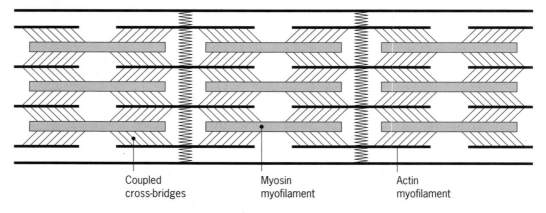

Coupled cross-bridges   Myosin myofilament   Actin myofilament

is developing tension as it lengthens against a resistance (rather than as it shortens against a resistance). This is sometimes called "negative work." A typical eccentric contraction occurs when slowly lowering a weight to its initial position (after lifting it), with a slow, sustained movement with (as opposed to against) gravity. Slowly walking down stairs is an example of negative work. In typical weight-lifting movements, eccentric contractions usually follow concentric contractions.

Isometric muscle contraction occurs when actual muscle shortening does not take place. Since no joint movement occurs, this type of contraction is sometimes referred to as a static contraction. During this type of muscular contraction, the tension developed within the muscle does not change because the muscle length does not change. An example of an isometric muscle contraction is holding a weight at arm's length or attempting to move an immovable object (e.g., exerting force outward against a door frame). The actual amount of tension developed by a muscle is directly related to the number of motor units stimulated by the nervous system. For example, more motor units will be stimulated to overcome a 10-pound resistance than a 2-pound resistance.

Isokinetic contractions, in outward appearance, look much like isotonic contractions. In this kind of contraction, however, tension within the muscle does not change even though the muscle length changes (shortens or lengthens) (Fig. 1.8b). To accomplish an isokinetic contraction, special equipment is required to alter the resistance offered the muscle as it contracts at a constant velocity. This approach is sometime referred to as "accommodating resistance" or "variable resistance" exercise. Isokinetic exercise enables maximal tension to develop in a muscle throughout its

entire range of motion; with isotonic exercise, the muscle can develop maximal tension only at its optimal length.

Muscular Response to Training

Three components of physical fitness warrant more discussion because they are directly related to the neuromuscular system. Muscular strength, muscular endurance and flexibility can be altered with regular exercise if some basic principles are applied. Consider how the principle of specificity applies to these three components of physical fitness.

Muscular Strength. Muscular strength refers to the maximal tension or force produced by a muscle or muscle group. Strength is usually measured by determining how much weight can be lifted in a single effort. The 1 repetition maximum (1 RM) test is determined through a trial-and-error procedure using either free weights (barbells and weights) or special machines (e.g., dynamometers, Hydra-gym, Nautilus, Universal apparatus). Most often 1 RM tests are completed for the following muscle groups: (1) the bench press for the muscles of the chest and upper arms; (2) the arm curl for the muscles on the anterior aspect of the upper arms; and (3) the leg press for the muscles of the upper legs and hips.

After testing, training programs can be developed to enhance muscular strength. To improve strength, training intensity should be high, the number of **repetitions** of each lift or movement should be kept relatively low, and the movements should be performed carefully at a controlled speed so that there is a consistent application of force throughout the movement. Good posture and body mechanics are extremely important. Movements requiring a high level of strength are performed primarily by the FT muscle fibers because

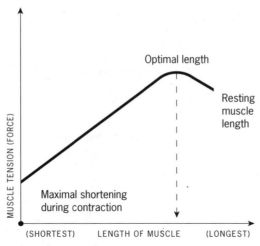

a. Isotonic contraction.

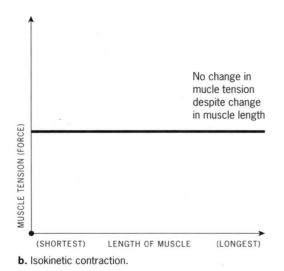

b. Isokinetic contraction.

Figure 1.8

The length-tension curve
during contraction.

they are capable of generating more force,
and are primarily anaerobic in nature.
Therefore, strength-training movements
do not require a high level of aerobic capacity because the muscles used require
anaerobic metabolism. Because strength
training is relatively stressful on the connective tissues and muscular structures of
the body, it is usually recommended that
heavy strength training be performed only
two or three times per week. It is important
that the muscles and supporting structures
be given time to recover sufficiently between workouts, but there is considerable
disagreement about the precise period of
time required.

In summary, training to improve
strength is characterized by the following
principles:

1. High resistance is used—often the
weight equivalent to the 6 to 10 repetition
maximum, or the maximum weight that
can be lifted 6 to 10 times.

2. Few repetitions are performed—
usually about 5 to 7 per set for three sets—
so muscles and joint structures are not
overstressed.

3. Movements are controlled and deliberate—emphasizing the movement speed
appropriate to the skill for which increased
strength is being developed.

After physical training, the physiological system that has been stressed alters its
state of homeostasis; that is, it adapts to
the demands that have been placed on it.
These adaptations result in a higher functional capacity, an improved ability to meet
physical demands. However, none of these
adaptations or changes in physiological response to exercise are permanent. According to the **reversibility principle**, training
adaptations will gradually decline if not
regularly reinforced by a "maintenance"
exercise program. Strength training causes
the following adaptations to occur in the
neuromuscular system:

1. Muscular **hypertrophy** is a general increase in the size or diameter of muscle
cells. Specifically, muscular hypertrophy
is the result of an increase in the muscle's
content of **contractile proteins**. Strength training stimulates a proliferation of myosin
and actin myofilaments within the myofibrils. Since strength training is largely performed by the FT fibers, these are the
fibers most capable of hypertrophy. People
with unusually large, muscular builds very
likely have a high percentage of FT fibers.
Generally, women do not experience muscular hypertrophy to the same extent as
men because the male hormone testos-

terone is important in synthesizing the contractile proteins. Nevertheless, women will increase substantially in strength in response to a progressive strength-training program. Thus, muscular hypertrophy is not absolutely required for improvement in strength. With muscle disuse, as in paralysis, muscle **atrophy** or wasting occurs.

2. Metabolic alterations in the strength-trained muscles include an enhancement of the phosphagen system. This occurs largely as a result of a higher production of the enzymes essential for the rapid resynthesis of ATP from CP.

3. Other changes occur that enhance the action of the FT motor units; however, these changes are beyond the scope of this manual.

Muscular Endurance. Endurance refers to the ability to repeatedly contract a muscle or muscle group against resistance. Tests of muscular endurance usually involve selecting a fixed percentage of the maximum strength, for example, 70 percent of the 1 RM, and counting the number of repetitions that can be completed without resting. Sit-up or pull-up tests are examples of muscular endurance tests (not of strength tests as often thought). It is usually recommended that muscular endurance training be completed three to five times per week for maximum results. This form of training is most specific to aerobic metabolism and to ST muscle fibers and motor units.

Training programs specific for muscular endurance should employ the following principles:

1. Moderate resistance is used.

2. Many (20 to 50) repetitions are completed because this is the aspect of performance being developed.

3. Speed of contraction is maintained at the same rate required for muscular endurance in performance.

4. Training frequency is usually three to five times per week.

After muscular endurance training, these neuromuscular adaptations are seen:

1. Increased muscle **vascularity** resulting in an enhanced blood supply and, consequently, oxygen delivery to the myofibrils.

2. Increased concentrations of oxidative enzymes, which extract oxygen from the blood, in the specific muscles trained. Increased concentration of oxidative enzymes coupled with increased vascularity means that the aerobic capacity of the trained muscles is improved.

3. Enhanced glycogen storage delays fatigue because more metabolic substrate is available.

These neuromuscular changes are specific to the ST muscle fibers and motor units, and are of particular relevance to aerobic exercise. Although aerobic exercise does not adhere precisely to the training principles mentioned earlier, regular participation in aerobic exercise generally enhances muscular endurance.

Flexibility. Flexibility refers to the range of motion possible about a joint. Flexibility is often relative to age; young children are usually extremely flexible, while the elderly gradually lose much of the flexibility they had as younger adults.

Range of motion (ROM) can be limited by the bony structure of a joint, the ligamentous structure of a joint, or the musculotendinous structure of the muscle(s) spanning the joint. The bony structure of a joint is a self-limiting factor that cannot be altered. A joint ligament (the fibrous band connecting bones) or joint capsule should not be stretched because to do so would lead to an unstable joint (joint laxity) and an increased risk of joint injury. Therefore, the only desirable way to alter range of motion is by gently stretching the musculotendinous structures controlling the move-

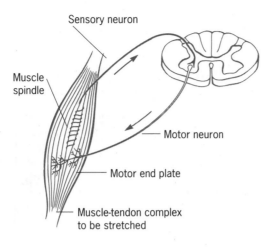

Figure 1.9

The muscle spindle and simple stretch reflex.

a. Simple muscle stretch reflex arc: the stretch of the muscle spindle causes reflex contraction.

b. Simple inverse stretch reflex arc: the stretch of Golgi tendon organ causes reflex inhibition (relaxation).

ment of the joint. Sometimes these structures can become extremely taut, causing a reduction in the normal range of motion.

Flexibility may be related to the incidence of acute muscle injury due to strenuous exercise and also to delayed muscle soreness. Acute muscle injuries, such as muscle pulls or tears, are more likely to occur if the muscle fibers or surrounding tissues are so taut and inflexible that a sudden stretch causes tissue injury. The exact cause of **delayed onset muscle soreness (DOMS)** which occurs 24 to 48 hours after strenuous exercise is not known. Current evidence suggests that DOMS is caused by microscopic damage to muscle cell ultrastructure due to excessive mechanical force exerted by the muscle and connective tissues. Delayed muscle soreness is particularly associated with the eccentric phase of a movement. Stretching exercises performed before and after an exercise session may help to prevent soreness and also to relieve soreness when it does occur, but not all evidence agrees.

There are two types of stretching to increase flexibility: static stretching and dynamic or ballistic stretching. **Static stretching** involves holding a static (nonmoving)

position so that a joint is immobilized in a position that places the desired muscles and connective tissues passively at their greatest possible length. A static stretch position should be held for 30 to 60 seconds to achieve optimal results. Static stretching is best characterized as low-force, long-duration stretching, and has repeatedly been shown to produce good results with little muscle soreness. In fact, static stretching is commonly used to reduce muscle soreness. Little risk of physical injury exists if static stretching is performed as described.

Dynamic or **ballistic stretching** is characterized by rhythmic bobbing or bouncing motions representing relatively high-force, short-duration movements. Ballistic stretching motions, while seemingly effective, actually invoke **stretch reflexes** that oppose the desired stretching. Muscle stretch reflexes are involuntary motor responses controlled by the **muscle spindle**, a sensory organ located within the muscle. When a muscle spindle is stimulated, an impulse is propagated over a sensory nerve fiber. The nerve fiber synapses in the spinal cord with a motor neuron that returns to the muscle containing the muscle spindle (Fig. 1.9a). This reflex causes the suddenly stretched muscle to respond with a corresponding contraction; the amount and rate of this contraction varies directly with the amount and rate of the movement causing the initial stretch. Thus, ballistic stretching evokes the opposite physiological response from that desired—an increase in muscle tension.

A firm static stretch, on the other hand, invokes an inhibition of the stretch reflex by stimulating another sensory organ (with a higher threshold level) called the **Golgi tendon organ**. When stimulated, this organ causes an inhibition not only of the muscle whose muscle spindle was stretched, but also of the entire muscle group (Fig. 1.9b). Thus, static stretching brings about a reduction in muscle tension—the desirable physiological response. In addition, static stretching is safer than ballistic stretching because it does not impose a sudden, possibly injurious force upon the tissues.

A third type of stretching, **proprioceptive neuromuscular facilitation** or **PNF**, is a relatively new technique originally developed for rehabilitative purposes in physical therapy. PNF involves statically stretching a muscle immediately after maximally contracting it. Carefully controlled experiments using PNF have found no advantage over regular static stretching techniques.

General flexibility exercises should be part of every physical fitness exercise program. Gentle stretching exercises should be included in every warm-up and cool-down phase of an exercise session. Some general principles specific to the enhancement of flexibility include the following:

1. A very easy general warm-up (such as walking and swinging the arms) should precede specific stretching exercises to increase blood flow to the area.

2. Stretching exercises should be performed without bouncing or jerking, which may injure connective tissues and stimulate the stretch reflex.

3. Attempts to stretch a muscle or muscle group beyond the normal ROM should never be made.

4. Excessive resistance should never be used. All stretching should be done gently and only to the extent that muscle tension is perceived. Muscle pain should not occur.

5. Instructors should understand that their students will vary greatly in flexibility and responsiveness to flexibility training.

With specific flexibility training, the muscles and connective tissues adapt by elongating slightly, thus increasing the range of motion.

THE CARDIOVASCULAR-RESPIRATORY SYSTEM

Cardiorespiratory endurance was defined earlier as the capacity of the heart and lung systems to deliver blood and, hence, oxygen, to the working muscles during sustained exercise. Oxygen is used to produce ATP to perform low-to moderate-intensity exercise for long periods. The production of ATP requires metabolic systems with a relatively unlimited capacity to produce ATP at a slow rate (Table 1.1). Physical activities classified as cardiovascular endurance activities (aerobic exercise) require aerobic metabolism, specifically aerobic glycolysis (carbohydrate as substrate) or fatty acid oxidation (fatty acids as substrate). One's capacity to perform aerobic exercise depends largely on the interaction of the cardiovascular system and the respiratory system to provide oxygen to the active cells so that carbohydrates and fatty acids can be converted to ATP for muscular contraction. These two systems are also important for the removal of metabolic waste products such as carbon dioxide and lactic acid, and for the dissipation of the internal heat produced by metabolic processes.

Consider how these systems accomplish

these tasks. Basically, there are three primary factors:

1. Getting oxygen into the blood—a function of the oxygen-carrying capacity of the blood and respiratory ventilation.

2. Delivering oxygen to the active cells—a function of cardiac output.

3. Extracting oxygen from the blood to complete the metabolic production of ATP—a function of the oxidative enzymes located in the active cells.

Oxygen-Carrying Capacity

The **oxygen-carrying capacity** of blood is determined primarily by two variables, the hemoglobin content of the blood and the ability to ventilate the lungs adequately. **Hemoglobin** (Hb) is a protein molecule in red blood cells that is specifically adapted to bond (carry) oxygen molecules. Persons with low hemoglobin concentrations cannot carry as much oxygen in their blood as persons with high hemoglobin concentrations. **Anemia** (less than 12 gm of Hb per 100 ml of blood), although relatively rare, limits the blood's oxygen-carrying capacity. In most healthy persons, however, the oxygen-carrying capacity of the blood is not a limiting factor in the performance of aerobic exercise.

Respiratory ventilation is a function of the depth of each breath **(tidal volume)** and the respiratory rate (breaths per minute). With exercise, both tidal volume and respiratory rate increase. Certain respiratory diseases may limit the ability to load oxygen onto the red blood cells. Persons with **asthma** (constriction of breathing passages) or **emphysema** (loss of normal elasticity of lung tissues) cannot move enough air through their lung tissues **(hypoventilation)** to interface adequately with the blood flowing through these tissues **(perfusion)**. As a result, the blood leaving the lungs is insufficiently loaded with oxygen.

At high levels of exercise, **hyperventilation** may occur. This means that more air is breathed in and out through the lung passages than is necessary for the existing metabolic rate (i.e., more air is supplied than is needed). When this happens, carbon dioxide is "blown off" faster than it is produced metabolically, resulting in a condition know as **hypocapnia**, which is a lowering of normal blood levels of carbon dioxide. Hypocapnia may be triggered by emotional excitement or fear, and is sometimes seen in the inexperienced exerciser. Symptoms include dizziness, lightheadedness, bluish lips and tingling of the fingers.

Oxygen Delivery

Probably the most important factor in cardiovascular-respiratory endurance, the delivery of blood to the active cells, is a function of cardiac output. **Cardiac output** is the product of **stroke volume** (the quantity of blood pumped per heartbeat) and heart rate (beats per minute):

Cardiac output = SV x HR

A full explanation of how cardiac output is regulated is beyond the scope of this manual. Basically, stroke volume (SV) is a function of the amount of blood filling the heart during its resting or diastolic period (venous return), and the force of the contraction of the heart during its contraction or systolic period. Static exercise (as in isometric exercise) or holding the breath while contracting the chest muscles (the **Valsalva maneuver**) increases thoracic pressure, hinders venous return of blood to the heart, and reduces stroke volume. On the other hand, rhythmic exercise characterized by alternating contraction and relaxation of large muscle groups favors the venous return of blood to the heart and enhances stroke volume.

The higher the stroke volume for any given level of cardiac output, the lower the heart rate needs to be. Because the heart gets more rest with a slower heart rate, delivery of blood is more efficient with a higher stroke volume and a lower heart rate. Outstanding endurance athletes usually have very high stroke volumes and rather low corresponding heart rates compared to sedentary persons.

Because humans have a limited quantity of blood (blood volume equals about 5 to 6 liters), all cells in the body are not perfused with blood at once. Blood is distributed according to metabolic need. At rest, cardiac output level is low (about 5 to 7 liters per minute depending on body size). Essential organs, such as the brain, heart, lungs, liver and kidneys, receive most of the blood, while tissues performing secondary functions receive relatively low quantities. For example, when eating a meal, our intestinal tract temporarily receives more blood to enhance digestion and absorption, and while sunbathing, skin blood flow increases so overheating does not occur. Normally, however, these tissues receive little blood flow.

As exercise intensity increases, blood-flow patterns change according to metabolic need. As the blood flow to the muscles (to produce ATP for contraction) and to the skin (to dissipate the metabolic heat produced) increases, the amount of blood flowing to less active organs, such as the kidney and intestinal tract, decreases. In this instance, one conserves water (less urine is formed) and delays digestion. Because muscles need so much oxygen to carry on their work, the net effect is a tremendous increase in cardiac output. One of the most significant factors in cardiovascular endurance, which represents the ability to perform aerobic exercise, is cardiac output. The larger one's capacity to increase cardiac output, that is, to deliver oxygen to the active muscle cells and to dissipate the internal heat of metabolism, the larger one's capacity for endurance (aerobic) performance.

Blood pressure is very important in blood-flow distribution because it drives the circulatory system. Blood pressure is influenced by many factors. Basically, blood pressure is a function of the force generated by the heart during its contractile phase (systole), and the resistance offered by the vessels to the blood flowing through them (peripheral resistance). Just as the strength of heart contractions can vary, some blood vessels (notably the smaller arteries called arterioles) can contract **(vasoconstriction)** or relax **(vasodilation)**, and thus alter their resistance to blood flow. This variable is important in determining patterns of blood flow. For example, during exercise, vasoconstriction occurs in the vessels of inactive organs (such as the intestine), and vasodilation occurs in vessels of active organs (muscles), thus redirecting blood flow to areas of the body where it is most needed.

Oxygen Extraction

A third factor important in cardiovascular respiratory endurance is the extraction of oxygen from the blood at the cellular level for the aerobic production of ATP. The amount of oxygen extracted is largely a function of muscle fiber type and the availability of specialized oxidative enzymes. As discussed earlier, the ST muscle fibers are specifically adapted for oxygen extraction and utilization due to their high levels of oxidative enzymes. The oxygen is used by the cells to produce ATP in the mitochondria.

RESPONSES TO AEROBIC EXERCISE

Aerobic exercise—whether dance-exercise, walking, jogging, running, cycling, swimming or cross-country ski-

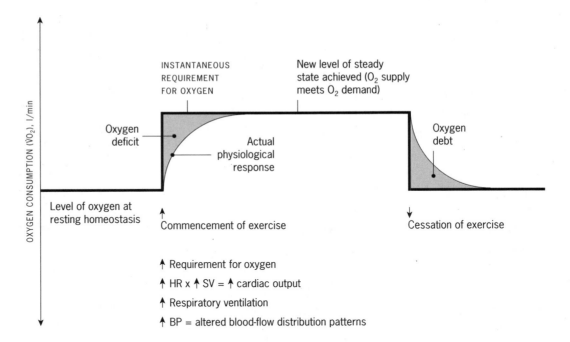

Figure 1.10

Oxygen consumption
during aerobic exercise.

ing—is best characterized as rhythmic, large muscle activity (i.e., alternating muscle contraction and relaxation) of low to moderately high intensity that can be sustained without undue fatigue for at least 10 to 15 minutes. Such movement patterns depend on oxidative or aerobic metabolic pathways to use the potential energy contained within carbohydrate or fatty acid substrates for ATP production. The other metabolic pathways (the phosphagen system and anaerobic glycolysis) are used only minimally to produce energy for muscular activity.

Physiological responses to aerobic exercise: (1) provide oxygen to the metabolically active cells, (2) rid the body of metabolic waste products (excess CO_2 and LA), and (3) dissipate the internal heat produced during energy production. For these functions to occur, respiratory ventilation, cardiac output, blood pressure and blood-flow distribution patterns must adequately meet the body's metabolic needs. In terms of **oxygen consumption (VO_2)**, the body is in a steady state, meaning that the delivery and utilization of oxygen is meeting metabolic

demands, and aerobic pathways are providing the energy required.

When aerobic exercise begins, the body rapidly responds to increase the quantity of oxygen required to produce the ATP necessary to meet elevated metabolic demands. Cardiac output must increase to deliver more blood to the active muscle cells. To meet this requirement, heart rate, stroke volume and systolic blood pressure increase immediately. Diastolic blood pressure either remains constant or decreases. Respiratory ventilation must increase to provide more oxygen to the red blood cells in the lungs as they release carbon dioxide produced by the oxidation of glucose or fatty acids in the muscles.

Fig. 1.10 graphically illustrates these responses. The heavy bold line indicates the level of oxygen consumption required at rest and the instantaneous increase that occurs with commencement of exercise (at upward arrow). The line returns to the resting level when exercise is abruptly stopped (at downward arrow). The actual oxygen consumption that results from the physiological responses to aerobic exercise

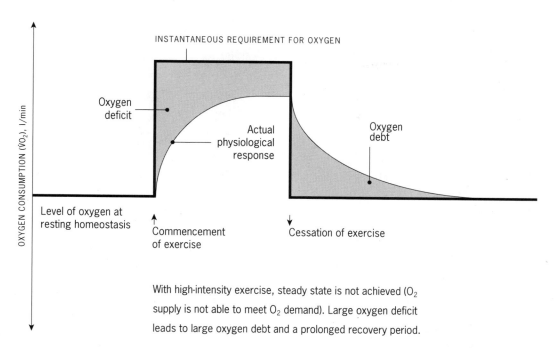

INSTANTANEOUS REQUIREMENT FOR OXYGEN

Oxygen
deficit

Actual
physiological
response

Oxygen
debt

Level of oxygen at
resting homeostasis

Commencement
of exercise

Cessation of exercise

With high-intensity exercise, steady state is not achieved (O_2
supply is not able to meet O_2 demand). Large oxygen deficit
leads to large oxygen debt and a prolonged recovery period.

Figure 1.11

Oxygen consumption
during anaerobic
exercise.

is indicated by the sloping line in the figure. Notice that the actual oxygen consumption does not immediately meet the physiological requirement for oxygen. Instead, an **oxygen deficit** occurs.

The physiological responses that occur with commencement of exercise take approximately 2 to 4 minutes to meet the increased metabolic demands for oxygen. During this time, the anaerobic metabolic systems—which are capable of producing energy more rapidly—produce the energy needed to carry out the exercise. During this period, the phosphagens are depleted, and excess LA is produced. When the cardiorespiratory systems have fully responded, a new level of oxygen consumption is achieved. If the exercise intensity is not too high relative to one's ability to provide oxygen to the muscles, a new steady state is achieved as shown in Fig. 1.10.

With cessation of exercise, the requirement of oxygen abruptly returns to the initial resting level. Again, however, the body responds more slowly. As cardiac output, blood pressure and respiratory ventilation return to resting levels, oxygen consump-

tion slowly declines as well. This temporarily elevated level of oxygen consumption, called **oxygen debt**, "pays back" the oxygen deficit. The energy produced during this time is used to replenish the depleted phosphagens, to eliminate accumulated LA if it has not already been cleared from the blood, and to restore other homeostatic conditions.

If exercise intensity is so high that the body cannot depend predominantly on aerobic pathways for ATP production, then the oxygen deficit and corresponding oxygen debt are extremely high, and exercise cannot be performed for more than a few minutes. Fig. 1.11 illustrates the typical oxygen consumption pattern during high-intensity anaerobic exercise. Extreme **dyspnea** (respiratory distress) and muscle pain (the "burn" of lactic acid or oxygen deficiency) are experienced. With high-intensity exercise, anaerobic metabolic pathways must be relied on heavily for ATP production. The result is phosphagen depletion, a high concentration of LA in the blood and muscles—and fatigue. In such a case, a homeostatic steady state cannot be achieved, and the recovery period is prolonged in proportion to the duration of exercise.

HEALTH BENEFITS OF AEROBIC EXERCISE FOR HEALTHY PARTICIPANTS

Regular exercise, particularly aerobic exercise, enhances a person's physiological or functional capacity and enables him or her to achieve an improved quality of life. With a heightened physiological reserve, the regular stresses and strains of life, whether physical or psychological, are taken in stride. More specifically, the musculotendinous and skeletal systems are maintained at a moderately high level of strength and endurance. Although aerobic exercise improves muscle tonus (firmness) and general body flexibility, it is not specific to the development of muscular strength and endurance. To develop high levels of muscular strength and endurance, weight training must be added to regular aerobic exercise. Recent studies have shown that weight-bearing exercise promotes improved bone density, an extremely important consideration in the prevention of osteoporosis after ages 50 to 60, particularly in women.

The benefits of aerobic exercise are most specific to the cardiovascular and respiratory systems. A regular program of aerobic exercise significantly improves the efficiency with which the body performs. Hand in hand with improvement in aerobic performance is improved cardiac efficiency (increased stroke volume, lowered heart rate), improved breathing capacity (increased capacity for respiratory ventilation), and improved capacity for dissipating metabolically produced heat. Further, regular participation in a progressive exercise program enhances the body's ability to use oxygen for the production of ATP (oxygen consumption). Generally, these physiological benefits occur with a well-planned, 12-week period of aerobic exercise performed a minimum of three times per week.

A long-term program of aerobic exercise produces favorable changes in body composition—an increase in lean body mass (muscle mass) and a decrease in body fat.

Obviously, exercise burns calories. Numerous studies on the psychological benefits of aerobic exercise have shown that persons who regularly perform aerobic exercise have increased vigor and decreased depression scores on basic psychological tests. Students of aerobic exercise claim to be invigorated by both the music and the exercise.

HEALTH BENEFITS OF AEROBIC EXERCISE FOR PERSONS WITH CHRONIC DISEASE

A well-planned aerobic exercise program will provide health benefits to persons with chronic diseases such as adult-onset diabetes, osteoarthritis, obesity, asthma and coronary heart disease.

Living with **adult-onset diabetes** (non-insulin-dependent diabetes mellitus or NIDDM) often requires a complete lifestyle change, including losing body fat, reducing stress and learning to monitor blood glucose levels. Exercise enables carbohydrates to be used more effectively by promoting glucose uptake from the blood, and thereby reducing the need for insulin secretions from the pancreas. Severe exercise, however, may induce hazardously low blood glucose levels. Research has shown that regularly performed moderate exercise can help a diabetic maintain normal blood glucose levels, but the guidance of a physician as well as a dietitian may be necessary. The diabetic needs to understand the interactions among exercise, glucose uptake, insulin, and carbohydrate consumption. A regular program of physical activity may help diabetics lose body fat, reduce tension and anxiety, and deal with stress.

Arthritis (osteoarthritis) is a gradual, progressive degeneration of joint structures that causes painful movement and sometimes severe aches and pains. The notion that severe exercise early in life contributes to the incidence of arthritis later on recently has been debunked. There is no association between exercise and the incidence of arthritis, other than the tendency for arthritic pain to occur in areas of the body that experienced earlier athletic injury. Persons with mild arthritic pain generally respond well to moderate levels of exercise. Maintenance of flexibility and moderate levels of muscular strength and endurance is important; movement should not be avoided because of general aches and pains. However, movements involving high-impact stress on the knees, hips and low back should be avoided. Low to moderate-intensity, low-impact movements are more productive than higher intensity movements requiring considerable jumping or hopping.

Obesity (having excess body fat) has become a severe nutritional and health-related problem in the industrialized world. Low to moderate-intensity aerobic exercise is the best method for obese persons to use energy and expend calories. The most effective way to lose body fat is to restrict caloric intake, particularly fat intake, and to perform regular aerobic exercise to increase caloric output (energy production). Dieting alone is ineffective. While severe dieting can lead to weight loss, the loss is frequently from the lean body mass (mainly the muscles) rather than from the fat mass of the body. Low to moderate-intensity, long-duration exercise allows the fatty acids from adipose

tissue to be used as energy substrate (fatty acid oxidation). Higher intensity exercise utilizes carbohydrate stores, not body fat stores, as the substrate for energy production. The mobilization of fatty acids from adipose tissue is a slow process requiring about 20 minutes of exercise; therefore, long-duration exercise is specifically prescribed for fat reduction.

Asthma occurs when the bronchi (large breathing passages) become constricted (bronchospasm). Although exact causes are unknown, the onset of symptoms is related to irritants such as tobacco smoke, animal dander and cold air. The labored breathing that occurs when the bronchi constrict discourages asthmatics from exercising. Some people experience exercise-induced asthma (EIA). The most widely accepted hypothesis is that airway cooling causes the bronchospasm. Nevertheless, an exercise program for asthmatics is not contraindicated. Asthmatics can learn to recognize symptoms and employ proper self-care steps to control the condition. A very gradual warm-up may prevent EIA. Asthmatics should be encouraged to exercise and to have bronchodilator medications readily available if symptoms become severe. Research has shown that increased aerobic fitness raises the exercise level at which asthmatic symptoms occur.

Coronary heart disease (CHD) is partial or total closure of the coronary arteries resulting in symptoms or signs of reduced or occluded coronary blood flow. The American Heart Association has identified a number of factors that increase the risk of cardiovascular disease. The primary risk factors are hypertension (elevated blood pressure), cigarette smoking, elevated blood lipid levels and physical inactivity. Secondary risk factors include family history of heart disease, obesity, diabetes, being male, age over 65, and a high level of emotional stress. Obviously, little can be done to change one's age, gender or family health history, but lifestyle changes can significantly alter other risk factors. Regular participation in a well-planned, aerobic exercise program has been shown to reduce high blood pressure, serum lipid levels, body fat and emotional stress.

ENVIRONMENTAL CONSIDER- ATIONS WHEN EXERCISING

A physiological function that is closely regulated is body temperature. Since most mechanisms used to maintain body temperature are directly or indirectly related to the cardiovascular system, exercising under extreme environmental conditions adds significantly to cardiovascular stress.

Exercising in the Heat

Considerable metabolic heat is produced during exercise. To reduce this internal heat load, venous blood is brought to the skin surface (peripheral vasodilation) to be dissipated to the cooler environment. Sweating also occurs; sweat glands secrete extracellular water onto the skin where the water can evaporate. If environmental conditions are favorable, these mechanisms will adequately prevent the body temperature from rising more than about 2 to 3 degrees during heavy exercise.

When exercising in the heat, however, dissipating internal body heat is difficult and external heat from the environment may significantly add to the total heat load. In an attempt to cool the body, extensive vasodilation reduces the venous return of blood to the heart and the stroke volume of the heart declines. The heart attempts to maintain cardiac output with a considerably elevated heart rate. To add to the physiological stress, profuse sweating re-

sults in a considerable loss of body water. If lost fluids are not replenished, dehydration eventually results, and blood volume declines. These conditions are also manifested by a very high heart rate.

The most stressful environment for exercising combines heat and humidity, **(wet bulb temperature)**. When the air contains a large quantity of water vapor, sweat will not evaporate readily. Since it is the evaporative process that cools the body, adequate cooling may not occur in humid conditions. The intensity of exercise lasting 30 minutes or more should be reduced whenever **relative humidity** (% RH) and air temperature create a dangerous situation. Careful heart-rate monitoring is particularly important in a hot, humid environment (Table 1.2). (See Chapter 14, Emergency Procedures, pages 425-427, for a further discussion of heat-related injuries.)

It is important to not impede heat loss from the body. When exercising in the heat, never wear anything or do anything that will interfere with heat loss.

1. Always wear lightweight, well-ventilated clothing. Cotton materials are cooler; most synthetics retain heat. Wear light-colored clothing if exercising in the sun; white reflects heat better than other colors.

2. Never wear impermeable or non-breathable garments. The notion that wearing nonbreathable leggings while performing exercise will result in fat loss from the legs is a myth. Wearing impermeable clothing is a dangerous practice that could lead to significant heat stress and heat injury.

3. Replace body fluids as they are lost. Drink lots of fluids (preferably water) at regular intervals while exercising. Don't wait until thirst occurs because thirst is not an adequate indicator of the need to replace body fluids.

4. Recording daily body weights is an excellent way to prevent accumulative dehy-

Table 1.2

ENVIRONMENTAL DANGER ZONE FOR SUSTAINED EXERCISE

Air Temperature (°F)	Relative Humidity (%)
70	80
75	70
80	50
85	40
90	30
95	20
100	10

dration. For example, if 5 pounds of body water is lost after aerobic exercise, this water should be replaced before exercising again the next day. If lost water has not been regained, exercise should be curtailed until the body is adequately rehydrated.

5. Heat acclimatization can occur quickly. Begin exercise in the heat gradually. Exercise for a short period each day for a week. Discomfort will decrease noticeably as the week progresses.

Exercising in the Cold

Generally, few temperature-regulation problems occur when exercising in cool environments. The environmental conditions favor the loss of internal body heat, and the body remains cool and refreshed while exercising. Following exercise, however, chilling can occur quickly if the body surface is wet with sweat and vasodilation continues to bring body heat to surface tissues. Therefore, when it is cool, wear warm-up clothing (including a hat) to retain body heat immediately after exercising.

Temperature regulation can become a problem when exposure is prolonged or when the body core temperature cannot

be maintained. Under these conditions, a general vasoconstriction results in an elevation in central blood volume. The kidneys increase urine production and the blood becomes more concentrated. To prevent dehydration while exercising, this lost body fluid must be replaced.

The following guidelines govern exercising in the cold:

1. Wear several layers of clothing. By layering clothing, garments can be removed and replaced as needed. When exercise intensity is high, remove outer garments. Then, during periods of rest, warm-up, cool-down or low-intensity exercise, put them back on. A head covering is also important because considerable body heat radiates from the head.

2. Allow for adequate ventilation of sweat. Sweating during heavy exercise can soak inner garments. If evaporation does not readily occur, the wet garments will continue to drain the body of heat during rest periods, when retention of body heat is important.

3. Select garment materials that allow the body to give off body heat during exercise, and retain body heat during inactive periods. For example, cotton is a good choice for exercising in the heat because it soaks up sweat readily and allows evaporation; for those same reasons, though, cotton is a poor choice for exercising in the cold. Even when wet, wool garments help maintain body warmth. When windchill is a problem, nylon materials are good for outerwear. Since water vapor cannot permeate nylon, however, inner garments can become quite wet. Remove outer garments during exercise and replace them during rest periods.

4. Replace body fluids in the cold, just as in the heat. There is a loss of body water in the cold due to both increased urine production and increased respiratory loss

because of the low relative humidity in cold air. This makes fluid replacement very important when exercising in the cold.

Exercising at Higher Altitudes

At moderate to high altitudes, the **partial pressure** of oxygen in the air is reduced. Because there is less pressure to drive the oxygen molecules into the blood in the lungs, the oxygen-carrying capacity of the blood is reduced. Therefore, a person exercising at high altitude will not be able to deliver as much oxygen to the exercising muscles, and exercise intensity will have to be reduced (compared to sea level). Generally, respiratory distress is the dominant symptom, and recovery from exercise is delayed. Persons who usually exercise at sea level may develop a headache when exercising at higher altitudes. This headache will eventually subside.

Remember: The usual level of exercise intensity will be more difficult to perform at higher altitude. For best results, reduce exercise intensity to a comfortable level. A more gradual warm-up and cool-down period is also desirable.

It generally takes longer to acclimatize to altitude than to heat or cold. Some adaptations occur within about one week, but other physiological adaptations may remain incomplete.

SUMMARY

This chapter is designed to provide the exercise instructor with basic principles of exercise physiology. Considerable space is devoted to the presentation of aerobic and anaerobic metabolism because the principle of specificity clearly dictates that physiological adaptations are specific to encountered stresses. The exercise instructor must understand the various methods of applying progressive overload and the physiological adaptations that result. Too often the exercising public falls victim to the poor advice of exercise teachers, coaches and other "experts" who fail to apply the concept of exercise specificity because they simply do not understand basic principles.

A large amount of information has been given in a relatively small amount of space. The emphasis has been on basic understanding rather than on detailed explanation. Students of this material are strongly encouraged to seek further knowledge of exercise physiology and the principles of physical fitness and human movement through more advanced study.

SUGGESTED READING

American College of Sport Medicine. (1991). *Guidelines for Exercise Testing and Prescription.* 4th ed. Philadelphia: Lea & Febiger.

American College of Sports Medicine. (1990). Position Stand on the Recommended Quantity and Quality of Exercise for Developing and Maintaining Cardiorespiratory and Muscular Fitness in Healthy Adults. *Medicine and Science in Sports and Exercise,* 22: 265-274.

Anderson, B. (1980). *Stretching.* Bolinas, California: Shelter Publishers.

Beaulieu, J.E. (1980). *Stretching for All Sports.* Pasadena: The Athletic Press.

Bowers, R.W. & Fox, E.L. (1992). *Sports Physiology.* 3rd ed. Philadelphia: Saunders College Publishing.

Katch, F.I., and W.D. McArdle. (1988). *Nutrition, Weight Control, and Exercise.* 3rd ed. Philadelphia: Lea & Febiger.

Sharkey, B.J. (1984). *Physiology of Fitness.* 2nd ed. Champaign, Illinois: Human Kinetics Publishers.

Chapter 2

Fundamentals of Anatomy

By Rod A. Harter

Anatomy is the study of the structure of organisms. It entails dissecting the parts of organisms to determine their location, function and relationship to one another. A fundamental understanding of human anatomy is necessary for the aerobics instructor whose professional responsibilities include exercise programming designed to achieve clients' cardiovascular and musculoskeletal personal fitness goals. The focus of this chapter is to provide an overview of the functional anatomy of three major systems operating within the human body: the cardiorespiratory system, the

Rod A. Harter, Ph.D., A.T.C., is currently assistant professor and program director of athletic training education in the Department of Exercise and Sport Science at Oregon State University in Corvallis. His areas of specialization are athletic training/ sports medicine and biomechanics. Dr. Harter is a fellow of the American College of Sports Medicine, and currently serves on the editorial boards of two sports medicine journals.

nervous system and the musculoskeletal system.

ANATOMICAL POSITION AND TERMINOLOGY

In order to describe body parts and their locations accurately, a standard reference point and a set of uniquely descriptive terms are required. The reference position for the human body, termed **anatomical position,** is a standing position with the feet together and the arms extended at the side (Fig. 2.1).

The Latin root for the word anatomy means dissection, and the descriptive terms used to divide the human body into sections require imaginary cutting of the body in anatomical position. These imaginary cuts divide the body into three planes—sagittal, frontal and transverse. A **sagittal plane** runs from front to back and divides the body or organ into left and right halves (Fig. 2.2a). A **frontal plane** is formed by an imaginary cut from left to right, dividing the body or organ into **anterior** (front) and **posterior** (back) sections (Fig. 2.2b). A **trans-**

verse plane** runs horizontally across the body and creates **superior** (above) and **inferior** (below) segments (Fig. 2.2c).

Studying anatomy for the first time, one will encounter descriptive terms that may not be familiar. It is important for a fitness professional to use the correct anatomical terms when describing a particular movement or exercise.

Most anatomical terms have their roots in the Greek and Latin languages and are usually quite descriptive. For example, some muscle names indicate location, size, shape and/or function. In the quadriceps femoris muscle, for example, quadriceps means "four-headed muscle" (quad = four, cephalad = head), while femoris means "of the femur." By knowing the meanings of these root words, one can now understand the meaning of this anatomical term; and in this case, one knows the configuration and location of the muscle. More specifically, the quadriceps femoris is the large muscle on the front of the thigh whose primary function is to extend the knee.

While there are more than 600 muscles

Figure 2.1a-b

Anatomical position and regional terms used to designate specific body areas.
Source: Redrawn from Marieb (1992).

a. Anterior view.

b. Posterior view.

a.

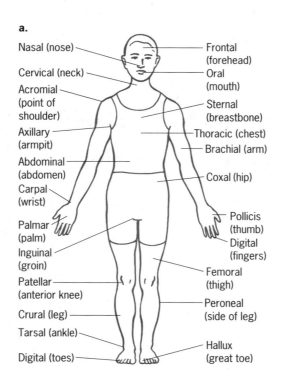

Nasal (nose)
Cervical (neck)
Acromial (point of shoulder)
Axillary (armpit)
Abdominal (abdomen)
Carpal (wrist)
Palmar (palm)
Inguinal (groin)
Patellar (anterior knee)
Crural (leg)
Tarsal (ankle)
Digital (toes)

Frontal (forehead)
Oral (mouth)
Sternal (breastbone)
Thoracic (chest)
Brachial (arm)
Coxal (hip)
Pollicis (thumb)
Digital (fingers)
Femoral (thigh)
Peroneal (side of leg)
Hallux (great toe)

b.

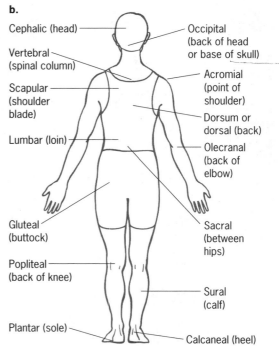

Cephalic (head)
Vertebral (spinal column)
Scapular (shoulder blade)
Lumbar (loin)
Gluteal (buttock)
Popliteal (back of knee)
Plantar (sole)

Occipital (back of head or base of skull)
Acromial (point of shoulder)
Dorsum or dorsal (back)
Olecranal (back of elbow)
Sacral (between hips)
Sural (calf)
Calcaneal (heel)

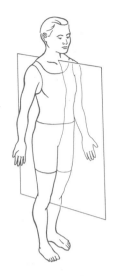
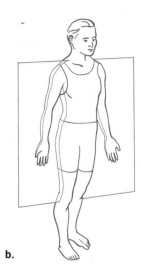
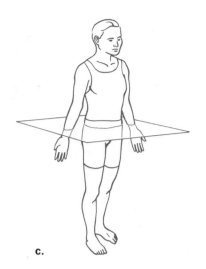

a.

b.

c.

Figure 2.2a-c
Anatomical planes of motion.
Source: Redrawn from Marieb (1992).

a. Sagittal plane

b. Frontal plane

c. Transverse plane

and 200 bones in the human body, some anatomical terms are used more frequently than others.

MAJOR ANATOMICAL SYSTEMS

In this section, the functions of three major systems in the human body most pertinent to aerobic exercise will be reviewed in a summary manner. These systems are the cardiorespiratory system, the nervous system and the musculoskeletal system.

THE CARDIORESPIRATORY SYSTEM

The cardiorespiratory system components include the blood, the blood vessels, the heart, the lungs and a series of passageways that lead to and from the lungs (mouth, throat, trachea and bronchi). Components of this system distribute oxygen and nutrients to the cells, carry carbon dioxide and metabolic wastes from the cells, protect against disease, help regulate body temperature and the acid-base balance (pH) of the body, and prevent serious blood loss through the formation of clots after an injury has occurred.

Oxygen is required for energy production and thus sustains cellular activity in all the organ systems in the human body. A by-product of this activity (cellular metabo-

lism) is carbon dioxide. High levels of carbon dioxide in the cells produce acidic conditions that are poisonous to cells, and therefore, must be rapidly eliminated.

Blood is composed of two parts, formed elements, which include white blood cells, red blood cells and platelets, and plasma, the liquid portion of blood. Plasma consists of approximately 92 percent water and 8 percent dissolved solutes. Blood volume in an average-sized woman is about 4 to 5 liters (approximately 4 to 5 quarts), while an average-sized man has about 5 to 6 liters of blood in the cardiorespiratory system.

There are two types of blood vessels— **arteries**, which carry blood away from the heart, and **veins**, which carry blood toward the heart. Arteries are stronger and thicker than veins, and their muscular walls help propel blood. Unlike arteries, veins contain valves to prevent the backflow of blood. The largest arteries are those nearest the heart; as blood flows farther away from the heart, smaller arteries called **arterioles** deliver the blood to the **capillaries**. Capillaries are microscopic blood vessels that branch to form an extensive network throughout the **distal** tissues. It is in the capillary beds that the critical exchange of nutrients and metabolic waste products

Figure 2.3

Anatomy of capillary bed circulation where delivery of oxygen and nutrients occurs and pickup of carbon dioxide and metabolic by-products takes place.

Source: Redrawn from Marieb (1992).

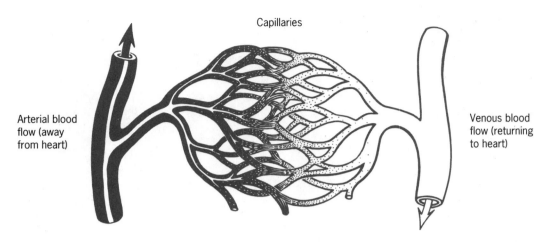

Capillaries

Arterial blood flow (away from heart)

Venous blood flow (returning to heart)

takes place (Fig. 2.3).

Depleted of its oxygen and nutrients on the way from the heart to the periphery, capillary blood now begins the journey back to the heart via small vessels called **venules.** The venules are a continuation of the capillaries, and join together to form veins. As the blood is transported back to the heart, the veins become larger, carrying a greater volume of blood. The major arteries and veins of the body are presented in Figures 2.4 and 2.5.

The human heart, a hollow muscular organ that pumps blood throughout the blood vessels is the "center" of the cardiorespiratory system. In an adult, the heart is about the same size as a closed fist, and lies to the left of center behind the sternum and between the lungs.

The heart is divided into four spaces (chambers) that receive circulating blood. The two upper chambers are called the right and left **atria;** the two lower chambers of the heart are known as the right and left **ventricles** (Fig. 2.6). The heart is, in reality, a series of four separate pumps: two "primer" pumps (the atria) and two "power" pumps (the ventricles).

Knowledge of the sequence of blood flow through the heart is fundamental to understanding the cardiorespiratory system. The right **atrium** receives blood from all parts of the body with the exception of the lungs. The superior vena cava, which drains blood from body parts superior to the heart (head, neck, arms) and the inferior vena cava, which brings blood from the parts of the body inferior to the heart (legs, abdominal region) transport blood to the right atrium. During contraction of the heart, blood accumulates in the right atrium.

With relaxation of the heart, blood from the right atrium flows into the right ventricle, which pumps it into the pulmonary trunk. The pulmonary trunk then divides into right and left pulmonary arteries which transport blood to the lungs where carbon dioxide is released and oxygen is acquired. This newly oxygenated blood returns to the heart via four pulmonary veins which empty into the left atrium. The blood then passes into the left ventricle, which pumps the blood into the ascending **aorta.** From this point, the blood is distributed to all body parts (except the lungs) by several large arteries (Fig. 2.4).

The Process of Respiration

Respiration is defined as the overall exchange of gases (oxygen, carbon dioxide, nitrogen) between the atmosphere, the blood and the cells. There are three general phases of respiration: external, internal and cellular. **External respiration** is the exchange of oxygen and carbon dioxide between the atmosphere and the blood within the large capillaries in the lungs. Internal respiration involves the exchange of these gases between blood and cells. The process of cellular respiration involves the utilization of oxygen and the production of carbon dioxide by the metabolic activity within cells.

Air enters the respiratory system usually via the nostrils of the nose. When air enters the nostrils, it is warmed as it passes through a series of nasal cavities lined by a mucous membrane with cilia (small hairs) which filter out small particles. From the nasal cavity, inspired air next enters the pharynx (throat), which lies just posterior to the nasal and oral (mouth) cavities. The

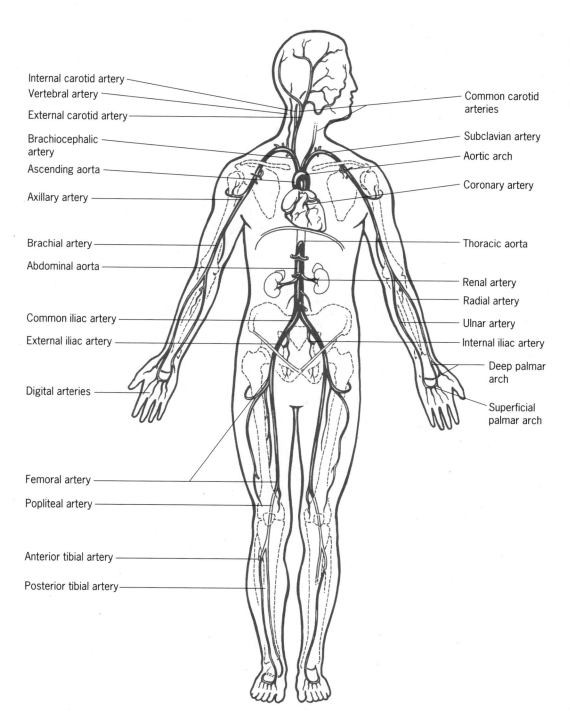

Internal carotid artery
Vertebral artery
External carotid artery
Brachiocephalic artery
Ascending aorta
Axillary artery
Brachial artery
Abdominal aorta
Common iliac artery
External iliac artery
Digital arteries
Femoral artery
Popliteal artery
Anterior tibial artery
Posterior tibial artery

Common carotid arteries
Subclavian artery
Aortic arch
Coronary artery
Thoracic aorta
Renal artery
Radial artery
Ulnar artery
Internal iliac artery
Deep palmar arch
Superficial palmar arch

Figure 2.4

Major arteries of the body (anterior view).
Source: Redrawn from Marieb (1992).

pharynx serves as a passageway for air and food, and also provides a chamber for creating speech sounds. During vigorous exercise, mouth breathing predominates and air taken in via the mouth is not filtered to the same extent as air taken in through the nostrils.

The larynx (voice box) is the enlarged upper (**proximal**) end of the trachea (windpipe) that conducts air to and from the lungs via the pharynx. An easy surface anatomy landmark used to locate the larynx is the thyroid **cartilage** (Adam's apple). The trachea extends from the larynx to approximately the level of the fifth thoracic vertebra, where it divides into the right

Figure 2.5

Major veins of the body (anterior view). *Source: Redrawn from Marieb (1992).*

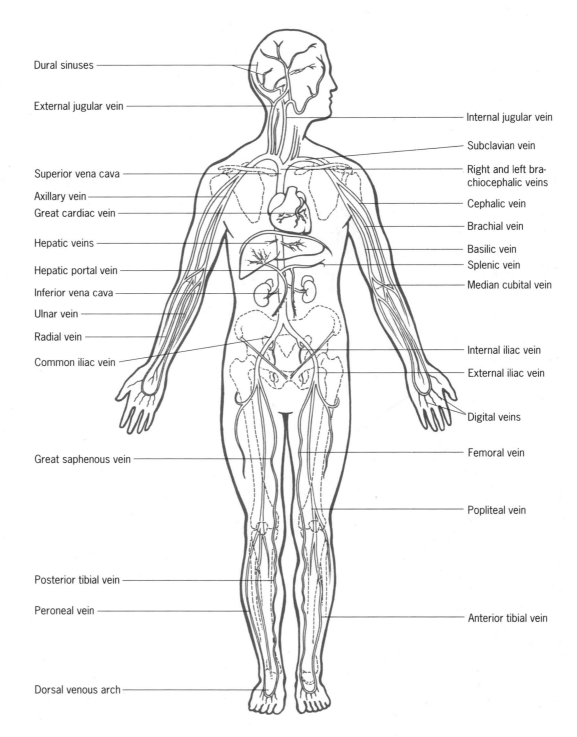

Dural sinuses

External jugular vein

Internal jugular vein

Subclavian vein

Right and left brachiocephalic veins

Superior vena cava

Axillary vein

Great cardiac vein

Cephalic vein

Brachial vein

Hepatic veins

Basilic vein

Hepatic portal vein

Splenic vein

Inferior vena cava

Median cubital vein

Ulnar vein

Radial vein

Common iliac vein

Internal iliac vein

External iliac vein

Digital veins

Great saphenous vein

Femoral vein

Popliteal vein

Posterior tibial vein

Peroneal vein

Anterior tibial vein

Dorsal venous arch

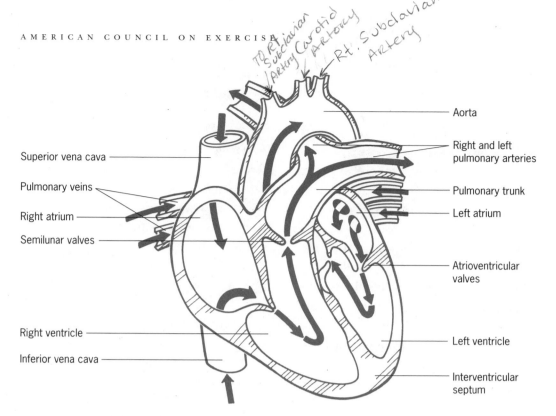

To Rt Jocular Artery
Subclavian Artery Carotid Artery
Rt. Subclavian Artery

- Aorta
- Right and left pulmonary arteries
- Pulmonary trunk
- Left atrium
- Atrioventricular valves
- Left ventricle
- Interventricular septum

Superior vena cava
Pulmonary veins
Right atrium
Semilunar valves
Right ventricle
Inferior vena cava

Figure 2.6
Structure of the heart and pattern of blood flow.

and left **primary bronchi.** The trachea is a 5-inch-long tubular passageway for air that is kept open by a series of C-shaped cartilages that function like the wire rings in a vacuum-cleaner hose.

After the trachea divides into the right and left primary bronchi, each primary bronchus then enters a lung and divides into smaller secondary bronchi, one for each lobe of the lungs. The secondary bronchi branch into many tertiary bronchi, and these branch several times further to eventually form tiny terminal **bronchioles.** The terminal bronchioles form microscopic branches called respiratory bronchioles that subdivide into several alveolar ducts (plural = **alveoli**).

The actual exchange of oxygen and carbon dioxide between the lungs and the blood occurs at this anatomic level. It is estimated that the lungs contain 300 million alveoli, which provide an extremely large surface area (approximately 230 square feet) for the exchange of gases. The continuous branching of the trachea resembles a tree trunk with its branches and is common-

ly referred to as the bronchial tree (Fig. 2.7).

The final components of the cardiorespiratory system to be noted are the lungs, two cone-shaped organs that lie within the thoracic cavity. The right lung has three lobes (superior, middle and inferior), while the left lung has only two (superior and inferior lobes). The diaphragm, the muscle that forms the floor of the thoracic cavity, contracts during inspiration and relaxes to allow expiration. The lungs are separated by a space known as the mediastinum. Most notably, the mediastinum contains the heart, the esophagus (food pipe), and part of the trachea.

THE NERVOUS SYSTEM

The nervous system is the body's control center and internal communication network. The nervous system has three primary functions: to monitor the changes (stimuli) occurring inside and outside the body by gathering information from millions of sensory receptors (sensory input); to analyze and interpret the sensory input and make decisions about what should oc-

Chapter 2
Fundamentals
of Anatomy

cur at each moment, and (3) to formulate a response (motor output) by activating muscles or glands.

For ease of discussion, the nervous system may be divided into two parts according to location: the central nervous system and the peripheral nervous system. The central nervous system (CNS) consists of the brain and the spinal cord. The CNS is fully enclosed within bony structures; the brain is protected by the skull while the spinal cord is protected within the vertebral canal of the spinal column. The CNS is the control center that receives input from the peripheral nervous system, integrates this information and formulates appropriate responses to the input.

The peripheral nervous system is composed of nerves that connect the outlying parts of the body (the extremities and trunk) with their receptors within the CNS. The peripheral nervous system includes 12 pairs (right and left) of cranial nerves, of which 2 pairs arise from the brain and 10 pairs originate from the brain stem; and

31 pairs of spinal nerves that arise from the spinal cord.

Spinal Nerves

The 31 pairs of spinal nerves include 8 cervical pairs, 12 thoracic pairs, 5 lumbar pairs, 5 sacral pairs and 1 coccygeal pair (Fig. 2.8). These nerves, which all have motor and sensory functions, are named and numbered according to region and the vertebral level from which they emerge from the spinal cord. For example, the sixth cervical nerve (written C6) exits the spinal cord at the level of sixth cervical vertebra.

The anterior (ventral) branches of the second through twelfth thoracic spinal nerves (written T2 through T12) individually supply muscles and abdominal organs. In all other cases, the ventral branches of the spinal nerves join with adjacent nerves to form a plexus, or a network of nerve branches. Only the ventral branches of these peripheral nerves form plexuses; the posterior (**dorsal**) branches are not in-

Figure 2.7a-b

a. Upper and lower respiratory pathways.

b. Terminal bronchiole into alveoli (enlarged view).

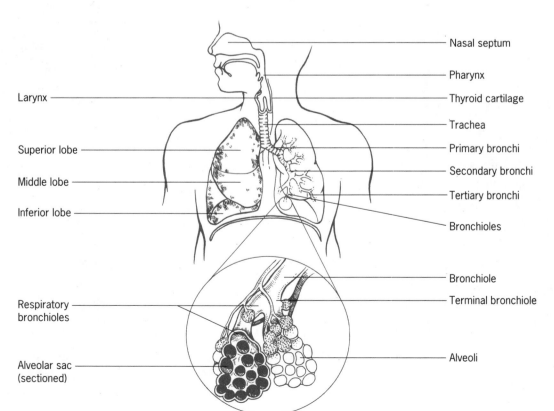

Nasal septum

Pharynx

Thyroid cartilage

Trachea

Primary bronchi

Secondary bronchi

Tertiary bronchi

Bronchioles

Larynx

Superior lobe

Middle lobe

Inferior lobe

Bronchiole

Terminal bronchiole

Respiratory bronchioles

Alveoli

Alveolar sac (sectioned)

volved. The configuration of spinal nerves into plexuses causes each resulting branch of a plexus to contain fibers from several spinal nerves, and thus provides a measure of protection against paralysis or loss of sensation if any single spinal nerve is damaged.

There are four main plexuses in the human body: the cervical plexus (C1 to C4 nerve roots), which innervates the head, neck, upper chest and shoulders; the brachial plexus (C5 to T1 nerve roots), supplying the shoulder down to the fingers

The nervous system

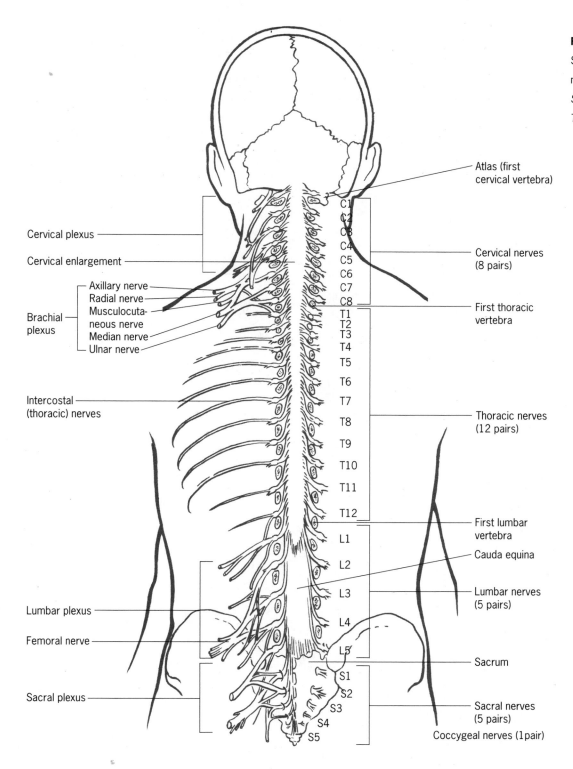

Figure 2.8

Spinal cord and spinal nerves (posterior view). *Source: Redrawn from Tortura (1992).*

of the hand; the lumbar plexus (L1 to L4 nerve roots), which supplies the abdomen, groin, genitalia and anterior and **lateral** thigh; and the sacral plexus (L4 to S4 nerve roots) (Fig. 2.8), which innervates the large muscles of the posterior thigh, and the entire lower leg, ankle and foot.

Sensory nerve cells carry nerve impulses from the peripheral **receptors** to the spinal cord and brain. Motor nerve cells carry impulses from the CNS to respond to the perceived changes in the body's internal or external environment. An example of how this system works may be illustrated by the

withdrawal reflex. If a hand encounters a very hot stimulus, say, scalding hot water, receptors in the skin send impulses to the spinal cord that communicate extreme heat and pain. In a matter of milliseconds, the appropriate muscles are activated to "withdraw" the hand from the hot water.

Similarly, when performing a complex physical activity, such as a step training routine, the central and peripheral nervous systems collaborate to initiate, guide and monitor all aspects of the specific activity. If someone previously learned how to perform the step-aerobics routine, it

Figure 2.9a-b
Skeletal system.

a. Anterior view.

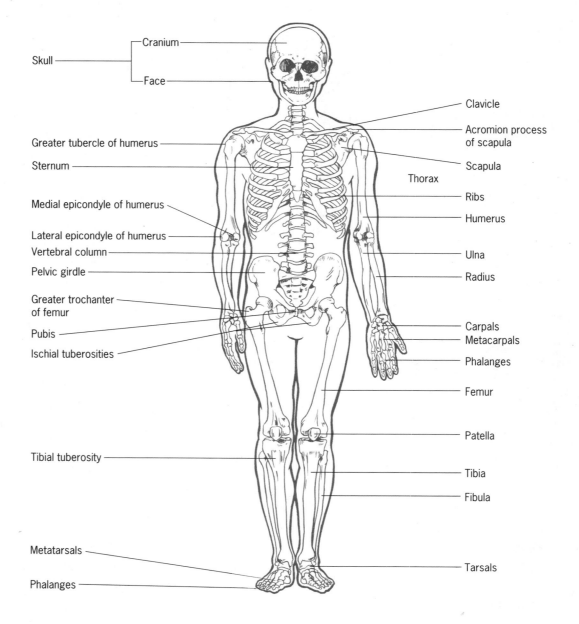

can be assumed that the CNS has stored in memory a sequential program of specific impulses to send to the muscles in order to perform the step routine in a coordinated manner. The nerve receptors in the periphery (in this example located in the lower extremity) provide constant information (feedback) to the CNS regarding the height of step, the cadence of the activity (musical rhythm), limb position, pressure sensed on the soles of the feet, and so on.

Communication between the central and peripheral nerve systems via the motor and sensory nerves is essential in order for one to learn, modify and successfully perform both the simple and complex physical activities of aerobic exercise.

THE MUSCULOSKELETAL SYSTEM

Aerobics instructors will develop numerous strengthening and flexibility exercise routines for clients. Essential to this task is a thorough understanding of the components of the human musculoskeletal system, in particular, the specific functions of bone and the locations and functions of

b. Posterior view.

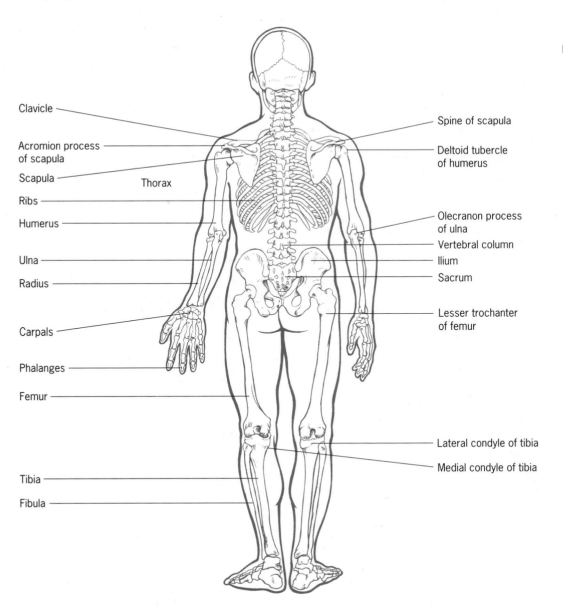

Clavicle

Acromion process of scapula

Scapula

Thorax

Ribs

Humerus

Ulna

Radius

Carpals

Phalanges

Femur

Tibia

Fibula

Spine of scapula

Deltoid tubercle of humerus

Olecranon process of ulna

Vertebral column

Ilium

Sacrum

Lesser trochanter of femur

Lateral condyle of tibia

Medial condyle of tibia

the muscles attached to the skeleton.

The Skeletal System

The human skeletal system (Fig. 2.9a-b), consisting of 206 bones, can be divided into two sections: the **axial skeleton,** with 80 bones that comprise the head, neck and trunk; and the **appendicular skeleton,** with 126 bones that form the extremities (Table 2.1).

Functions of Bone. The bones that form the skeleton combine to provide five basic, yet essential, functions. First, the skeletal system provides protection for many of the vital organs, such as the heart, brain, kidneys and spinal cord. Second, the skeleton provides support for the soft tissues so that erect posture and the form of the body can be maintained. Third, the bones provide a system of levers to which skeletal muscles are attached. The shapes of bones and joints to which these muscles attach determine the types of movement possible. Fourth, the red marrow of certain bones is responsible for the production of red blood cells, some types of white blood cells, and platelets. Finally, bones serve as key storage areas for calcium and phosphorus, as well as potassium, sodium and other minerals. Because of their high mineral content, bones remain intact for many years after death.

Composition of Bone. Bone is composed of two main ingredients: an organic component made of **collagen**, a complex protein that is found in various forms within other **connective tissues**; and an inorganic component of mineral salts, primarily calcium and phosphorus.

Many assume that once people reach their full height their bones become static structures that remain unchanged throughout their adult lives. Nothing could be further from the truth, for bones are dynamic structures that are constantly changing (remodeling) throughout life.

According to **Wolff's law**, bone is capable of adjusting its strength in proportion to the amount of stress placed upon it. If stresses are applied over long periods of

Table 2.1

THE 206 BONES OF THE HUMAN SKELETON

	Axial Skeleton	Number of Bones
Skull	Cranium	8
	Face	14
	Hyoid	1
	Vertebral column	26
Thorax	Sternum	1
	Ribs	24
	Auditory ossicles*	6
Total	Axial Skeleton Bones	80

	Appendicular Skeleton	Number of Bones
Lower Extremity	Phalanges	28
	Metatarsals	10
	Tarsals	14
	Patella	2
	Tibia	2
	Fibula	2
	Femur	2
Pelvic Girdle	Hip or pelvic bone (os coxae)	2
Shoulder Girdle	Clavicle	2
	Scapula	2
Upper Extremity	Phalanges	28
	Metacarpals	10
	Carpals	16
	Radius	2
	Ulna	2
	Humerus	2
Total	Appendicular Skeleton Bones	126

The auditory ossicles, three per ear, are not considered to be part of the axial or appendicular skeletons, but rather a separate group of bones. They were placed in the axial skeleton group for the sake of convenience.

time by such activities as aerobic exercise, resistance exercise and running/walking, bones with adequate blood supply and nutrition will become more dense through increased collagen fibers and mineral salts. If bone is not subjected to stress, as in individuals with a sedentary lifestyle or in the absence of gravity (as in space flights), bones will become less dense as mineral salts are gradually withdrawn from bone.

An easy way to remember Wolff's law is with the phrase, "form follows function." Simply stated, the form that bone will take (strong or weak) is in direct response to the recent function of that bone.

The current prevalence of **osteoporosis** among some **amenorrheic** and many **post-menopausal** women should underscore to aerobics instructors the importance of the unique ability of bone to respond to the stresses (or lack of stresses) placed upon it.

The causes of osteoporosis are multi-factorial, including genetics (gender and race), dietary calcium intake, level of physical activity and reproductive hormone (estrogen) status. The fitness professional must always have the bone health of the client in mind when designing and implementing specific aerobics programs.

Classifications of bone. Bones may also be classified according to their shape: long, short, flat or irregular.

Long bones are those bones whose length exceeds their width and thickness. Most of the bones in the lower and upper extremities are long bones. They include the femur, tibia, fibula and metatarsals in the lower limb; and the humerus, radius, ulna and metacarpals in the upper extremity.

Each long bone has a shaft called a diaphysis and two ends that are usually wider than the shaft, known as epiphyses (singular = epiphysis) (Fig. 2.10). The diaphysis of a long bone is surrounded by a sheath of connective tissue called periosteum. The periosteum has two layers, an outer fibrous layer that provides attachment sites for tendons and ligaments, and an inner layer that contains osteoblasts (bone-forming cells). As new bone is being formed by the periosteum, bone is also being reabsorbed by osteoclasts (bone-destroying cells) that line the medullary cavity, the middle section of the diaphysis of long bones. Fat is also stored within the medullary cavity (Fig. 2.10).

Short bones do not have a long axis, but are approximately equal in length and width. Short bones are found in the hands (carpals) and the feet (tarsals). Flat bones

Figure 2.10

Long bone gross anatomy.

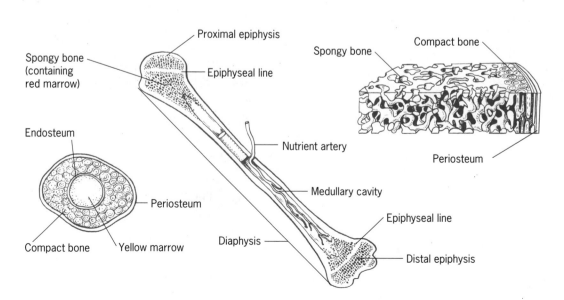

Spongy bone (containing red marrow)

Proximal epiphysis

Epiphyseal line

Endosteum

Periosteum

Compact bone

Yellow marrow

Diaphysis

Nutrient artery

Medullary cavity

Epiphyseal line

Distal epiphysis

Spongy bone

Compact bone

Periosteum

are thin but tend to be curved rather than flat. Examples of flat bones include the bones of the skull, the ribs, sternum and scapulae (shoulder blades). Irregular bones are defined as bones of various shapes that do not fit into the other three categories of bones. The hip bones, the **vertebrae**, and many of the bones of the skull are examples of irregular bones.

The Axial Skeleton. As previously stated, the **axial skeleton** consists of the 80 bones that form the skull, the vertebral column and the thorax. This portion of the skeletal system provides the main structural support for the body and protects the central nervous system and vital organs of the thorax (brain, heart, lungs). Of primary interest is the vertebral column, consisting of 33 vertebrae divided into five subgroups according to the region of the body. Start-

ing at the head and moving downward, the first seven vertebrae are called **cervical** vertebrae, followed by twelve thoracic vertebrae, five lumbar, five sacral vertebrae and four **coccygeal** vertebrae. Children and adolescents have 33 movable vertebrae; adults have only 26 movable vertebrae as the sacral vertebrae fuse to form the sacrum, while the coccygeal vertebrae fuse to become the **coccyx** (Fig. 2.11).

The Appendicular Skeleton. The appendicular skeleton is composed of the bones of the lower and upper limbs, and the bones by which the legs and arms attach to the axial skeleton—the pelvic (hip) and pectoral (chest) girdles. The pelvic girdle consists of two large hip bones known collectively as the os coxae, with right and left sides comprising an ilium, an ischium and a pubis (Fig. 2.9). Much of the weight supported by the os coxae is transferred to the bones of the lower limbs.

The right and left pectoral girdles, each consisting of a clavicle (collarbone) and scapula (shoulder blade), attach the bones of the upper extremities to the axial skeleton at the sternum (Fig. 2.9). The sternoclavicular joints are the only bony attachments of the upper extremity to the axial skeleton. The configuration of the pectoral girdle permits a wide range of movement at the shoulder, making this the most mobile joint in the body. Unfortunately, the anatomical trade-off for increased **mobility** is decreased stability, and thus, injuries to the shoulder joint are quite common.

Articulations (Joints)

Joints link bones together to form the functional units that permit body movement. An **articulation** (joint) is the point of contact or connection between bones, or between bones and cartilage. The stability of each joint is maintained by **ligaments**—

Figure 2.11

Vertebral column
(lateral view).

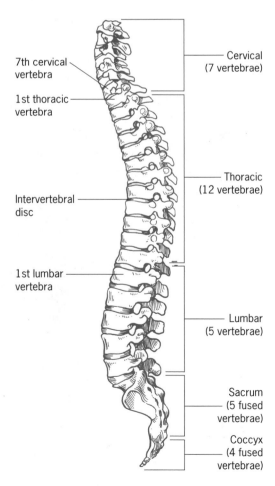

7th cervical
vertebra

1st thoracic
vertebra

Intervertebral
disc

1st lumbar
vertebra

Cervical
(7 vertebrae)

Thoracic
(12 vertebrae)

Lumbar
(5 vertebrae)

Sacrum
(5 fused
vertebrae)

Coccyx
(4 fused
vertebrae)

dense, fibrous strands of connective tissue that link the bony segments together. Some joints permit a large **range of motion** in several directions, while other joints permit no motion whatsoever. The numerous joints in the human body can be described by two general characteristics: according to structure and according to the type(s) of movement possible.

Structural Classification of Joints. Two major characteristics differentiate the types of joints in the body: the type of connective tissue that holds the bones together and the presence or absence of a joint cavity. There are three major structural categories of joints—fibrous, cartilaginous and synovial.

Fibrous joints have no joint cavity and include all joints in which the bones are held tightly together by fibrous connective tissues, ligaments and interosseous membranes. Very little space separates the ends of the bones of these joints, and as a result, little or no movement occurs. Examples of fibrous joints include the joints (sutures) between the bones of the skull, the joint between the distal tibia and fibula, and between the radius and ulna (Fig. 2.12).

Cartilaginous joints are those in which the bones are united by cartilage. No joint cavity exists, and, like fibrous joints, little or no motion occurs. Familiar examples of cartilaginous joints include the joints formed by the articular cartilages that connect the ribs to the sternum (breastbone) (Fig. 2.13) and the fibrocartilages that separate the vertebrae in the spinal column.

The majority of joints in the body are synovial joints. In these joints, a space exists between the bones that form the joint. The movement of a synovial joint is limited only by the shapes of the bones and the soft tissues (ligaments, joint capsules, tendons, muscles) that surround it.

Synovial joints have four distinguishing features that structurally set them apart

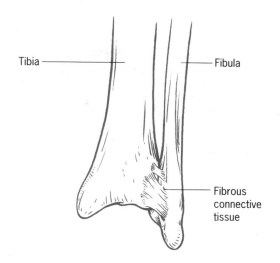

Tibia

Fibula

Fibrous connective tissue

The musculoskeletal system

Figure 2.12

Example of a fibrous joint: distal tibiofibular joint at the ankle.

from the other types of joints. First, the ends of the bones are covered with a thin layer of articular (hyaline) cartilage. While this type of cartilage covers the surfaces of the articulating bones, it does not attach the bones together. Second, all synovial joints are surrounded by a joint capsule made of dense, fibrous connective tissue. Third, the inner surface of the joint capsule is lined with a thin synovial membrane. The synovial membrane's primary function is the secretion of synovial fluid, the fourth distinguishing characteristic of this type of joint. Synovial fluid acts as a lubricant for the joint and provides nutrition to the articular cartilage. Normally, only a very small amount of synovial fluid (3 to 5 milliliters) is present in even the largest joints, such as the knee. However, overuse of a synovial joint can stimulate the synovial membrane to secrete excessive synovial fluid, which typically affects function due to swelling and pain.

In addition to these four features, some synovial joints have fibrocartilage disks called meniscii (singular = meniscus). When present in a joint, these meniscii may divide the joint cavity into two separate spaces. In a large, weight-bearing joint such as the knee, these fibrocartilages help to absorb shock, increase joint stability, and aid in joint nutrition by directing the flow of syn-

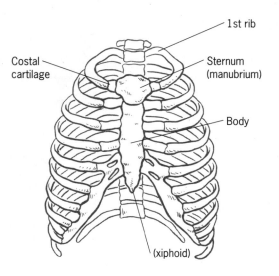

Costal cartilage
1st rib
Sternum (manubrium)
Body
(xiphoid)

Figure 2.13

Example of cartilaginous joint: attachment of the ribs to the sternum. *Source: Redrawn from Luttgens (1992).*

ovial fluid. A torn meniscus is one of the most common knee injuries, and will be discussed in Chapter 13.

Functional Classification of Joints. Functional classification of joints is based upon the amount and type of movement they allow. Fibrous joints are classified as **synar-**

throses (syn = together, arthro = joint; "an immovable joint") (Fig. 2.12). Cartilaginous joints, which fall into the category of **amphiarthroses** (amphi = on both sides, arthro = joint; "cartilage on both sides of the joint"), are slightly movable (Fig. 2.13). Finally, the largest functional category of joints, **diarthrodial** (di = apart, arthro = joint; "apart joint"), are synovial joints. Diarthroses are freely movable joints and many different movements are possible.

Unlike joints classified according to the way the bones are connected, synovial joints are defined based upon the movements they allow. Typically, the shapes of the bony structures that form a synovial joint are the primary factors in limiting that joint's movement. Other factors that limit motion in synovial joints are: ligament/capsule tension, muscle/tendon tension, and apposition (touching) of the

Table 2.2

MAJOR JOINTS OF THE BODY

	Joint	Type	Axes of Rotation	Movement(s) Possible
Lower Extremity	Metatarsophalangeal (feet and toes)	synovial	2	Flexion-extension; abduction-adduction; circumduction
	Subtalar	synovial	1	Inversion-eversion
	Ankle	synovial	1	Plantarflexion-dorsiflexion
	Knee (femur and tibia)	synovial	2	Flexion-extension; medial-lateral rotation
	Hip	synovial	3	Flexion-extension; abduction-adduction; circumduction; medial-lateral rotation
Upper Extremity	Metacarpophalangeal (hands and fingers)	synovial	2	Flexion-extension; abduction-adduction; circumduction
	Thumb	synovial	3	Flexion-extension; abduction-adduction; circumduction; opposition
	Wrist	synovial	2	Flexion-extension; abduction-adduction; circumduction
	Proximal Radioulnar	synovial	1	Pronation-supination
	Elbow (ulna and humerus)	synovial	1	Flexion-extension
	Shoulder	synovial	3	Flexion-extension; abduction-adduction; circumduction; medial-lateral rotation
	Ribs and sternum	cartilaginous	0	Slight movement possible

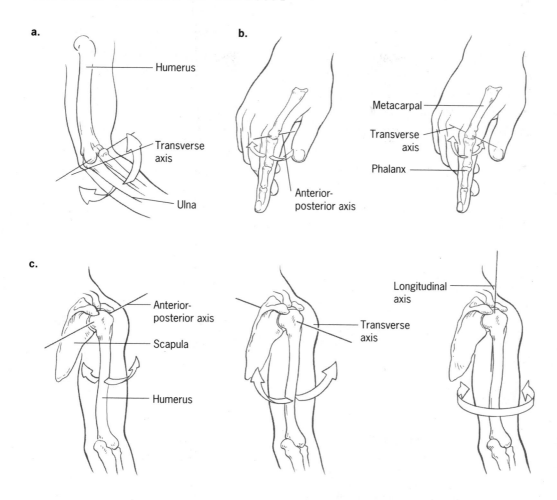

a.

Humerus

Transverse axis

Ulna

b.

Metacarpal

Transverse axis

Phalanx

Anterior-posterior axis

c.

Anterior-posterior axis

Scapula

Humerus

Transverse axis

Longitudinal axis

Figure 2.14a-c

Movement of synovial joints.

a. Uniaxial: Flexion and extension of the elbow (sagittal plane).

b. Biaxial: Abduction and adduction about an anterior-posterior axis in the frontal plane. Flexion and extension about a transverse axis (sagittal plane).

c. Multiaxial: Abduction and adduction around anterior-posterior axis (frontal plane). Flexion and extension around transverse axis (sagittal plane). Medial and lateral rotation around longitudinal axis (transverse plane).

soft tissues (e.g., a bodybuilder's forearm against her biceps limiting elbow flexion).

A summary of the major joints in the body, classified by the type and movements possible at each, is presented in Table 2.2.

Movement of Synovial Joints. All motions at joints are described as occurring in an anatomical plane (sagittal, frontal or transverse) about an axis of rotation (Fig. 2.2). An axis of rotation is an imaginary line perpendicular (at right angles to) the plane of movement about which a joint rotates. Many joints have several axes of rotation that allow movement in the various anatomical planes (Fig. 2.14a-c).

Uniaxial joints have one axis of rotation and permit movement on one anatomical plane. Uniaxial joints are also known as hinge joints, as the hinges on a door work only in one plane. The ankle (talocrural) and elbow (ulnohumeral) joints are the best examples of uniaxial joints. Some joints have two axes of rotation, allowing motion in two planes. These biaxial joints are common throughout the body and include the knee (tibiofemoral) joint, the metacarpal-phalangeal joints (linking the hands and fingers), and the metatarsal-phalangeal joints (linking the feet and toes). Multiaxial joints are defined as having at least three axes of motion and permitting movement in three planes. Examples include the hip joint, the shoulder (glenohumeral) joint and the thumb (first metacarpal-phalangeal) joint.

Two basic types of movements occur in the various synovial joints: angular and circular. Angular movements increase or decrease the angle between bones and are most frequently called flexion, extension, abduction and adduction.

Flexion and **extension** occur in the sagittal plane of motion. Flexion usually involves a decrease in the angle between the anterior surfaces of articulating bones while extension most often describes an increase in this angle. Exceptions to these definitions occur at the knee and toe joints, at which the reference points for flexion and extension are the posterior articulating surfaces of the joints. Additionally, in the anatomical position the palms face forward and, therefore, wrist flexion is anterior.

Abduction and **adduction** movements always occur in the frontal plane and are defined with respect to the midline of the body. When an arm or leg is moved away from the midline of the body, abduction occurs. Adduction is the return motion from abduction, and involves movement of the body part toward the midline of the body to regain anatomical position.

In addition to the four primary angular movements, four circular movements occur at some synovial joints. Forearm **supination** and **pronation** are motions that occur in the transverse plane. Supination is the term that specifically describes the **lateral (outward) rotation** of the forearm causing the palms of the hands to face anteriorly. The radius and the ulna are parallel in this position, the anatomical position for the forearms (Fig. 2.1). Pronation describes the **medial (inward) rotation** of the forearm in which the radius crosses diagonally over the ulna and the palms of the hand face posteriorly.

Rotation is defined as the motion of a bone around a central axis, and is described as being either **medial** or lateral rotation of the anterior surface of the bone involved. Rotation occurs in the transverse plane about an imaginary axis that runs the length of the bone(s). The fourth circular movement, **circumduction**, is the sequential combination of flexion, abduc-

tion, extension and adduction. Similar to rotation, circumduction commonly occurs at the hip and shoulder joints.

The fundamental movements at some synovial joints are given specialized names in order to indicate the joint at which the motion occurs and to clarify their action. These movements, along with the primary angular and circular movements, are presented in Table 2.3. Chapter 3, "Biomechanics and Applied Kinesiology," presents examples of movements within the anatomical planes.

The Muscular System

As the bones and joints provide the framework for the body, muscular activity produces the forces that enable people to move. Knowledge of the location, functions and interrelationships of muscles and muscle groups is critical for the aerobics instructor.

Types of Muscle Tissue. There are three general types of muscle tissue: skeletal, cardiac and visceral. Skeletal muscle tissue is voluntary muscle, i.e., it can be stimulated or relaxed by conscious effort. Both ends of a skeletal muscle are attached to bone via **tendons** (dense cords of connective tissue). In some cases, skeletal muscles are attached to bone by an aponeurosis, a broad, flat type of tendon. The wide, flat insertion of the rectus abdominis is an excellent example of an aponeurosis.

Cardiac muscle tissue forms the walls of the heart and is involuntary by nature. The third type of muscle, visceral muscle, is found in the walls of internal organs, like the stomach and intestines, and in blood vessels. The contraction of visceral muscle is also involuntary and not subject to conscious control.

Given that there are more than 600 muscles in the body, only the major muscles can be discussed in this chapter. In naming muscles, several criteria are employed to describe particular characteristics of the muscle being identified. Muscles are named according to their location (posterior tibialis, subscapularis), shape (deltoid, trapezius, rhomboid), action (flexor digitorum longus, adductor magnus), number of divisions (biceps femoris, triceps brachii, quadriceps femoris), size (pectoralis major, pectoralis minor) and bony attachments (coracobrachialis, iliocostalis).

When skeletal muscle is stimulated, it develops force either by shortening (**concentric muscle action**) or by lengthening (**eccentric muscle action**). Muscle tissue also has elastic properties, so that with proper techniques, muscles may be safely stretched. From a functional perspective, most muscles of the extremities and trunk are arranged in opposing pairs, so that when one muscle is acting to achieve a desired movement (the **agonist**), its opposite muscle (the **antagonist**) is being stretched. For example, when contracting the hip flexor muscles during the upward phase of a step-aerobics routine, one's hip extensor

The musculoskeletal system

Table 2.3

FUNDAMENTAL MOVEMENTS FROM ANATOMICAL POSITION

Plane	Action	Definition
Sagittal	Flexion	Decreasing the angle between two bones.
	Extension	Increasing the angle between two bones.
	Dorsiflexion	Moving the top of the foot toward the shin (ankle only).
	Plantarflexion	Moving the sole of the foot downward; "pointing the toes" (ankle only).
Frontal	Abduction	Motion away from the midline of the body (or part).
	Adduction	Motion toward the midline of the body (or part).
	Elevation	Moving to a superior position (scapula).
	Depression	Moving to an inferior position (scapula).
	Inversion	Lifting the medial border of the foot (subtalar joint only).
	Eversion	Lifting the lateral border of the foot (subtalar joint only).
Transverse	Rotation	Medial (inward) or lateral (outward) turning about the vertical axis of bone.
	Pronation	Rotating the hand and wrist medially from the elbow.
	Supination	Rotating the hand and wrist laterally from the elbow.
	Horizontal flexion	From a 90-degree, abducted arm position, the humerus is flexed in toward the midline of the body in the transverse plane.
	Horizontal extension	The return of the humerus from horizontal flexion.
Multiplanar	Circumduction	Motion that describes a "cone"; combines flexion, abduction, extension and adduction in sequential order.
	Opposition	Thumb movement unique to primates and humans.
	Pronation (foot)	Combination of ankle joint dorsiflexion, subtalar joint eversion and forefoot abduction.
	Supination (foot)	Combination of ankle joint plantarflexion, subtalar joint inversion and forefoot adduction.

Table 2.4

ACTIONS OF MAJOR LOWER-EXTREMITY MULTIJOINT MUSCLES

Muscle	Hip	Knee	Ankle
Rectus Femoris	flexion	extension	
Biceps Femoris	extension (long head); lateral rotation	flexion; lateral rotation	
Semitendinosus	extension; medial rotation	flexion; medial rotation	
Semimembranosus	extension; medial rotation	flexion; medial rotation	
Gracilis	adduction; medial rotation	flexion; medial rotation	
Sartorius	flexion; lateral rotation	flexion; medial rotation	
Gastrocnemius		flexion	plantarflexion

muscles are stretched.

At most joints several muscles combine to perform the same anatomical function; these muscles are functionally known as **synergists.** For example, the synergistic contractions of, among others, the gastrocnemius, soleus and posterior tibialis muscles, produce **plantarflexion** at the ankle joint.

The forces produced by muscular contraction create human motion and maintain posture. Locomotion (walking, running) is the result of the complex, combined functioning of the bones, joints and muscles attached to the bones. A by-product of muscle activity is the creation of heat that plays a critical role in maintaining normal body temperature. Shivering uncontrollably from being too cold is the body's automatic effort to produce much-needed heat through muscular contractions.

From a functional perspective, a skeletal muscle can be viewed as a "rope and pulley" system. The "rope" in this analogy is the cord-like tendon attached near a joint, and the "pulley" is the force applied by a muscle through its tendon.

By knowing the origins and insertions of the major skeletal muscles, one can readily determine the anatomical motions these muscles produce. The term origin is used

to describe the location of attachment of a muscle to a fixed or nonmovable bone. There is often more than one origin for a given muscle. For example, the psoas major originates from each of the five transverse processes of the lumbar vertebrae. The term insertion is used in anatomy to describe a muscle's attachment to a movable bone via its tendon. Typically, the origin is the proximal attachment of the muscle while its insertion is the distal attachment.

Muscles of the Lower Extremity

The major links of the lower extremity are the ankle joint, formed by the distal tibia, distal fibula and talus; the knee joint, composed of the tibiofemoral and patellofemoral joints; and the hip joint, linking the femur with the hip.

Compared to the muscles of the upper extremity, the muscles of the lower extremity tend to be larger and thus are more able to develop force. Many of the muscles of the lower extremity cross two joints (either the hip and the knee or the knee and the ankle). The major muscles of the lower extremity that act at more than one joint are listed in Table 2.4.

Muscles of the Leg. The muscles of the leg are grouped into three compartments

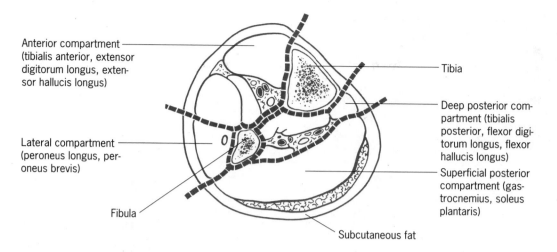

Anterior compartment (tibialis anterior, extensor digitorum longus, extensor hallucis longus)

Lateral compartment (peroneus longus, peroneus brevis)

Fibula

Tibia

Deep posterior compartment (tibialis posterior, flexor digitorum longus, flexor hallucis longus)

Superficial posterior compartment (gastrocnemius, soleus plantaris)

Subcutaneous fat

Figure 2.15

Muscular compartments of the left lower leg (transverse section cut just below the knee).

(anterior, lateral, posterior) divided by fascia and an interosseous membrane (inter = "between," os = "bone") between the tibia and fibula. The tibial compartments are associated with the anatomical functions of the muscles, for the location of a muscle in relation to the joint in which it acts dictates its function (Fig. 2.15).

The anterior tibial compartment muscles extend the toes and **dorsiflex** (flex) the ankle. These muscles include the anterior tibialis, extensor digitorum longus and extensor hallucis longus. The peroneus longus and brevis muscles are located in the lateral tibial compartment and act to cause **eversion** (abduction) of the foot and plantarflexion of the ankle. The muscles of the posterior tibial compartment are divided into three superficial compartment muscles (gastrocnemius, soleus, plantaris) and four deep compartment muscles (popliteus, posterior tibialis, flexor hallucis longus, flexor digitorum longus). The primary functions of these posterior muscles

Table 2.5

MAJOR MUSCLES THAT ACT AT THE ANKLE AND FOOT

Muscle	Origin	Insertion	Primary Functions
Anterior Tibialis	proximal two thirds of lateral tibia	medial aspect of 1st cuneiform and 1st metatarsal	ankle dorsiflexion; foot inversion
Peroneus Longus	head of fibula and proximal two thirds of lateral fibula	inferior aspects of 1st cuneiform and 1st metatarsal	ankle plantarflexion; foot eversion
Peroneus Brevis	distal two thirds of lateral fibula	base of the 5th metatarsal	ankle plantarflexion; foot eversion
Gastrocnemius	posterior surfaces of the femoral condyles	posterior surface of calcaneus via Achilles tendon	ankle plantarflexion
Soleus	proximal two thirds of posterior surfaces of tibia and fibula	posterior surface of calcaneus via Achilles tendon	ankle plantarflexion
Posterior Tibialis	posterior surface of the tibia-fibular interosseous membrane	lower medial surfaces of medial tarsals and metatarsals	ankle plantarflexion; foot inversion

Table 2.6

MAJOR MUSCLES THAT ACT AT THE KNEE JOINT

Muscle	Origin	Insertion	Primary Function(s)
Rectus Femoris	anterior-inferior spine of ilium	patella and tibial tuberosity	knee extension
Vastus medialis, intermedius and lateralis	proximal two thirds of anterior femur at midline	patella and tibial tuberosity	knee extension
Biceps Femoris	ischial tuberosity	lateral condyle of tibia and head of the fibula	knee flexion and lateral rotation
Semitendinosus	ischial tuberosity	proximal anterior-medial aspect of tibia	knee flexion and medial rotation
Semimebranosus	ischial tuberosity	posterior aspect of medial tibial condyle	knee flexion and medial rotation

are plantarflexion (extension) of the ankle, flexion of the toes and **inversion** of the foot. The Achilles tendon, the largest tendon in the body, attaches the gastrocnemius and soleus to the calcaneus (heel bone). The origins, insertions and primary functions of the muscles of the leg that act at the ankle and foot are presented in Table 2.5.

Muscles of the Thigh. Similar to the muscles of the leg, muscles of the thigh can be divided into three functional and anatomical compartments (anterior, medial, posterior). Many of these muscles act at both the knee and hip joints (Table 2.4). The four major muscles on the front of the thigh are located in the anterior compartment. The primary function of these muscles is to extend the knee. These muscles are typically grouped together and referred to as the quadriceps, although each muscle has its own individual name. The quadriceps, in descending order from largest to smallest cross-sectional size, are the rectus femoris, vastus lateralis, vastus medialis and vastus intermedius (Fig. 2.16). The quadriceps insert via a common tendon known as the patellar tendon, which attaches to the tibia just below the knee at the tibial tubercle. The rectus femoris is the only muscle of

the quadriceps group that crosses the hip joint, and given its location in front of the hip joint, acts as a hip flexor.

The muscles in the medial compartment of the thigh are the adductor muscles, named for their function at the hip joint. These muscles bring the thigh toward the midline of the body and include the adductor magnus, adductor longus and adductor brevis. The adductor muscles originate on the pelvis and insert all along the medial aspect of the femur. The adductor magnus laterally rotates the femur, while the adductor longus and adductor brevis medially rotate the femur.

The muscles in the posterior compartment of the thigh are the biceps femoris, semitendinosus and semimembranosus. These muscles, collectively known as the hamstrings, are two-joint muscles that cross the knee and hip joints to cause flexion of the knee and extension of the hip. This group of large muscles has its common origin at the ischial tuberosity (Fig. 2.17). In the normally active individual, the hamstrings are about one half the size and force-generating capacity of the quadriceps. This agonist/antagonist muscle imbalance makes the hamstrings vulnerable to muscle injuries.

The biceps femoris attaches laterally to the head of the fibula, while the semitendinosus and semimembranosus attach on the medial aspect of the tibia. Between the hamstring tendons lies the popliteal space, a triangular area on the posterior aspect of the knee joint (Fig. 2.17).

When the knee is fully extended ("locked"), no rotation is possible. When the knee is flexed, both medial rotation (by the semitendinosus and semimembranosus) and lateral rotation (by the biceps femoris) are possible. Maximum rotation of the knee joint occurs when the knee is bent at 90 degrees.

A fourth major group of muscles on the thigh is the pes anserine ("goose's foot") group, which includes the sartorius and the gracilis and the previously mentioned semitendinosus. These muscles are grouped together due to their common tendinous attachment, shaped like a goose's foot, on the medial tibia just below the knee. The sartorius, the longest muscle in the body, originates on the ilium and courses diagonally across the anterior aspect of the thigh to its insertion on the proximal tibia. Although it is an anterior muscle, concentric muscle action of the sartorius produces knee flexion. As a group, these three muscles medially rotate the tibia when the knee is flexed.

The origins, insertions and primary functions of the major muscles of the thigh that act upon the knee are presented in Table 2.6.

Muscles of the Hip. Most of the muscles that cross the hip joint have their origins on the pelvis. The psoas major and the psoas minor, located on the anterior aspect of the hip, originate from the five lumbar vertebrae. These two muscles, along with the iliacus, attach to the lesser trochanter on the medial femur, and work together as powerful flexors of the hip.

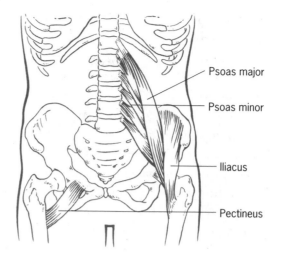

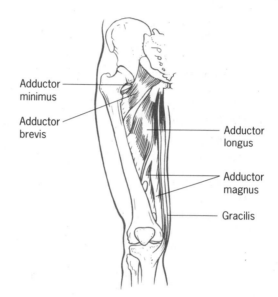

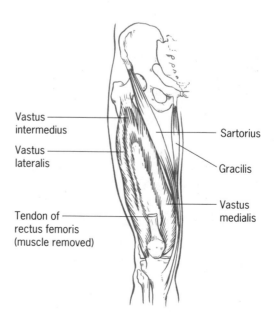

The musculoskeletal system

Figure 2.16a-c
Anterior lower extremity muscles.
Source: Redrawn from Luttgens (1992).

a. Hip.

b. Thigh.

c. Knee.

This group of three muscles is commonly referred to as the iliopsoas muscle (Fig. 2.16).

Posteriorly, three large muscles combine to give shape to the buttocks and serve as powerful mobilizers of the hip joint. The gluteus maximus, the largest and most superficial of the three gluteal muscles, extends and externally rotates the hip. Underlying the gluteus maximus are the gluteus medius and gluteus minimus, which work together to abduct and medially rotate the femur (Fig. 2.17).

The origins, insertions and primary actions of major muscles of the hip are presented in Table 2.7.

Muscles of the Trunk

Discussion of the muscles of the trunk will be limited to the major muscles associated with the spinal column and the walls of the abdomen. Concentric and eccentric actions of these muscles, in their agonist/antagonist relationships, result primarily in flexion and extension of the trunk.

Posteriorly, three major muscles are responsible for movement of the trunk: the iliocostalis, the longissimus and the spinalis. These muscles are better known by their functional name as extensors of the trunk—the erector spinae. These vertical, column-like muscles originate on the pelvis and are found on both the right and left sides of the spine.

Most medial of the three muscles is the spinalis; the longissimus is the long, intermediate muscle and the iliocostalis (extending from the pelvis to the neck) is the most lateral. In addition to extending the trunk, unilateral contraction of the iliocostalis muscle will produce **lateral flexion** to that side (Fig. 2.18).

Concentric muscle action of the erector spinae produces trunk extension, while eccentric muscle action of the erector spinae helps control the action of bending forward at the waist (e.g., to touch the toes, by resisting the downward pull of gravity on the body). The walls of the abdominal cavity are supported entirely by the strength of the muscles located there, as no bones provide support for this region. To make up for the lack of skeletal support, the three layers of muscles in the abdominal wall run in different directions, thus providing additional support (Fig. 2.19). In the outermost (superficial) layer is the external oblique muscle, whose fibers run anteriorly downward and toward the midline. In the second layer, the fibers of the internal oblique muscle run posteriorly and downward. An easy way to remember the orientation of the external obliques is to place the palms on the sides of the ribs and slide the hands forward into the front pockets of a pair of jeans. Conversely, to trace the path of the internal obliques, again place the hands on the sides of the chest, sliding them diagonally backward into the rear pockets.

Unilateral (one-sided) tension in the lateral fibers of the obliques (external and internal) produces lateral flexion of the

Figure 2.17

Posterior lower extremity muscles of the hip and thigh.

Source: Redrawn from Luttgens (1992).

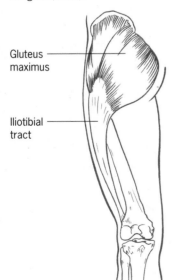

Gluteus maximus

Iliotibial tract

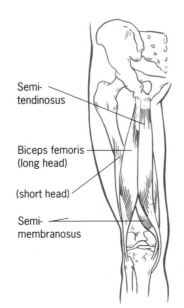

Semi-tendinosus

Biceps femoris (long head)

(short head)

Semi-membranosus

Table 2.7

MAJOR MUSCLES THAT ACT ON THE HIP JOINT

Muscle	Origin	Insertion	Primary Function(s)
Iliacus	inner surface of the ilium and base of sacrum	lesser trochanter of femur	hip flexion and lateral rotation
Psoas Major and Psoas Minor	transverse processes of all five lumbar vertebrae	lesser trochanter of femur	hip flexion and lateral rotation
Rectus Femoris	anterior-inferior spine of ilium	superior aspect of patella and tibial tuberosity	hip flexion
Gluteus Maximus	posterior one fourth of iliac crest and a sacrum	gluteal line of femur and iliotibial band	hip extension, abduction, adduction and lateral rotation
Gluteus Medius and Gluteus Minimus	lateral surface of ilium	greater trochanter of femur	hip abduction
Biceps Femoris	ischial tuberosity	lateral condyle of tibia and head of the fibula	hip extension and lateral rotation
Semitendinosus	ischial tuberosity	proximal anterior-medial aspect of tibia	hip extension
Semimembranosus	ischial tuberosity	posterior aspect of medial tibial condyle	hip extension
Adductor Magnus	pubic ramus and ischial tuberosity	medial aspects of femur	hip adduction and lateral rotation
Adductor Brevis and Longus	pubic ramus and ischial tuberosity	medial aspects of femur	adduction, flexion and medial rotation

trunk on that side. Trunk rotation is produced by concentric muscle actions of opposing external and internal oblique muscles (e.g., contractions of the left internal oblique and right external oblique produce left rotation of the trunk). Contraction of the right and left external and internal obliques compresses the abdominal cavity; these muscles are active during forced exhalation, defecation and urination.

The transverse abdominis muscle is the deepest muscular layer in the abdominal wall. The fibers of this thin muscle run horizontally, encircling the abdominal cavity. Contraction of this muscle also compresses the abdomen. The rectus abdominis is a narrow, flat muscle on the anterior aspect of the abdominal wall that flexes the trunk. The fibers of the rectus abdominis

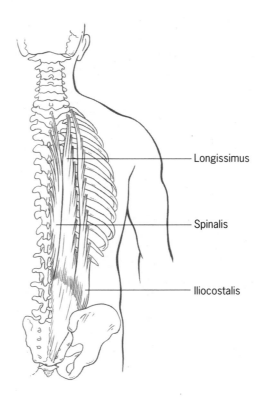

Longissimus

Spinalis

Iliocostalis

Figure 2.18

The erector spinae muscles (posterior view). *Source: Redrawn from Daniels & Worthingham (1986).*

Table 2.8

MAJOR MUSCLES THAT ACT ON THE TRUNK

Muscle	Origin	Insertion	Primary Function(s)
Rectus Abdominis	pubic crest	cartilage of 5th through 7th ribs & xiphoid process	flexion and lateral rotation of the trunk
External Oblique	anterolateral borders of lower eight ribs	anterior half of ilium, pubic crest and anterior fascia	lateral flexion of the trunk and trunk rotation
Internal Oblique	iliac crest	cartilage of last three to four ribs	lateral flexion of the trunk and trunk rotation
Transverse Abdominis	iliac crest, lumbar fascia and cartilages of last six ribs	xiphoid process of sternum, anterior fascia and pubis	compresses abdomen
Erector Spinae	posterior iliac crest and sacrum	angles of ribs, transverse processes of all ribs	extension of trunk

are vertically oriented, run from the pubis to the rib cage, and are crossed by three transverse fibrous bands called tendinous inscriptions (Fig. 2.19).

The origins, insertions and primary functions of the muscles that act on the trunk are presented in Table 2.8.

Muscles of the Upper Extremity

When studying the musculature of the upper extremity, concentrate on understanding the motions (and muscles responsible for producing motion) at the four major links: the shoulder joint, consisting of the proximal humerus and the glenoid fossa of the scapula; the scapulothoracic articulation; the elbow joint, formed by the proximal ulna and the distal humerus; and

the wrist joint, composed of the distal radius and ulna, and proximal carpal bones. The connection between the scapula and the thorax is not a bony joint, but an important soft tissue (muscle and fascia) link between the scapula and the trunk (Fig. 2.9). Many muscles in the upper extremity act at two joints. These muscles are identified in Table 2.9.

Muscles of the Shoulder. This chapter covers seven major muscles of the shoulder (glenohumeral) joint. The two largest muscles that act at the shoulder, the pectoralis major and the latissimus dorsi, have their origins on the thorax. Most people are familiar with the anterior location of the pectoralis major, which makes up the contour of the chest. The pectoralis major has several important functions at the shoulder: flexion, adduction and medial rotation. The latissimus dorsi, the primary extensor of the shoulder joint, arises posteriorly from the pelvis and lumbar and lower thoracic vertebrae. Although a posterior chest muscle, the latissimus dorsi, thanks to its insertion on the medial humerus near the pectoralis major, shares two functions with the pectoralis: adduction and medial rotation (Fig. 2.20).

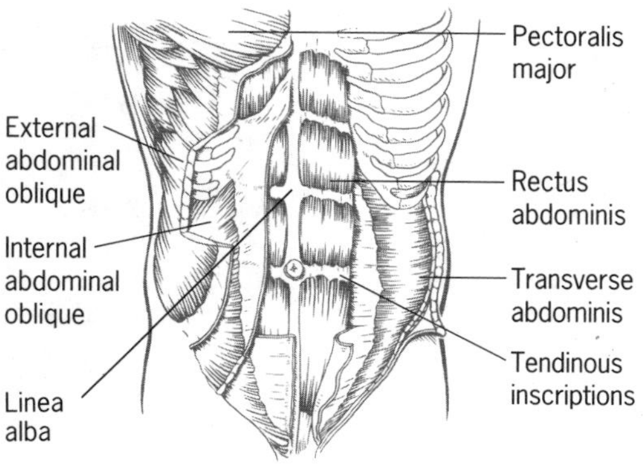

Figure 2.19

Muscles of the abdominal wall.

Labels: Pectoralis major; External abdominal oblique; Internal abdominal oblique; Linea alba; Rectus abdominis; Transverse abdominis; Tendinous inscriptions

The remaining shoulder joint muscles have their origins on the scapula. The deltoid muscle, a superficial muscle located on the superior aspect of the shoulder joint, resembles its name several ways. The deltoid is shaped like a triangle (Greek letter delta = Δ) and is divided into three functional sections. The anterior deltoid fibers flex and medially rotate the arm. The middle portion of the deltoid is the primary abductor of the arm, while the posterior fibers extend and laterally rotate the arm (Fig. 2.21).

The rotator cuff muscles, a group of four small muscles, are functionally very important. These muscles act to stabilize the head of the humerus within the shoulder joint, as well as cause medial and lateral rotation of the humerus. The muscles are frequently inflamed and injured due to overuse or improper or insufficient warm-up.

The rotator cuff muscles are easily remembered as the "SITS" muscles: supraspinatus, which abducts the arm; the infraspinatus and teres minor, which externally rotate the arm; and the subscapularis, which, as its name describes, is located on the inferior surface of the scapula and medially rotates the arm (Fig. 2.22).

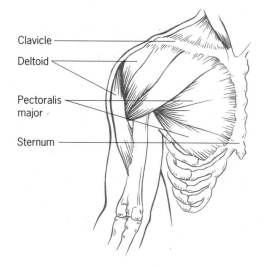

Figure 2.20

Anterior upper-extremity muscles of the chest and shoulder.

Clavicle

Deltoid

Pectoralis major

Sternum

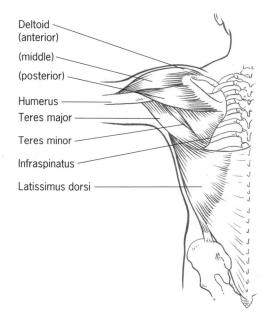

Figure 2.21

Posterior upper-extremity muscles of the shoulder. *Source: Redrawn from Luttgens (1992).*

Deltoid (anterior)

(middle)

(posterior)

Humerus

Teres major

Teres minor

Infraspinatus

Latissimus dorsi

Table 2.9

ACTIONS OF MAJOR UPPER-EXTREMITY MULTIJOINT MUSCLES

Muscle	Shoulder	Elbow	Forearm	Wrist
Biceps Brachii	flexion	flexion	supination	
Brachioradialis		flexion	pronation & supination	
Triceps Brachii	extension (long head)	extension		
Flexor Carpi Radialis		flexion		flexion; abduction
Flexor Carpi Ulnaris		flexion		flexion; adduction
Extensor Carpi Radialis (Longus and Brevis)		extension		extension
Extensor Carpi Ulnaris		extension		extension; adduction

Table 2.10

MAJOR MUSCLES THAT ACT AT THE SHOULDER

Muscle	Origin	Insertion	Primary Function(s)
Pectoralis Major	clavicle, sternum, and 1st costal cartilages	greater tubercle of the humerus	flexion; adduction and medial rotation
Deltoid	anterolateral clavicle, border of the acromion, spine of the scapula	deltoid tubercle of humerus on the midlateral surface	abduction; flexion (anterior fibers); and extension (posterior fibers)
Latissimus Dorsi	lower six thoracic vertebrae, crests of ilium and sacrum, lower four ribs	medial side of the intertubercular groove of the humerus	extension; adduction and medial rotation
Rotator Cuff Muscles (4)	various aspects of scapula	all insert on the greater tubercle of the humerus except for the subscapularis, which inserts on the lesser tubercle of the humerus	abduction; lateral and medial rotation; humeral head stabilization

Figure 2.22a-b

Rotator cuff muscles: supraspinatus, infra-spinatus, teres minor, and subscapularis.

Source: Redrawn from Luttgens (1992).

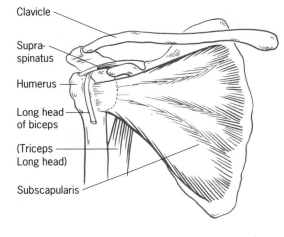

a. Anterior view.

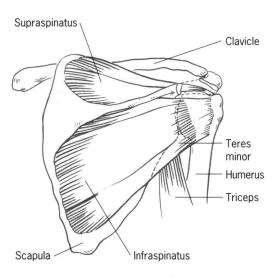

b. Posterior view.

The origins, insertions and primary functions of the muscles that cross the shoulder joint are presented in Table 2.10.

Muscles of the Scapula. The primary function of the muscles and fascia that connect the scapula (shoulder blade) and the trunk is to stabilize the scapula during movement of the humerus. The muscles that anchor the scapula are named for their shape (trapezius, rhomboid major and minor) and function (the levator scapulae elevate the scapulae) (Fig. 2.23).

Anatomists partition the trapezius into three sections based upon the direction of pull of its fibers. The upper portion of the trapezius is responsible for **elevation** of the scapula (example = shrugging the shoulders). The levator scapulae muscle assists the upper trapezius in elevating the scapula. The middle section of the trapezius has horizontal fibers, and when it shortens during concentric action, it pulls the scapula medially toward the midline (adduction). Concentric action of the lower portion of the trapezius results in **depression** and adduction of the scapula.

Beneath the trapezius are the rhomboid major and minor, which work in unison to produce adduction and elevation of the scapula. Good muscle tone in the rhomboids sustains good upper-back posture and helps prevent the "rounded shoulders" posture. The origins, insertions and primary functions of the muscles of the scapula are listed in Table 2.11.

Muscles of the Elbow. The elbow (ulno-humeral) joint is a hinge joint, and as such, permits motion in only one plane (sagittal). The flexors of the elbow, the bi-ceps brachii, brachialis and brachioradialis ("the three B's"), are located on the anterior aspect of the humerus (Figure 2.24).

The primary extensor of the elbow, the triceps brachii, is located on the posterior aspect of the arm. As its name suggests, the triceps has three heads: one on the scapula and two on the proximal humerus. All three heads converge and insert via a common tendon into the olecranon process of the ulna at the posterior elbow (Fig. 2.24). The

Table 2.11

MAJOR MUSCLES THAT ACT UPON THE SCAPULA

Muscle	Origin	Insertion	Function(s)
Trapezius	occipital bone, spines of cervical and thoracic vertebrae	acromion process and spine of scapula	elevation (upper trapezius); adduction (middle trapezius); and depression (lower trapezius)
Levator Scapulae	upper four or five cervical vertebrae	vertebral border of the scapula	elevation of scapula
Rhomboids (Major and Minor)	spines of 7th cervical through 5th thoracic vertebrae	vertebral border of scapula	adduction and elevation of scapula

Table 2.12

MAJOR MUSCLES THAT ACT ON THE ELBOW AND FOREARM

Muscle	Origin	Insertion	Primary Function(s)
Biceps Brachii	long head from tubercle above glenoid cavity; short head from coracoid process of the scapula	radial tuberosity and bicipital aponeurosis	elbow flexion; forearm supination
Brachialis	anterior humerus	ulnar tuberosity and coronoid process of ulna	elbow flexion
Brachioradialis	distal two thirds of lateral humerus	radial styloid process condyloid ridge of humerus	elbow flexion
Triceps Brachii	long head from the lower edge of glenoid cavity of scapula; lateral head from posterior humerus; short head from distal two thirds of posterior humerus	olecranon process of ulna	elbow extension
Pronator Teres	distal end of medial humerus and the medial aspect of the ulna	middle one third of the lateral radius	forearm pronation

Chapter 2
Fundamentals
of Anatomy

Figure 2.23

Muscles of the scapula.
Source: Redrawn from Luttgens (1992).

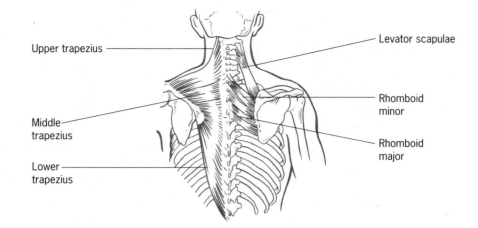

Figure 2.24a-c

Muscles of the elbow.
Source: Redrawn from Luttgens (1992).

a. Anterior view (superficial).

b. Anterior view (deep).

c. Posterior view.

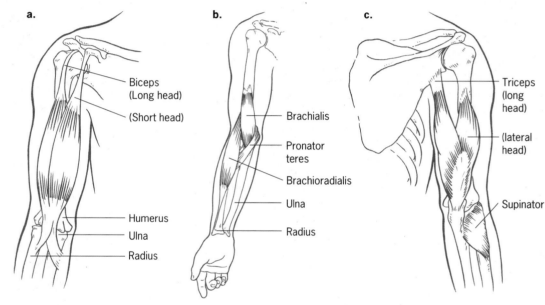

Figure 2.25a-b

Muscles of the wrist.
Source: Redrawn from Luttgens (1992).

a. Flexors.

b. Extensors.

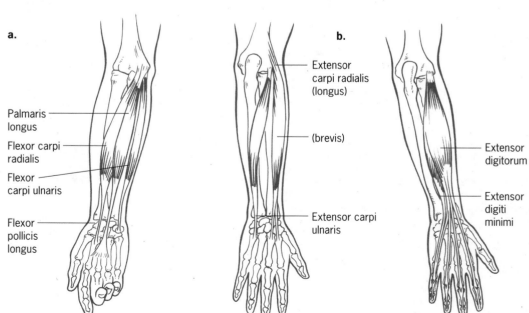

Table 2.13

MAJOR MUSCLES THAT ACT AT THE WRIST

Muscle	Origin	Insertion	Primary Function(s)
Flexor Carpi Radialis	medial epicondyle of humerus	2nd and 3rd metacarpals	wrist flexion
Flexor Carpi Ulnaris	medial epicondyle of humerus	5th metacarpal	wrist flexion
Extensor Carpi Radialis Longus and Brevis	lateral epicondyle of humerus	2nd metacarpal	wrist extension
Extensor Carpi Ulnaris	lateral epicondyle of humerus	5th metacarpal	wrist extension

origins, insertions and primary functions of the muscles that act at the elbow joint are listed in Table 2.12.

Muscles of the Wrist. The muscles that act at the wrist joint can be grouped according to their origin and function. The wrist flexor-pronator muscles originate at the elbow on the medial epicondyle of the humerus and produce flexion of the wrist and pronation (palm-down position) of the forearm. The flexor carpi radialis, palmaris longus and flexor carpi ulnaris are the primary wrist flexors. The names of the pronators of the forearm tell their function: the pronator teres muscle (located at the elbow) and the pronator quadratus muscle (located at the wrist) (Fig. 2.25). The antagonist muscle group to the flexor-pronators is the extensor-supinators, which arises from a common tendon on the lateral humeral epicondyle at the elbow. As their names indicate, these muscles extend the wrist and supinate (palm-up position) the forearm. The major wrist extensors are the extensor carpi radialis longus and extensor carpi radialis brevis, and the extensor carpi ulnaris. The supinator muscle, with help from the biceps brachii, is responsible for supination of the forearm (Fig. 2.25).

The origins, insertion and primary functions of the muscles that act at the wrist and forearm are presented in Table 2.13.

SUMMARY

Aerobics instructors are required to provide exercise programs that are appropriate and effective and accomplish the desired fitness goals of clients. Without a fundamental understanding of human anatomy, this is nearly an impossible task. To that end, the three major anatomical systems—cardiorespiratory, nervous and musculoskeletal—were discussed in considerable detail in this chapter. In the next chapter, on kinesiology, the functional aspects of the musculoskeletal system will be presented, applying much of the information detailed in this chapter.

Chapter 3

Biomechanics and Applied Kinesiology

By Deborah Ellison

Posture and muscle balance

- Abnormal and fatigue postures
- Muscular balance and imbalance

Human movement terminology

Biochemical factors and movement

- Inertia
- Acceleration and momentum
- Impact and reaction forces
- Linear and rotary motion
- Levers and torque

Muscle contraction and movement

- Contraction types
- Muscle coordination and movement

Neurological factors affecting movement

- The all-or-none principle
- Stretch and tendon reflexes
- Kinesthetic awareness
- Reciprocal innervation and inhibition
- Principles of muscular strength training

Principles of muscle endurance training

Principles of flexibility training

Kinesiology of the lower body

- Pelvis and lumbar spine
- Muscles acting at the hip joint
- Muscles acting at the knee joint
- Muscles acting at the ankle

Kinesiology of the upper body

- Shoulder girdle muscles
- Muscles of the shoulder joint proper

Exercise design, instruction and correction

- Exercise analysis and substitution of risky exercises
- Components of a balanced exercise program
- Body mechanics of lifting

Kinesiology is the study of human motion. It blends the sciences of anatomy, physiology, neurology and biomechanics into an appreciation of the movement capabilities of the human body. The human body and its movements are beautiful and astounding—orderly, synchronized, adaptable, quick and precise. The body is like an incredible machine. It actually improves with use if its movement is compatible with its design and the physical laws of motion. However, if movement occurs repetitively that is incompatible with the body's design, a breakdown

Deborah Ellison, PT, is a physical therapist and ergonomic consultant in San Diego. Debby trains fitness instructors internationally as a member of Nike's training team, Body Elite, and presents frequently for IDEA and IHRSA. Former education director for the American Council on Exercise, she has written several texts and articles on biomechanics and kinesiology as well as scripts for exercise videos. Her book and video series, Movement That Matters, was released in 1993.

results, either as an acute injury or degeneration over time. Therefore, it is vital that aerobics class activities not only enhance the body's performance, but also prevent injury in and out of the classroom.

Physical educators employ **kinesiology** when they coach and teach athletic skills. Therapists use kinesiology to restore function and to compensate for impairments so that patients can perform their activities of daily living. Fitness instructors use kinesiology to promote fitness. Therefore, they need to think in terms of preparing clients to do the physical activities of their lives more effectively and healthily. They must combine rhythmic activities of large muscle groups to promote cardiovascular endurance and aerobic metabolism. Likewise, they must design exercises to meet the specific strength, flexibility and alignment needs of clients. Also, to avoid injury, they need to avoid movements that go against joint structure or go beyond an individual's present capability.

Kinesiology provides the tools to analyze movement and its components to improve function and prevent injury. To use these tools, consider the body's daily activities, postures and the physical stresses it undergoes in those positions. Next, identify possible areas of weakness or tightness caused by those habitual positions and activities. Then, design activities to improve the body's function under those performance conditions. The result will be a balanced fitness program including not only cardiovascular endurance, but also muscular balance, neutral alignment and good body mechanics.

POSTURE AND MUSCLE BALANCE

Because of variations in body types, there is considerable disagreement about what comprises "ideal posture."

However, a **neutral spinal alignment** minimizes excessive stress on the spine and soft tissues. In neutral posture there is a slight inward curve at the neck and low back, and a slight outward curve of the thoracic spine connected to the ribs (Fig. 3.1).

Instructors can assess muscular balance by having a client stand in neutral and observing him or her from the side and from the back. If a person stands in neutral alignment and is viewed from the side, a plumb line would pass through the midline of the ear, the center of the shoulder joint, center of the hip joint, just behind the kneecap and just in front of the ankle joint. If these points do not align, look for muscle imbalances. When viewed from behind, is the spine straight from the base of the skull to the tailbone? Is the pelvis level? Are the shoulders level? Is the muscle bulk equal on the left and right sides of the spine? Are the shoulder blades flat on the back? Are the shoulder blades parallel and equally distant from the spine? Do the shoulders round forward, pulling the shoulder blades away from the spine?

Aerobics classes can promote good posture and muscular balance by having clients perform all activities with neutral spinal alignment. Effective cueing and correction techniques, as well as oral and visual feedback, help clients to be more aware of their posture. Good posture is a neuromuscular skill that can by acquired by practice and retraining.

Abnormal and Fatigue Postures

Deviations from the neutral position can be temporary or permanent. They may be caused by fatigue or soft-tissue (muscle, ligament, tendon, fascia) imbalance, which exercise can improve. They may be due to structural abnormalities of the bones that are not affected by exercise. There are three primary postural deviations—lordo-

Figure 3.1

Neutral spinal alignment with slight inward curve at neck and low back.

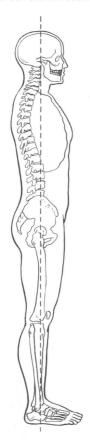

sis, kyphosis and scoliosis (Fig. 3.2). **Lordosis** is an increase in the normal inward curve of the low back, often accompanied by a protruding abdomen and buttocks, rounded shoulders and forward head. **Kyphosis** is an increase in the normal outward curve of the thoracic spine. It is often accompanied by rounded shoulders, a sunken chest and forward head with neck hyperextension. Scoliosis is a lateral curve of the spine. In scoliosis, the vertebrae may rotate, causing a backward shift of the rib cage on one side. The pelvis and shoulders often appear uneven. If a client is unable to actively assume a neutral posture, refer him or her to a physician.

A temporary lordosis (in standing) and kyphosis (in sitting) occur every day in the bodies of clients when they are tired—so-called fatigue postures. Fatigue postures cause physical stress, muscle imbalance and eventually pain. Over time, the bones

of the spine may adapt to these postures, causing the deviations to become structural and irreversible.

Muscular Balance and Imbalance

Careful analysis of poor sitting and standing postures reveals the areas of the body that become imbalanced as a result (Fig. 3.3). With poor standing alignment (lordosis), the abdominals may be weak; the neck and low back, hip flexors, hamstrings and calf muscles may be tight and the head is too far forward. With poor sitting posture, the head is again too far forward; the neck, chest, shoulders, hamstrings, and hip flexors may be tight; the middle back muscles are overstretched and weak, and the low back is too flat (forward flexed).

When muscular balance is present, neutral alignment can occur. However, a problem in one muscle group often produces another in an opposing muscle group. If

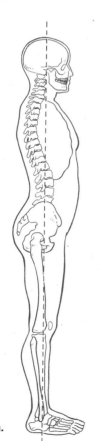
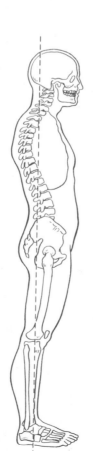
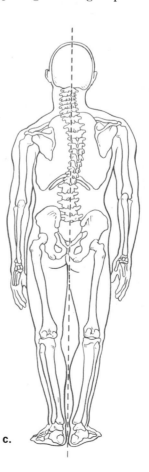

Figure 3.2
Postural deviations.

a. Lordosis: Increased inward lumbar curve from neutral.

b. Kyphosis: Increased outward thoracic curve from neutral.

c. Scoliosis: Lateral spinal curves with possible vertebral rotation.

a.

b.

c.

one muscle group is too tight, it passively pulls the body out of neutral, and causes increased stress and tendency toward imbalance on the opposite side of the spine. If one muscle group is weak and overstretched, it causes the body to fall out of alignment in the opposite direction. That misalignment in turn stresses other areas. Accordingly, muscle imbalances often occur in pairs.

The term muscular balance refers to balance within the interrelated components of muscle and connective tissue. It involves several elements:

1. Muscle groups are balanced in strength and flexibility on right and left sides.

2. There is balance front to back in terms of spinal alignment. For example, the chest muscles are of normal length and the mid-back muscles are sufficiently strong.

3. There is a balance in strength ratios in opposing muscle groups, although they may not be exactly equal in strength.

4. There is balanced flexibility around a joint so that motion is not restricted, or allowed to go too far.

HUMAN MOVEMENT TERMINOLOGY

Because the human body has so many movable parts, all of which move in several directions, it can be overwhelming at first to decipher everything that is going on. The key is to look at one segment at a time, and see how a segment has moved from a given starting position.

The anatomical position is the starting position from which human movement is described. In the anatomical position, the joints and body segments are in neutral position (not flexed, hyperextended or rotated), except the forearm, which is **supinated** (palms facing up) (see Chapter 2, "Fundamentals of Anatomy").

Several terms are basic to a discussion about movement. The first ones are positional or directional terms, like north, south, east and west in three dimensions. They are important in describing body segments or positions in relation to other parts of the body or positions (Table 3.1).

Human motion occurs in three dimensions as body parts move around joints. The second group of terms identifies the three planes of movement in which joint action occurs. The anterior-posterior plane is called the **sagittal plane**. Flexion and extension occur in the sagittal plane. **Flexion** usually involves a decrease in the angle between two bones; **extension** is the movement that returns the segment to the neutral (anatomical) position. **Hyperextension** is a continuation of the extension movement past the neutral position. The medial-lateral plane is called the **frontal plane.** Abduction and adduction occur in the frontal plane. **Abduction** is a lateral movement away from the midline of the body, usually at the hip or shoulder. **Adduction** is a medial movement returning the limb toward the midline of the body. The **transverse plane** is horizontal and would divide the body into

Figure 3.3a-d
Correct and incorrect sitting and standing postures.

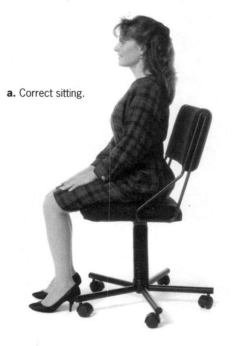

a. Correct sitting.

superior (top) and **inferior** (bottom) parts. **Medial and lateral rotation** occur around an axis that runs the length of the body segment. Rotation is medial when the rotation is inward toward the midline of the body. Rotation is lateral when it is outward, away from the midline of the body. **Supination** of the forearm turns the hand forward, or palm up, when the elbow is flexed. **Pronation** of the forearm turns the hand to the back, or palm down, when the forearm is flexed (see Chapter 2, "Fundamentals of Anatomy").

The third group of terms describes movement of body parts. It includes the general terms mentioned above, and a few terms that are unique to particular joints. The movements are summarized in Table 3.1. The movements and the ranges of motion at each joint are pictured in Figs. 3.4-3.6.

BIOMECHANICAL FACTORS AND MOVEMENT

To accurately analyze human movement, one must first understand the physical laws that apply to the motion of all objects. Sir Isaac Newton is famous for formulating three important ones, which are summarized here.

Inertia

Newton's first law is the **law of inertia**. It states that a body at rest stays at rest. It also states that a body in motion stays in motion with the same velocity and direction, unless acted on by unbalanced forces.

A body's inertia is proportional to its mass. Therefore, it is harder to start moving a dense object than a light one. Also, if moving at the same velocity, it is harder to stop the denser object than the lighter one. For example, a lead weight has more inertia than a piece of plastic of the same dimensions.

Acceleration and Momentum

Newton's second law is the **law of acceleration**. It states that the force (F) acting on a body in a given direction equals the body's mass (m) multiplied by the body's acceleration (a) in that direction (**F = ma**).

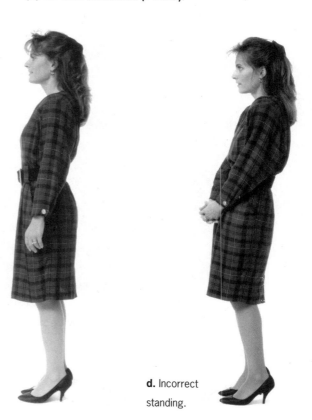

b. Incorrect sitting.

c. Correct standing.

d. Incorrect standing.

Table 3.1

FUNDAMENTAL MOVEMENTS (FROM ANATOMICAL POSITION)

Plane	Action	Definition
Sagittal	Flexion	Decreasing the angle between two bones.
	Extension	Increasing the angle between two bones.
	Hyperextension	Increasing the angle between two bones beyond anatomical position (continuing extension past neutral).
	Dorsiflexion	Moving the top of the foot toward the shin (ankle only).
	Plantarflexion	Moving the sole of the foot downward (ankle only).
Frontal	Abduction	Motion away from the midline of the body (or part).
	Adduction	Motion toward the midline of the body (or part).
	Elevation	Moving to a superior position (scapula).
	Depression	Moving to an inferior position (scapula).
	Inversion	Lifting the medial border of the foot (subtalar joint only).
	Eversion	Lifting the lateral border of the foot (subtalar joint only).
Transverse	Rotation	Medial (inward) or lateral (outward) turning about the vertical axis of bone.
	Pronation	Rotating the hand and wrist medially from the elbow.
	Supination	Rotating the hand and wrist laterally from the elbow.
	Horizontal flexion (horizontal adduction)	From a 90-degree abducted arm position, the humerus is flexed in toward the midline of the body in the transverse plane.
	Horizontal extension (horizontal abduction)	The return of the humerus from horizontal flexion (adduction) to 90-degree abduction.
Multiplanar	Circumduction	Motion that describes a "cone"; combines flexion, abduction, extension and adduction in sequential order.
	Opposition	Thumb movement unique to primates and humans that follows a semicircle toward the little finger.

The second law also relates to a moving body's momentum. A body's **linear momentum** is equal to its mass multiplied by its velocity. For a given mass, increased force will accelerate the body to a higher velocity; therefore, it creates greater momentum. For a given velocity, momentum will increase if the mass of the body increases. **Angular momentum** is the same with respect to angular motion, as when body segments rotate around joints. So, when holding a given weight in the hand and moving to faster tempo music will create greater momentum. Also, at the same tempo of movement to music (velocity), the momentum will be higher if the mass increases (e.g., holding a 5-pound weight as opposed to a 3-pound weight).

Momentum can play a positive role in human movement, and it plays an important role in sports such as football and judo. However, excessive momentum can cause injury, especially when working with weights. As momentum increases, stopping the motion requires more force. Movements with weights should occur at speeds that are under complete muscular control. If too much momentum is created by "swinging" the weight (instead of "lifting" with muscular contraction), the force needed to decelerate may exceed the muscle's ability to stop the motion. Then the motion is stopped by connective tissues and joint structures. This leads to risk of injury.

Momentum can also be a problem in very fast arm movements with extended elbows. The arms are moving rapidly at the end of the range of motion, and the motion is not under muscular control. The ligaments and joint structures must absorb the force created by the momentum to stop the movement. This can cause injury to the shoulder joint.

Impact and Reaction Forces

Newton's third law says that for every force applied by one body to a second, the second applies an equal force on the first in the opposite direction. Thus, for every action there is an equal and opposite reaction. This law has bearing on the impact forces that the body must absorb during activities such as running, jumping or high-impact aerobics. According to Newton's third law, the Earth exerts a force against the body equal to the force that the body applies to the Earth as it runs or jumps.

Combine Newton's second law (force equals the mass multiplied by the acceleration) with this law, and the magnitude of the impact of the force on the feet and body becomes evident. The body's mass multiplied by the downward acceleration equals the reaction force from the Earth that the body must overcome by equal and opposite muscular forces.

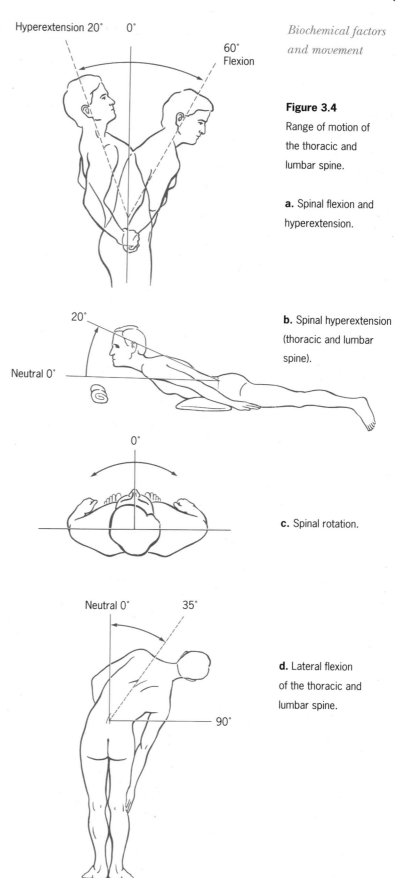

Biochemical factors and movement

Figure 3.4
Range of motion of the thoracic and lumbar spine.

a. Spinal flexion and hyperextension.

b. Spinal hyperextension (thoracic and lumbar spine).

c. Spinal rotation.

d. Lateral flexion of the thoracic and lumbar spine.

Chapter 3
*Biomechanics
and Applied
Kinesiology*

Such forces can multiply quickly in high-impact activities. These high forces can cause overuse and stress injuries, such as shin splints, stress fractures, knee and back problems. Proper footwear and flooring, such as suspended wood that has some flexibility, can help reduce the forces that the body must dissipate. However, the best approach to injury prevention is to vary the moves in aerobic exercise to decrease the total impact forces.

Linear and Rotary Motion

There are two basic types of movement, linear and rotary. The whole body moves in linear motion as it moves forward or back or side to side across the floor. Rotary or angular motion occurs at the joints of

Figure 3.5a-f

Lower extremity movements and range of motion.

a. Hip flexion range of motion without pelvic rotation 120°; extension (to 0°).

b. Hip extension and hyperextension (<30°).

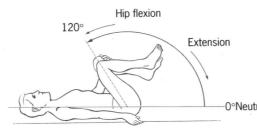

a.

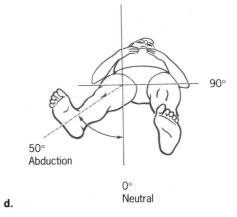

b.

c. Range of motion for rotation at the hip.

d. Range of motion of hip abduction.

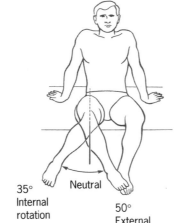

c.

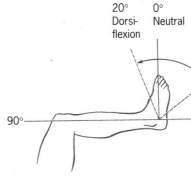

d.

e. Range of motion of the knee: flexion-extension, hyperextension.

f. Ankle range of motion with knee flexed.

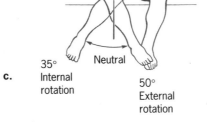

e.

f.

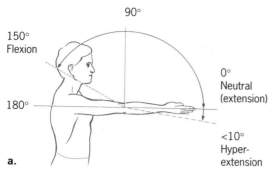

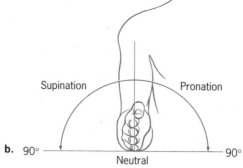

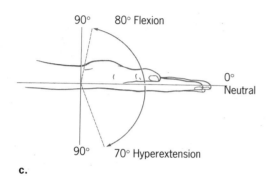

Figure 3.6a-j

Upper extremity movements and ranges of motion.

a. Elbow range of motion: flexion 150°; extension (to 0°); hyperextension (<10°).

b. Forearm range of motion: pronation 90°; supination 90°.

c. Wrist range of motion: flexion 80°; extension (to 0°), hyperextension 70°.

d. Range of motion of the wrist: radial deviation 20°, ulnar deviation 30°.

the body. Linear and rotary motion occur simultaneously in aerobics class as various arms movements are performed while walking forward or performing a grapevine to the side.

Levers and Torque

Body segments move in rotary motion like a system of levers. A **lever** is a rigid bar that rotates around a fixed point when an external force is applied. Body segments (thigh, forearm, lower leg) are considered rigid bars. The fixed points around which they rotate are the joints.

Forces on the lever system can be **internal** or **external.** Muscular contraction is considered an internal force when speaking of the body as a whole. Muscular contraction is considered an external force when speaking of joint motion, since the muscle is external to the joint.

For motion to occur at a joint, an external **force** must act on the segment (lever) at some distance from the center of the joint. A **motive force** is an external force that causes an increase in speed or change in direction of movement. A **resistive force** is an external force that resists the motion of the motive force. Motion occurs when the motive and resistive forces acting on a body segment are unequal. When the motive and resistive forces are equal, no motion occurs: the lever system is either at rest (if the forces pass through the center of the joint), or an isometric contraction occurs in which the force of the muscle matches the force of the resistance.

A force lever arm is the perpendicular distance from the center of the joint to the point where the force acts (Fig. 3.7). The lever arm length of the motive force (F) is the **force arm** (Fa). The lever arm length of the resistance (R) is the **resistance arm** (Ra). **Torque** is the turning effect of a force applied to a body segment (lever) at some distance from the center of the joint. It is the product of the force multiplied by the length of the lever arm (F x Fa). The lever

Chapter 3
Biomechanics
and Applied
Kinesiology

is in balance if the torque of the motive force (F x Fa) is equal and opposite in direction to the torque of the resistance (R x Ra) (F x Fa = R x Ra). It also stays in balance at rest if the force passes directly through the center of the joint. (This is an-

other reason for neutral posture: the pull of gravity goes through the center of several joints allowing them to be in balance without any force necessary from muscular contraction.)

Joint motion occurs when the motive

e. Shoulder abduction 180°; adduction (to neutral); hyperadduction 75° (frontal plane).

f. Shoulder range of motion in sagittal plane: flexion 180°; extension (to 0°); hyperextension 60°.

g. Shoulder range of motion in the transverse plane: horizontal adduction (flexion) 130°; horizontal abduction (to 0°); horizontal extension 45° past neutral.

h. Shoulder rotation range of motion in the transverse plane (shoulder is adducted to neutral): extend rotation 90°; internal rotation 90°.

i. Shoulder rotation range of motion in sagittal plane external (outward) rotation 90°; internal rotation 70° (shoulder joint is abducted to 90°).

j. Rotation with arm at side, rotation with arm in abduction, internal rotation posteriorly.

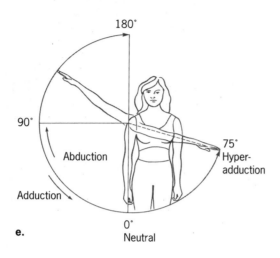

e.

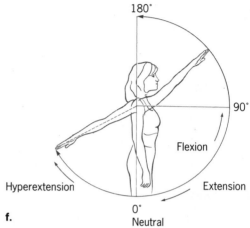

f.

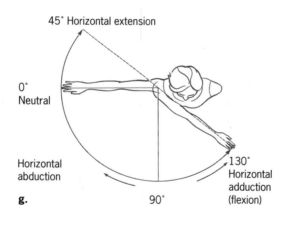

g.

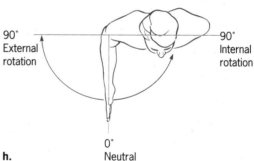

h.

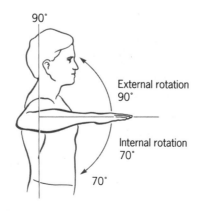

i.

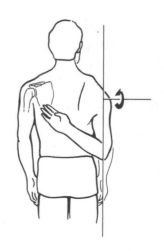

j.

torque (F x Fa) overcomes, or is greater than, the resistance torque (R x Ra). Consider the force required for a biceps curl with a 10-pound hand weight. For example, say the biceps attaches 0.5 inches from the center of the joint. The resistance of the weight acts in a perpendicular line 12 inches from the center of the joint. The force of the biceps contraction necessary to overcome the torque of the resistance is calculated as follows: R x Ra = 10 x 12 = 120; F = R x Ra/Fa = 120/.5 = 240. So, when the muscle attaches closely to the joint and the resistance acts far away, the force in the muscle required to overcome the resistance may be many times that of the weight itself.

MUSCLE CONTRACTION AND MOVEMENT

Body segments rotate at the joints when the acting torques (force times lever arm length) are unequal. Muscles may produce force to overcome a resistive force. Muscles may resist or give into gravity or another motive force. No movement occurs if the muscles match another external force. Look at the example of the biceps action at the elbow in Fig. 3.7. Note the locations of the joint center, motive force and force of resistance. A muscle contracts to develop force. However, the word contract may be misleading in regard to muscles since it usually means to shorten or become smaller. Individual muscle fibers can only contract (shorten); however, when a muscle as a whole (group of muscle fibers) contracts, it may shorten (come together), lengthen (away from the middle), or remain the same length. This may be due to different recruitment patterns of the individual muscle fibers. A muscle shortens when it acts as a motive force. It lengthens when it resists another external motive force, such as gravity. The muscle length

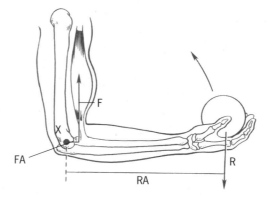

Figure 3.7

An example of a lever system in the human body. X-axis of rotation. F (biceps contraction) = motive force; R (weight in hand) = resistance; Fa (biceps force x distance of biceps attachment from axis) = lever arm of the motive force; Ra (weight x distance from axis) = lever arm of the resistance.

stays the same when it matches another external force, as in an isometric contraction.

Concentric (shortening) Contraction

When a muscle acts as a motive force, the force generated by the muscle is greater than that of the applied resistance. The muscle shortens as it contracts and motion occurs at the joint. For example, the biceps contracts concentrically in the up-phase of a biceps curl with a dumbbell. The biceps force overcomes the force of the resistance. Movement occurs in the direction opposite the resistance.

Eccentric (lengthening) Contraction

An **eccentric contraction** occurs when the external force exceeds the contractile force generated by the muscle. In an eccentric contraction the muscle is producing a resistive force but "gives in" to the motive force of gravity. The muscle as a whole is also returning to its resting length from a shortened position. For example, the biceps contracts eccentrically in the return phase of a biceps curl with a dumbbell. It slows the natural fall that gravity would cause if there were no muscle contraction. Movement occurs in the same direction as the external motive force.

So, although the elbow joint extends, the triceps (elbow extensor) does not contract. The biceps (elbow flexor) controls elbow extension when it occurs in the same direction as gravity.

An understanding of concentric and eccentric contractions is crucial to exercise design and analysis. Joint motion alone does not accurately predict the muscle causing the motion. The body's position and the direction of the resistance must be considered (Fig. 3.8a-b).

If the movement occurs upward against gravity (antigravity movement), the muscle located superior to the moving joint contracts concentrically. If the movement is slow and downward in the same direction as gravity (gravity-assisted movement), the muscle superior to the joint contracts eccentrically. When the movement occurs parallel to the floor (neither against nor with gravity—a gravity-eliminated movement), opposing muscle groups contract concentrically unless elastic resistance is

used. When elastic tubing is used as resistance, the same principles apply in all planes: concentric if the motion occurs against the resistance, eccentric if the motion occurs in the same direction as the resistance.

As an illustration, first consider hip abduction and adduction performed side-lying (Fig. 3.9a). Second, analyze the hip abduction and adduction performed supine with the hips flexed and knees extended (Fig. 3.9b). Third, look at hip abduction and adduction performed in supine position with the hips and knees extended (Fig. 3.9c). Fourth, consider the same position with an elastic band around the ankles (Fig. 3.9d).

1. In Fig. 3.9a the initial action is hip abduction occurring against gravity. Therefore, the agonists (the hip abductors) are contracting concentrically. In the return phase of the side leg raise, the joint action is hip adduction. However, the motion occurs slowly in the same direction as gravity. Therefore, hip adduction is controlled by the hip abductors contracting eccentrically.

2. In Fig. 3.9b the first action is horizontal abduction of the hip as the legs move apart. However, since the movement occurs in the same direction as gravity, the hip adductors control the motion by eccentric contraction. In bringing the legs together again, the hip adduction occurs against gravity by concentric contraction of the adductors.

3. In the third example, Fig. 3.9c, the joint actions are hip abduction and adduction performed supine with the hips and knees extended. The actions occur neither against nor in the same direction as gravity. They occur in the plane perpendicular to the pull of gravity; therefore, the effect of gravity is not a factor. The muscle contractions are concentric of the hip abductors as the hip abducts and concentric of

Figure 3.8

Example of the effect of body position on muscle contraction.

a. Hip adduction is sometimes controlled by eccentric contraction of the hip abductors, when the movement occurs in the same direction as gravity.

Down phase:
Adduction in same direction as gravity=eccentric contraction of hip abductors

Up phase: Antigravity abduction=concentric contraction of hip abductors

Down phase of leg lift   Up phase of leg lift

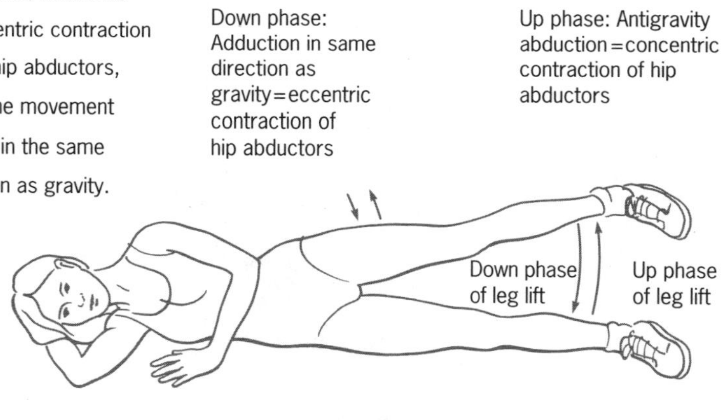

b. When gravity is eliminated, (when lying on one's back) muscle contractions are all concentric.

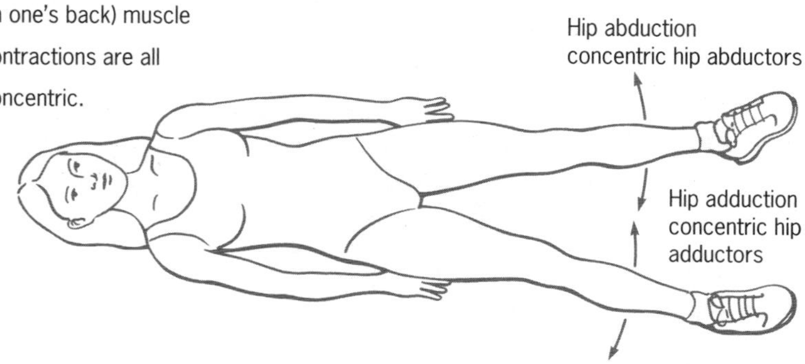

Hip abduction concentric hip abductors

Hip adduction concentric hip adductors

the adductors as the hip adducts. The resistance is small in this position, so it is not a good position for exercising these muscle groups unless elastic resistance is used.

4. In the last example, (Fig 3.9d), hip abduction occurs against the resistance of the band (concentric hip abductors). In the return phase, the band exerts an elastic force to bring the legs together, so the abductors may contract eccentrically until there is slack in the band.

Isotonic Contraction

When a muscle contracts concentrically or eccentrically to move or resist the movement of a fixed amount of weight or resistance such as an elastic band, the contraction is known as **isotonic**. "Isotonic" is a poor descriptor since it implies that the tone (force) in the muscle stays the same (iso-). It does not. In reality, the muscle force changes as the movement occurs.

Static or Isometric Contraction

When the torque generated by the muscle is less than (as in pushing against a wall or attempting to lift a weight that is too heavy) or matches the torque of the resistance and no visible movement occurs, the contraction is **isometric**. The resistance may come from the opposing muscle group (co-contraction), or another force, such as gravity, an immovable object or weight-training equipment.

Body-builders use isometric co-contraction to strike a pose to show their muscle development. Physical therapists use isometrics in rehabilitation following an injury, when the joint must not move, or in certain stretching techniques. Fitness instructors may include them in conditioning programs (see Chapter 9, "Variations: From Step to Strength Training"). They are an important component in training the stabilizing muscles, described below.

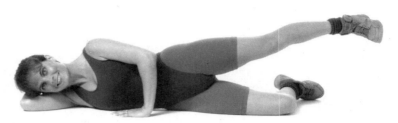

a. Side-lying leg lifts.

Figure 3.9

Hip muscle actions.

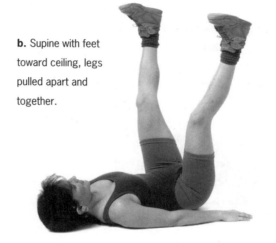

b. Supine with feet toward ceiling, legs pulled apart and together.

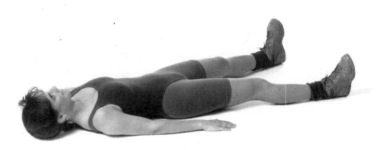

c. Moving apart: concentric of hip abductors, moving together: concentric of hip adductors.

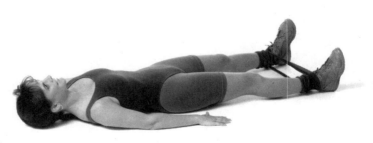

d. Concentric and eccentric of hip abductors with elastic resistance.

Examples are brief holds in the up phase of a trunk curl or push-up, or holding the shoulder blades squeezed together while performing a set of triceps kickbacks.

Isokinetic Contraction

Isokinetic contraction refers to a contraction in which the joint is moving (kinetic) at a constant (iso) angular velocity. The external resistance torque varies at different points in the range of motion. This type of contraction is only possible with specialized, electronic resistance equipment capable of varying the resistance and maintaining a constant angular velocity. It is not applicable to a dance-exercise class.

Muscle Coordination and Movement

The muscle group responsible for a particular joint motion is the **agonist** (like the hero of a book or play). The opposing muscle group is the **antagonist.** Muscle groups are classified in agonist/antagonist pairs on either side of a joint according to their function at that joint. Muscle balance needs to be developed and/or maintained between agonists and antagonists.

In any given joint movement, several things happen simultaneously. Some agonist muscles function as **prime movers.** They are the ones primarily responsible for that motion. In addition, the prime movers have helpers, called **synergists,** which assist in the movement. Synergists are muscles that help each other to produce a single movement, often when high forces are required.

Finally, some muscles contract isometrically and function as **stabilizers.** Stabilization occurs to protect the joint from unwanted movement. Stabilization also occurs at other joints to enable the motion to occur when and where it is wanted and to maintain alignment. In designing

exercise combinations, it is important to include activity for the stabilizing muscles.

NEUROLOGICAL FACTORS AFFECTING MOVEMENT

Voluntary movement is regulated and coordinated by complex interactions among sensory receptors (muscle, joint, skin, labyrinthine and neck proprioceptors), reflexes and various parts of the brain and central nervous system.

The All-or-none Principle

Muscle contractions occur with varying intensity. For example, the biceps can contract to lift 2 ounces or 25 pounds. Within the muscle, however, there are groups of muscle fibers that work together called motor units. These units contract maximally or not at all, depending on the strength of the nerve stimulus. If the stimulus is less than a certain threshold value, the motor unit does not fire. If it is greater than the threshold value, the whole unit contracts completely. This is known as the all-or-none principle.

The gradations in muscle contractions depend on the number of motor units recruited and the frequency of stimulation. To get a maximal contraction of a muscle, the impulses must occur at high frequency and stimulate the maximum number of motor units. In an aerobics class with low resistance available, instructors must use all means possible to recruit as many motor units as possible.

The all-or-none principle does not apply when the muscle fibers in the motor unit are fatigued. Once the fibers are fatigued, even a very high stimulus will not cause a contraction.

Proprioceptors

Effective coordination of movement patterns depends on input from the sensory pathways to the brain. This information is interpreted and determines motor response in regard to the degree, direction and rate of change of body movements. Sensory receptors that gather information about body position, direction and velocity are called **proprioceptors**. They are located in the muscles, tendons, joints, connective tissue (ligaments, fascia) and in the labyrinth of the inner ear. They give a conscious awareness of body and limb position and are involved in unconscious reflexes.

Stretch and Tendon Reflexes

Two types of proprioceptors are located in muscles (muscle spindles) and tendons (Golgi tendon organs). The **muscle spindles** are sensitive to a strong, quick stretch of a muscle and causes a reflex contraction of the muscle to prevent tearing. The **Golgi tendon organs** respond to tension in the tendon, usually caused by a strong muscle contraction. The reflex response is muscle relaxation to prevent the tendon from tearing when the tension is extreme.

Kinesthetic Awareness

Kinesthesis is the conscious awareness of the position of body parts and the amount and rate of joint movement. It comes primarily from proprioceptors located in the joint capsules and ligaments. Such perception allows a person to initiate and modify movement patterns. It also affects his or her perception of his or her posture. When poor postures are habitual, the person may perceive that alignment as feeling "right." To change that perception, additional input must be given to the sensory receptors. For example, to correct a forward head posture, the person must practice head retraction repeatedly.

Reciprocal Innervation and Inhibition

One of the neurological mechanisms that contributes to coordinated movement is reciprocal innervation (stimulation) and inhibition. In this mechanism, as impulses stimulate one muscle group (agonist) to contract, the motor neurons to the opposite muscle group (antagonist) are simultaneously inhibited. Therefore, the antagonists remain relaxed, and the agonists contract without opposition.

Principles of Muscular Strength Training

To increase strength, the muscle must be overloaded. Overload means over and above the usual load. Early increases in strength may be largely neurological so clients become stronger without a change in muscle size.

An instructor can use a series of modifications to progressively overload muscles to build strength, using the principles of biomechanics presented in this chapter:

1. Change the body position from one in which gravity is not a factor to an anti-gravity position.

2. Increase the lever arm of the resistance, such as lifting the leg with the knee extended instead of flexed.

3. Add additional external resistance, as in manual resistance, elastic bands or tubing, or free weights.

PRINCIPLES OF MUSCLE ENDURANCE TRAINING

Several muscle groups function primarily as stabilizers, and as such, need to be able to contract at low levels throughout the day. These are primarily postural muscles (abdominals and posterior shoulder girdle muscles). These muscle groups would benefit from endurance training as well as strength training. For endurance training, the overload comes from increased repetitions or being able to hold a contraction for a longer period of time. To progressively overload a muscle to build endurance, there are several modifications and variations of exercises:

1. Perform consecutive sets of different exercises that work the same muscle group. For example, push-ups followed by pectoral presses, followed by pectoral flies.

2. Use a series of concentric, eccentric and isometric contractions of the same muscle group.

3. For the stabilizing muscles of the torso, especially the posterior shoulder girdle muscles, perform several sets of isotonic contractions, then hold an isometric contraction while performing a set of isotonic contractions of other arm muscles (e.g., triceps kickback, biceps curl).

PRINCIPLES OF FLEXIBILITY TRAINING

When a person stretches a "muscle," the interrelated components of muscle and connective tissue are stretched. To stretch a muscle effectively, keep in mind the muscle's line of pull, and position the muscle so that the fibers seem to pull apart. Another way to think of it is to place the body segment in a position that opposes all the functions of the muscle. For example, the pectoralis major flexes, adducts and internally rotates the arm. To stretch it most effectively, place the arm behind the plane of the body abducted and externally rotated.

A safe and effective stretch must also occur from a neutral spine position. For example, the pectorals stretch best in

supine with an active pelvic tilt to maintain a neutral low back (Fig. 3.10). Otherwise, a person with tight pectorals will arch the back to achieve the arm position.

An effective stretch should be in an unloaded position. That is, make sure not to ask the muscle to contract and stretch simultaneously. A hamstring stretch is ineffective in a standing position if the stretching leg is weight-bearing.

Stretches are more effective when the muscles are warm, i.e., after the warm-up. They are also more effective when the person is mentally and emotionally relaxed. This suggests that the most effective sequencing for flexibility training would be warm-up, aerobics, strengthening, relaxation, then stretching.

Understanding the biomechanical and neurological factors affecting movement as well as principles of effective strengthening and flexibility are crucial to effective exercise design. The next step is to learn muscle locations, lines of pull as they cross the joints, and their resulting contribution to joint movement.

KINESIOLOGY OF THE LOWER BODY

Movements of the lower body are those of the lumbar spine and pelvis (considered together) and movements at the hip, knee and ankle joints. Table 3.2 summarizes the muscles of the lower body.

Pelvis and Lumbar Spine

A central focus of applying kinesiology in an exercise class is teaching clients to maintain their spine in the **neutral posture** during all activities. It is particularly important in a progressive exercise program as the muscles of the upper or lower body are overloaded with weights. The spine must be in neutral to avoid injury. In neutral the pelvis is upright, not tilted in any direction.

Figure 3.10

Pectoral stretch: Supine on bench, hands behind head, pelvic tilt. Press elbows below bench level.

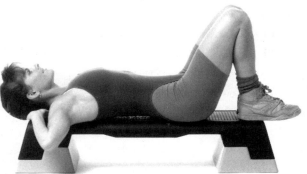

The lumbar spine is neutral, not flexed or hyperextended, with a slight inward curve at the low back.

The lumbar spine can flex (bend forward), extend (return to neutral), hyperextend (extend past neutral), flex laterally (bend side to side) and rotate. Pelvic motion corresponds to motion of the lumbar spine, but in the opposite direction. As the lumbar spine flexes forward the pelvis tilts backward **(posterior pelvic tilt)**. As the lumbar spine extends or hyperextends backward, the pelvis tilts forward **(anterior pelvic tilt)** (Fig. 3.11).

Lumbar and pelvic motion can be passive (due to fatigue or the downward pull of gravity) or active (caused by muscular contraction). Lumbar flexion is passive in fatigue sitting posture as the upper body leans forward. It occurs actively by using the abdominal muscles to perform a posterior pelvic tilt or abdominal-curl exercise.

Lumbar extension occurs as the spine returns to neutral from a flexed position. It is usually active, caused by contracting the lumbar extensors. Lumbar hyperextension (anterior pelvic tilt) happens passively if the hip flexors are too tight (see section on iliopsoas). It also occurs passively if a client leans on anterior hip ligaments when standing. Or, it can occur actively by contracting lumbar erector spinae, as in arching the back when lying face down on the floor.

In an aerobics class it is important to maintain the spine as close to neutral as possible in standing, sitting and performing progressive resistance exercises. For activities performed in upright standing, the abdominals must tilt the pelvis back to counteract the effects of gravity and retain the normal lumbar lordosis. For activities performed in sitting or in standing with a forward bend at the hips (i.e., squats, lunges), contract the erector spinae to

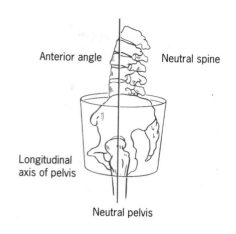

Figure 3.11

Lumbar motion with corresponding pelvic motion. The bucket of water is used to illustrate the direction of the pelvic tilt.

a. Neutral lumbar spine with neutral pelvis.

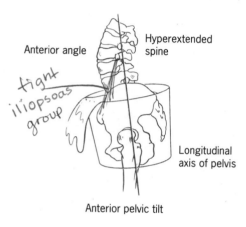

b. Lumbar hyperextension with anterior pelvic tilt.

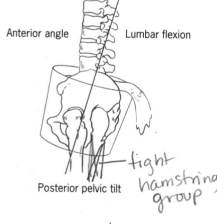

c. Slight lumbar flexion with posterior pelvic tilt.

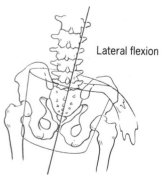

d. Lateral lumbar flexion with lateral pelvic tilt.

Table 3.2

LOWER BODY MUSCLES — FUNCTIONS AND SELECTED EXERCISES

Muscle	Primary Function	Selected Exercises
Erector spinae	Trunk extension, hyperextension, lateral flexion	S/E: Prone back hyperextension (Fig.3.14a), squats, good sitting posture. F: Supine knees to shoulders (Fig. 3.14c).
Rectus abdominis	Flexion and lateral flexion of the spine	S/E: Standing and supine pelvic tilts with resistance, supine abdominal curl-ups, straight reverse abdominal curls, abdominal crunches.
External oblique	Lateral flexion of the spine	S/E: Oblique abdominal curls, straight and oblique reverse abdominal curls, resisted pelvic tilts, straight abdominal curls with feet away from buttocks.
Internal oblique	Lateral trunk flexion	S/E: Side-lying torso raises, supine pelvic tilts, oblique abdominal curls, reverse abdominal curls.
Transverse abdominis	Compresses abdominal viscera	S/E: Forceful expiration while lifting.
Iliopsoas	Hip flexion and lateral rotation	S/E: Straight leg raises, bench-stepping, knee lifts. F: Forward lunge with back knee bent, posterior pelvic tilt (Fig. 3.20).
Rectus femoris	Hip flexion and knee extension	S/E: Squats, bench-stepping, lunges, lunge walk, standing straight leg raise. F: Standing, passive knee flexion holding to ankle, posterior pelvic tilt.
Sartorius	Hip flexion, abduction and lateral rotation; knee flexion and medial rotation	S/E: Knee lift with hip external rotation, wide stance onto bench.
Tensor fasciae latae	Hip flexion, medial rotation, abduction	S/E: Side-lying leg lifts with the hip slightly flexed, and internally rotated. F: Side-lying, hips extended; let top leg drop behind.
Gluteus maximus	Hip extension and lateral rotation	S/E: Bench-stepping, squats, lunges, resisted hip extension in standing, jumping.
Biceps femoris (hamstring)	Hip extension and knee flexion	S/E: Knee flexion with hip held in extension, standing or elbows and knees. F: (Fig. 3.24) sitting stretch.
Semitendinosus	Hip extension and knee flexion	S/E: Hamstring curls with knee in media, rotation and hip in extension.
Semimembranosus	Hip extension and knee flexion	S/E: Same as for semitendinosus.
Hip external rotators	Hip lateral rotation	S/E: Side leg lifts with knee flexed and hip flexed to 90 degrees (Fig. 3.26a). F: (Fig. 3.26b) Supine crossover stretch.
Adductor magnus, brevis and longus	Hip adduction and rotation	S/E: Side-lying bottom leg raises, supine resisted adduction with hips flexed (Fig. 3.28).

Table 3.2 (Continued)

LOWER BODY MUSCLES — FUNCTIONS AND SELECTED EXERCISES

Muscle	Primary Function	Selected Exercises
Gracilis	Hip adduction, knee flexion and medial rotation	S/E: Same as for adductors.
Pectineus	Hip flexion and internal rotation	S/E: Sitting, lift flexed knee toward opposite shoulder.
Gluteus medius and minimus	Hip abduction, medial rotation	S/E: Standing leg raises to the side (Fig. 3.30), side-lying leg raises, supine hip abduction against elastic resistance.
Quadriceps: Vastus medialis, intermedius and lateralis	Knee extension	S/E: Resisted knee extension, straight leg raises, squats, one-legged squats, lunges, bench-stepping. F: Same as rectus femoris.
Gastrocnemius	Ankle plantarflexion and assists with knee flexion	S/E: Bilateral heel raises, unilateral heel raises. F: Sitting hamstring stretch position + active dorsiflexion.
Soleus	Ankle plantarflexion	S/E: Same as for gastrocnemius, bent-knee resisted heel raises, bi- & unilateral. F: Same as for gastrocnemius with knee flexed.
Posterior tibialis	Foot inversion, assists with ankle plantarflexion	S/E: Resisted inversion with plantarflexion using elastic resistance.
Anterior tibialis	Ankle dorsiflexion, foot inversion	S/E: Resisted dorsiflexion with inversion, toe-tapping side to side.
Peroneus longus	Plantarflexion and eversion	S/E: Resisted eversion, alternate toe-and-heel lifts moving right and left.
Peroneus brevis	Plantarflexion and eversion	Same as for peroneus longus.

Key to selected exercises:
S/E: (Strength/Endurance): Exercises to improve strength and/or endurance of the muscle, depending upon the resistance and repetitions. Each exercise is not isolated to that particular muscle, as muscles work in groups to cause movement; however, the exercises listed would include the designated muscle as a prime mover. The exercises listed are ones that can be performed in the context of an aerobics class.
F: (Flexibility): Exercises to improve the flexibility of the designated muscle. Flexibility exercises do not stretch the muscle fiber itself, but are designed to lengthen the connective tissue associated with each particular muscle group. For maximum effectiveness, they should be performed after the muscle group is thoroughly warmed.

counteract the effect of gravity and maintain the normal lumbar lordosis (Fig. 3.12).

Lumbar Extensors: Erector Spinae

The erector spinae extend, hyperextend and laterally flex the spine (Fig. 3.13). The muscle is large in the lumbosacral region, but divides into several segments (iliocostalis, longissimus and spinalis) as it continues upward toward the head. In normal standing with neutral alignment, the muscle activity is very low. However, in forward lumbar flexion in standing or sitting, the erector spinae contract eccentrically. Because of the torque (F x Fa) of the upper body, the erector spinae muscles must generate tremendous force with a short lever arm to match it. Therefore, the low back muscles are easily strained by forward flexion in standing or sitting. It is even more

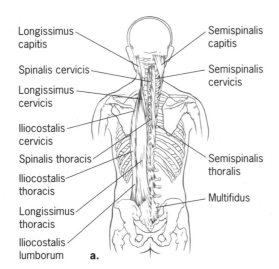
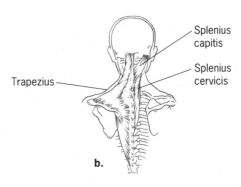

Figure 3.13

The erector spinae muscles extend, hyperextend and laterally flex the spine.

dangerous when lifting or lowering additional weight, such as a heavy box or a child.

The erector spinae in the lumbar area can no longer contract effectively past about 60 degrees of forward flexion. At that point the lower back ligaments support the full weight of the trunk. Poor sitting postures may stretch lumbar ligaments. Overstretched ligaments are less protective of the lumbar discs. Therefore, potentially harmful torque and shearing forces directly stress the discs in this position.

The potential harm is even greater if trunk rotation is added to the forward flexed position. This happens when twisting to place a box to the side or twisting to take a child out of a crib. The internal pres-

sure of the intervertebral discs is already very high, and the unprotected rotation can cause tearing of the outer fibers of the disc. Discs can then herniate or rupture (commonly called "slipped discs") as a result. This is why toe-touches, opposite toe-touches, opposite elbows to knees and windmill-type movements must be avoided.

To strengthen this muscle group, slowly hyperextend the back from the prone (face down) position (Fig. 14a). Another example is to lift the opposite arm and leg simultaneously. This will cause the erector spinae to assist and function as stabilizers while keeping the spine in neutral position (Fig. 3.14b). To stretch this muscle group, lie face up on the floor and pull the knees up toward the shoulders (Fig. 3.14c).

Lumbar Flexors: Abdominal Muscles

The abdominal muscles flex and rotate the lumbar spine. Flexion can be forward (posterior pelvic tilt or abdominal curl-up) or lateral to either side. Lateral flexion and rotation occur when the abdominals contract in various combinations with the quadratus lumborum and spinal rotators. The abdominal muscle group is composed of the rectus abdominis, external obliques, internal obliques and transverse abdominis (Fig. 3.15).

Figure 3.12

Squat showing neutral spine, less than 90° of knee flexion, heels on floor, feet shoulder-width apart.

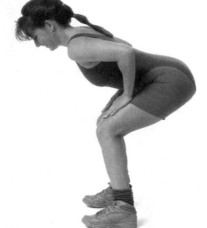

External Obliques. The external oblique fibers run diagonally (like putting hands in pockets). They originate on the ribs and insert into the iliac crest and the aponeurosis covering the rectus abdominis. When left and right sides contract together, they forward flex the lumbar spine as in a backward pelvic tilt (standing or supine). They also flex the lumbar and thoracic spine, as in an abdominal curl with hips and knees partially flexed and feet on the floor. Right and left sides can contract independently to cause lateral flexion and rotation of the trunk to the opposite side. An example is an oblique abdominal curl (shoulder toward opposite hip).

They are also active along with the internal obliques in forced expiration and bearing down when the breath is held. The best exercises for the external obliques are standing pelvic tilts (one-legged for more resistance), supine pelvic tilts and straight abdominal curls with hips and knees partially extended so that the feet are away from the buttocks (Fig. 3.16), oblique abdominal curls and straight and oblique reverse abdominal curls.

Internal Obliques. Internal obliques are deep to the external obliques. Their fibers are also diagonal, but in the opposite direction (like an inverted V). They originate on the iliac crest, and fan upward, inward and forward to insert on the lower ribs and the aponeurosis covering the rectus abdominis. They flex the lumbar and thoracic spine, laterally flex the spine and rotate to the same side. The best exercises for the internal obliques are supine pelvic tilts, oblique abdominal curls, straight and oblique reverse abdominal curls (lifting knees overhead until buttocks lift from the floor) and side-lying torso raises (Fig. 3.17). The abdominal muscles act as a group so the obliques will also participate in exercises listed for the rectus abdominis, especially

when heavier resistance is used.

Rectus Abdominis. The rectus abdominis fibers run longitudinally from the lower part of the chest to the pubis. This muscle forward flexes the lumbar spine against resistance by concentric contraction. It controls a backward lean of the trunk in standing or sitting by contracting eccentrically. Right and left sides can contract independently to laterally flex the spine. The best exercises for this muscle are resisted pelvic tilts (standing and supine) (Fig. 3.18), supine abdominal curls, straight reverse abdominal curls and abdominal crunches.

Transverse Abdominis fibers run hori-

Figure 3.14
Strength and flexibility
exercises for the lumbar
extensors.

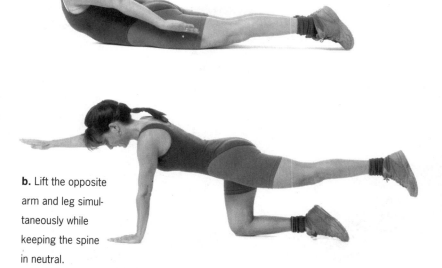

a. Prone hyperextension.

b. Lift the opposite arm and leg simultaneously while keeping the spine in neutral.

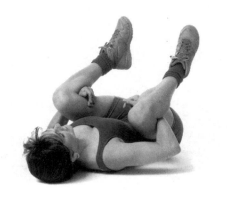

c. Flexibility exercise for the erector spinae: supine, pelvic tilt, knees to shoulders.

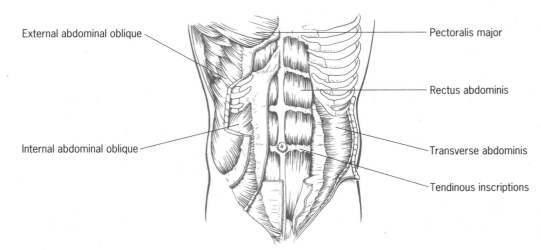

Figure 3.15

Abdominal muscles contract to tilt pelvis posteriorly and flex the thoracolumbar spine against resistance.

zontally around the torso from the thoracolumbar fascia to the linea alba. They do not participate in spinal motion, but pull inward on the abdominal viscera. They contract in forceful expiration and stabilize the trunk in activities requiring extreme effort, such as lifting a very heavy object.

Ways to vary the resistance for abdominal exercises include:

1. Change body positions relative to gravity: e.g., pelvic tilt on hands and knees, standing, supine; partial abdominal curl in supine; partial abdominal curl on incline

bench (head down).

2. Change the length of the lever arm of resistance: abdominal curl with arms lightly touching thighs, with arms crossed over chest or with arms behind the head.

3. Change which end of the muscle is stabilized and which one moves: e.g., abdominal curl with shoulders lifted, or reverse curl with hips lifted.

4. Add weights: abdominal curls with weights in hands or on chest; resisted pelvic tilts with ankle weights.

An instructor can also emphasize endurance training for the abdominals by the following methods:

1. Emphasize different types of muscle contractions: e.g., concentric (curl-up or resisted pelvic tilt); eccentric (curl down); isometric (hold full curl with varying arm positions).

2. Hold the abdominal curl at various points in the arc of motion and perform exercises for the pectorals, quadriceps or hip adductors.

Muscles Acting at the Hip Joint

The hip joint is a triaxial joint allowing motion to occur in all three planes. The movements that occur at the hip joint are flexion and extension, hyperextension, abduction and adduction, internal and external rotation, and circumduction.

Figure 3.16

Strength and endurance (S/E) for external obliques: abdominal curl.

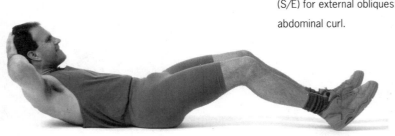

Figure 3.17

S/E for lateral internal and external obliques: side-lying torso raise.

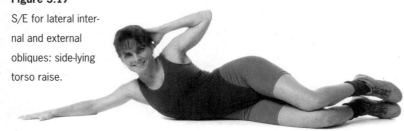

It is important to remember that where the muscle crosses the hip joint determines its function. If the muscle crosses in front of the joint, it will flex and/or internally rotate the hip; if it crosses behind the joint, it will extend and hyperextend and/or externally rotate the hip; if it crosses laterally (to the outside), it will abduct; if it crosses medially (to the inside), it will adduct. Note that all the muscles acting at the hip connect the lower extremity to the pelvis, except the iliopsoas, which also attaches to the anterior surface of the lumbar spine (Fig. 3.19).

Anterior Hip Muscles: Hip Flexors

The hip flexors are the iliopsoas, rectus femoris (one of four parts of the quadriceps), sartorius, tensor fasciae latae, and pectineus. They act to flex the hip, as in a straight leg raise or knee lift. However, they often act eccentrically to control hip extension, such as in a leg-lowering exercise or in leaning back from a seated position.

Iliopsoas. The iliopsoas is actually two muscles, the psoas major and the iliacus, that function as one (Fig. 3.19). It crosses in front of the hip joint connecting the front of the lumbar spine and the inside surface of the ilium to the top of the femur. It flexes the hip when the lumbar spine is stabilized, such as in a straight leg raise in supine. The hip flexor moves the trunk toward the thighs if the femur is stabilized, such as in a sit-up when the legs are held down. Because it attaches high on the femur (short lever arm), it must contract with tremendous force to raise or lower a straight leg. It must resist the long lever arm and large mass of the leg. In most people, the abdominals are not strong enough to balance the strong pull of the iliopsoas to keep the spine in neutral. This is precisely why leg-lowering and straight sit-ups are not recommended. To strengthen the iliopsoas, tilt the pelvis (using abdominals) to stabilize the lumbar spine, then lift one leg against gravity with the knee straight.

Because of its attachment to the lumbar spine, iliopsoas tightness can cause passive lumbar hyperextension or lordosis. Tightness of the iliopsoas is due to poor standing and sitting postures. To stretch the iliopsoas, stand in a forward

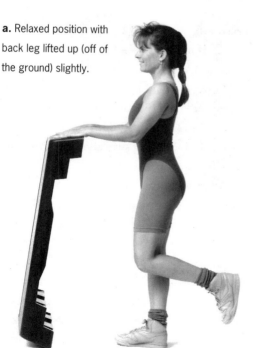

a. Relaxed position with back leg lifted up (off of the ground) slightly.

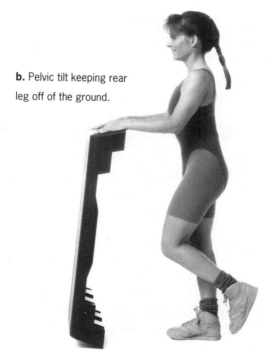

b. Pelvic tilt keeping rear leg off of the ground.

Figure 3.18
Resisted pelvic tilt, standing.

Figure 3.19

Anterior muscles of
the hip and knee.

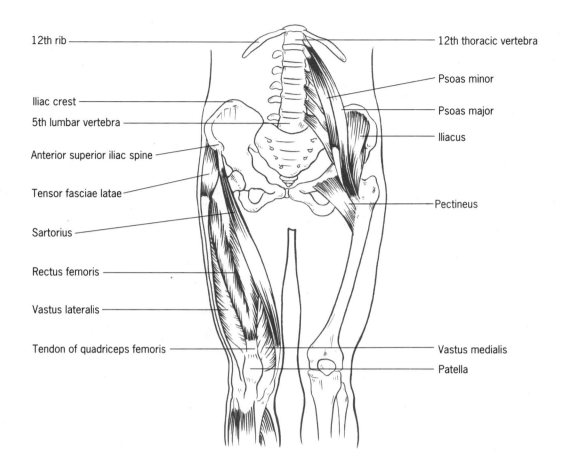

12th rib

Iliac crest

5th lumbar vertebra

Anterior superior iliac spine

Tensor fasciae latae

Sartorius

Rectus femoris

Vastus lateralis

Tendon of quadriceps femoris

12th thoracic vertebra

Psoas minor

Psoas major

Iliacus

Pectineus

Vastus medialis

Patella

lunge position, knee flexed and heel off the floor. Then contract the abdominals to tilt the pelvis and flex the lumbar spine (Fig. 3.20a-b).

Next, look at how muscle function changes as the body position changes. To discern which muscle is contracting, decide whether the motion is antigravity or gravity-assisted. If the movement is antigravity, it is a concentric contraction of the muscle. This is the muscle located superior to the joint. If the movement is gravity-assisted, the antagonist to the movement is contracting eccentrically (lengthening to put the brakes on). Again, this is the muscle located superior to the joint in that particular position.

For example, in a straight leg raise in supine, the hip is flexing and the leg is lifting against gravity. Hence, a concentric contraction occurs of the hip flexors. How-

ever, forward flexion of the hip in standing would not involve the hip flexors, but would instead be an eccentric contraction of the hip extensors (Fig. 3.21). This is one reason that the old standing hamstring stretch is ineffective—the muscle cannot relax and stretch, it is working hard to keep the body from falling forward! Also, if the person bends forward at the waist, the low back could be injured due to harmful torque and shearing stresses on the lumbar discs (see lumbar extensors).

All muscles crossing in front of the hip joint contribute to hip flexion. In addition to the iliopsoas are the rectus femoris, sartorius, tensor fasciae latae and pectineus (Fig. 3.19).

Rectus Femoris. The rectus femoris is one of four heads of the quadriceps muscle of the anterior thigh. It crosses in front of the hip and knee joints. Concentric contraction against gravity causes hip flexion, knee extension or both. The best strengthening exercise is to perform a straight leg raise in standing. To stretch the rectus, perform the iliopsoas stretch, then lower the body so the back knee bends. To stretch the muscle to its maximum, the hip must be extended and the knee bent (Fig. 3.20a-b).

Sartorius. The sartorius originates on the anterior superior iliac spine and inserts on the medial side of the knee. Another two-joint muscle, it flexes, abducts (as the line of pull shifts laterally) and externally rotates the hip and flexes and inwardly rotates the knee.

Tensor Fasciae Latae. This muscle originates near the sartorius on the outer surface of the anterior superior iliac spine and the anterior part of the iliac crest. It inserts into the iliotibial tract of fascia latae about one third of the distance down the femur. It flexes, internally rotates and abducts the hip, tenses the fascia latae and may contribute to the stability of the extended knee.

Pectineus. The pectineus originates on the pubic bone and inserts along the an-

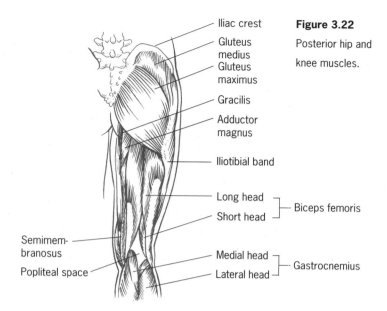

Figure 3.22

Posterior hip and knee muscles.

- Iliac crest
- Gluteus medius
- Gluteus maximus
- Gracilis
- Adductor magnus
- Iliotibial band
- Long head
- Short head
- Biceps femoris
- Semimembranosus
- Popliteal space
- Medial head
- Lateral head
- Gastrocnemius

teromedial surface of the femur. It assists with hip flexion and adduction.

Posterior Hip Muscles: Hip Extensors

The hip extensors are the gluteus maximus, biceps femoris, semitendinosus and semimembranosus. They extend the hip joint against gravity, such as in a prone leg lift. However, they often function eccentrically to control hip flexion, such as in the down phase of a squat or lunge.

Figure 3.21

In forward hip flexion hamstrings contract eccentrically, a potentially harmful position for the lumbar spine.

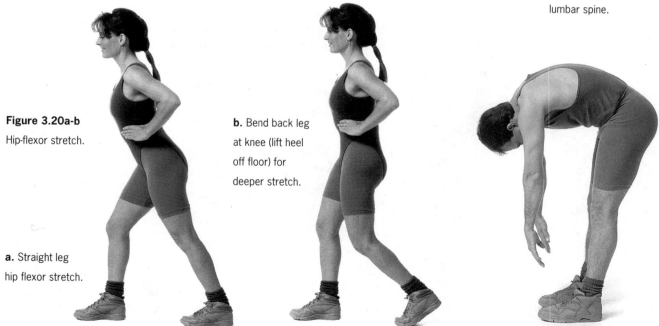

Figure 3.20a-b
Hip-flexor stretch.

b. Bend back leg at knee (lift heel off floor) for deeper stretch.

a. Straight leg hip flexor stretch.

Gluteus Maximus. The largest and most superficial hip extensor, the gluteus maximus attaches to the pelvic rim at one end and broadly along the iliotibial tract (IT band) at the other. This muscle is a good example of why a single function is seldom assigned to a muscle (Fig. 3.22).

Remember, a muscle's function depends on its line of pull across a joint. Looking at the fibers of the gluteus maximus, one sees that, for the most part, it crosses behind the hip. Therefore, it extends the hip. But, some fibers cross superiorly to the center of the joint and others cross inferiorly to the joint. That means that those fibers contribute to abduction and adduction, respectively, but only against strong external resistance. It is also an external rotator of the hip when the hip is extended.

Besides extension, abduction and adduction against resistance, researchers have found the greatest activity of the gluteus maximus is during the following activities: walking up an inclined plane, stair-climb-

ing, jumping, hyperextending the hip against resistance from the erect standing position and isometric contractions. The most effective exercises for this muscle in aerobics class would include these activities.

Hamstrings. The other major hip extensors are the hamstring muscle group. The hamstrings are two-joint muscles crossing the hip and knee. Their origin (except the short head of the biceps femoris) is on the ischial tuberosity ("sitz" bone) (Fig. 3.22). They also cross the knee joint, the semimembranosus and semitendinosus attaching medially and the biceps femoris laterally. Because they cross posteriorly to both joints, they extend the hip and flex the knee. They are also important stabilizers of the knee.

The hamstrings often contract eccentrically in activities of daily life. For example, when bending forward at the hip in standing, the hips are flexing in the same direction as gravity (Fig. 3.21). As noted earlier, the hamstrings are contracting eccentrically (lengthening contraction to hold the body against the pull of gravity). Since the hamstrings are contracting strongly, this is a very poor position for a hamstring stretch.

The hamstrings often show two imbalances – they are weak in relation to the quadriceps and are short in many clients. Hamstrings are difficult to overload in a class setting, but an instructor can take

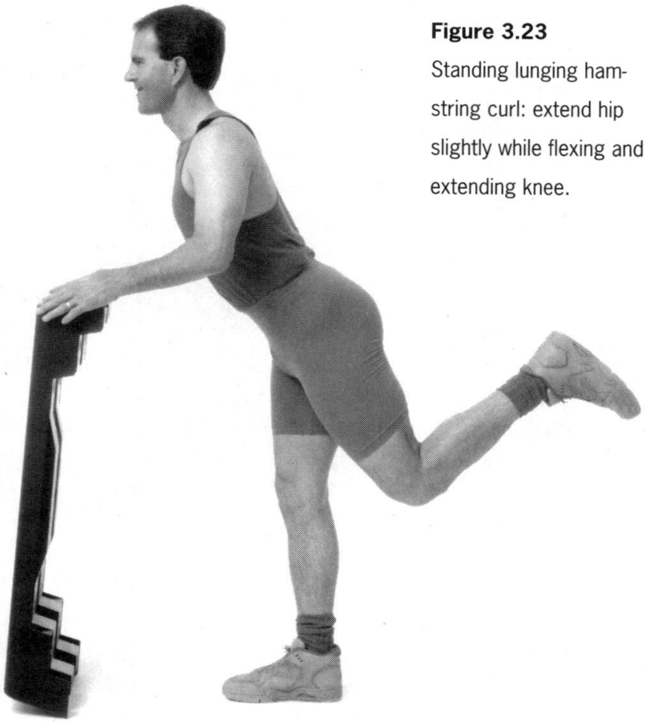

Figure 3.23
Standing lunging hamstring curl: extend hip slightly while flexing and extending knee.

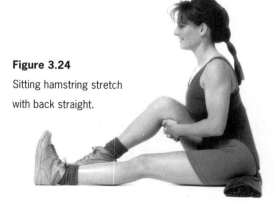

Figure 3.24
Sitting hamstring stretch with back straight.

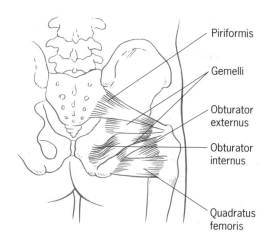

Piriformis

Gemelli

Obturator
externus

Obturator
internus

Quadratus
femoris

Figure 3.25
Deep rotators of the hip.
Avoid overloading these
muscles with long lever
arm exercises.

advantage of the fact that it is a two-joint muscle. Hold the hip in extension, then bend and straighten the knee. More of the exercise is against gravity if performed in standing (Fig. 3.23).

To stretch the hamstrings effectively, position the muscle in hip flexion and knee extension. In sitting position, tilt the pelvis forward to position the low back in neutral. Bend one knee with the other knee straight. Keep the chest pressed to the thigh of the bent leg and slowly slide the foot down until a stretch is felt in the opposite hamstring. This position isolates the stretch to the hamstring and avoids overstretching the back (Fig. 3.24).

Hip External Rotators

The gluteus maximus is primarily a hip extensor, but it also externally rotates the hip because it crosses behind the joint. The gluteus medius also has fibers crossing posteriorly to the joint. That portion of the muscle laterally rotates the hip and may assist with extension.

Six small rotators are located deep to the gluteus maximus (Fig. 3.25). Their order, from top to bottom, is: piriformis, gemelli superior, obturator internus, gemelli inferior, obturator externus and quadratus femoris. The direction of their fibers is horizontal and cross behind the

joint. Their attachment to the femur is very close and behind the joint. Therefore, they rotate the hip externally, and they help the femoral head to stay in its socket. They are very small with a short lever arm. They are not designed to resist large forces alone.

To exercise these muscles safely, keep the lever arm short by bending the knee (Fig. 3.26a). Performing this exercise with the knee straight is too much overload on these muscles for the average client. Also, support the spine in neutral alignment.

To stretch and relax these muscles, simply position the hip in internal rotation (opposite to the muscle's concentric function). A client can achieve greater range of motion if he or she also flexes the hip (Fig. 3.26b).

**Medial Hip Muscles: Hip Adductors
and Internal Rotators**

The muscles that adduct the leg (bring it more closely to the midline) cross the joint toward the inside (medially). They are the pectineus, adductor magnus, gra-

Figure 3.26
Strength and flexibility
exercises for the hip
rotators.

a. S/E for hip rotators
with short lever arm:
avoid leg lifts with top leg
straight in front of torso.

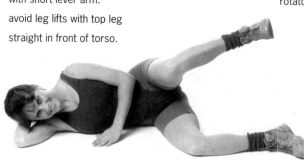

b. Stretching hip external
rotators. Keep shoulders
and back flat; pull flexed
hip and knee across torso.

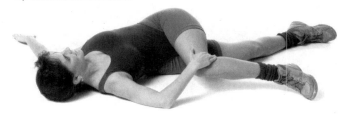

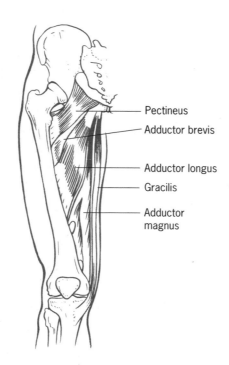

Pectineus

Adductor brevis

Adductor longus

Gracilis

Adductor magnus

Figure 3.27

Adductors muscles of the hip.

cilis, adductor brevis and adductor longus (Fig. 3.27). Because of the anatomy of the femur and hip joint, these muscles sometimes function as internal rotators and sometimes as external rotators. Which one depends on the angle of the joint at the time. They may also help as hip flexors at certain angles. Because of this, these muscles act as synergists and stabilizers in many weight-bearing movements not generally thought of as adductor exercises.

A resistive exercise for the hip adductors is pictured (Fig. 3.28). The starting position is side-lying with top leg flexed at the hip and knee. The knee should be lifted so as to stay in the same plane with the hip joint. Maintain a neutral spine position. The weight of the top leg is on the inside edge of the foot. Lift the bottom leg with the knee extended.

The inner thigh is an area of concern for many female clients. They consistently want to lose the fat deposits along the medial thigh, and want to "tone" the adductors. It is important to educate clients that spot-reducing does not work. To decrease body fat stores along the inner thigh or anywhere else, they must exercise aerobically on a regular basis (4 to 5 times per week).

Lateral Hip Muscles: Hip Abductors

The muscles causing abduction of the hip joint are the gluteus medius and minimus (Fig. 3.29) and the tensor fasciae latae. The attachments are superior to the joint; therefore, as these muscles contract, the femur will be pulled out to the side, away from the midline of the body (abduction).

Gluteus medius and minimus. The attachments of the gluteus medius and minimus are also slightly anterior to the joint, so these muscles also internally rotate the hip. Note that these muscles are located high on the hip, not on the outer thigh. Therefore, the most effective exercises would incorporate abduction and internal rotation.

Besides the common side-lying leg raise, another effective position for exercising the abductors is a side leg lift in the standing position (Fig. 3.30). Though the lift is not antigravity through the full range of motion, this position works the left and right abductors simultaneously. The abductors of the leg being lifted contract concentrically and eccentrically to raise and lower the leg. The abductors of the standing leg contract isometrically to stabilize the pelvis. Standing exercises for the abductors better prepare them for their primary function—walking.

Tensor fasciae latae. This muscle abducts the hip when the hip joint is flexed. People with weak gluteus medius and minimus pull the leg forward as they perform a side leg lift. Then they use the tensor to abduct

Figure 3.28

Antigravity exercise for hip adductors. Keep top knee even with the hip. Weight of top leg is on inside edge of foot.

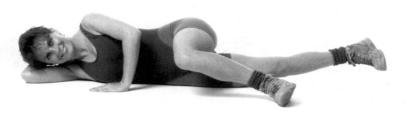

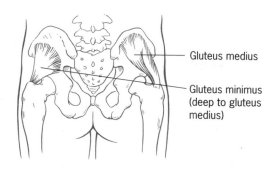

Gluteus medius

Gluteus minimus (deep to gluteus medius)

the leg. To isolate the gluteal muscles, keep the hip in extension.

Muscles Acting at the Knee Joint

The knee is a hinge joint, so the primary motions for the instructor's purposes are flexion and extension. It is supported medially and laterally by ligaments. The muscles controlling knee motion are anterior (the extensors) and posterior (the flexors).

Anterior Knee Muscles: Knee Extensors

The anterior muscles of the thigh control knee extension when the leg is moving freely against gravity. However, when the foot is on the ground, muscle controls knee flexion (eccentrically), as in a squat or lunge.

Quadriceps. The quadriceps is composed of four muscles that act together to extend the knee: the rectus femoris (which also crosses the hip joint), vastus medialis, vastus intermedius and vastus lateralis (Fig. 3.31). Obviously, this large muscle group can produce large forces.

There is little activity in the quadriceps during relaxed standing. In daily function, strong quadriceps are needed in lifting heavy objects, stair-climbing and in walking downhill. To exercise the muscle in a way that prepares it for its daily function, overload it with body weight. Use eccentric contractions, as in squats or lunges. Use concentric contractions to lift the body weight against gravity, as in climbing a step.

There is controversy among the ex-

perts regarding safe strengthening exercises for the quadriceps. It has to do with the stability of the knee when performing a squat or deep knee bend. During a squat the hip and knee flex in the same direction as gravity. Therefore, antagonists to the movement contract eccentrically (hamstrings and gluteus maximus at the hip and quadriceps at the knee). Clearly, large forces are involved. As the knee flexes more, the direction of pull changes. The muscle forces tend to dislocate rather than stabilize the joint. Also, in some women, the patella may be pulled off track because of the quadricep's more diagonal line of pull. In addition, the force acting on the knee increases dramatically with increased knee flexion.

Squats, lunges and stepping are important elements in preparing the quadriceps for daily function. Some experts say the safest approach in a class setting is to limit knee flexion in a weight-bearing position to 90 degrees. The angle between the thigh and shin during a squat or lunge would not be less than 90 degrees (Fig. 3.12). However, to lift objects from the

Kinesiology of the lower body

Figure 3.29

Posterior hip abductors.

Figure 3.30

Standing side leg lift exercises hip abductors bilaterally. Lift to 45° and keep pelvis level.

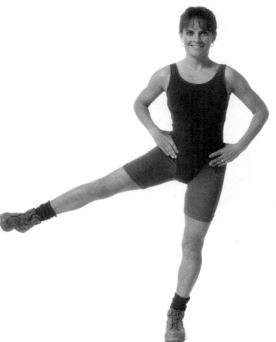

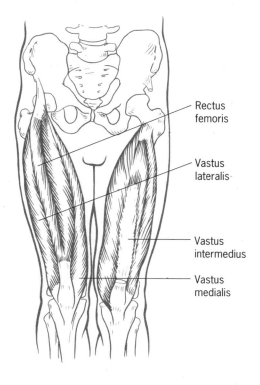

Figure 3.31

Quadriceps muscle.

Rectus femoris

Vastus lateralis

Vastus intermedius

Vastus medialis

floor correctly, the knees must be flexed more than 90 degrees, and often the weakest part of the range of motion is at the beginning of the lift. Figure 3.32 shows correct lifting technique with a neutral spine, using the legs, not the back, to lift by flexing and extending the knees and hips.

Posterior Knee Muscles: Knee Flexors

Figure 3.32a-d

Correct lifting technique.

The primary knee flexors are the hamstrings that were discussed previously with the hip extensors. Secondary knee flexors include the sartorius, gracilis and popliteus (Figs. 3.19, 3.27, 3.33). The popliteus is a stabilizer, but unlocks the knee by inward rotation from the anatomical position and helps to prevent dislocation when a squatting position is maintained. The gastrocnemius, though primarily an ankle muscle, acts in certain instances to stabilize or flex the knee.

Posterior Muscles Acting at the Ankle: Plantarflexors

The gastrocnemius and soleus group make up the bulk of muscle on the posteri-

or calf (Fig. 3.33). Both muscles cross posteriorly to the ankle joint, therefore, they plantarflex the ankle. The gastrocnemius, a two-joint muscle, has a large angle of pull. It can create large forces.

Because it is designed to support body weight, one way to provide resistance is using body weight against gravity. Overload it by performing multiple sets of heel raises on both feet progressing to one foot. Increase the range of motion by dropping the heel, such as over the edge of a step.

Gastrocnemius. The gastrocnemius and soleus muscles are often tight, particularly in clients who wear high heels. To stretch the gastrocnemius effectively, keep in mind that it is a two-joint muscle. Therefore, extend the knee and dorsiflex the ankle preferably in a position that does not require the muscle to support body weight, such as sitting or supine. The hip should be extended so that a tight hamstring does not interfere with the gastrocnemius stretch.

Soleus. The soleus acts with the gastroc-

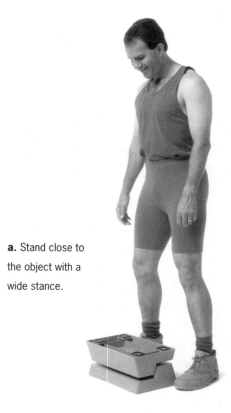

a. Stand close to the object with a wide stance.

nemius at the ankle (plantarflexes) but does not cross the knee. Therefore, to isolate the muscle for strengthening or stretching, the knee must be flexed. For strengthening, perform heel raises with knees flexed. To stretch, the position would be the same as for a gastrocnemius stretch except with the knee flexed and the passive stretch applied more at the ball of the foot.

Posterior Tibialis. This is one of the deep muscles of the calf, located between the tibia and fibula, and connecting to several bones of the foot. It inverts the foot and participates in plantarflexion. It is important in maintaining the longitudinal arch of the foot.

Anterior Muscles Acting at the Ankle: Dorsiflexors

The anterior muscles of the lower leg, the primary one being the tibialis anterior, are pictured in Figure 3.34. Its line of pull operates anterior to the ankle joint, so its function is to dorsiflex the ankle. This muscle, along with the others located along the shin, are the first line of defense for shock absorption in high-impact activities with heel-strike impacts (running). They are also important to balance in walking and running, particularly on uneven ground. It is important to adequately prepare them for the job with a thorough warm-up before impact activities. A common method of warming these

muscles is toe raises (tapping), straight and side to side.

Lateral Muscles Acting at the Ankle and Foot

The **peroneus longus and brevis** are the muscles that compose the lateral compartment of the lower leg (Fig. 3.35). Their tendons curve around the lateral malleolus of the ankle and attach to the first and fifth metatarsal, respectively. Their common functions are plantarflexion and eversion. They are active in walking and are also important in maneuvering on uneven ground. Alternate heel and toe raises moving to the side to warm these muscles.

KINESIOLOGY OF THE UPPER BODY

Upper-body movement includes movement of the head and neck, scapulae, shoulders, arms and hands, and the cervical and thoracic spine. Movement of the lumbar spine impacts upper-body movement and alignment. Table 3.3 sum-

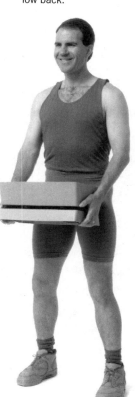

d. When upright, pivot with feet. Do not twist low back.

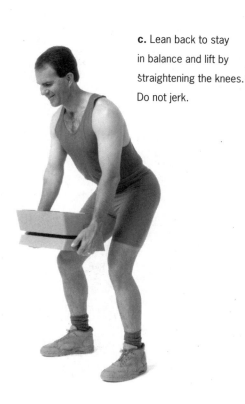

c. Lean back to stay in balance and lift by straightening the knees. Do not jerk.

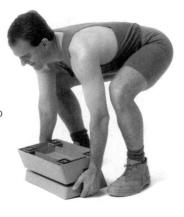

b. Bend knees to go down to the object and keep the curve in the low back.

Chapter 3
Biomechanics
and Applied
Kinesiology

marizes the muscles of the upper body. The shoulder joint or glenohumeral joint is the articulation between the humerus and the glenoid fossa of the scapulae. It is a triaxial joint, allowing movement in three planes.

Therefore, many motions are possible: flexion and extension in the sagittal plane, abduction and adduction in the frontal plane, external and internal rotation and horizontal flexion and extension in the transverse plane, and circumduction occurring in a combination of planes.

Movements of the upper arm are the result of motion at several joints. However, only movements of the scapulae and the

glenohumeral joint will be addressed within the scope of this chapter.

The scapulae and glenohumeral joints work together and use highly coordinated, synchronized movements to perform most functions of the upper extremities. One such coordinated effort is called scapulohumeral rhythm. Studies have shown that in 90 degrees of shoulder abduction, 30 degrees of the motion are due to scapular motion and 60 degrees are due to glenohumeral joint movement (Fig. 3.36).

Shoulder Girdle Muscles

In activities of daily living, the scapular muscles function primarily as stabilizers,

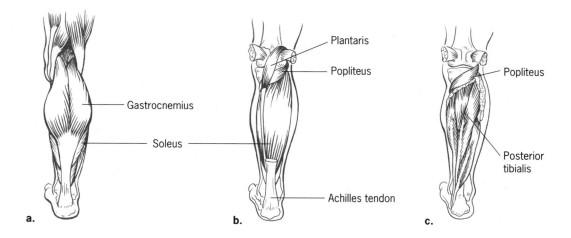

Figure 3.33
Posterior calf muscles.

Figure 3.34 (left)
Anterior muscles of
the lower leg.

Figure 3.35 (right)
Lateral muscles of
the lower leg.

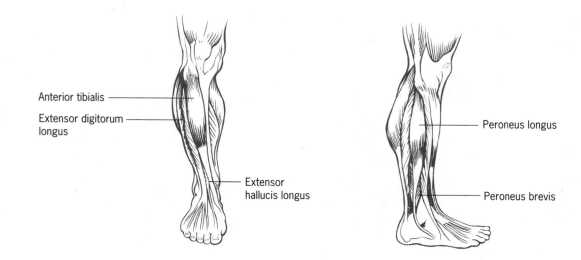

Table 3.3

UPPER BODY MUSCLES — FUNCTIONS AND SELECTED EXERCISES

Muscle	Primary Function	Selected Exercises
Trapezius: upper	Scapular elevation, stabilizer for scapular adduction, upward rotation of the scapula, with insertion fixed, acting bilaterally, head and neck extension; unilaterally, head extension, lateral flexion and rotation to the opposite side	S/E: Upright rows, shoulder shrugs with shoulder joint hyperextended (Fig. 3.39). Avoid arms held at or above horizontal for long periods. F: Depress shoulder, tilt head diagonally to opposite side (Fig. 3.40).
Trapezius: middle	Scapular adduction, stabilizer for upward rotation	S/E: Prone or simulated prone for antigravity position; bilateral or unilateral scapular adduction (double- or single-arm row with elbow straight) (Fig. 3.41); Standing scapular adduction against elastic resistance (Fig. 3.42). F: Usually overstretched already.
Trapezius: lower	Scapular depression, stabilizer for scapular adduction, upward rotation	S/E: Upright with elastic resistance: pull scapulae down and toward the middle (Fig. 3.43).
Rhomboids (major and minor)	Scapular adduction and elevation, downward rotation of scapula	S/E: Prone or simulated prone for antigravity position: arms extended and adducted; pull scapulae up and together; upright, same motion with elastic resistance under feet (Fig. 3.44).
Levator scapulae	Scapular elevation, downward rotation; with insertion fixed— rotates and laterally flexes the cervical vertebrae to the same side	S/E: Upright with elastic resistance under feet: elevate scapulae; prone: rotate head to the side and extend neck. F: Depress scapulae, tuck chin and flex head forward.
Serratus anterior	Upward rotation of scapula, holds scapula flat on thorax, scapular abduction	S/E: Push-ups, bench press, scapular abduction at end of supine pectoral fly; upright anterior shoulder press against elastic resistance around midback.
Pectoralis minor	Tilts scapulae anteriorly; with scapulae stabilized in adduction, may lift chest and assist with forced inspiration	S/E: Squeeze scapulae together, then lift chest. F: Must be stretched manually.
Deltoid (anterior)	Shoulder flexion and internal rotation, stabilizer for shoulder abduction	S/E: Anterior shoulder raise, bringing backs of hands together at the end of the range of motion.
Deltoid (middle)	Shoulder abduction	S/E: Lateral shoulder raises with weights or elastic resistance under feet. Avoid abduction with internal rotation to protect the rotator cuff from impingement.
Deltoid (posterior)	Shoulder extension and external rotation, stabilizer for shoulder abduction	S/E: Forward lunge position: arms down toward the floor. Abduct, extend and externally rotate the arm (Fig. 3.47).
Supraspinatus (rotator cuff)	Shoulder abduction, stabilizes humeral head in glenoid fossa	S/E: Lateral shoulder raises in neutral rotation.
Infraspinatus (rotator cuff)	Shoulder external rotation, stabilizes numerus in glenoid fossa during shoulder motion	S/E: Holding elastic resistance in front at waist level, arms adducted, pull hands apart, rotating back.

Table 3.3 (Continued)

UPPER BODY MUSCLES—FUNCTIONS AND SELECTED EXERCISES

Muscle	Primary Function	Selected Exercises
Teres minor (rotator cuff)	Shoulder external rotation, stabilizes humeral head in glenoid fossa during shoulder motion	S/E: Same as for infraspinatus.
Subscapularis (rotator cuff)	Shoulder internal rotation, stabilizes humeral head in glenoid fossa during shoulder motion	S/E: Holding elastic resistance in back at waist level, arms adducted and elbows flexed, cross hands in front, rotating inwardly at the shoulder.
Latissimus dorsi	Shoulder adduction, extension and internal rotation	S/E: Pulling the arms downward against elastic resistance held overhead; one arm dumbbell row.
Teres major	Shoulder adduction, extension and internal rotation	S/E: Same as for latissimus dorsi.
Pectoralis major	Shoulder adduction and internal rotation; upper fibers: shoulder flexion and horizontal adduction to opposite shoulder; lower fibers: horizontal adduction toward opposite iliac crest	S/E: Push-ups, standing horizontal adduction against elastic resistance around midback; supine "bench press" or "fly"; incline bench press or fly using bench with unequal risers. F: Supine on bench, clasp hands behind head and press elbows back (maintain flat back) (Fig. 3.10).
Coracobrachialis	Shoulder flexion and adduction	S/E: Shoulder flexion and adduction with elbow deltoid tuberosity held flexed and forearm supinated.
Biceps brachii	Shoulder flexion; long head assists with shoulder abduction if the humerus is externally rotated; elbow flexion and forearm supination	S/E: Biceps curls adding supination with weights or elastic resistance under feet; upright rows.
Brachialis	Elbow flexion	S/E: Biceps curls without supination using weights or elastic resistance under feet; upright rows with resistance.
Brachioradialis	Elbow flexion; assists with supination to midposition; assists with pronation to midposition	S/E: "Hammer curls": curls with forearm in neutral position (not pronated or supinated).
Triceps brachii	Elbow extension; long head may assist in shoulder adduction and extension	S/E: Push-ups; dips from bench; bench press; triceps kickbacks.
Pronator teres	Forearm pronation; assists with elbow flexion	Curls with pronation and supination.

Key to selected exercises:
S/E (Strength/Endurance): Exercises to improve strength and/or endurance of the muscle, depending upon the resistance and repetitions. Each exercise is not isolated to that particular muscle, as muscles work in groups to cause movement; however, the exercises listed would include the designated muscle as a prime mover. The exercises listed are ones that can be performed in the context of an aerobics class.
F (Flexibility): Exercises to improve the flexibility of the designated muscle. Flexibility exercises do not stretch the muscle fiber itself, but are designed to lengthen the connective tissue associated with each particular muscle group. For maximum effectiveness, they should be performed after the muscle group is thoroughly warmed.

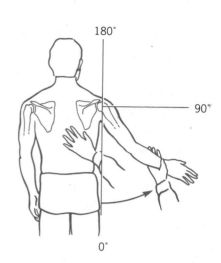

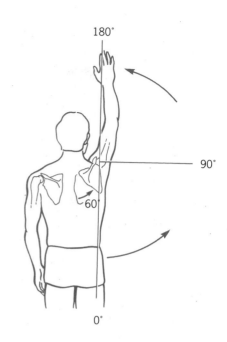

Figure 3.36
Scapulohumeral rhythm.

a. Shoulder joint abduction to 90° is 30° scapular rotation and 60° abduction of the glenohumeral joint.

b. As the arm is abducted overhead, the scapula outwardly (upwardly) rotates to 60°.

but also are powerful muscles in upper-limb movements. They hold the upper body in position so that one can reach, push or pull with the arms and hands. If trained and used correctly, they can also provide increased strength of those arm movements.

Scapular muscles are divided into two groups by their location and stabilizing function: posterior shoulder girdle and anterior shoulder girdle muscles. Posterior shoulder girdle muscles connect the scapula to the back of the torso (trapezius, rhomboids, levator scapulae). Anterior shoulder girdle muscles connect the scapulae to the front of the torso (serratus anterior, pectoralis minor).

Scapular movements are pictured in Fig. 3.37a-f. They include adduction and abduction (sometimes called retraction and protraction), elevation and depression, and upward and downward rotation.

Posterior Shoulder Girdle

Trapezius. The trapezius is the largest and most superficial of the posterior shoulder girdle muscles, and it attaches along the base of the skull, all the cervical vertebrae and all the thoracic vertebrae (Fig. 3.38). At the other end, it attaches to the scapular spine and the lateral third of the clavicle. Note that because the muscle's origin is very broad, the fibers travel in three very different directions, and as such, function as three different muscles.

If the upper fibers contract, the diagonal line of pull causes the scapula to move up and toward the spine (elevate and adduct) (Fig. 3.37). The fibers of the middle trapezius are horizontal between the spine and the scapula. When they contract, the scapula moves toward the spine (adducts). The lower trapezius fibers are on a diagonal, with the origin along the lower thoracic spine moving up and outward to the spine of the scapula. Lower trapezius contraction causes the scapula to move down and in (depress and adduct) (Fig. 3.37b&d).

The trapezius fibers alternately contract and relax to rotate the scapula. If the arms lift in front or out to the side, the shoulder blades rotate with the lower corner moving upward and away from the spine. This is upward rotation of the scapula. Upward rotation occurs as the upper and middle trapezius, rhomboids and ser-

Chapter 3
Biomechanics
and Applied
Kinesiology

Figure 3.37
Scapular movements.

a. Elevation

b. Depression

c. Adduction (retraction)

d. Abduction (protraction)

e. Upward rotation

f. Downward rotation
(return to neutral position).

ratus anterior (Fig. 3.37e) pull on different edges of the scapula. Lower trapezius fibers return the scapula to neutral position (downward rotation), assisted by the rhomboids and levator scapulae (Fig. 3.37f).

Upper Trapezius. To effectively design exercises for this muscle group, consider what it needs and the stresses it encounters every day. In typical sitting and standing postures the upper trapezius is in a shortened position, and must contract isometrically in this shortened position to support the arms and head. It is also active when a heavy weight is held down by the side, or a heavy bag over the shoulder. It typically needs stretching and strengthening through the full range of motion. The trapezius does NOT need long, isometric contractions. Therefore, avoid holding the arms out to the side or overhead, or making little arm circles with the arms extended at shoulder level. When

the arms are held out to the side or overhead, the upper trapezius contracts isometrically to hold the scapula in upward rotation. The deltoid muscle is at a mechanical disadvantage in the higher arm positions. So, the upper trapezius tries to help by contracting even harder to elevate and rotate the scapula.

The upper trapezius is strengthened in upright standing or sitting by shrugging the shoulders with the arms extended behind (Fig. 3.39). To effectively stretch the upper trapezius, position the muscle opposite a shoulder shrug, with the shoulder blade depressed and the head tilted slightly forward and to the opposite side. To achieve a better stretch, press gently on the shoulder and side of the head (Fig. 3.40).

Middle Trapezius. In the typical round-shouldered sitting posture this muscle is usually overstretched and weak. Therefore, it does not need to be stretched in a

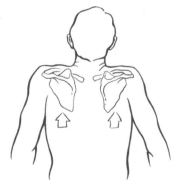

a.

b.

c.

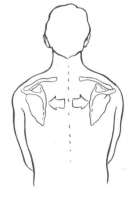

d.

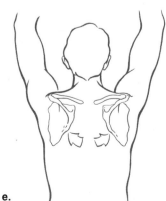

e.

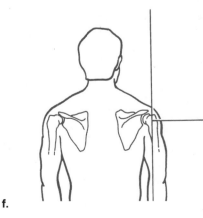

f.

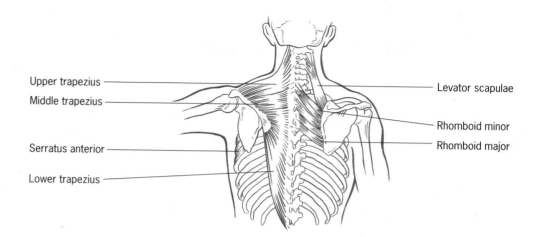

Upper trapezius
Middle trapezius
Serratus anterior
Lower trapezius
Levator scapulae
Rhomboid minor
Rhomboid major

Figure 3.38
Posterior shoulder
girdle muscles.

balanced exercise program. It does need to be strengthened in an antigravity position. That is, the muscle must lift some resistance against gravity. Adducting the shoulder blades in standing does not strengthen it because there is no resistance. An antigravity position is prone (face down) or a simulated-prone position, such as a forward lunge or half-kneeling with the torso supported on the front thigh. The movement in the prone position would be to squeeze the shoulder blades together causing the arms to lift against gravity (Fig. 3.41).

To ensure isolation of the middle trapezius, make sure no movement occurs at the shoulder or elbow. The middle trapezius can also be strengthened in standing, but only with elastic bands or tubing as resistance (Fig. 3.42).

Lower Trapezius. The simplest way to strengthen the lower trapezius is using elastic resistance. Hold the band up and in front of the body, pull the shoulder blades down and toward the middle. Don't let the shoulder or elbow joints move. Like the other scapular adductors, this muscle does not generally need to be stretched (Fig. 3.43).

Rhomboids. The rhomboids (major and minor) are located beneath the middle and upper trapezius (Fig. 3.38). Note that the fiber direction is not horizontal like the middle trapezius. The fibers run diagonally from the spine to the scapula along its inside (medial) edge. Their function, then, judging from the fiber direction, is to adduct and elevate the scapula. They also participate in downward rotation of the scapula. When these muscles are weak and overstretched, the scapulae tilt and pull away from the spine. This is due to the unopposed pull of the pectoralis minor and serratus anterior. To get the strongest contraction of the muscle, one must be in an antigravity position with the arms down by the sides. The action is to elevate and squeeze the shoulder blades together (Fig. 3.44).

Levator Scapulae. This muscle attaches to the transverse process of the cervical vertebrae and the upper inside corner of the scapula. Its primary functions are elevation and downward rotation of the scapulae.

Anterior Shoulder Girdle

The anterior shoulder girdle muscles attach the scapulae to the front of the thorax. They are the serratus anterior and the pectoralis minor (Fig. 3.45).

Serratus Anterior. The serratus anterior attaches underneath the scapula along the medial border and inserts onto the front part of ribs one through nine. The muscle meshes with the upper attachments of the external obliques of the abdominals. The serratus anterior abducts the scapula and works with the trapezius to upwardly rotate the scapula. It enables forceful forward motion of the arm, such as a boxer's knockout punch, and reaching forward. Strengthen the serratus by lying supine with the shoulder flexed, elbow extended, and holding a weight. Then, push the weight toward the ceiling without bending the elbow. This movement is effective at the end of a shoulder press or pectoral fly. The serratus also contracts strongly in a push-up and bench press.

Pectoralis Minor. Its origin is on the coracoid process of the scapula and its insertion is on the third, fourth and fifth ribs. It can have a positive or negative effect on posture, depending on the condition of the scapular adductors (middle trapezius and rhomboids). If the adductors are weak or overstretched, it tilts the

shoulder blades forward and down, worsening the rounded-shoulder position. If the scapular adductors are stabilizing the shoulder blades, the pectoralis minor exerts its pull on the ribs to lift the chest. This is another reason to condition the scapular adductors.

Muscles of the Shoulder Joint Proper

The next muscle group consists of muscles that attach the humerus to the torso or scapula and cause movement at the glenohumeral joint. It includes the deltoid, rotator cuff muscles, pectoralis major, coracobrachialis, latissimus dorsi and teres major (Fig. 3.46). Because each muscle has several functions, depending on joint angle, they are not listed in groups as flexors, abductors, etc.

Deltoid. Similar to the trapezius, the deltoid has fibers running in three different directions, and has three names, according to fiber location relative to the joint (Fig. 3.46). The anterior deltoid at-

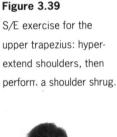

Figure 3.39
S/E exercise for the upper trapezius: hyperextend shoulders, then perform a shoulder shrug.

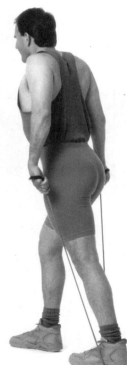

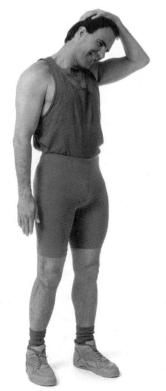

Figure 3.40
Stretch for upper trapezius: stretch: depress scapula, diagonally flex and rotate head to the opposite side.

Figure 3.41
S/E antigravity exercise for the middle trapezius: maintain neutral spine, pull scapula toward spine keeping elbow straight and arms hanging down.

taches in front of the joint along the lateral third of the clavicle. It acts with the posterior deltoid as a stabilizer and synergist during shoulder abduction. Also, because it crosses the shoulder joint anteriorly, it flexes, horizontally adducts and internally rotates the arm at the shoulder joint. The most effective position to strengthen the anterior deltoid is sitting or standing. Raise the arms straight ahead to 90 degrees. Bring the backs of the hands together as they approach 90 degrees to incorporate horizontal adduction and internal rotation.

The middle deltoid's line of pull passes above (superiorly) the joint. As it contracts concentrically, its function is shoulder abduction (raising the arm up and out to the side, away from the torso). In standing or sitting, the middle deltoid also controls shoulder adduction as the arm returns to the torso in a lengthening (eccentric) contraction. Here, the muscle is controlling a movement that occurs in the same direction as gravity. When perform-

ing a lateral raise to isolate the middle deltoid, it is important to hold the shoulder joint in neutral or external rotation. Abducting with internal rotation can damage the rotator cuff muscles as they become impinged between the acromion (the shelf of bone forming the top of the shoulder) and the greater tubercle of the humerus (Fig. 3.48).

The fibers of the posterior deltoid pass behind the joint, attaching to the inferior edge of the spine of the scapula. This muscle stabilizes shoulder abduction. Contracting alone, it extends and externally rotates the shoulder. To effectively strengthen the posterior deltoid, stand in a forward lunge position with a neutral spine. Begin with the shoulder flexed, adducted and internally rotated, then extend, abduct and externally rotate (Fig. 3.47).

In a class setting, large amounts of weight are not available to overload a muscle and recruit muscle fibers to contract. Therefore, instructors must design the ex-

Kinesiology of the upper body

Figure 3.43a-b
S/E exercise for the lower trapezius.

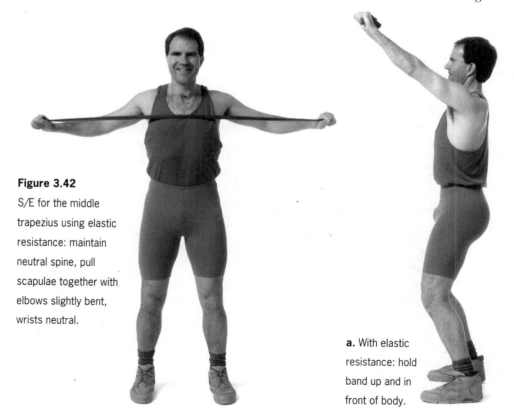

Figure 3.42
S/E for the middle trapezius using elastic resistance: maintain neutral spine, pull scapulae together with elbows slightly bent, wrists neutral.

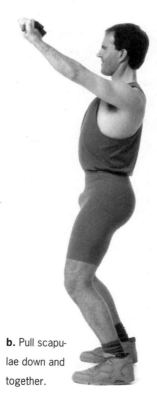

a. With elastic resistance: hold band up and in front of body.

b. Pull scapulae down and together.

Therefore, instructors must design the exercises to incorporate multiple muscle functions in antigravity positions.

Rotator Cuff Muscles

The other posterior muscles originate on the scapula and act at the glenohumeral joint. They serve primarily as stabilizers and rotators. They are the rotator cuff muscles, because they rotate the shoulder joint. Their tendons form a cuff around the glenohumeral joint. They are sometimes called the "SITS" muscles: supraspinatus, infraspinatus, teres minor and subscapularis. They attach to the humerus in that "SITS" order: starting at the top of the humerus and moving toward the back, then around underneath to the front (Fig. 3.48).

Their names tell where they are located. Supraspinatus is above (supra) the spine (spinatus) of the scapula. Infraspinatus is below (infra) the scapular spine. The name teres minor doesn't tell much, but it is located inferior to the infraspinatus. The subscapularis is located on the anterior sur-

face of the scapula. It attaches to the front of the humerus. The subscapularis passes anterior to the joint—it is an internal rotator. The infraspinatus and teres minor cross posterior to the joint; therefore, they are external rotators of the shoulder. One way to strengthen the external rotators is with elastic resistance. Stand with your elbows flexed and close to your sides (i.e., shoulders adducted). Wrap the tube or band around your hands until your hands are about four inches apart. Keeping your lower arms parallel with the floor, externally rotate the shoulders to a comfortable limit of your range of motion (Fig. 3-49).

Impingement of the rotator cuff tendons occurs when the shoulder is abducted and internally rotated simultaneously. When this happens the humerus bumps into the acromion. The rotator cuff tendons are impinged between the two bones and can fray and become inflamed over time. For injury prevention, make sure the shoulder is in neutral or external rotation any time the arms are lifted out to the side.

Latissimus Dorsi and Teres Major. The position and fiber direction of the latissimus dorsi and teres major muscles are pictured in Figure 3.46c. The fiber directions of the upper latissimus dorsi and teres major are very similar. The teres major attaches to the lower corner of the scapula. The latis-

Figure 3.44

S/E for the rhomboids with elastic resistance: forward lunge with band beneath rear foot, pull scapulae up and together.

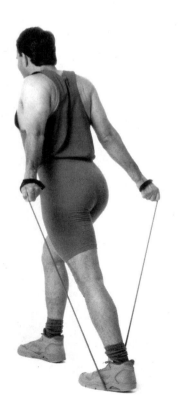

Figure 3.45

Anterior shoulder girdle muscles.

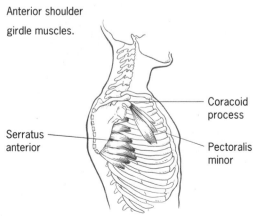

Serratus anterior

Coracoid process

Pectoralis minor

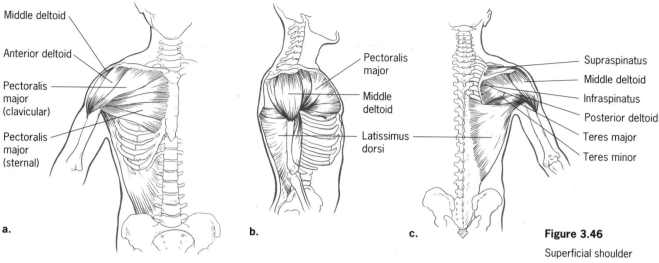

Middle deltoid

Anterior deltoid

Pectoralis major (clavicular)

Pectoralis major (sternal)

a.

Pectoralis major

Middle deltoid

Latissimus dorsi

b.

c.

Supraspinatus

Middle deltoid

Infraspinatus

Posterior deltoid

Teres major

Teres minor

Figure 3.46

Superficial shoulder muscles.

a. Anterior deltoid and pectoralis major.

b. Latissimus dorsi pectoralis and deltoid, lateral view.

c. Posterior muscles of the shoulder (glenohumeral) joint.

simus has a much broader attachment along the lower thoracic spine and all the lumbar vertebrae.

In the class setting, strengthen the latissimus by adducting and extending the arm against elastic bands or tubing held overhead by the opposite hand (Fig. 3.50). Lifting the body up in a sitting push-up on a bench would also strengthen these muscles. This move differs from a triceps dip in that the arms are away (abducted) from the torso. Here, the muscle would have to lift body weight against gravity to adduct and extend the shoulder.

A common mistake in class is to perform a "lat pull down" movement with hand-held weights (no elastic resistance). However, this movement does not involve a contraction of the latissimus. Because the shoulder adduction is occurring in the same direction as gravity, an eccentric contraction of the deltoid and upper trapezius control the motion. Be sure the muscle to be strengthened is working against gravity if hand weights are used as resistance.

Pectoralis Major. The pectoralis major is another adductor and internal rotator of the humerus at the shoulder joint. It inserts on the humerus very near the inser-

tion of the latissimus dorsi. Its origin is very broad along the medial half of the clavicle, the anterior surface of the sternum and cartilages of the first six through seven ribs and the aponeurosis of the external oblique (Fig. 3.46). As a whole, the muscle serves to flex and horizontally adduct the arm. It also adducts and internally rotates the arm against resistance. To strengthen the pectorals effectively in a class with hand weights, get into the antigravity position (lying supine). In sitting or standing, a pectoral fly overloads the deltoids and upper trapezius (holding the weight of the arm against gravity), but does nothing to overload the pectoral. It is virtually useless and a time-waster.

The push-up is an important exercise to strengthen the pectorals. The pectoralis major, serratus anterior and triceps contract eccentrically to lower the weight of the body in the same direction as gravity. Then, they contract concentrically to lift the body weight against gravity. Take care to maintain the spine in a neutral position. Neutral position refers to maintaining the natural curves of the back without flexion, extension, rotation or excessive anterior pelvic tilt. For example, Figure 3.51a shows unsafe alignment of the neck and low back while performing a push-up. The head is jutted forward and the low back is out of alignment. Figure 3.51b shows safe, neutral alignment, with the head retracted and the abdominals tilting the pelvis posteriorly against gravity. To stretch the muscle effectively, put the arms in a position that opposes all the functions of the muscle. The pectoralis adducts, flexes and internally rotates the arm. Therefore, to stretch it, place the arm in abduction, hyperextension and external rotation behind the plane of the body (Fig. 3.10). Pelvic tilt to hold the spine flat on the bench to stabilize the other end of the muscle.

Biceps Brachii and Coracobrachialis. The lines of pull of these muscles are anterior to the joint, so they flex the arm (along with the pectoralis major and anterior deltoid) (Fig. 3.52).

The biceps brachii acts at the shoulder and elbow joints. It has a long and short head that cross the shoulder joint at dif-

ferent places. Unless the shoulder is externally rotated, the long head crosses in front and helps flex the arm at the shoulder. In external rotation, the long head moves to a superior and lateral position, so its function changes from flexion to abduction. The biceps will participate more as a shoulder abductor when external resistance is applied.

The long head of the biceps lies in a shallow groove in the humerus as it crosses the shoulder. Fast, repeated long lever arm movements of the arms, either in flexion or abduction, can cause tendinitis in the biceps. To prevent injury, go through a smaller range of motion if the arms are straight, or bend the elbows to shorten the lever arm or slow the movement down.

Besides shoulder motion, the biceps flexes the elbow and supinates the forearm. A biceps curl can be more challenging if it is started with the palm down, then turn the palm up (supinate) while flexing the elbow. Also, if the shoulder joint is supported in a flexed position, it is more difficult for the muscle to lift the same external resistance (Fig. 3.53).

In addition, with the insertion fixed, the biceps flexes the elbow, moving the humerus toward the forearm as in a pull-up or chinning exercise.

Triceps. The triceps is also a two-joint muscle, crossing posteriorly to the shoulder and elbow (Fig. 3.54). Therefore, it extends the arm at the shoulder and the forearm at the elbow. This muscle can be placed into an antigravity position in several ways. The simplest position is to stand in a slight forward lunge, hold the shoulder in hyperextension (muscle is shortened over one joint), then extend the elbow. Another would be to lie supine, point the elbow toward the ceiling and extend the elbow.

Avoid the position of shoulder abduc-

Figure 3.47

S/E exercise for the posterior deltoid.

a. Maintain a neutral spine—shoulders flexed and internally rotated (back of hands together).

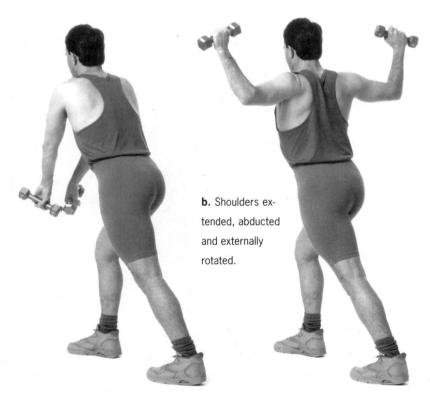

b. Shoulders extended, abducted and externally rotated.

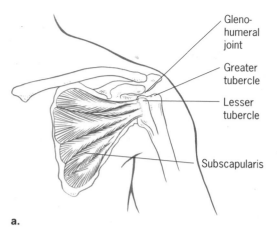

Gleno-
humeral
joint

Greater
tubercle

Lesser
tubercle

Subscapularis

a.

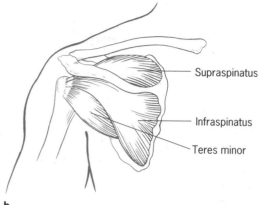

Supraspinatus

Infraspinatus

Teres minor

b.

Figure 3.48

Rotator cuff muscles.
Avoid shoulder abduc-
tion with internal rotation
to prevent impingement.

a. Anterior view.

b. Posterior view.

tion to 90 degrees, extending the elbow out to the side. This is an antigravity position for the triceps, but it is NOT recommended for two reasons: (1) it requires a sustained isometric contraction of the deltoid and upper trapezius that is better avoided, and (2) it also involves internal rotation of the arm with abduction that causes impingement of the rotator cuff.

To prevent shoulder injury, drop the arm to 70 degrees of abduction.

EXERCISE DESIGN, INSTRUC-TION AND CORRECTION

The successful fitness instructor must demonstrate five basic skills to apply kinesiology successfully in the aerobics class:

1. Design movements that effectively

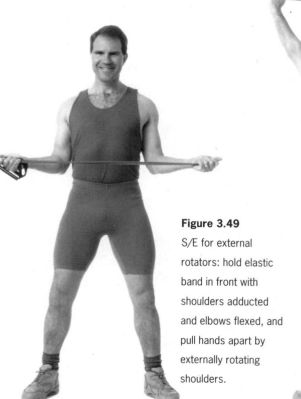

Figure 3.49

S/E for external rotators: hold elastic band in front with shoulders adducted and elbows flexed, and pull hands apart by externally rotating shoulders.

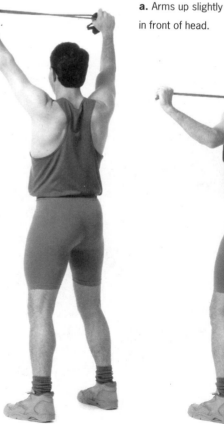

a. Arms up slightly in front of head.

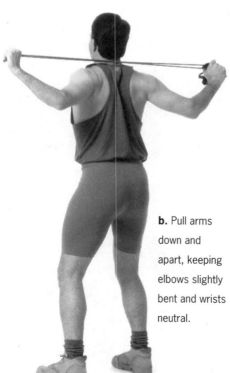

Figure 3.50

S/E for latissimus dorsi with elastic resistance.

b. Pull arms down and apart, keeping elbows slightly bent and wrists neutral.

Figure 3.52

Biceps and
coracobrachialis.

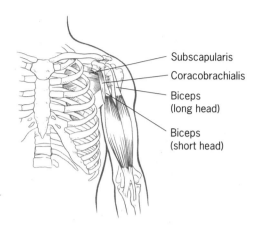

Subscapularis

Coracobrachialis

Biceps
(long head)

Biceps
(short head)

isolate and strengthen or stretch a particular muscle group.

2. Properly execute a movement.

3. Verbally cue a movement and explain it so that the clients can do the movement correctly.

4. Recognize improper alignment and/or execution.

5. Correct improper alignment and/or execution.

Exercise design is a very important factor in a successful exercise program. However, instructors must also orally express the movement accurately and concisely. Just as with dance-type choreography, start with simple movements. Then, add to and modify the movement. Gradually increase the overload and incorporate all the functions of the muscle. But even when an instructor can show and orally cue a movement correctly, some clients just don't get it. In seeking to correct poor form, check first that their spinal alignment is neutral—that alone may line everything up so the exercise can be done correctly. Then if more correction is need-

ed, do not push the body part to where it should be—the person's reflexes will naturally resist.

The instructor should hold his or her own hand where the body part should be, then have the the client move to touch it. Thus, the client is using the right muscles to establish the correct neurological pathways.

Exercise Analysis and Substitution of Risky Exercises

The following exercises involve some risk to most clients in an aerobics class. Therefore, it is recommended that they be excluded from programming. The following are explanations of the risks involved and modifications that achieve the benefit without compromising safety.

Double Leg Raises, (also known as leg-lowering exercise). This movement requires a strong contraction of the hip flexors on both sides as well as a very strong contraction of the abdominals to stabilize the spine. Most people do not have the abdominal strength to balance the force of the hip flexors as they lift the weight of the extended legs (long lever arm). An acceptable substitute would be a pelvic tilt with one leg bent and one leg straight. Then slowly raise and lower the straight leg alone, carefully maintaining the pelvic tilt (Fig. 3.55).

Full Squats (extreme knee flexion while bear-

Figure 3.51

Push-up alignment.

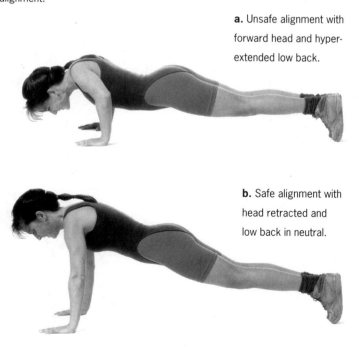

a. Unsafe alignment with forward head and hyperextended low back.

b. Safe alignment with head retracted and low back in neutral.

ing weight). Full squats put the knees in a position of deep flexion while bearing weight. As discussed in the section on quadriceps, several risks are involved. At 120 degrees of knee flexion, the forces on the joint itself can be eight times body weight. These forces are acting to pull the joint apart because of the angle of pull. In addition, the tracking of the patella in its groove can be adversely affected, causing irritation and wearing down of the cartilage on the underside of the kneecap.

In a class setting, it is advisable to limit squats to 90 degrees of knee flexion. The angle between the thigh and the shin should not be less than 90 degrees (Fig. 3.12).

Full Neck Circles. The problem with full neck circles comes in the area between lateral flexion and hyperextension of the neck. With the head back at a diagonal, the weight-bearing surfaces of the spine change from the vertebral body to the small facet joints. These joints are not designed to bear weight. In addition, many people have small misalignments of the

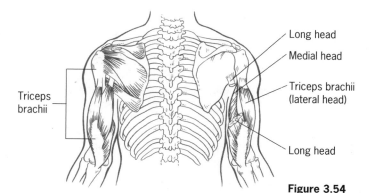

Figure 3.54

Triceps: long, medial and lateral heads.

cervical vertebrae that can be made worse in this position. They may compress the spinal nerves in this position.

They are ineffective to strengthen neck muscles because standing and sitting would not be an antigravity position for any of them. There are better stretch positions without risk if stretches are done with individual muscle fiber direction in mind.

Do all head and neck movements slowly, under muscular control, and from a neutral spine (head retracted) position. Most people hold their heads forward with hyperextension of the neck. The muscles in the back, then, tend to be tight and need stretching. To stretch effectively, first retract the head by tucking the chin, then tilt the head forward and actively press the head against the hand. If a client is not actively pressing, the muscles he or she is trying to stretch are contracting eccentrically to counter the resistance of the weight of the head (Fig. 3.56).

Hurdler's Stretch. In a stretching program, the aim is to stretch the connective tissue and fascia associated with muscle. Exercisers do not want to stretch the ligaments that protect the joints by limiting undesirable motion. There are two common versions of the hurdler's stretch. One aims to stretch the adductors on one leg and hamstrings on the other (Fig. 3.57a). The second aims to stretch the quadriceps (Fig. 3.57b). However, both of these can

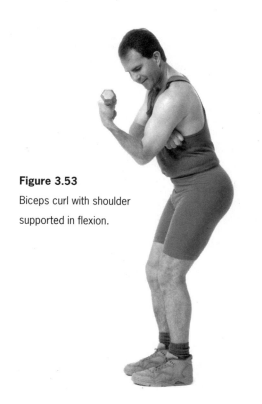

Figure 3.53

Biceps curl with shoulder supported in flexion.

also stretch the medial collateral ligament of the knee. Therefore, they can cause medial instability of the knee joint. The back can be strained trying to get into the position as the iliopsoas contracts eccentrically to extend the hip joint.

The quadriceps can be stretched safely and effectively in standing, prone or sidelying positions. Take care to keep the lumbar spine in neutral and extend the hip joint actively with the gluteals. Do not allow the back to arch. Safe alternatives for the contralateral adductor and hamstring stretch are pictured in Fig. 3.57c & d.

Plough Exercise. This exercise is probably intended to stretch the low back. However, there are several problems with this movement: people tend to go too far back and bear their weight on the cervical spine, and the position demands eccentric contractions of the muscles. It tries to stretch as one lowers the extended legs overhead, and the area of the thoracic spine does not usually need to be stretched. To stretch the low back a better position would be knees to armpits, with an active pelvic tilt (Fig. 3.14c).

Unsupported Forward Flexion of the Lumbar Spine (with or without rotation). As previously discussed, unsupported forward lumbar flexion is potentially harmful to the low-back ligaments and discs. Flexion with rotation increases the risk even more. The original purpose of the exercise was per-

haps to stretch the low back and hamstrings, but again these very muscles contract eccentrically as one forward flexes, so it is very ineffective as a stretch. Because of the high risk to the lumbar spine, it is recommended that the movement be excluded from a fitness class.

Back Hyperextension. Back hyperextension is only a problem if it is done ballistically, using momentum rather than muscular control. It is to be avoided as a substitution for hip hyperextension. Both problems can be seen in poor execution of hip extension exercises on hands and knees, elbows and knees, or in standing position. It is something to watch for and correct during hip-extension exercises or in hip-flexor stretches.

Back hyperextension may be contraindicated for people with certain back conditions. However, most people would benefit from back-extension exercises performed slowly under muscular control (Fig. 3.14a).

Components of a Balanced Exercise Program

A balanced exercise program consists of a variety of activities that promote the following:

1. Aerobic (cardiovascular) conditioning.

Figure 3.55

Substitute for double leg raise: keep one leg flexed and pelvis tilted back (angle of hip doesn't change).

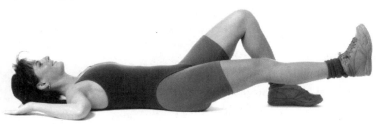

Figure 3.56

Posterior neck stretch: head retracted and flexed, press forward against hand.

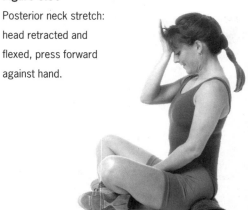

2. Muscle strengthening activities that are compatible with ways the muscle is required to function in daily activities.

3. Instruction in proper body mechanics of lifting.

4. Flexibility of connective tissue allowing full range of motion of all joints.

5. Balance—static and dynamic.

6. Kinesthetic awareness—resulting in the ability to maintain neutral alignment and proper form in the execution of exercises.

Such a program would include exercises for pelvic and scapular stability. That is, the pelvic and scapular muscles must be strengthened through their full range of motion, but they must also be required to function as stabilizers. It is beneficial to simulate movements required in daily tasks so there is a direct carryover out of the classroom.

For example, teach pelvic tilts in standing since that is the position in which people need a pelvic tilt to maintain neutral alignment of the spine. Pelvic and lumbar spine stability is crucial for neutral alignment and proper execution of almost all strengthening or stretching exercises.

The importance of scapular stability can hardly be overstated. Improving kinesthetic (not just cognitive) awareness of neutral alignment of the upper body is the first step. Strengthening the scapular muscles, particularly the posterior shoulder girdle, is the second. Recognizing and reinforcing proper alignment of the shoulder girdle, head and neck is the third.

Regarding kinesiology in the cardiovascular conditioning segment of class, design choreography so that the time spent not only provides aerobic conditioning but also:

1. Provides safe, neutral alignment of the spine;

2. Minimizes high reaction forces on

Figure 3.57
Safe and higher risk lower extremity stretches.

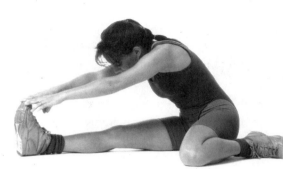

a. Risky hurdler's stretch for hamstring and adductors.

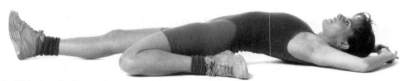

b. Risky hurdler's stretch for quadriceps.

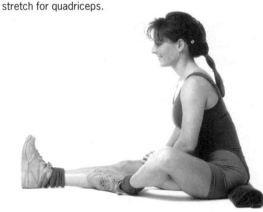

c. Safe adductor and hamstring stretch. Bend forward from hips keeping inward curve of lumbar spine.

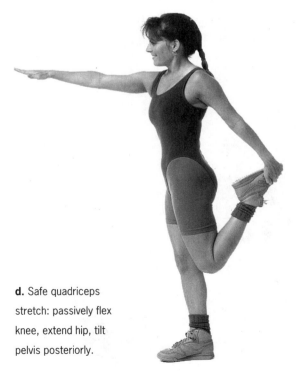

d. Safe quadriceps stretch: passively flex knee, extend hip, tilt pelvis posteriorly.

the joints (knees, hips, back) by varying the impact;

3. Decreases risk to neck and shoulders by limiting fast movements of the extended arms through full flexion or abduction; avoiding abduction with internal rotation of the shoulder joints; avoiding prolonged segments with the arms held at or above the horizontal; and avoiding ballistic movements of the head, neck and shoulders.

Body Mechanics of Lifting

A primary need in daily living for muscle strength, conditioning and knowledge of proper technique is in the ability to safely lift heavy objects. The fitness class is a natural place to instruct and practice proper technique and strengthen the muscle groups necessary to do this task.

Proper lifting techniques include several basic steps:

1. Stand close to the object with a wide stance.

2. Use the low back extensors to actively stabilize and maintain the curve in the low back (lordosis).

3. Bend the knees to go down to the object and keep the back neutral with the head up. Squat or lunge, depending on leg

strength, the heaviness of the object and which angle will get one closest to the object.

4. Get a secure grip and hold the object as close as possible.

5. Lean back to stay in balance and lift the object by extending the knees and hips.

6. Make the lift a smooth, steady motion, not a quick jerk.

7. Exhale during the lift.

8. When upright, pivot with the feet to turn. Do not twist the torso.

Duplicate the necessary movement pattern in class by squats or lunges to pick up a small object from the floor (a dumbbell) (Fig. 3.58). Make the movement slow and controlled. Use this time to educate the clients verbally about proper lifting technique so they can more readily apply it to lifting children, groceries, luggage, etc.

Many back injuries occur when people twist to put an object down in a different place. To prevent such injuries, people need to learn to lift and then pivot before putting the object down. In class, simulate

Figure 3.58
Body mechanics training.

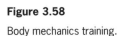

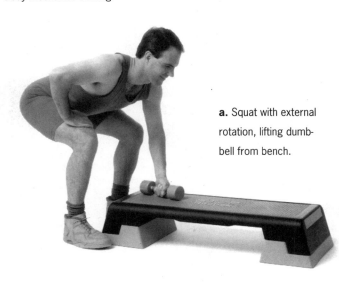

a. Squat with external rotation, lifting dumbbell from bench.

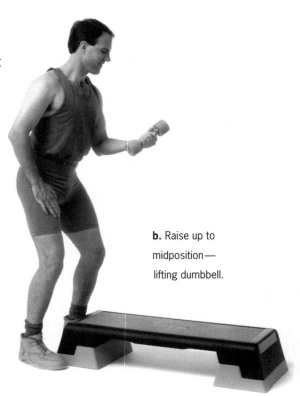

b. Raise up to midposition— lifting dumbbell.

this in a squat-pivot combination so people can learn safe lifting techniques kinesthetically, not just cognitively. It is very important that people practice good lifting mechanics so the neuromuscular pathways are reinforced. Many people know how to lift properly, but still do not use good body mechanics because they have not developed the proper patterns of movement.

SUMMARY

This chapter has presented the tools to design safe, effective exercise programs for aerobic and muscle conditioning classes. The neurological and anatomical factors that affect human movement have been explained. Effects of outside forces, such as gravity and applied resistance, have been examined. The primary muscle groups addressed in group exercise have been discussed, with suggestions for strengthening and stretching exercises. The mechanical principles necessary to create a progressive exercise program have also been reviewed.

A list of the most effective exercises for each muscle group is a good reference tool to keep variety in programs. A graded series for each muscle group is also important in gradually progressing the beginning student.

REFERENCES

Ellison, D. (1991). Biomechanics and Applied Kinesiology. In M Study (Ed), *Personal Trainer Manual: The Resource for Fitness Instructors*, San Diego: American Council on Exercise.

Ellison, D. (1993). *Movement That Matters*, San Diego: E & C Productions.

Luttgens, K.; Deutsch, H., & Hamilton, N. (1992). *Kinesiology: Scientific Basis of Human Motion*. Dubuque, Iowa: Brown and Benchmark.

Kapit, W., & Elson, L. (1977). *The Anatomy Coloring Book*. New York: Harper & Row.

Kendall, H.; Kendall, F., & Wadsworth, G. (1971). *Muscles: Testing and Function*. Baltimore: Williams & Wilkins.

Kreighbaum, E., & Barthels, K. (1981). *Biomechanics*. Minneapolis: Burgess.

Rasch, P. (1989). *Kinesiology and Applied Anatomy*. Philadelphia: Lea & Febiger.

Chapter 4

Nutrition and Weight Control

By Karen S. Newton

well-selected diet is a key factor in health and athletic performance. It is important for instructors to have basic knowledge of nutrition because they, too, are endurance athletes and because they are frequently asked to provide guidance on nutrition by participants in their classes. People in aerobics classes are interested in improving their health and physical appearance and are often willing to try any dietary regimen or nutritional supplement in their search for weight loss, improved athletic performance or better health. Some may go beyond good sense

Karen S. Newton, M.P.H., R.D., is a nutrition and health-promotion consultant in Lexington, Kentucky. She has lectured and trained extensively in the field of lifestyle management and obesity treatment. She is the co-author of People Karch International's texts for the Weight Control for Life and Lighter Living Weight Management Programs.

and try dietary practices that contribute nothing to their goals for improved fitness and health. The worst scenario is they may adopt dietary habits that are harmful.

Nutrition is a science and an art. The science of nutrition is relatively new and began with the discovery of vitamins in this century. Research and interest have exploded since then, and nutrition information is currently doubling every 18 months. This sometimes overwhelming amount of information has reinforced the old adage: "You are what you eat."

Nutrition scientists now generally agree that diet is directly and causally related to development of degenerative diseases. The abundance of information has also created an arena for misinformation, and instructors frequently hear participants complain that it is difficult to sort out nutrition fact from fiction and to make knowledgeable food choices. The first part of this chapter provides a foundation of accurate, current knowledge about the science of nutrition. The art of nutrition (the application of nutrition theories and facts) is covered later in this chapter.

In addition to being a positive role model, the instructor should be able to provide solid information on nutrition, guidance on the intensity and duration of exercise most effective for weight control, and motivating encouragement for each individual's goals in the class. Instructors should not attempt to counsel participants on their personal nutrition needs, prescribe diets, or suggest supplements. Participants should be encouraged to contact a qualified professional to discuss their specific nutritional questions or medical problems. Registered Dietitians (RDs) are uniquely qualified to assess nutritional status and provide counseling. Check the Yellow Pages, local hospitals, or call the American Dietetic Association to obtain

a list of local RDs who provide nutrition consultation services.

OVERVIEW OF TERMS

What is **energy**? The ultimate source of energy is the sun. This energy is captured in the chlorophyll in plants, the plants are consumed by animals, and the energy is condensed in their tissues. We consume foods from both plant and animal sources to obtain the necessary energy to fuel all body processes. Energy is available in the body in two forms: active and storage (or potential) energy. Active energy is readily available to fuel metabolic processes. Storage energy is the body's reserve and is stored as fat or as glycogen (sugar).

What are **calories**? The units by which the energy in food is measured are called kilocalories (kcal). Kilocalorie is often mistakenly shortened to "calorie" in discussions of nutrition and exercise but 1 kilocalorie actually equals 1,000 calories. A 100-calorie plain potato actually contains 100 kcal. Calories with a capital "C" refers to kilocalorie. All calories (energy) used by the body originate from dietary protein, carbohydrates, fat or alcohol. Vitamins, minerals and water do not contain calories (energy).

What is **metabolism**? The sum total of all chemical processes that convert food and its components into the fundamental chemicals the body uses for energy and for the repair, maintenance and growth of tissues is called metabolism. Metabolism is a constant process; energy is produced during sleep, eating, exercise, sitting or work. The amount of energy used will vary, however, depending on the individual's metabolic rate and activity level. Metabolic rate is the measure of how rapidly the body burns calories. A high metabolic rate means the body quickly burns calories, a slow metabolic rate means the body conserves calories and is more likely to store the excess as fat in fat tissue.

NUTRITION BASICS

A basic principle of healthful **nutrition** is balance. A well-selected variety of foods will provide the nutrients needed for health and physical activity. This section describes the nutrients and suggests a system for balanced eating.

Nutrients

In physiological terms, food satisfies three fundamental body needs: (1) the need for energy, (2) the need for new tissue growth and tissue repair, and (3) the need to regulate the metabolic functions constantly occurring in the body. These needs are met by the components of foods called **nutrients**. There are six classes of nutrients: water, vitamins, minerals, protein, fats and carbohydrates.

Water. **Water** is the most important, yet most frequently forgotten, nutrient. The body can survive for weeks or months without food, but even a few days without water will result in death. Adequate intake of water is essential for all energy production in the body, for temperature control (especially during vigorous exercise), for transportation of all nutrients and waste products in and out of the body, and for the lubrication of joints and other structures. Failure to consume adequate water **(dehydration)** results in impaired exercise, fatigue, faulty regulation of body temperature, and the risk of heat exhaustion and heat stroke. The tendency toward fluid retention common among chronic dieters is often complicated by inadequate consumption of water. Ironically, it is relieved by increased fluid intake.

Thirst is not a good indicator of the need for fluids. The recommended eight glasses of water per day is probably adequate for a sedentary person, but is not enough in hot temperatures or for a very active person who should consume about 1 quart of water for every 1,000 Calories burned. Any beverage (except those with alcohol and caffeine, which are dehydrating) will meet this requirement.

Vitamins. **Vitamins** are organic (carbon-containing) compounds that are required in the body in minute amounts to function as metabolic regulators of biochemical reactions, including energy production, growth, maintenance and repair. The body cannot manufacture them, which is why they must be obtained from the diet. For a substance to be called a vitamin, inadequate intakes of the substance must produce a deficiency disorder that is corrected when the vitamin is returned to the diet. Vitamins provide no calories and, therefore, cannot be used as fuel.

Thirteen vitamins have been identified and are categorized as either fat-soluble or water-soluble (Table 4.1). Each has a special function in the body and also works in complicated ways with other nutrients. The fat-soluble vitamins (A, D, E and K) are stored in the body fat, principally in the liver. Adequate daily intake of the water-soluble vitamins is important since the body excretes excesses in the urine and stores very little for later use.

The best source for vitamins is the daily diet since food enhances availability. However, optimal vitamin status may be difficult on a diet that contains less than 1,600 to 1,800 Calories per day. The question, "Who should take vitamin-mineral supplements?" is answered later in this chapter.

Minerals. **Minerals** are inorganic compounds that enter the food chain via plants that absorb minerals from soil and water. Essential minerals are required in small amounts from the diet to sustain life and promote health. Fifteen minerals are recognized as essential (Table 4.2). Mineral status is very dependent on balance: many minerals compete in the intestine for absorption, and over consumption of one mineral can restrict the absorption of a competing mineral. For example, a large supplemental dose of iron can cause a secondary deficiency of copper or zinc, unless these minerals are supplemented concurrently (Simmer, 1987). The proper balance between minerals also enhances their use in the body. For example, calcium absorption and utilization are dependent on magnesium and zinc.

Minerals serve a variety of functions in the body. For example, calcium and phosphorous are used to build bones and teeth. Others are important components of hormones, such as zinc in insulin. Iron is essential in the formation of hemoglobin, the oxygen-carrying pigment within the

Table 4.1

VITAMINS: SOURCES AND ADULT RECOMMENDED DIETARY ALLOWANCES (RDAs)

	Vitamin	Sources	Adult RDAs
Fat-soluble	A	Liver, carrots, sweet potato, spinach, apricots, beets greens, winter squash, cantaloupe, broccoli, peaches, dark green lettuce, egg yolk, peas, fortified milk	4,000–5,000 IU*
	D	Fish oils, fortified milk, fortified cereals, egg yolk and sunlight (absorbed through skin)	400 IU
	E	Vegetable oils, wheat germ, whole grains, nuts	30 IU
	K	Leafy green vegetables, broccoli, cabbage, cauliflower, tomatoes, wheat bran, (adults also produce vitamin K in the intestines)	65–80 mcg**
Water-soluble	C	Citrus fruits, strawberries, collard greens, broccoli, melons, tomatoes, potatoes, green peppers	60 mg***
	B_1 (Thiamine)	Pork, organ meats, oysters, green peas, collard greens, oranges, cooked dried beans and peas, wheat germ, nutritional yeast, fish, peanuts, whole grains	1.0–1.5 mg
	B_2 (Riboflavin)	Milk and dairy products, organ meats, avocado, chicken, fish, leafy green vegetables, broccoli	1.2–1.7 mg
	Niacin	Lean meat, chicken, fish, cooked dried beans and peas, nutritional yeast, peanuts, milk, cheese, soybeans, nuts	13–19 mg
	B_6 (Pyridoxine)	Lean meat, poultry, fish, soybeans, cooked dried legumes, peanuts, bananas, avocado, cauliflower, cabbage	1.6–2.0 mg
	B_{12}	Lean meat, poultry, fish, shellfish, organ meats, cheese, eggs, fermented soybean products	2.0 mcg
	Folacin (Folic Acid)	Dark green leafy vegetables, organ meats, nutritional yeast, orange juice, avocado, beets, broccoli, lentils	180–200 mcg
	Pantothenic Acid	Whole grain breads and cereals, organ meats, fish, chicken, eggs, avocado, canned mushrooms, cauliflower, green peas, legumes, nuts, potatoes	4–7 mg****
	Biotin	Organ meats, oatmeal, eggs, soybeans, nutritional yeast, bananas, mushrooms, peanuts	30–100 mcg****

* I.U.= International Units   ** mcg= micrograms   *** mg= milligrams   **** No RDA has been established—these are "safe and adequate ranges."

Table 4.2

MINERALS: SOURCES AND ADULT RECOMMENDED DIETARY ALLOWANCES (RDAs)

	Mineral	Sources	Adult RDAs
Major Minerals (*Needed in amounts greater than 100 mg per day*)	Calcium	Milk and milk products, dark green leafy vegetables, broccoli, tofu, canned sardines and salmon with bones, shrimp, oysters	800–1,200 mg*
	Phosphorus	Meat, fish, poultry, eggs, milk and milk products, legumes, soft drinks	800–1,200 mg
	Magnesium	Nuts, cooked dried beans and peas, whole grains, dark green leafy vegetables, seafood	280–350 mg
Electrolytes	Potassium	Citrus fruits, bananas, milk, avocados, potatoes, lean meats	2,000 mg***
	Sodium	Table salt, seafood, (abundant in most foods except fruits)	500 mg***
	Chloride	Table salt, seafood, (abundant in most foods except fruits)	750 mg***
Trace Minerals (*Needed in amounts less than 100 mg per day*)	Iron	Organ meats, lean red meats, dean poultry, dried cooked legumes, dried fruits, dark green leafy vegetables, fish, prunes, oysters, whole grain breads and cereals, green peas, strawberries, tomato juice, winter squash, broccoli	10–15 mg
	Copper	Organ meats, shellfish, oysters, whole grains, nuts, legumes	1.5–3.0 mg****
	Zinc	Lean meats, oysters, poultry, fish, organ meats, whole grain breads and cereals	10–15 mg
	Iodine	Iodized table salt, seafood, water	150 mcg**
	Selenium	Whole grains, poultry, dairy products, lean meats, (content can vary by 200-fold, depending on soil)	55–70 mcg
	Fluoride	Fluoridated water (content in food and water varies)	1.5–4.0 mg****
	Manganese	Spinach, tea, whole grains, carrots, broccoli, blueberries, cooked dried legumes	2.0–5.0 mg****
	Chromium	Whole grains, nutritional yeast, molasses, lean meats, cheeses	50–200 mcg****
	Molybdenum	Hard tap water, lean meats, whole grains (content in food and water varies)	75–250 mcg****

* mg=milligram   ** mcg=microgram   *** No RDA has been established—these are minimum requirements.   **** No RDA has been established—these are "safe and adequate ranges."

red blood cells. Minerals are also part of the body's regulation of muscle contraction, conduction of nerve impulses, clotting of blood, and heart rhythm. The terms "major" and "trace" refer to the required amounts and do not reflect the importance of a mineral in maintaining optimal health. Like vitamins, daily food intake is the best source, although certain individuals may benefit from supplements.

Macronutrients: The Energy Nutrients. Three nutrient categories supply energy (calories). The energy supplied by these nutrients fuels billions of processes that sustain life, including maintenance of body temperature, and growth and repair of all organs and tissues. Excessive intake of calories from any of the energy nutrients is converted and stored as fat. In other words, protein, carbohydrate, and fat are all "fattening" if eaten in excess. However, fat is the most concentrated form of Calories. For example, 1 tablespoon of salad dressing contains more Calories than 3 cups of lettuce/vegetable salad. Sour cream has three times more Calories than the same amount of plain yogurt.

The energy nutrients provide the following Calories:

Protein. . . . . 4 Calories / gram or
112 Calories / ounce

Carbohydrate. . . . . . 4 Calories / gram or
112 Calories / ounce

Fat. . . . . 9 Calories / gram or
252 Calories / ounce

Traditionally, fat has been estimated to supply 9 Calories/gram. Recent research shows fat might contain even more calories than previously thought or approximately 11 Calories/gram (308 Calories/ounce). This evidence is preliminary, however, and more documentation is required before changes in calorie contents of foods can be made (Donald & Hegsted, 1985).

Protein. **Proteins** are large molecules made up of long strands of approximately 23 different amino acids. Eight to ten of these amino acids are essential; that is they must be obtained from the diet since the body cannot manufacture them. Proteins are major structural components of all body tissue, are needed for growth and repair, and are also necessary components of hormones, enzymes and blood-plasma transport systems. Examples of protein-rich foods include fish, poultry, meat, milk, cheese, eggs and tofu. Combination vegetarian dishes are also good sources of protein; examples are grains with cooked dried beans/peas (such as split pea soup and cornbread) and grains with milk (such as pasta with cheese or cereal with milk).

Fats. **Dietary fats** (also called **lipids**) are actually a family of water-insoluble compounds that includes triglycerides, cholesterol and lecithin. **Triglycerides**, most synonymous with "fat," are found in all "fatty" foods, supply calories and can be used for

energy, and are the storage form of fat in the body. Although fats are the "bad guys" of the nutrition field because of their roles in cardiovascular disease and their concentration of calories (**caloric-density**), they are as essential to health as the other nutrients. Fat insulates and protects the body's organs, is involved in the absorption and transportation of the fat-soluble vitamins, and is the source of essential fatty acids.

Triglycerides are organized into two categories: saturated and unsaturated fats. **Saturated fats** (fats that are solid at room temperature) are found primarily in foods of animal origin, such as meat, dairy products and eggs, but also are components of shortening, margarine and coconut oil. **Unsaturated fats** (fats that are liquid at room temperature) can be further divided into **polyunsaturated** and **monounsaturated fats**. These fats are found primarily in foods of plant origin, such as vegetable oils, nuts, seeds, avocados olives, soybeans and wheat germ. Fish and chicken also contain some unsaturated fats.

Cholesterol is another type of fat, however, it does not supply calories and cannot be used for energy. Cholesterol is found only in foods of animal origin, such as meat and cheese, and is stored in relatively small amounts in the body as compared to triglycerides. Cholesterol also floats in the bloodstream and high levels of this type of fat are a prime risk factor for the development of cardiovascular disease.

Lecithin is a type of fat called a **phospholipid**, which means it contains a fatty portion and a water-soluble portion. It is manufactured by the body and does not supply calories.

All fat, with the exception of linoleic acid, can be manufactured in the body. The only **"essential" fat** that must be supplied by the diet is linoleic acid, a polyunsaturated fat found in vegetable oils, nuts, seeds, wheat germ and other foods that contain polyunsaturated fat.

Carbohydrates. **Carbohydrates** are organized into two categories: simple and complex. **Simple carbohydrates** include the refined sugars, such as table sugar, honey, brown sugar, corn syrup and the naturally occurring sugars in milk and fruit. Refined sugars supply little more than calories. Excessive consumption of foods high in added refined sugars may lead to dietary deficiencies if they replace more nutritious foods. Naturally occurring simple sugars in fruits and milk are found in combination with vitamins and minerals, protein or fiber and are healthful food choices.

In contrast, **complex carbohydrates** are the starches or long chains of sugars in whole grain breads and cereals, vegetables, fruits, and dried peas and beans. Complex carbohydrates, like naturally occurring sugars, are packed with essential vitamins, minerals, protein and fiber.

Carbohydrates are the most readily available source of food energy. During digestion and metabolism, all carbohydrates are broken down to the simple sugar glucose for use as the body's principal energy source. **Glucose** is the form of sugar in the blood and is the primary fuel used by the nervous system, as opposed to other tissues that use both fat and glucose. Glucose is stored in the liver and muscle tissue as **glycogen**. A carbohydrate-rich diet is necessary to maintain muscle glycogen, the preferred fuel during aerobic exercise. Therefore, a healthful diet is rich in carbohydrates, especially the complex "carbs" and naturally occurring sugars.

Alcohol

Alcohol supplies calories (7 kcal/gram) but is not a nutrient since it does not contribute to growth, maintenance or repair of body tissues. Indeed, alcohol intake may displace more nutritious foods and can be damaging to tissues if consumed in even moderate amounts or for long periods of time. Alcohol can be converted to fat when total daily calorie intake from protein, carbohydrate, fat and alcohol exceeds daily needs.

The Well-balanced Diet

The optimum diet provides adequate amounts of each of the 40-plus nutrients considered essential. The National Research Council of the National Academy of Sciences first defined the daily nutrient requirements for Americans in the 1940s as **Recommended Dietary Allowances (RDAs)**. The 10th revision of the RDAs was published in 1989. The RDA represents the daily amount of a nutrient recommended for practically all healthy persons to maintain optimal health. The recommendations include a large margin of safety. For example, although the body needs only 10 mg of vitamin C to prevent the deficiency disease scurvy, the RDA for vitamin C is 60 mg (Tables 4.1 and 4.2).

Dietary Guidelines for Americans

Since 1910, fat intake has increased, complex carbohydrate and fiber consumption has decreased, and refined sugar consumption has increased. Physical activity has also decreased 75 percent.

The American diet was evaluated in 1977 by the Senate Select Committee on Nutrition and Human Needs and it was determined to be out of balance: too high in total calories, sugar, sodium and fat (especially saturated fat), and too low in complex carbohydrates and fiber. This evaluation resulted in a set of recommendations called Dietary Guidelines for Americans (Fig. 4.1).

The major health-related associations and experts, including the American Heart

Chapter 4
Nutrition and
Weight Control

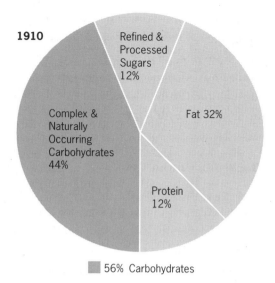

56% Carbohydrates

Figure 4.1

Dietary Guidelines for Americans. The goal is to have at least 48 percent of the calories consumed as complex carbohydrates, no more than 30 percent of calories as fat, about 12 percent in protein, and no more than 10 percent in refined and processed sugars. *Source: Nutrition Resource Manual. People Karch International, Chantilly, VA, 1988.*

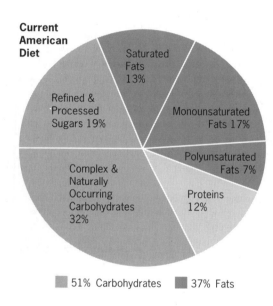

51% Carbohydrates   37% Fats

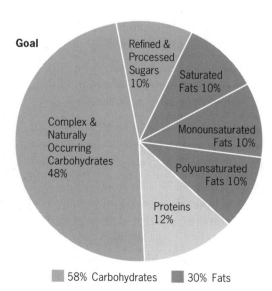

58% Carbohydrates   30% Fats

Association (Grundy et al, 1985), the American Cancer Society (1987), the American Institute for Cancer Research, the American Diabetes Association, the Senate Select Committee on Nutrition and Human Needs (USDA, 1980), the Surgeon General for the United States (1979), and the National Cholesterol Education Program (1988), recommend similar dietary guidelines for the promotion of optimal health and well-being as well as the prevention of many diseases, including cardiovascular disease, hypertension, diabetes, cancer and obesity.

Translating Fig. 4.1 into practical terms, the Dietary Guidelines recommend that Americans:

• Decrease consumption of foods high in fat: (a) oils, shortening and margarine, (b) fatty meats and dairy products, and (c) convenience or prepared foods that are high in fats and oils.

• Limit consumption of meat, choose only extra-lean cuts, and substitute with skinned poultry, fish, and plant proteins.

• Decrease consumption of cholesterol-rich foods, such as eggs and organ meats.

• Decrease consumption of refined sugars and processed foods high in sugar.

• Decrease consumption of salt, sodium-containing additives and salty foods.

• Increase consumption of fresh fruits and vegetables, whole grain breads and cereals, and cooked dried beans and peas.

• If alcoholic beverages are consumed, do so in moderation.

• Consume only enough calories from nutrient-dense foods to maintain a healthy body weight.

Even though these recommendations are simple and require, in most cases, only moderate changes in current eating habits, many people despair, thinking that there is nothing "good" left to eat. These people can be reassured that no one food is harmful and their favorite foods are not "bad";

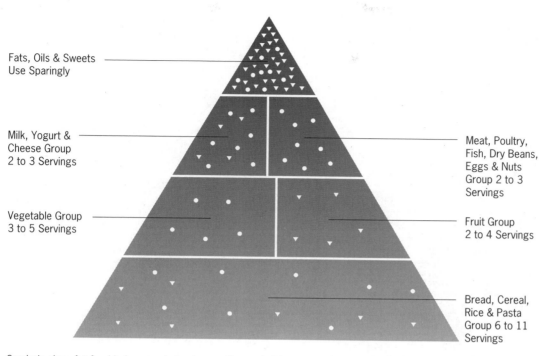

Fats, Oils & Sweets
Use Sparingly

Milk, Yogurt &
Cheese Group
2 to 3 Servings

Meat, Poultry,
Fish, Dry Beans,
Eggs & Nuts
Group 2 to 3
Servings

Vegetable Group
3 to 5 Servings

Fruit Group
2 to 4 Servings

Bread, Cereal,
Rice & Pasta
Group 6 to 11
Servings

Symbols show fat & added sugars in foods.   ▼ Sugars (added)   ● Fat (naturally occurring & added)

Figure 4.2

The Food Guide Pyramid
Source: U.S. Depart-
ment of Agriculture\U.S.
Department of Health &
Human Services.

but rather that it is the total diet that de-termines risk as well as promotes health.

The Food Guide Pyramid

The RDAs and the Dietary Guidelines for Americans provide valuable informa-tion but the average person cannot trans-late them into guidelines for food choices and meal planning. The Food Guide Pyra-mid was published in August 1992 and is fast replacing the old four food groups. It serves as a guide to daily food choices that will accomplish the dietary goals (Fig. 4.2 and Table 4.3).

The pyramid approach is a big step forward and instructors can confidently recommend this food choice guide to participants. However, the pyramid also has limitations: it probably does not pro-vide enough information for people who already know a lot about nutrition. Individ-uals still have to develop their "fat aware-ness" to make the best choices from groups that have put french fries and spinach in the same group, meats grouped together

with beans, and ice cream in the same group with skim milk.

To build "fat awareness," instructors can recommend that the Food Guide Pyra-mid be used in conjunction with a system for counting fat grams (described in the Pyramid booklet) and/or calculating the percentage of calories from fat in various foods. (See the "Resources" section for in-formation on ordering Food Guide Pyra-mid booklets, Fat Finder calculators, and Health Counts: A Fat and Calorie Guide.) Many people find that when they reduce fat and refined sugars in their diets, the other Dietary Guidelines easily fall into place. An even simpler plan is the Five-A-Day Plan, which strives to increase Amer-icans' consumption of fruits and vegetables.

NUTRITION AND EXERCISE

Well-balanced nutrition combined with exercise is a preventive and corrective approach to reducing risks for a variety of diseases. Fortunately, in the '90s, the same nutritional guidelines apply to

Table 4.3

SAMPLE DIETS FOR A DAY AT THREE CALORIE LEVELS

	Lower (about 1,600[1])	Moderate (about 2,200[2])	High (about 2,800[3])
Bread Group Servings	6	6	11
Vegetable Group Servings	3	4	5
Fruit Group Servings	2	3	4
Milk Group Servings	2-3[4]	2-3[4]	2-3[4]
Meat Group[2] (ounces)	5	6	7
Total Fat[3] (grams)	53	73	93
Total Added Sugars[4] (tsp)	6	12	18

[1] 1,600 calories is about right for many sedentary women and some older adults.
[2] 2,200 calories is about right for most children, teenage girls, active women and many sedentary men.
Women who are pregnant or breast-feeding may need somewhat more.
[3] 2,800 calories is about right for teenage boys, many active men and some very active women.
[4] Women who are pregnant or breast-feeding, teenagers and young adults to age 24 need 3 servings.

Table 4.3

How to Make the
Pyramid Work for You
*Source: U.S. Department
of Agriculture\U.S.
Department of Health
& Human Services.*

most diseases as well as the general population. Even for well-trained athletes, high-quality food choices are necessary if they are to perform to their full potential. This section describes the art of nutrition: the application of nutrition theories and facts to exploration of the complementary roles played by nutrition and exercise in reducing risk for disease and enhancing athletic performance.

Reducing Risk for Disease

The statistics are startling: one out of every two Americans will die from heart disease, cancer strikes three out of every four families, almost 12 million Americans have diabetes, and 58 million people have hypertension. More than 32 million adults are overweight, and more than 11 million are severely obese. Childhood obesity also is escalating; between the mid-60s and late '70s the incidence of obesity increased 54 percent in 6- to 11-year-olds and by 39 percent in the 12- to 17-year-olds. The rates continue to rise and it is estimated that more than 11 million American children are obese (Gortmaker et al, 1987). Changes in dietary and exercise patterns

since the turn of the century mirror the increased rates of illness and death from the "diseases of overconsumption."

Cardiovascular disease (CVD) is a general term for any disease of the heart (cardio) and blood vessels (vascular). Diseases in this category include: **atherosclerosis** and **coronary heart disease (CHD)**. Hypertension is a symptom of CVD. Heart attack or myocardial infarction, stroke, peripheral artery disease and congestive heart failure result from CVD and claim more American lives than all other causes of death combined (AHA, 1992). Coronary heart disease (CHD) accounts for more that half of the deaths from cardiovascular disease, making it the number one cause of death in the United States. CHD is almost always the result of atherosclerosis, a gradual buildup of fatty deposits, called **plaques**, in the arterial walls. As the plaques enlarge, the artery loses its elasticity and the passages become narrower, decreasing the blood flow. Atherosclerosis may involve the arteries to many areas of the body. If a blood clot develops, the flow can be stopped entirely. When the disease affects the arteries leading to the heart, a heart attack can result. When the arteries leading to the brain are affected, a stroke is the result.

Hyperlipidemia/hypercholesterolemia (elevated blood fats, especially cholesterol) and a sedentary lifestyle are key risk factors for CVD. Other factors that contribute to the risk are: cigarette smoking, hypertension, poorly controlled diabetes, excessive and prolonged stress coupled with a pessimistic or antagonistic attitude, obesity, family history, and gender (male gender after 35-years-old and female after menopause).

One of the major culprits in CVD is cholesterol, which is found in foods of animal origin and is also produced in the body. Cholesterol is an essential component of cell structures and hormones but a diet that is too high in fat, particularly saturated fat, may elevate cholesterol, which ends up as artery-clogging plaque.

As a result of recent research, doctors no longer use only a person's total cholesterol level to predict the risk of cardiovascular disease. Instead, they look at the relative proportion of two different types of cholesterol that are named according to molecules called **lipoproteins** (fat and protein), that distribute cholesterol throughout the body. **Low density lipoproteins (LDLs)** carry cholesterol (LDL-C) into the system, leaving a residue in the arterial walls, thus earning the reputation as "bad" cholesterol. **High density lipoproteins (HDLs)** remove cholesterol from the system, including the arterial walls, and transport it to the liver where it is reprocessed or eliminated. Therefore, the cholesterol carried by high density lipoproteins (HDL-C) is "good" because it removes fatty plaque deposits from arterial walls. Premenopausal women have higher HDL-C levels than men of the same age, which may account, in part, for their lower rate of CVD.

The ratio of HDL-C to total cholesterol is the single most important factor in determining risk for heart disease. Participants who have been told that they have "high cholesterol" but were not told the ratio of HDL-C to total cholesterol, should be encouraged to get that vital information from a health-care provider.

Diet and exercise are primary keys to lowering total cholesterol and raising HDL-C (Arntzenius, 1985). Research has shown that people at high risk for cardiovascular disease, including those who have already suffered heart attacks, may actually reverse the buildup of plaque in their arteries. This breakthrough research suggests that significant changes in diet, exercise and attitude will improve quality of life and life expectancy (Ornish, 1990).

What does all this mean for aerobics instructors? These findings mean that even though participants cannot change their gender or family history, they can indeed change their health status by making permanent diet and lifestyle changes. However, research shows that while change is possible, it will not be quick or without the discomfort associated with any significant change. Talking vitamin-mineral supplements will not alter the **HDL-C to total cholesterol ratio**, nor will an eating program that lasts only a few months. Instructors should emphasize gradual, healthful changes in lifestyle habits and diet (as outlined in the Food Guide Pyramid, Fig. 4.2 and Table 4.3).

Participants concerned about their cholesterol should be encouraged to focus on reducing all fats in their diets to achieve 30 percent or less of calories coming from fat. (Fig. 4.1) Table 4.4 outlines tips for achieving a low-fat diet.

What about exercise? Of course, diet is only one part of the fitness equation. Numerous studies have shown that although exercise does not decrease total choles-

Table 4.4

TIPS FOR ACHIEVING A LOW-FAT DIET

Prepare small meat portions and choose chicken, turkey and fish* more often than beef and pork. (Note: some cuts of beef and pork are now available that are as lean as poultry; ask the grocery store manager to stock these items.)

Trim all visible fat before cooking and broil, roast or stir-fry with flavored stock instead of frying.

Choose nonfat or very low-fat dairy products.

Reduce fats called for in recipes and use mono- or polyunsaturated oils (safflower, soybean, sunflower, corn, canola or olive oil) instead of butter or margarine.

Limit egg yolks to three or fewer per week.

Increase consumption of fruits, vegetables, whole grains and legumes. Not only are these foods low-fat, they also provide fiber, vitamins and minerals associated with low risk for heart disease, cancer and diabetes.

* The type of polyunsaturated fat (omega-3 fatty acids) found in cold-water fish, such as salmon, albacore tuna, mackerel, sardines and trout, may help lower serum cholesterol.

terol, it does favorably alter the HDL-C to total cholesterol ratio. Some benefits of aerobic exercise will be seen fairly quickly but other important changes will occur only over an extended time period. Williams et al (1982) compared a supervised running group and a sedentary control group at three-month intervals. They found: (1) the HDL-C to total cholesterol ratio did not begin to change until a threshold exercise level of 10 miles per week was maintained for nine months or more, and (2) fitness increased and percent body fat decreased sooner and at lower exercise levels than required for changes in the concentration of LDL-C and HDL-C. A similar study by Wood et al (1986) over a two-year period showed a significant decrease in total cholesterol at six months, but an increase in HDL-C was not seen until 12 months.

Unrealistic expectations undermine motivation. Participants should be warned against plunging into a frenzied period of exercise; their hopes to achieve rapid and miraculous health benefits will quickly be replaced by frustration and disappointment. A participant's exercise program should not be an additional stress factor! As with diet, the instructor should constantly stress the benefits of a realistic and long-term exercise commitment. Likewise, exercise "prescriptions" should include a gradual increase of activity to achieve long-term goals.

Smoking cigarettes is also a major risk factor for cardiovascular disease. Smoking lowers HDL-C and raises LDL-C, and that ratio is related to the number of cigarettes smoked per day. People who stop smoking can achieve HDL-C levels similar to non-smokers. Fortunately, an aerobic exercise program often helps smokers to cut back on the number of cigarettes they smoke or to stop smoking completely. Smokers often cite their fear of weight gain as the reason for continuing to smoke. Engaging in aerobic exercise will not only help avoid the weight gain but will provide an outlet for the stress associated with smoking cessation.

Hypertension (high blood pressure) damages the heart, kidneys and nervous system and increases the risk for heart attack, stroke, peripheral artery disease and kidney disease.

In most cases, high blood pressure is caused by the interaction between genetic predisposition and lifestyle choices, including high-salt diets, alcohol, smoking and obesity. High blood pressure is more common among African-American adults than white adults and is especially high in African-American women.

The best defense against hypertension is early detection and prevention. The second best choice is to control existing hypertension with diet, exercise, smoking cessation and medication. Body weight is a prime risk factor. In fact, achieving and maintaining a healthy body weight often eliminates the need for medications. Other nutritional factors may affect blood pressure:

Excessive salt (sodium chloride) intake is linked to increased risk for hypertension for susceptible individuals, estimated to be about 40 percent of diagnosed hypertensives. The only way to determine whether a hypertensive person is sodium sensitive is to reduce the salt intake for a period of time and monitor the results. Likewise, certain people are alcohol sensitive and can reduce their blood pressure by greatly reducing or eliminating alcohol.

Potassium, chloride, calcium, magnesium and the omega-3 fatty acids found in fish oils are also strongly linked to blood pressure regulation. The good news is that the low-fat diet described earlier (Fig. 4.2 and Table 4.3) not only provides these nutrients but is also appropriate for weight loss and control of hypertension.

Cancer is a group of diseases that have one thing in common: groups of cells multiplying out of control. Certainly diet is not the only factor playing a role in the development of cancer. (Cigarette smoking is the significant factor in lung cancer.) However, diet does seem to affect the development of a number of cancers, including cancers of the esophagus, stomach, colon, rectum, breast, lung, liver, pancreas, endometrium, ovaries, bladder and prostate. Several countries with eating patterns similar to the Dietary Guidelines (Fig. 4.1) have about one half the U.S. mortality rates for cancers associated with diet (Woteki & Thomas, 1992). Particular attention should be paid to adequate consumption of foods rich in vitamins A, C, E, folic acid, selenium and zinc (fruits, vegetables and whole grains). Cruciferous vegetables (broccoli, cauliflower, cabbage, brussels sprouts and kohlrabi) contain indoles, which are associated with reduced risk of cancers of the

stomach, colon and respiratory tract. Salt-cured, smoked and nitrite-containing foods should be avoided or consumed in limited amounts. Individuals, of course, should also reduce dietary fat.

Some studies have shown that the risk of colon cancer in men diminished as the level of physical activity increased. Statistically, sedentary women are three times as likely to develop breast cancers as active women (McArdle, 1987). Although there is no level of physical activity directly associated with reducing cancer risk, exercise is a powerful health-promoting factor, without which optimal health cannot be achieved.

Diabetes mellitus, like cancer, is a group of diseases with a common biochemical characteristic: abnormal metabolism of carbohydrates, particularly glucose. This can lead to kidney disease, atherosclerosis, heart attack, stroke, gangrene and blindness. All types of diabetes involve insulin, a hormone which helps control the levels of glucose in the blood. In about 10 percent of diabetics, the body loses its ability to produce insulin and the person must receive regular injections of insulin to survive. This is called **insulin-dependent diabetes.** The most common form of this disease is **non-insulin-dependent diabetes mellitus (NIDDM).** The major risk factors for this type of diabetes are genetics and obesity, especially fat stored in the abdomen.

Diet and exercise have long been the standard prescriptions for NIDDM. The guidelines shown in Figure 4.1 are also appropriate for the control of diabetes. Achieving and maintaining a more healthy body weight is extremely important for control of NIDDM. Instructors should welcome diabetic participants into their classes because exercise improves how the body uses insulin and aids in the regulation of blood sugar levels. However, a person with diabetes should work closely with a physician, dietitian and exercise specialist to establish a diet and exercise program.

Obesity is a risk factor for all the diseases discussed so far in this section. Because instructors are frequently asked questions about weight control, it will be discussed in more detail later in this chapter.

Well-balanced nutrition and aerobic exercise can also reduce the risk of **osteoporosis**, a condition in which bone mass decreases and susceptibility to fracture increases. Weight-bearing exercise, such as aerobic dance and walking, increases bone mass. Like muscle, bone responds to stress by becoming stronger. Studies of the elderly show that bone mineral loss is not always a function of age and that mineralization can increase with activity. Bone atrophy occurs in sedentary people and bone hypertrophy occurs with sufficient physical activity (Smith, 1982). Therefore, weight-bearing aerobic exercise plus an adequate calcium intake (more on this in the following section) is the best approach to preventing and treating osteoporosis.

This section has established the complementary roles played by nutrition and exercise in reducing risks for disease. It is important to note that the dietary guidelines discussed are appropriate for people who want to stay healthy as well as those trying to regain their health. However, doing it "because it is good for you" is not specific enough to motivate most people! Table 4.5 summarizes the benefits derived from healthful eating habits. The next section will focus on the application of nutrition theories and facts to special populations, including athletes.

NUTRITIONAL NEEDS OF SPECIAL POPULATIONS

Certain populations of people have special nutritional needs. Women, children and adolescents, older adults and

Table 4.5

BENEFITS OF HEALTHFUL EATING

Improve resistance to colds and infection.

Reduce the risk for developing cardiovascular disease, cancer, diabetes, hypertension, osteoporosis and other degenerative diseases.

Increase resistance to stress and stress-related disorders.

Help maintain a feeling of well-being.

Aid in the prevention of premature aging.

Help maintain a healthy appearance.

Maintain a healthy body weight.

Maximize energy level so one may enjoy life and perform necessary work.

Enhance athletic performance.

Aid in the maintenance of a stable emotional and social life.

frequent exercisers each face a number of discreet nutritional issues. Exercise instructors should have a general knowledge of the nutritional adjustments that people in these groups may need to make. Properly satisfying their nutritional requirements could be particularly important for those among them who exercise regularly. The following summarizes these special groups' nutritional needs.

Women

Women are at particular risk for developing osteoporosis and iron-deficiency anemia. Women also have special nutritional needs during pregnancy and lactation.

Calcium, the most abundant mineral in the body, is critical for the conduction of nerve impulses, heart function, muscle contraction and operation of certain enzymes. The bones and teeth contain 99 percent of the body's calcium; the remaining 1 percent circulates in the bloodstream. When the supply of calcium in the blood is too low, the body withdraws calcium from the bones.

An inadequate supply of calcium is one of the major factors contributing to osteoporosis, a degenerative bone disease characterized by long-term loss of calcium from the bones.

Bones gradually become porous, brittle and break easily. Women are at particular risk for developing osteoporosis because of their lifestyle and dietary habits as well as their small body size relative to men. Women are more likely than men to follow calorie-restricted diets that contain inadequate amounts of nutrients, especially calcium and vitamin D. Frequent consumption of diet soft drinks that contain phosphoric acid and avoidance of dairy products that contain calcium and vitamin D upsets the ratio of calcium to phosphorus and contributes to bone loss.

Osteoporosis is a serious health problem primarily among postmenopausal women, but also among younger female athletes who have stopped having regular menstrual periods. Both groups of women lack adequate estrogen, a hormone that helps to maintain bone density. Osteoporosis affects an estimated 15 to 30 million people and 25 to 35 percent of women past menopause. It is called the "silent disease" because it usually is not detected until a fracture occurs, often in the hip, wrist or spine.

Women can reduce the risk of developing osteoporosis with a lifelong, calcium-rich diet and regular exercise program, especially weight-bearing activities. Unfortunately, the typical 25- to 40-year-old woman consumes only 600 milligrams (mg) of calcium daily, less than the current RDA of 800 mg. The National Institutes of Health (NIH) suggests that the calcium needs of women are well above the 800 mg level. These experts recommend that adolescent women consume 1,200 mg of calcium per day; premenopausal women

Table 4.6

TIPS TO BOOST CALCIUM INTAKE

Add nonfat milk powder to casseroles, soups, meat loaf, cheese sauces, or milkshakes.

Add nonfat milk powder to recipes for French toast, muffins, dips, puddings, pie fillings, homemade breads, mashed potatoes, creamy salad dressings or creamed soups.

Cook rice, hot cereals, or other grains in nonfat or low-fat milk.

Use nonfat or low-fat yogurt as a partial substitute for sour cream in recipes and in place of sour cream in dips and on baked potatoes.

Increase the daily consumption of calcium-rich foods of plant origin (broccoli, dark green leafy vegetables and soy products, such as tofu).

Refer to Table 4.2 for a list of foods highest in calcium.

Source: The Essential Guide to Vitamins and Minerals by E. Somer. See "Suggested Reading" section.

consume 1,000 mg; and postmenopausal not on estrogen consume 1,500 mg. Premenopausal women who are amenorrheic should increase protein, calories and calcium to restore their menstrual periods and protect their bones.

Dairy products are the best sources of calcium, but other foods are also good sources. Table 4.6 provides guidelines on how to increase calcium in the diet. Fortunately, more women are becoming aware of their calcium needs. Aerobics instructors may be asked for advice on food sources and calcium supplements. In most cases, calcium supplements are a poor alternative to calcium-rich foods because the calcium from pills is absorbed less effectively than from food. Also, the calcium-rich foods supply other nutrients. Typically a person who does not eat dairy products is not getting enough calcium and also has a poor riboflavin intake. Before taking a supplement, a woman should consult a registered dietitian who will evaluate her whole diet and recommend the proper supplement, if necessary.

Table 4.7

TIPS TO BOOST IRON INTAKE

Eat foods rich in vitamin C with each meal. Vitamin C enhances iron absorption from the intestine. A glass of orange juice with breakfast can increase iron absorption nearly 300 percent.

Do not drink tea and coffee with meals. Substances in these beverages interfere with iron absorption.

Use cast iron cookware often. The more acidic the food and the longer it is cooked in a cast iron container, the higher the iron content. For example, the iron content of 1/2 cup of spaghetti sauce increases from 3 mg to 88 mg when simmered in a cast iron pot for 3 hours.

Animal protein provides the best and most readily absorbed source of iron. Examples are the dark meat of chicken and turkey, and lean beef, pork and lamb.

Combine poorly absorbed vegetarian sources of iron (10 percent absorption rate) with animal sources (40 percent absorption rate). Examples are a meat-and-bean burrito, broccoli with beef, spinach with chicken and lentil soup with turkey.

Increase consumption of iron-rich fruits and vegetables, such as dark leafy green vegetables, legumes, strawberries, watermelon, raisins, dried apricots and prunes.

Refer to Table 4.2 for a list of foods highest in iron.

Iron deserves special attention because **iron-deficiency anemia** is the nation's most common nutritional deficiency, affecting approximately 40 percent of women between the ages of 20 and 50 (Aftergood, Alfin-Slater, 1982).

Iron is needed to form hemoglobin, an iron-containing protein that carries oxygen in the blood and releases it to the tissues. When the total hemoglobin concentration drops, the muscles do not receive as much oxygen. A hemoglobin level below 12 mg/dl for women and below 14 mg/dl for men is considered anemic. An anemic person has less endurance and cannot exercise as strenuously because the maximum oxygen uptake, or aerobic capacity, is reduced due to the decreased oxygen-carrying capacity of the blood caused by low hemoglobin levels. Iron also strengthens the immune system and increases resistance to colds,

infections and disease. Iron deficiency in women is usually the result of inadequate dietary intake and menstrual blood loss. There is also evidence that strenuous training accelerates the destruction of red blood cells, increases iron loss in sweat and decreases iron absorption. The RDA for iron is 15 mg for premenopausal women and 10 mg for men and postmenopausal women, but the average woman consumes only 10 mg per day. Table 4.7 outlines ways to increase iron intake and correct this deficiency.

Because obtaining 15 mg of iron each day is a challenging task, and because many women are concerned about anemia, the supplement question again arises. Self-supplementation with iron is particularly dangerous. That "tired, listless feeling" can be caused by numerous conditions, and an iron deficiency can only be determined by measuring **serum ferritin** (storage iron) and checking the hemoglobin level. Iron supplementation will not improve the health or performance of an individual with normal iron stores. On the other hand, excessive intake can produce an iron overload and cause deficiencies of the trace minerals copper and zinc. In addition, excessive iron intake is now being considered a risk factor for heart disease (Monsen, 1992). The best advice to give a participant who believes that her iron intake is inadequate is to see her physician for a check-up and request a referral to a dietitian who can provide personalized dietary instructions.

Women have special nutritional needs during pregnancy and lactation. Providing nutrients for herself and the growing child requires increased calories and, in many cases, additional nutrient supplements. A woman should be in contact with her doctor as soon as she suspects pregnancy. There usually is no problem with continuing to exercise, but a pregnant participant should be encouraged to get specific guidance from her physician regarding exercise intensity and frequency, especially if she was unaccustomed to aerobic exercise prior to pregnancy.

Concerns about weight gain, losing muscle tone, and the ability to resume physical activities after the baby arrives are often greater among very physically fit women. Current recommendations suggest that gaining 30 to 35 pounds is associated with the fewest complications for both mother and baby. This is an awesome thought for a woman who has struggled to maintain her weight. Instructors can reassure her that the same guidelines for healthy eating still apply…just add more servings of nutrient-dense foods. Several nutrient requirements increase during pregnancy, including protein, calcium, folic acid and iron. (Refer to the section on vitamin-mineral supplements.) Adequate fluid intake is always important, but even more so when exercising during pregnancy, to avoid dehydration and hyperthermia. In addition, extra fluid is needed during lactation to replace what is used in milk and lost in perspiration.

Many women find that their motivation to eat well and maintain physical activity is even higher during pregnancy. Instructors can also encourage women to resume their exercise classes as soon they get their doctor's approval. Perhaps a savvy instructor can arrange for postpartum "Mom and Me" classes that allow new mothers to bring their infants to exercise with them. Breast-feeding is certainly the best nutritional choice for the baby and may also help the mother return to pre-pregnancy weight. However, some mothers find that they do not lose the last 5 to 10 pounds until they cease lactation. Instructors can help the lactating participant to keep her

perspective (there is life after breast-feeding) and keep exercising, the most powerful antidote for postpartum blues.

Older Adults

Senior citizens are one of the most nutritionally vulnerable groups. Due to sedentary lifestyles, their caloric intake is often very low and yet their requirements for essential nutrients are the same or higher than in their younger years. Many older adults consistently consume less than the RDA for essential nutrients while their nutrient requirements may be increased due to chronic medications or illness.

Participation in aerobics classes may positively affect the nutritional status of seniors by increasing their caloric requirements and, therefore, increasing the intake of other essential nutrients that come along with wholesome foods. Due to high incidence of osteoporosis among older adults, they should be encouraged to engage in weight-bearing activities and consume adequate calcium. (Refer to the previous section on osteoporosis.)

Children and Adolescents

Children and adolescents are another of the most nutritionally vulnerable groups. They are constantly growing rapidly, from birth until the end of adolescence. In addition to the nutrients needed to maintain their present selves, they also need nutrients to build new tissues. Ninety percent of bone development occurs by age 18. Recent studies suggest that children may need more than the current RDA for calcium (800 mg for 1 to 10 years and 1,200 mg for 11 to 18 years). In relation to body size, a child's requirements for nutrients are greater than an adult's. This means that the calories consumed by children and adolescents should be densely packed with nutrients. But this group also loves to eat high-fat and sugary foods which are calorie-dense but nutrient-poor.

Activity has a lot to do with appetite, body weight and the nutritional status of children and adolescents. The amount of time spent watching television is directly related to the level of obesity among young people. Parents cannot force their children to eat all healthy foods, but they can decide to not bring certain foods into the house. They also can display a commitment to healthy food choices and regular physical activity. The whole family can follow the Food Guide Pyramid (Fig. 4.2 and Table 4.3), and follow the guidelines for increasing calcium in Table 4.6.

Nutrition and Athletic Performance

Nutritional status is an important complement to physical training for both the beginning exerciser and the accomplished athlete. Most publications aimed at recreational and competitive athletes are full of advertising that suggests special formulas and pills are essential for top athletic performance. There is no evidence, however, that the nutritional needs of the active person are different from those of the sedentary population. In fact, physically active people have the potential for better nutritional status since they burn more calories and, therefore, may be able to consume larger quantities and a wider variety of foods. Aerobics instructors are often in this category. This section will address four areas of nutritional impact on athletic performance: maintenance of glycogen stores, eating before exercising, hydration, and injury prevention/recovery.

Maintenance of glycogen stores. Carbohydrates are the source of glycogen, the most efficient fuel for aerobic exercise. The high-carbohydrate, low-fat food plan discussed earlier is the best regimen for both overall health and aerobic exercise. Gone

are the days when "carbohydrate loading" was a requirement for endurance athletes. Most competitive athletes now follow a high complex-carbohydrate diet on a daily basis.

When muscle glycogen stores are reduced to low levels, an aerobic-exercise participant will become exhausted and will either have to stop exercising or reduce exercise intensity. Muscle glycogen decreases progressively during high-intensity exercise exceeding 90 minutes, such as running a marathon. However, glycogen stores can also be depleted gradually over several days of heavy exercise, such as teaching a grueling schedule of aerobics classes. As the glycogen stores decrease, aerobic exercise becomes more difficult and less enjoyable. Instructors with a heavy teaching load may experience this phenomenon. Instructors should be alert to this problem in beginning exercisers who attempt too ambitious a program or advanced participants who may take three to five classes per week and also engage in other physical activities, such as jogging, cycling or racquetball. Over several days, the participant becomes increasingly tired and unable to maintain even a normal exercise program. Exercise should be enjoyable, not stressful.

This chronic state of fatigue and staleness can be prevented by taking periodic rest days and consuming a diet rich in carbohydrates. Complex carbohydrates promote glycogen storage better than refined carbohydrates. Refined sugars can give fast energy because they enter the bloodstream quickly, but that energy does not last. Complex carbohydrates are absorbed more slowly, providing energy over a longer time and also supplying fiber and essential nutrients with their calories. Bread, cereal, pasta, potatoes, rice, vegetables and fruit are good sources of complex carbohydrates. The high-protein, high-fat diet typical of many Americans will not replace the glycogen lost during heavy exercise.

Eating before exercising. There are several good reasons for not eating just before exercising. During exercise, the body relies on existing stores of muscle glycogen and body fat. A meal just before exercise will not increase muscle glycogen stores, and when blood is diverted to the working muscles, food remaining in the stomach can cause nausea. In addition, a large meal will distend the stomach and may restrict breathing.

Although a pre-exercise meal will not contribute energy for the workout, it may help ward off feelings of weakness and fatigue. The best solution is to eat a light, high-carbohydrate meal/snack several hours before prolonged exercise so the stomach and upper bowel are empty before exercise begins. The meal/snack should be low in protein which takes approximately 24 hours to move through the digestive system as compared to approximately 3 hours for carbohydrates. Fat also slows food transit time. A breakfast meal that meets these guidelines might contain cooked or dry cereal (low in sugar) with nonfat or 1-percent milk and fresh fruit. Individuals can be encouraged to experiment with different foods to determine which provides the best and longest-lasting energy.

Hydration. Water is the most commonly overlooked endurance aid. Proper **hydration** is essential for any good athletic performance because fluids have important roles: (1) fluid in blood transports glucose to working muscles and carries away metabolic by-products, (2) fluid in urine eliminates metabolic waste products, (3) and fluid in sweat dissipates heat through the skin. During exercise in a warm environment, the body relies primarily on the evaporation of sweat to dissipate heat. This loss of body fluids gradually compro-

mises the body's ability to circulate blood and regulate body temperature, because the blood transferring oxygen to muscle tissue must be diverted to the skin to transfer heat from the body's core to the environment. This competition for blood between the muscles and the skin places a greater demand on the cardiovascular system. As a person becomes dehydrated, the heart rate increases, the blood flow to the skin decreases, and the body temperature rises. Performance begins to decline and exercise becomes labored. If the body temperature continues to rise, the participant may suffer heat exhaustion or heat stroke. (Refer to Chapter 14, for a discussion of heat illnesses.)

An adequate intake of fluids is obviously the best way to prevent dehydration. Normally, a person's water intake is governed by the thirst mechanism. However, thirst is not an accurate indicator of the body's need for water when exercising, especially in a hot environment. High humidity causes even more rapid fluid loss. A person who is exercising vigorously may become dehydrated before feeling thirsty. Therefore, fluids should be consumed regularly and before thirst occurs.

Instructors should inform their classes of the importance of fluid intake, especially during hot and humid weather, and should model stopping periodically to drink water. A person planning to exercise in hot weather should drink 2 to 3 cups of water about 2 to 3 hours before exercise, and another 1 to 2 cups about 15 minutes before exercise (some experts suggest 1 1/2 hours before). This technique, known as **hyperhydration**, helps to lower the body's core temperature and to reduce the added stress placed on the cardiovascular system. During exercise, the participant should drink 4 to 8 ounces of fluid every 10 to 20 minutes to replace sweat losses and to maintain blood volume.

Cold water is the best fluid for exercisers. Cold drinks empty more rapidly from the stomach than warm drinks and also help to lower the body's core temperature. (The exception is skiing, hiking or ice skating in cold weather when a warm beverage is preferable.) Drinks containing too much sugar are absorbed into the system more slowly and, therefore, function less effectively as a fluid replacement. Commercial sport drinks with a high sugar content (glucose, fructose or sucrose) may actually harm athletic performance. Fifteen minutes after drinking 1 cup of water, 60 to 70 percent of the water has been absorbed into the system. However, if the 1 cup of fluid contains 10 percent sugar (the sugar content of a soft drink), 95 percent of the fluid will still be in the stomach 15 minutes later. Commercial sport drinks containing more than 2.5 percent sugar should be diluted to 2.5 percent before being consumed–or rejected in favor of plain cold water. Advice regarding sports drinks is different for high-intensity athletes (those exercising at 70 percent or more of capacity for 90 minutes or more, [such as distance runners]). Recent research has shown that these endurance athletes may experience less fatigue when drinking fluids with carbohydrates rather than plain water. The electrolytes and sugar supplied by these beverages are not needed by the average aerobics participant or instructor. Water is a much more effective and less expensive fluid for aerobic exercisers.

Injury Prevention and Recovery

Periodic rest days are important not only to avoid the fatigue associated with glycogen depletion but also to avoid injury. If an injury that prevents exercise does occur, the most important nutritional advice is to adjust caloric intake to avoid weight gain during the recovery period. Certain intensities of aerobic exercise have an appetite-reducing effect and a suddenly-sedentary participant may experience tremendous appetite surges. The loss of that sense of control provided by an exercise program can also leave participants feeling adrift. Instructors can provide reassurance that this is normal and can encourage them to try other types of exercise, until the injury is healed.

NUTRITIONAL MISINFORMATION, MISCONCEPTIONS AND CLARIFICATIONS

There are many myths and misconceptions about how to enhance nutritional status and exercise performance. Instructors are likely to hear the following questions and can draw on this section for appropriate answers.

Q. Does a physically active person need vitamin and mineral supplements to maintain a high energy level?

A. No. Vitamin-mineral supplements do not supply energy and exercising does not "burn" vitamins. Physically active people do not necessarily need more vitamin and mineral supplements than sedentary people. There is no evidence that vitamin-mineral supplements improve athletic performance of people who already follow nutritionally adequate food plans.

Q. Are supplements good "health insurance?"

A. Not if taking supplements is an attempt to compensate for poor dietary habits. Other misguided reasons for taking supplements include inadequate sleep, crash diets, overtraining, chronic stress, frequent "fast food" meals, and fasting. There is no pill or tablet that can restore an out-of-balance lifestyle. The best approach to health and enjoyable physical activity is a well-balanced diet. On the other hand, there is no harm in taking a single multivitamin-mineral supplement that supplies no more than 100 percent of RDAs. There are, however, reasonable situations where supplements may be necessary for optimal health.

Q. Who should take vitamin-mineral supplements?

A. There are some individuals at risk for nutritional deficiencies. Supplements may be appropriate for people in the following categories:

• Restricted calories. It is difficult to get all the essential nutrients on a diet providing less than 1,600 to 1,800 Calories per day, even with careful menu-planning that includes only nutrient-dense foods. People in this category include senior citizens, and "energy efficient" individuals: formerly-obese people, chronic dieters and certain high-intensity or endurance athletes who consume far fewer calories than one would predict based on their activity levels.

• Allergic to or intolerant of certain foods. People who cannot eat certain types of foods, such as wheat, fruits and milk products, may miss out on some important nutrients. Note: the calcium provided in a multivitamin-mineral tablet may not be adequate for an individual who is lactose intolerant (unable to digest milk sugar, most common among blacks, Hispanics and Asians) and entirely avoids milk products.

• Pregnant or lactating. Specific prenatal formulations are prescribed by the physician during the first trimester. However, nutritional status prior to pregnancy, e.g., folic acid intake, also affects the health of mother and fetus and should be considered by women intending to become pregnant.

• Total vegetarian or avoids entire food group. People who completely eliminate animal products or "just hate vegetables" may benefit from a supplement.

• Chronic medications or illness. Drug-nutrient interactions should be discussed with the physician.

• Heavy smokers or drinkers. These individuals are not likely to show up in exercise classes, but if they do, they may be deficient in vitamin C, thiamine, niacin, B-6 and folacin.

Participants who fall into any of these descriptions should be referred to their physician or a registered dietitian who can assess specific needs and risks.

"Megadosing" with supplements is like overdosing on any pharmacological product: at the very least it strains the liver and kidneys and, in the extreme, may cause long-term damage. A megadose is generally considered five times the RDA of fat-soluble vitamins (A, D, E, K) or 10 times the RDA of water-soluble vitamins.

Q. What are the "power foods?"

A. The most often overlooked "power food" is not a food at all. It's water! Dehydration reduces energy and is usually unnecessary because water is readily available. The other "power foods" for exercisers are very low-fat complex carbohydrates, such as pretzels, rice cakes, bagels, cooked dried beans, pasta and fruits.

Q. Will caffeine enhance endurance?

A. Caffeine is a stimulant to the central nervous system. It is found in coffee, chocolate, colas and some aspirin medications. A study by Costill in 1978 suggested that 2 cups of coffee (330 mg caffeine) 1 hour prior to an exhaustive running event enhanced the runner's endurance. Subsequent studies, however, have failed to substantiate this claim and have suggested that a carbohydrate-rich diet is a better **"ergogenic"** (energy- enhancing) aid for endurance athletes (Weir et al, 1987). Caffeine is a drug banned by the U.S. Olympic Committee. Side effects include nausea, muscle tremors and headache. Caffeine is also a diuretic and will contribute to fluid loss.

Q. Will eating sugar before exercising provide an extra energy boost?

A. No, and in fact, it will probably impair performance. Sugar enters the blood quickly, producing a rapid increase in blood sugar and stimulating insulin production. The insulin inhibits the metabolism of fatty acids by the muscles, forcing the muscles to rely more heavily on glycogen stores. As the insulin also lowers the blood sugar levels, the exerciser may experience weakness and fatigue. Again, complex carbohydrates consumed several hours before exercising are the best source of energy.

Q. Will bee pollen give me more energy?

A. No. Some athletes may experience a placebo effect when taking bee pollen, ginseng, spirulina or desiccated liver pills but there is no evidence to support the claims that these substances enhance performance. The mind is a very powerful influence on any athletic performance and the belief in the power of these substances can seem to make a real difference in performance. However, instructors can support an equally powerful belief in the value of a low-fat, high complex-carbohydrate food plan!

Q. Should exercisers take salt tablets to replace the salt lost in sweat?

A. The American diet provides more than enough sodium for physically active people. Salt tablets are potentially dangerous because the excess sodium draws water out of the body's cells, dehydrating them and impairing their functions. Concentrated doses of salt can also irritate the stomach lining and cause nausea. The best way to replace sweat is with plain water and the salt provided through foods.

Q. Will protein supplements help meet the demands of a heavy exercise schedule?

A. Protein requirements increase only slightly with activity, even bodybuilding. The amount of protein typically consumed by active people more than meets the protein requirement. There is no evidence that protein powders improve strength or endurance.

Most Americans already eat two to three times more protein than they need. The RDA for protein is calculated according to the ideal body weight and, as with all RDAs, provides a generous allowance to meet the needs of nearly all healthy people. The daily protein requirement for a 138-pound woman is 50 grams. This reference woman can get more than the 50 grams by eating three high-protein foods, such as 2 cups of skim milk (17 grams), 3 ounces of tuna (24 grams) and 3/4 cup of cooked lentils (12 grams). The requirement for a 174-pound man, which is 63 grams, can be met by adding 1/2 cup of cottage cheese (15 grams). Vegetarians can easily satisfy their protein requirements using nonanimal foods: 1 cup cooked spaghetti contains 6.5 grams, one banana contains 1.3 grams, and 1/2 cup cooked kidney beans contains 7.2 grams protein.

Protein supplements are not only unnecessary, they may be harmful. Any excess calories, including those from protein, are stored as fat. Too much protein, whether from foods or powder supplements, produces extra nitrogen. This puts unnecessary strain on the kidneys and liver to eliminate the excess nitrogen, increases risk for dehydration and may cause calcium loss. Exercise, not protein, is the key to developing bigger muscles.

Q. Can vegetarians get enough protein to be healthy?

A. Yes. However, there is confusion about protein quality because of the terms "complete" and "incomplete." Animal sources of protein (meats and dairy products) have been called "complete" proteins because they contain the right proportions of all the essential amino acids (protein building blocks) required by the human body. Plant sources (dried peas and beans, grains, seeds, nuts, fruits and vegetables) are referred to as "incomplete" protein because the essential amino acid contents of these foods are not in ideal proportions for use by the human body. However, as long as a variety of plant proteins are being consumed on a regular basis, the body will have an adequate supply of all the essential amino acids from its amino acid pool. The best method for ensuring availability of all the essential amino acids is to consume plant proteins in combinations, such as beans with grains or seeds. Some vegetarians consume milk products, which adds these combination possibilities: cereal with milk, pasta with cheese, and grains with cheese. As discussed in the previous question, getting adequate protein is fairly easy to do. Vegetarians are more at risk for low iron and zinc than for protein deficiency.

Rarely, an instructor may encounter a participant who has shunned all meats and trades most protein calories for carbohydrates. This person is at risk for deficiency of protein, zinc, calcium, iron and several other nutrients and should be referred to a dietitian for diet instruction.

Q. Is beer a good aid for proper hydration during aerobic exercise?

A. Alcohol is the most commonly abused drug in our country and a major contributor to accidents and disease. Drinking alcohol before aerobic exercise may harm performance because alcohol is a central nervous system depressant that impairs balance and coordination. Alcohol redirects blood flow away from the heart and toward the periphery which means a person with heart disease may be at risk during exercise. Alcohol also decreases the liver's output of glucose, leading to low blood sugar **(hypoglycemia)** several hours after exercise.

Both the American College of Sports Medicine (1982) and the American Dietetic Association (1980) have concluded that alcohol does not contribute to performance, and, in most cases, appears to be detrimental, if not risky. An instructor who suspects that a participant has been drinking should advise the person of the potentially harmful effects and advise that the person not drink before coming to class.

"But I've heard that beer is a good sports drink because it's full of carbohydrates, potassium and B vitamins."

Wrong! The alcohol in beer is dehydrating so it causes fluid loss rather than replacement. Most of the calories in beer and wine come from the alcohol, not carbohydrates, and the calories from alcohol can not be used to replace glycogen. Finally, beer is a poor source of B vitamins. It would take 11 cans of beer to get the RDA for riboflavin. Choose water for a sports drink.

Q. Are artificial sweeteners a valuable part of a healthy diet because they help one avoid sugar?

A. The jury is still out on establishing the actual value of sugar and fat substitutes. It seems that many people consume these products to justify consuming additional calories from other foods. Some people experience increased appetite after consuming sugar substitutes. It has been established that certain individuals are sensitive to the most widely used non-nutritive sweetener, aspartame (NutraSweet®), and should avoid it if headaches result.

Q. Can physically active people eat whatever they want because exercise "burns up" cholesterol and fat?

A. Cholesterol is not used as a fuel source and diets high in fat do not provide the best fuel sources for physically active people. In addition, high levels of fat circulating in the blood create a risk for disease. This question is a perfect lead-in to the next section on weight control; an exercise program motivated primarily as an excuse to "eat whatever I want" is doomed to fail.

WEIGHT CONTROL

Many participants come to aerobics classes for the purpose of controlling or reducing their weight. An uninformed instructor can perpetuate an already negative and repetitive cycle of weight loss followed by weight gain. On the other hand, a knowledgeable instructor can guide participants toward realistic goals and selection of safe, long-term approaches to maintaining healthy body weight and body composition.

Several terms will be used in the discussion of nutrition and weight control. **Overweight** means that a person weighs more than the average for his or her weight, height and frame size, as determined by standard scales. The scale, however, cannot differentiate between fat pounds, bone pounds and muscle pounds. An extremely fit person with a high muscular density and/or bone density may be classified as overweight while a sedentary person of normal weight can be at risk for health problems because a high percentage of that weight is fat. It is estimated that 40 percent of Americans are overfat.

Obesity is a condition characterized by excessive, generalized storage of fat. In 1985, the NIH Consensus Panel told the nation that obesity is not just a matter of appearance; it is a disease that increases risk for heart disease, cancer and diabetes. It is the nation's most serious nutritional problem since approximately 25 percent of Americans are obese.

Underweight is a condition in which lack of body fat and/or lean muscle tissue puts the individual at health risk or at a disadvantage for certain competitive sports.

Body composition is the percentage of total body weight that is fat mass compared with the percentage that is lean body mass (muscles, bones, skin, organs and water). Refer to Chapter 6 for discussion on methods for determining body composition. For men, 3 to 6 percent is essential, 15 percent body fat is considered healthy, and over 23 percent is obese. For women, 8 to 12 percent is considered essential, 25 percent is healthy, and over 30 percent is obese.

Regional fat distribution refers to the locations of fat storage (hips, thighs, abdomen). This may be as important a variable as the degree of overweight (ACSM, 1992). Since the fat stored in the abdominal area is the most risky, ratios of waist to hip measurements can be correlated to health risk.

Energy balance is characterized by body weight remaining in a stable range and is achieved when the caloric intake is closely matched to caloric output.

Energy imbalances result in underweight, overweight and obese. They are caused by overeating or undereating, overexercising or underexercising, and/or medical conditions.

Caloric deficit is required to lose weight. A deficit of 3,500 kcal is required to lose 1 pound of stored fat. Therefore, a woman who consumes an average of 2,500 kcal per day and reduces her daily consumption by 500 kcal/day would lose 1 pound per week. That woman could also reduce her caloric intake by 250 kcal/day and increase her physical activity by 250 kcal/day to lose 1 pound per week.

Yo-yo dieting is characterized by periodic weight reduction followed by often rapid weight gain. Since both fat and muscle tissue are lost during dieting but mostly fat is added back during rapid regain, the yo-yo dieter becomes progressively fatter (percentage of body fat) and finds it even more difficult to avoid further weight gain. It also appears that people who lose weight repeatedly start overproducing an enzyme called **lipoprotein lipase**, that stimulates fat storage.

Achieving Healthy Energy Balance

Instructors frequently hear from participants, "I'm here because I want to lose weight." Sadly, that is what they have often repeatedly done: lost weight—and regained it. Many people are still caught in wishful thinking; wanting to weigh less but to also continue eating and exercising (or not exercising) just as they are. Until they understand that what they really need is to achieve energy balance at a lower body weight, they will continue to engage in yo-yo dieting. An imbalance between expenditure and intake will cause a change in body weight. Chronic dieters have become quite skilled at creating short-term imbalances which result in weight loss. Successful weight maintainers are also skilled at re-establishing energy balance at a lower weight.

What is the best method for weight loss? The best way to accomplish weight loss is by reducing calories consumed and concurrently increasing calories burned by physical activity. The benefits to combining exercise with moderate caloric reduction to achieve weight loss are listed below.

Lean body tissue is maintained. Research has shown that caloric reduction alone results in loss of lean body tissue as well as fat. Extreme caloric restrictions with no concurrent exercise may result in up to 25 to 45 percent of the weight loss coming from lean body mass. Even a moderate deficit that produces a loss of 1 or 2 pounds per week may include some loss of lean body weight. However, since muscle mass is "metabolically active" (it burns calories even at rest), the goal should be to maintain as much lean mass as possible.

Nutritional status is improved. Dieters who pair a physical activity plan with moderate caloric restriction can lose weight while eating more calories than by dieting alone. More calories equals more nutrients.

Muscle tone is improved. Not only is muscle preserved, the improved muscle tone contributes to a healthier, more fit appearance and ability to enjoy physical activities.

Metabolic rate is increased. Exercise builds muscle mass which increases the metabolic rate even during inactivity and, of course, the activity itself uses calories (energy). Proportionally, more fat is burned relative to carbohydrates as the duration of exercise increases; activities of moderate intensity and long duration are usually more effective for "burning" calories.

More positive attitude and better long-term motivation. Physical activity is mood-lifting and provides opportunities for dieters to see and appreciate the positive benefits of their efforts in action.

Physical activity is essential to weight maintenance. Any successful long-term maintainer will talk you about the importance of exercise. After all, lack of exercise is a key factor in the obesity epidemic: Americans have reduced physical activity 75 percent since 1900! All body systems work best when regular physical activity is part of the lifestyle.

Incorporates lifestyle changes into the weight-loss process. Americans have seriously experimented with dieting for almost 40 years and the results are clear: short-term caloric reduction without significant lifestyle changes, such as regular physical activity, is doomed to fail.

Models positive behavior for children. As discussed earlier, American children are becoming fatter. The most powerful message adults can give their children is to develop a commitment to healthy food choices and regular physical activity.

Ideal Body Weight Versus Realistic Body

Weight. Asking, "What should a person weigh?" is not as important as "What is a realistic weight goal, based on health status and self-esteem?" The terms "ideal" and "desirable" are not even used by the Metropolitan Life Insurance Company anymore. The 1983 tables are simply called Height and Weight Tables. The validity of these tables has been challenged but people want guidelines for healthy weights. These are the standard methods to determine how a person's weight compares to standards for health and mortality, height-weight tables, scale and body composition.

In the absence of an individually determined weight goal, people are likely to still latch on to those "ideal" weights posted on charts in doctor's offices and by scales in fitness centers. Fortunate is the individual who finds a health professional to guide him or her through a process to determine a realistic body weight goal! Refer to Fig. 4.3 which includes key factors to be included in such a discussion. Notice that periodic re-evaluation of body weight goals is included. Waist to hip ratio might be one of the additional considerations under "Personal Health Concerns." Instructors should refer participants with questions about "ideal body weight" to health professionals who will help them select realistic goals and will not prescribe weights from a chart.

Safe and Effective Weight Loss Methods. The American College of Sports Medicine (ACSM) has provided sound guidelines for healthful weight loss:

• A Caloric intake not lower than 1,200 for normal adults (unsupervised) combined with an endurance exercise program of 20 to 30 minutes at least three days per week.

• The Caloric deficit may range from 500 to 1,000 kcal per day, resulting in a rate of sustained weight loss not to exceed 2 pounds per week. Instructors may recommend use of the Dietary Guidelines and Food Guide Pyramid.

Additional factors which influence successful weight loss and maintenance:

• Role of water and other fluids. Water positively affects weight loss by aiding the efficient utilization of fat as fuel. People who easily put on "water weight" often mistakenly restrict water which actually contributes to fluid retention. Water helps minimize the frustrating weight gain caused by fluid retention by stimulating excretion of excess sodium and fluids.

• Role of physical activity (Table 4.8). The instructors can play a key role by providing motivation and reinforcement for exercise and suggesting alternative activities if a participant is "burning out" and needs more variety.

• Group support versus doing it alone. Many people find it motivational to join a group dedicated to similar goals. Aerobics classes may actually serve as this support group since exercise is often the most challenging piece of lifestyle to change. Consulting dietitians frequently assist support groups to deal with nutrition-related questions.

• Lifestyle appraisal and gradual habit change. Before making changes, it is wise to assess one's current set of habits which impact weight and fitness. The key to lifestyle change is making choices one can live with: choosing to keep "useful" behaviors and gradually replacing "not-so-useful" behaviors with reasonable alternatives. Heavy-handed imperatives to change are rarely effective long-term.

• Medical clearance and ongoing support from health professionals, including a dietitian and exercise specialist.

Exercise for Weight Maintenance

The elusive goal of achieving long-term weight maintenance hinges on re-establishing energy balance: learning how much

Figure 4.3

SAMPLE FORM: SETTING INITAL WEIGHT-LOSS GOALS

The Lighter Living Program® will help you achieve a healthy weight you realistically can maintain. One of the most common reasons for discouragement and difficulty with weight maintenance is having unrealistic expectations of what you "should" weigh. There are variety of factors that influence your rate of weight loss. These factors also might influence your most appropriate maintenance weight range.

You will not set your final goal weight today, only an initial weight-loss goal. Approaching and achieving this initial goal will be your signal to review your progress, celebrate your success and set new goals.

Today you will consider some of the factors that will influence your personal weight-loss patterns and your personal weight-management range. You periodically will re-examine these factors as you lose weight and refine your maintenance weight-range goal.

Factors That Influence Weight-loss and Maintenance Goals

1. Dieting History: How often have you lost and regained more than 10 pounds? _____ times

How long have you been overweight 10 pounds or more? _____ years

2. Current Age _____

3. Motivation to modify lifestyle habits (circle one number)

1	2	3	4	5	6	7	8	9	10
LOW									HIGH

4a. Motivation to be physically active (circle one number)

4b. Ability to be physically active ("X" out one number)

1	2	3	4	5	6	7	8	9	10
LOW									HIGH

5. Level of social support from friends, family and co-workers

1	2	3	4	5	6	7	8	9	10
LOW									HIGH

6. Personal health concerns based on you and/or your family's medical history: _____

_____

(Note: Even a relatively small reduction in body weight has positive health benefits. It is not necessary to achieve "ideal body weight" to experience improvements in your health!)

7. Other (Perhaps factors discovered by completing the Participant Questionnaire): _____

_____

Initial Goal Weight: _____ pounds

The participant understands the need to periodically re-examine his or her weight and fitness goals and to establish realistic, progressive goals based on personal experience in the program.

Date _____ Approximate date for goal review _____

Staff member _____

Source: Participant Questionnaire for the Weight Control for Life! and Lighter Living Programs. People Karch International, Chantilly, VA, 1989.

Table 4.8

AEROBIC EXERCISE FOR WEIGHT LOSS AND MAINTENANCE

Participants should be instructed to consider these four components:

Mode	Low or moderate impact activities involving large muscle groups
Intensity	Moderate intensity using perceived exertion or 60–80% of maximum heart rate*
Duration	40+ minutes per session at moderate intensity to lose weight*
	20+ minutes per session at moderate intensity to maintain weight*
Frequency	4–6 times per week to lose weight
	3–4 times per week to maintain weight

*Note: participants exercising at lower intensities (40–60%) should increase duration to achieve desired caloric expenditure. Increases in aerobic fitness will be minimal at lower intensities. However, the instructor should remember that her 60% pace may be an 80%+ pace for some participants in the class.

Stanforth (1992).

exercise is required to balance the calories consumed. This is a method for roughly estimating caloric needs for weight maintenance: multiply body weight in pounds by a factor between eight and fifteen to estimate the total calories needed each day to maintain that weight. Sedentary people, older women, or formerly-obese-recently-reduced people will use the lower factor. The higher values (12 to 15) are appropriate for very active, young or male individuals. Calories required for physical exercise beyond normal daily activities are in addition to these factors.

These rough estimates emphasize the importance of physical activity for long-term maintenance. The additional calories "burned" during exercise make the difference between a reasonable food intake and a highly restricted food intake. Would-be weight maintainers face these choices: 1) exercise regularly and eat reasonably; or 2) try to maintain weight by calorie restriction and risk frequent hunger; or 3) avoid exercise, eat "normally," and regain the weight.

Minimum exercise requirements for weight maintenance are 20 to 30 minutes of aerobic exercise four times per week or about 2,000 kcal per week from deliberate physical activity, such as aerobics classes and walking (Table 4.8). Using exercise to "correct" excessive caloric consumption can be a dangerous pattern and will be discussed in the next section.

Dangerous and Ineffective Weight-Loss Methods

Weight loss is a big business and the American public is bombarded with unrealistic models of thinness selling appetite suppressants, fad diets and exercise gimmicks that promise to make the process "quick and easy." At best, these techniques are ineffective; at worst, they are potentially harmful. The aerobics instructor can provide a valuable service by offering accurate, scientifically based information to counter false advertising claims.

Spot-reducing is often promoted to eliminate the so-called cellulite in specific areas of the body. **Cellulite** is just another name for **subcutaneous fat** that has a dimpled appearance. The only way to remove fat deposits is through diet and exercise. The energy for exercise, even when using localized muscle groups, draws from fat stores throughout the body, not from selected fat deposits in the area being worked. Sit-ups will increase the muscle tone for the abdomen, for example, but will not burn off the "tummy roll."

Diet pills, drugs and laxatives should be avoided entirely. Diet pills usually contain a stimulant to suppress the appetite. However, this is a temporary effect and tapers off with time. More importantly, these stimulants can be addictive and cause insomnia, high blood pressure, headaches and dizziness. Phenylpropanolamine, another appetite-suppressing ingredient, can cause high blood pressure, irregular heart rhythm and liver damage. Laxatives disrupt the electrolyte balance, prevent absorption of essential nutrients and can inhibit normal functioning of the bowel system.

Unsupervised low-calorie diets (less than 1,200 kcal/day) and very-low-calorie diets (less than 800 kcal/day) may put the dieter at medical risk. According to the American Medical Association and the American Dietetic Association, these diets may be appropriate for seriously obese individuals who are already at medical risk due to their obesity, but should be used only under close medical supervision. Complete fasting is never appropriate for weight loss and is life-threatening.

Vibrating belts, elastic belts, electric muscle stimulators, and rubber or plastic suits are all ineffective methods for weight loss because no caloric deficit is created by any of these devices. Methods which dramatically reduce body fluids, such as the rubber suit and lengthy saunas, may lead to dehydration.

Fad diets come and go but are generally characterized by promises of "rapid and easy" weight loss. They tend to be very specific and often restrictive food plans. They claim that exercise is unnecessary, and they emphasize weight loss with a dis-regard for the lifestyle change process required for maintenance. The impact of these diets on the participant is perpetuating the myth that the "diet" (losing the weight) takes care of the problem.

SUMMARY OF NUTRITION AND WEIGHT CONTROL

Body weight is the result of a complex set of factors including genetic predisposition (inherited tendency to be overweight or thin), the culture in which the individual lives, physical activity, nutrition, behavioral patterns (many established in early years), and thinking patterns. With the exception of genetics, these are learned lifestyle patterns which means they are open to modification. Weight management is an educational process. People can learn to attain and maintain lower, healthier, fit body weights by focusing on the factors that are within their personal control (Nunn et al, 1992). Instructors can provide solid information, positive exercise experiences and reinforcement for this challenging process.

EATING DISORDERS AND BODY IMAGE

Eating disorders and distorted body image are serious, widespread problems of our society, affecting primarily women but also extending to men and adolescents. These problems stem from unrealistic standards for body weight and body proportions. Dancers, wrestlers and other athletes who strive for low body fat are particularly vulnerable. These problems affect not only participants in aerobics classes but are often real issues for the instructors and health professionals working in the diet/eating disorders field. An instructor cannot treat a person with an eating disorder. However, by providing sound nutritional advice, supporting realistic weight goals and promoting realistic time frames for weight loss, the instructor can play a role in the prevention of eating disorders.

Anorexia nervosa (lack of appetite due to intense fear of obesity and severe disturbance of body image) is self-imposed starvation to the point of emaciation. Anorexics often lose up to 25 percent of their body weight. Because of an extremely distorted body image, however, they still feel heavy and "see" a heavy image when looking in a mirror. Obviously anorexics are at great risk for nutritional deficiency and health complications. Research has shown that most anorexics are intelligent, high achievers who are encouraged to lose weight as children or adolescents, either for the sake of appearance alone or for the purpose of athletic competition. They lose the weight and feel in control. Normal eating feels out of control and normal body weight "feels fat." Anorexics are obsessed with resisting food and often engage in vigorous exercise as a way to atone for consuming a few calories. Their goals for thinness are unrelated to health and fitness.

Bulimia ("ox hunger") is characterized by a binge-purge cycle in which huge amounts of food are eaten over a short period and then vomiting is induced or laxatives or diuretics are used in an attempt to control weight. These episodes of binging, followed by feelings of shame and then purging, are usually carried out secretly, and even family and close friends remain unaware of the problem. Like the anorexic, the bulimic is trapped by an obsession with thinness and a preoccupation with food. Unlike the anorexic, the bulimic is usually either normal weight or slightly overweight. The anorexic can be identified by her low weight, excessive exercise patterns and sometimes a downy arm hair. The bulimic may go for years before exhibiting noticeable physical symptoms,

such as decaying tooth enamel and frequent throat irritations.

In a recent study of female collegiate athletes, 32 percent reported that they practiced one or more weight-control behaviors defined as pathogenic (disease-producing), including binging, self-induced vomiting, and using laxatives, diet pills or diuretics (Rosen et al, 1986). Unfortunately, these practices impair health and performance. The complications of eating disorders can be serious and life-threatening, including malnutrition, electrolyte imbalances, dehydration, irregularities in heartbeat, fatigue, fainting, seizures and even death. The emotional toll is equally unhealthy.

Compulsive overeating and/or overexercising, while not as life-threatening as anorexia nervosa and bulimia, are emotionally destructive, physically draining and may progress to the two most serious eating disorders already discussed. Compulsive overeating or overexercising are often linked to unrealistic goals for body weight and athletic performance. These individuals are overwhelmed with thoughts about food: when they will eat, what they will eat, remorse about what they've eaten, calculating how many hours they must exercise to make up for a normal meal with friends, or how many meals they must skip to atone for a slip. Food has become an enemy and exercise has become a punishment. They cannot enjoy a meal nor appreciate the nourishment that food provides. They ignore the physiological fact that recovery time is an important component of any exercise program.

On the surface, it may not be easy to tell the difference between a participant's healthy concern for body composition and athletic performance and an obsessive, destructive concern for being thin. A highly motivated exerciser may exhibit some of the compulsive behaviors common among persons with eating disorders. Both share the drive to excel and to control mind and body. Both set goals just beyond reach and experience anxiety and depression when their exercise routines cannot be maintained. However, an instructor who observes the following symptoms should suspect an eating disorder:

1. Repeated complaints about feeling fat, even when the person is of normal weight or underweight.

2. A drive to exercise excessively, beyond requirements of health and fitness.

3. Wide fluctuations in weight over short periods.

4. Edema or bloating of the face, hands, or ankles, not related to menstrual periods.

5. Complaints of dizziness, light-headedness, fatigue and muscles cramps.

6. Questions about the use of laxatives, diuretics or diet pills.

7. More than average dental problems (caused by erosion and decay from repeated vomiting of highly acidic stomach contents).

8. Frequent throat irritations (also caused by repeated induced vomiting).

9. Loss of hair and/or growth of fine body hair.

10. Extreme distress over missing a workout or failure to meet a weight-loss goal.

What is the role of the aerobics instructor? First, instructors should be healthy role models, with positive and realistic self-images. An instructor who is frequently complaining about his or her weight will only feed the obsession of a participant with an eating disorder. Secondly, instructors should openly address the general problem of eating disorders in class, stressing realistic goals for weight and nutrition. Thirdly, instructors should communicate positive messages about areas of the body that are focused on in class. For example, "Let's work on strengthening those powerful thighs which carry us around all day," instead of "Let's work those ugly thighs." Instructors can also provide a list of professional resources for anyone who has, or knows someone who has, the problem.

Finally, an instructor who suspects a participant (or another instructor) is anorexic or bulimic should speak privately to that person in a supportive, nonjudgmental way. By expressing concern as a fitness professional and a caring person, the individual may be willing to talk and accept referrals to physicians, dietitians or psychologists who specialize in eating disorders. If the person denies the problem, keep channels of communication open and let him or her know that help is available when needed. It is normal to feel hesitant about approaching someone, but ignoring the problem increases the danger to the participant. Undiagnosed and untreated eating disorders may lead to permanent physical injury.

Body image and self-esteem are closely linked to eating disorders. The ultimate role for an aerobics instructor is to promote exercise as a form of self-care and a source of joy that builds positive feelings about life.

SUMMARY

Fitness-oriented people often seek the secret ingredient that will improve their health and physical performance. Thus, nutritional extremes are prevalent in the world of fitness centers and health clubs. Expensive vitamin and mineral supplements, diets and exercise gimmicks may be promoted to boost performance and reduce body fat. The fact remains, however, that there is no quick and easy way to lose weight, get fit or become a better athlete.

The instructor has a great opportunity to contribute to the health and fitness goals of aerobics participants by serving as a positive role model and by providing them with solid, basic information on nutrition and weight control. A diet high in complex carbohydrates and low in fat is the best regimen for serious athletes and overweight, beginning exercisers. The best way to lose and maintain weight is to combine a modest reduction in calories with moderate aerobic exercise. To that end, the instructor should be a source of positive reinforcement for achievement of realistic fitness goals.

REFERENCES

Aftergood, L & Alfin-Slater, P. (1980). *Women and Nutrition.* Contemporary Nutrition (General Mills, Inc.).

American College of Sports Medicine . (1992). Regional Fat Distribution: Metabolic Implications and Effects of Exercise. American College of Sports Medicine. Indianapolis, IN.

American Cancer Society. (1987). *Cancer Facts and Figures.* New York, NY.

American Diabetes Association. (1981). *The Exchange Lists for Meal Planning.*

American Heart Association. (1982). *Heart Facts* 1983. Dallas, TX.

American Heart Association. (1982). Report of AHA Nutrition Committee: Rationale of the diet-heart statement of the American Heart Association. *Arteriosclerosis.* 2:177-191.

American Institute of Cancer Research. (1992). *Dietary Guidelines to lower cancer risk.* Washington, D.C.

Arntzenius, A.C., et al; (1985). Diet, Lipoproteins, and the Progress of Coronary Atherosclerosis. *New England Journal of Med.* 312:805-811.

Department of Health, Education & Welfare. (1979). *Healthy People: The Surgeon General's Report on Health Promotion and Disease Prevention.* Publication No. 79-5501.

Donald, K. & Hegsted, D. (1985). Efficiency of utilization of various sources of energy for growth. *Procedures of the National Academy of Sciences.* 82:4866.

Gortmaker, S, et al; (1987). Increasing pediatric obesity in the United States. *American Journal of Diseases in Childhood.* 141:535-540.

Grundy, S, et al; (1985). Coronary risk factor statement for the American public: A statement of the Nutrition Committee of the American Heart Association. *Arteriosclerosis,* 5:A678-A682.

McArdle, W. (1987). *Building Endurance.* Time Life Books. New York.

Monsen, E. (1992). Iron and serum lipids in pathogenesis of heart disease. *Journal of the American Dietetic Association* 92, 12:1502.

National Cholesterol Education Program. (1988). The Expert Panel: Report of the National Cholesterol Education Program expert panel on detection, evaluation and treatment of high blood cholesterol in adults. *Archives of Internal Medicine.* 148:36-69.

Nunn, R, et al; (1992). 2.5 Years Follow-Up of Weight and Body Mass Index Values in the Weight Control for Life! Program. *Addictive Behaviors, International Journal,* Vol 17.

Ornish, D. (1990). *Dr. Dean Ornish's Program for Reversing Heart Disease.* Random House, New York.

Rosen, L, et al; (1986). Pathogenic Weight Control Behavior in Female Athletes. *The Physician and Sportsmedicine,* January: 79-86.

Stanforth, P. & Stanforth, D. (1992). Burning Fat: The Rest of the Story, *Certified News,* Vol. 2. ACSM, Indianapolis, IN.

Simmer, K, et al; (1987). Are iron-folate supplements harmful? American Journal of Clinical Nutrition. 45:122-125.

Smith, E. (1982). Exercise for Prevention of Osteoporosis: A review. *The Physician and Sportsmedicine.* March:72-83.

U.S. Dept. of Agriculture. (1980). *Dietary Guidelines for Americans.* Washington D.C.

Weir, J. et al; (1987). A high carbohydrate diet negates the metabolic effects of caffeine during exercise. *Medicine and Science in Sports and Exercise.* 19:100-105.

Williams, P. et al; (1982). The Effects of Running Mileage and Duration on Plasma Lipoprotein Levels. *Journal of the American Medical Association.* 247:2674-79.

Wood, P. et al; (1985). Metabolism of Substrates: Diet, Lipoprotein Metabolism, and Exercise. *Federation Proceedings.* 44:358-63.

Woteki, C. & Thomas, P. (1992). *Eat for Life.* National Academy Press. Washington D.C.

SUGGESTED READING

Center for Science in the Public Interest. Nutrition Action Healthletter. 1875 Connecticut Ave., NW, Suite 300, Washington DC, 20009. (202) 667-7483.

Clark, N. (1990). *Sports Nutrition Guidebook*. Champaign, IL: Leisure Press.

Colvin, R., & Olson, S. (1989). *Keeping It Off: Winning at Weight Loss*. Arkansas City, KS: Gilliland Press.

Natow, A., & Heslin, J. (1990). *The Fat Attack Plan*. New York: Simon & Schuster.

Ornish, D. (1990). *Dr. Dean Ornish's Program for Reversing Heart Disease*. New York: Random House.

Rodin, J. (1992). *Body Traps*. New York: William Morrow and Co., 1992.

Shape Magazine. 21100 Erwin St., Woodland Hills, CA 91367.

Somer, E. (1992). *The Essential Guide to Vitamins and Minerals*. New York: Harper Collins.

Tribole, E. (1992). *Eating on the Run*. Champaign, IL: Leisure Press.

Woteki, C. & P. Thomas. (1992). *Eat for Life*. Washington D.C.: National Academy Press.

RESOURCES

Food and Nutrition Board, Commission on Life Sciences, National Research Council. Recommended Dietary Allowances, Tenth Edition. Washington DC: National Academy Press, 198.

Kaiser Permanente, Dept. of Health Education and Health, Promotion. Health Counts: A Fat and Calorie Guide. New York: John Wiley & Sons, 199.

The National Center for Nutrition and Dietetics, The American Dietetic Association, 215 West Jackson Boulevard, Suite 800 Chicago, IL 60606-6995, (312)899-4853 or (800)366-1655, Contact for: referrals to dietitians and to order nutrition education material.

The Produce for Better Health Foundation, (302)738-7100, to order: Five-A-Day Plan.

U.S. Government Printing Office, Consumer Information Center-2D, P.O. Box 100, Pueblo, CO 81002, to order The Food Guide Pyramid booklet and Dietary Guidelines for Americans booklet.

Vitaerobics, 41-905 Boardwalk, Suite B, Palm Desert, CA 92260, (619)773-5576, to order the Fat Finder Calculator.

Part II
Assessment, Programming and Instruction

Chapter 5

Health Screening

By Steven Van Camp

Medical disorders and conditions that may make exercise unsafe

- Cardiovascular—coronary heart disease, hypertension

- Pulmonary—asthma, emphysema, chronic bronchitis

- Musculoskeletal—arthritis

How to screen participants; risk factors that warrant referral of someone to a physician for medical evaluation and clearance

- Health history form
- Medical clearance form

The effects of medications and other drugs on the heart-rate response to exercise

- Beta blockers
- Diuretics
- Antihypertensives
- Antihistamines
- Cold medications
- Tranquilizers
- Antidepressants
- Diet pills
- Alcohol
- Caffeine
- Nicotine

An exercise class should be beneficial and enjoyable. If instructors screen participants properly, conduct exercise sessions safely, and learn how to respond to emergencies properly, aerobic exercise should also be safe. This chapter will discuss the important role health screening plays in an aerobic exercise program and offer practical screening procedures. These procedures are appropriate for traditional, general classes in an environment where elaborate fitness testing is not the norm. This chapter cannot qualify instructors to be health care deliverers, nor can it prepare

Steven P. Van Camp, M.D., a cardiologist in private practice in San Diego, is medical director of the exercise physiology laboratory and the Adult Fitness Program at San Diego State University. Dr. Van Camp is a fellow of the American College of Cardiology and the American College of Sports Medicine. He has served on the American Council on Exercise's board of directors and the IDEA board of advisors.

Chapter 5
Health Screening

instructors for all possible health contingencies for participants in an exercise class. However, the screening process presented here will help instructors identify persons who need special attention or who should be exercising in special classes, as well as persons who should not be exercising at all until they obtain **medical clearance** from their physicians.

The health screening process has other positive features as well. It can: (1) help instructors become more familiar with the physical abilities of their students, (2) enhance the credibility of the instructor as a concerned professional, (3) help protect instructors against potential legal problems, and (4) open lines of communication between physicians and aerobic instructors, thus helping instructors gain exposure in their communities as concerned professionals.

MEDICAL DISORDERS THAT AFFECT EXERCISE

While it appears that appropriate exercise will add to the quality and, most likely, to the length of life, exercise does carry a health risk for persons with certain medical disorders of the cardiovascular, pulmonary and musculoskeletal systems. The most significant condition that may make exercise unsafe is coronary heart disease, also known as coronary artery disease and atherosclerotic heart disease.

Coronary heart disease is the result of **atherosclerosis,** a thickening and hardening of the walls of the arteries by deposits of cholesterol. Atherosclerosis may result in narrowing of the arteries, including the coronary arteries that supply the heart with blood and, therefore, oxygen.

During exercise the heart beats faster and more forcefully (the heart rate and systolic blood pressure are elevated), which means that the myocardium (heart muscle) needs more oxygen. If the arteries that supply the myocardium with oxygen are significantly narrowed by the cholesterol and calcium deposits of atherosclerosis, the flow of blood is restricted. When the myocardium's demand for oxygen exceeds the supply available through the coronary arteries, **myocardial ischemia** (deficiency of blood supply to the heart muscle) occurs. Myocardial ischemia, in turn, may lead to **angina pectoris** (a feeling of pressure, usually in the center of the chest), cardiac **arrhythmias** (abnormal heart rhythms), or even **cardiac arrest** (the heart stops). In addition, people with atherosclerotic narrowing of coronary arteries are at risk for **myocardial infarctions** (heart attacks).

Clearly, vigorous exercise is potentially unsafe for people with coronary heart disease, and they should exercise only in accordance with their physician's recommendations. In most cases, participants with diagnosed (known) coronary heart disease should not exercise in aerobic exercise programs designed for the general population.

Unfortunately, coronary heart disease is not always obvious to those who have it. Some people either are asymptomatic (i.e., have no symptoms), or they may misinterpret or not understand the significance of their symptoms. Therefore, not only do persons with known heart disease need medical clearance before exercising, persons who are at significant risk for coronary heart disease should also be evaluated by their physicians. Medical research has identified certain **risk factors** associated with increased likelihood of disease. Risk factors can be hereditary or the product of lifestyle, or a combination of the two. The more risk factors one possesses and the more severe they are, the greater the chance of having or developing the disease

Figure 5.1

SAMPLE FORM: THE HEALTH FORM

Name _____ Date _____

Sex _____ Age _____

What is the present state of your general health? _____

_____

Physician's name _____ Physician's telephone number _____

Person to contact in case of an emergency?

Name _____ Phone number _____

Are you presently taking any medications? (please list) _____

_____

Are you now or have you been pregnant within the past three months? _____

Does your physician know you are participating in an aerobic exercise program? _____

Do you now or have you had within the past year:	Yes	No
1. History of heart problems?	_____	_____
2. High blood pressure?	_____	_____
3. Difficulty with physical exercise?	_____	_____
4. A chronic illness?	_____	_____
5. Advice from a physician not to exercise?	_____	_____
6. Muscle, joint or back disorder that could be aggravated by physical activity?	_____	_____
7. Recent surgery (within the past three months)?	_____	_____
8. History of lung problems?	_____	_____
9. History of diabetes?	_____	_____
10. Cigarette-smoking habit?	_____	_____
11. Obesity (more than 20 pounds overweight)?	_____	_____
12. High blood cholesterol?	_____	_____
13. History of heart problems in immediate family?	_____	_____

What regular physical activity do you presently do? _____

with which they are associated.

The most significant risk factors for a particular disease are termed **primary risk factors.** Less important risk factors are **secondary risk factors.** Generally accepted as primary risk factors for coronary heart disease are cigarette smoking, hypertension, sedentary lifestyle, and abnormal blood cholesterol levels (either high total cholesterol or low high-density lipoprotein [HDL] cholesterol). Secondary risk factors are obesity, age over 65, being male, family history of coronary heart disease in relatives younger than 65 years, diabetes mellitus, and possibly, psychosocial stress. A person with a risk-factor profile that indicates a significant possibility of coronary heart disease should, therefore, be evaluated by a physician before beginning an exercise program.

Exercise may also present a health risk for persons with disorders of the lung, or pulmonary system, such as **asthma, emphysema** or chronic **bronchitis.** Each of these conditions may result in **dyspnea** (difficult or labored breathing), making exercise difficult. Exercise may aggravate the condition for some people and improve the condition for others. The important point is that anyone with a disorder of the pulmonary system should have a medical evaluation before beginning or continuing an exercise program.

Similarly, people with disorders of the musculoskeletal system can experience difficulty with exercise, and exercise may aggravate their disorders. These disorders—involving any problem with muscles, joints or the back—include **arthritis, bursitis** and **tendinitis.** After proper medical evaluation, people with these conditions can usually participate in some type of exercise class, although a typical aerobics program may aggravate an existing condition. Some participants may be able to exercise in a standard class by modifying their activities in accordance with their physician's recommendations.

HEALTH SCREENING PROCESS

A health form (Fig. 5.1) contains information that should be obtained from participants before they begin an exercise class. Ideal forms are brief enough to be practical and simple enough that participants can complete them without referring to their medical records. The sample included here is only a model; it may be modified according to the needs of each program and the recommendations of that program's medical and legal advisors. The information on the form should be updated on a regular basis, for example, every six to twelve months, and whenever a participant has problems during an exercise program.

Information gathered by this process will help instructors become familiar with new participants. Information about current activity patterns, although not crucial to the health-screening process, will help instructors understand the participant's present fitness level and identify the most appropriate type of exercise program. It will also help instructors to decide an appropriate rate of progression for each participant.

When a participant's health history or medical symptoms indicate a condition that would make exercise unsafe, referral to a physician for evaluation and clearance is appropriate. To facilitate communication among the instructor, the participant and the physician, the instructor can submit a medical clearance form (Fig. 5.2) to the physician. The form describes the class, including the mode and intensity of exercise, the duration of the class, and how often it meets. This approach helps the physician accurately assess the risks of a

Figure 5.2

SAMPLE FORM: MEDICAL CLEARANCE FORM

Date _____

Dear Dr. _____

Your patient _____

wishes to exercise with _____ exercise programs.

The activity will involve the following: _____
                                       (type, frequency, duration, and intensity of activities)

_____

If your patient is taking medications that will affect his or her heart-rate response to exercise, please indicate the manner of the effect (raises, lowers, or has no effect on heart-rate response):

Type of medication _____

Effect _____

Please identify any recommendations or restrictions that are appropriate for your patient in this exercise program:

_____

_____

Thank you.
Sincerely,

Jane Jones
Super-Duper Aerobics
Address Phone

_____ has my approval to exercise in _____

_____ the program with the recommendations or restrictions stated above.

_____   _____
Physician's Signature   Date

particular class for a certain participant. The instructor should keep the medical clearance in a file along with the health-history records.

When an instructor notices any of the following risk factors, it is appropriate to refer the participant to a physician and to require a written medical clearance before the person begins or continues an exercise program:

1. Age over 40 years for men and over 50 for women. Older participants will have increased risk of conditions that would make exercise hazardous or difficult.

2. Pregnancy or childbirth within the previous three months. It is important to obtain a written clearance from the participant's physician before allowing a pregnant or recently pregnant woman into an aerobic exercise program (see Chapter 12, "Exercise and Pregnancy").

3. History of heart disease. The eligibility of a participant with a history of heart problems depends on the type and severity of the condition. Heart conditions may range from inconsequential to severe, but any such history requires evaluation and clearance by the participant's physician.

4. **Hypertension** (high blood pressure). In general, participants with medically controlled high blood pressure will be allowed to exercise by their physicians. However, these participants should avoid exercise with significant isometric components. Such exercises may produce a potentially dangerous rise in blood pressure. Medications used to treat high blood pressure will be discussed later in this chapter.

5. Past difficulty with physical exercise. If the difficulty was mild, or if it is explainable by factors no longer present (e.g., pregnancy, anemia or an infectious disease), referral to a physician may still be appropriate, but it is not absolutely necessary.

6. A chronic illness.

7. Advice from a physician not to exercise.

8. Musculoskeletal problems, including muscle, joint or back disorders, that could be aggravated by physical activity.

9. Recent surgery (within the past three months). The extensiveness of the surgical procedure, the patient's recovery and the time since the surgery will be important in a physician's decision to allow or encourage exercise.

The presence of any of the following indicates that referral to a physician is appropriate, but not absolutely necessary.

1. Age of 35 to 40 years old for men, 45 to 50 for women. These people are in an age range in which medical referral is not absolutely necessary, but in which there begins to be a possibility (usually small) of problems with exercise.

2. History of lung problems, including chronic bronchitis, emphysema or asthma.

3. Persons with diabetes mellitus. Referral is especially important if the participant is receiving insulin. Participants with diabetes mellitus, an abnormality of glucose metabolism, may significantly benefit from regular exercise. However, each person's situation and exercise program should be discussed carefully with his or her physician to maximize the program's benefits and minimize the problems.

4. Cigarette-smoking habit.

5. Obesity (over 20 percent above ideal weight, or more than 30 percent body fat for women and more than 23 percent body fat for men).

6. High blood cholesterol.

7. History of heart problems in the immediate family.

Persons with the last four characteristics have increased risk of heart disease, even if they have no symptoms. The risk increases with the severity of the factors. In other words, a person who smokes four packs of cigarettes per day is at greater risk than someone who smokes half a pack. In most cases, referral to a physician may not be crucial, but in all cases it benefits the person, and is therefore recommended.

In summary, medical clearance should be required for men over 40 years old, women over 50 years old or pregnant, and anyone answering yes to one of the first seven questions on the health-history form (Fig. 5.1). Medical referral should be carefully considered for men 35 to 40, women 40 to 50, and anyone answering yes to one of the questions 8 through 13 on the form.

The health-screening process should also note any medications that class participants are taking. An instructor who knows which participants are taking medications can observe them carefully for exercise-related difficulties or unusual heart-rate responses. Certain situations may require further assessment. Instructors and studio owners should discuss their approach to medication-related issues with their program's medical consultants.

Once the health history has been collected, it should be used and not just filed away and forgotten. The information can be helpful in designing an exercise class and providing support and guidance for participants. The information obtained from a health-history form should be supplemented by observation of participants.

MEDICATIONS

Many participants in exercise classes take prescription and nonprescription (over-the-counter) medications that affect their heart-rate response to exercise. These medications may be identified by the participant directly or through the health-screening process, or they may be brought to the instructor's attention when a participant has an unusual heart-rate response to exercise (15 or more beats per minute higher or lower than would

be considered normal).

It is important to understand the effects of these medications on heart-rate response to assist participants in their exercise programs. A medication may be referred to by its manufacturer's brand name or by its scientific generic name. For example, Inderal is a brand name for the beta blocker propranolol. Lasix is a brand name for the diuretic furosemide. To understand the probable effects of a specific medication, an instructor needs to identify the general category to which it belongs. Table 5.1 shows the general effects of several categories of medications on heart-rate response. These are the typical effects that may be seen in most persons. To use the table, consult the participant, the participant's physician or a medical reference to find the correct category for a participant's medication.

When evaluating a participant's response to medications and exercise, it is important to remember that individual responses will vary. For example, the effects of many medications are dose-related, which means that greater effects occur with larger doses. An important factor in this dose-related response is the time the medication was administered in relation to the exercise session. For instance, if a small dose of medication is taken a long time before an exercise session, the effect will probably be small. On the other hand, if a large dose is taken shortly before exercise, the effect will probably be larger. In addition, some classes of medications have variable effects. For instance, as shown in the table, **calcium channel-blocking drugs** may either increase, decrease or have no effect on the heart rate. Therefore, while it is important to understand the general effects of different types of medications, it is equally important to remember that individual responses can vary widely.

Table 5.1

EFFECTS OF MEDICATIONS ON HEART-RATE (HR) RESPONSE

Medications	Resting HR	Exercise HR	Maximal Exercising HR	Comments
Beta-adrenergic blocking agents	↓	↓	↓	Dose-related response
Diuretics	↔	↔	↔	
Antihypertensives	↑, ↔ or ↓	↑, ↔ or ↓	usually ↔	Many antihypertensive medications are used. Some may decrease, a few may increase and others do not affect heart rates. Some exhibit dose-related response.
Calcium channel blockers	↑, ↔ or ↓	↑, ↔ or ↓	↓ or ↔	Variable & dose-related responses
Antihistamines	↔	↔	↔	
Cold medications: without sympathomimetic activity (SA))	↔	↔	↔	
with sympathomimetic activity (SA)	↔ or ↑	↔ or ↑	↔	
Tranquilizers	↔, or if anxiety reducing may ↓	↔	↔	
Antidepressants and some antipsychotic medication	↔ or ↑	↔	↔	
Alcohol	↔ or ↑	↔ or ↑	↔	Exercise prohibited while under the influence; effects of alcohol on coordination increase possibility of injuries
Diet pills: with SA	↑ or ↔	↑ or ↔	↔	Discourage as a poor approach to weight loss; acceptable only with physician's written approval.
containing amphetamines	↑	↑	↔	
without SA or amphetamines	↔	↔	↔	
Caffeine	↔ or ↑	↔ or ↑	↔	
Nicotine	↔ or ↑	↔ or ↑	↔	Discourage smoking; suggest lower target heart rate & exercise intensity for smokers

↑ = increase   ↔ = no significant change   ↓ = decrease

Note: Many medications are prescribed for conditions that do not require clearance. Don't forget other indicators of exercise intensity, e.g., participant's appearance, rating of perceived exertion.

Beta Blockers. Among the most commonly administered medications are **beta-adrenergic blocking agents** or **beta blockers,** which may be used to treat a variety of cardiovascular and other disorders. These medications exert their effects by blocking beta-adrenergic receptors and limiting adrenergic (sympathetic) stimulation. In simpler terms, they block the effects of catecholamines (adrenalin or epinephrine and norepinephrine) throughout the body and reduce the resting, exercise and maximal heart rates.

Patients have similar general responses to beta blockers. However, the size of the response may vary from patient to patient because beta blockers are competitive, reversible blockers of sympathetic activity.

Therefore, the effects are dose-related, temporary (usually lasting for hours), and dependent on a person's own catecholamine levels.

If any exerciser is taking a beta blocker as treatment for angina pectoris, high blood pressure, a previous heart attack, or abnormal heart rhythm, then a medical clearance must be obtained before exercising. It is important to understand the effects of beta blockers because in some exercise participants taking beta blockers will be appropriately cleared by their physicians. These medications are also used for conditions that do not require medical clearance, such as migraines and familial tremors. (See Chapter 11, "Special Populations and Health Concerns" for a discussion of appropriate ways to monitor heart rates for participants on beta blockers.)

Diuretics. Diuretic medications have no effect on the heart rate. However, because they produce excretion of water and electrolytes (including sodium) from the kidney, diuretics may decrease blood volume and, thus, predispose an exerciser to dehydration. Therefore, participants taking diuretics should be especially careful to maintain adequate fluid intake before, after and sometimes during an exercise session. Fluid intake is especially important when exercise is prolonged or done in a warm, humid environment.

Antihypertensives. Several medications are available for treating hypertension, including beta-adrenergic blocking agents and calcium channel blockers. As shown in Table 5.1, those medications can vary widely in their effects on heart-rate response. Any medication affecting the resting or exercising heart rate may require adjustment in desired target heart-rate range.

Cold Medications. Cold medications may contain an antihistamine or a medication with sympathomimetic activity or both. Those with antihistamines alone generally have no significant effect on heart rates. Those with sympathomimetic activity may increase heart rates at rest and possibly during exercise.

SUMMARY

Health screening is a crucial first step in maintaining the safety of an aerobic exercise program. Health screening also enhances an instructor's credibility and opens lines of communication with physicians. After initial screening at the beginning of an exercise program, periodic reassessment is important. Instructors should use screening information when designing and conducting classes and should back up this information with careful observation. Any participant who is identified as at-risk, either during the initial screening or as a result of symptoms exhibited during an exercise program, should be referred to a physician.

Chapter 6

Fitness Testing and Aerobic Programming

By Larry S. Verity

P reventive and rehabilitative exercise programs have long considered fitness assessment an important element of comprehensive exercise programming. Although fitness testing can be divided into either skill-related or health-related elements, health-related fitness is the premier goal for the industry to embrace. Those elements comprising health-related fitness are cardiorespiratory fitness, musculoskeletal fitness and body composition (Fig. 6.1). Assessment of each health-related fitness element is presented in this chapter. Whenever health-related fitness testing is conducted, sound

Larry S. Verity, Ph.D., is associate professor of physical education and director of the Adult Fitness Program at San Diego State University. He is certified by the American College of Sports Medicine and is the director of the ACSM Health Fitness Instructor™ and Exercise Specialist™ workshops held in San Diego.

rationale should precede administration: "why" is this person being tested?, or "how" will these results be used? Moreover, aerobic instructors who administer all or portions of the fitness assessment should possess knowledge and skills about the various tests to be used, as well as their interpretation.

Aerobics instructors should conduct fitness tests for a number of reasons (Table 6.1). From a public health perspective, the nation is focused upon preventive care and is striving to improve the nation's physical activity by the year 2000. From the practical point of view, evaluating health-related fitness affords the exercise leader with information to develop safe, effective and individualized exercise programs.

Selection of Fitness Tests

In addition to the purposes of comprehensive fitness testing, aerobics instructors should also consider four criteria for implementing fitness tests: validity, reliability, norms and economy (Table 6.2). Health-related fitness tests that meet these criteria can yield accurate and consistent information which can be compared to similar groups of clients (e.g., age, sex and activity

level), and can be easily and inexpensively administered.

Although the purpose of fitness testing should be identified and test selection criteria should be addressed, it may not always be possible to meet each of the criteria when selecting a fitness test. Often, test norms have not yet been developed for comparisons to be made, even though the test has practical value (e.g., **flexibility** assessment). Regardless, the aerobics instructor should be aware of the limitations when using health-related fitness tests. In this chapter, purposes and criteria will be presented, for each of the components of fitness testing, along with other tests that may be useful for the aerobics instructor to evaluate clientele.

Pre-testing Procedures

Prior to fitness testing or programming, it is important to ensure the welfare and safety of clientele. Consequently, pre-participation health screening, as well as possible medical screening, are required to assess the risk for cardiovascular heart disease and physical health of each individual prior to participating in health-related fitness testing (see Chapter 5, "Health Screening").

Before implementing any exercise tests, an **informed consent** should be obtained. All fitness professionals are legally required to inform the client of the purpose(s) of the testing and its process, along with all potential risks (e.g., muscular soreness, injury, death) and discomforts of the testing procedures (see Chapter 15, "Legal and Professional Responsibilities").

Emergency Procedures

All fitness facilities should ensure that the staff are well informed of the established emergency plan prior to conducting any fitness testing. In addition, all staff should be well-qualified to not only con-

Figure 6.1

Elements of health-related fitness assessment.

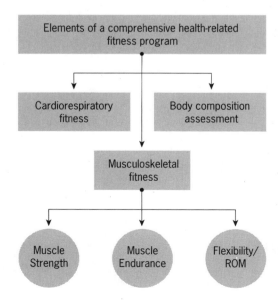

duct fitness tests, but also implement the emergency plan. Knowing that risks of injury and health problems exist when participating in exercise, an emergency plan should be written within the operating procedures and policies of the facility that delineates staff responsibilities in the event an unexpected injury or health problem arises. Emergency plans should be made available to all staff and should be practiced routinely (see Chapter 14, "Emergency Procedures").

CARDIORESPIRATORY FITNESS ASSESSMENT

Tests for **cardiorespiratory fitness** (CRF) measure the amount of continuous work the body can undertake, or the ability of the body to sustain aerobic activity, and either directly or indirectly determine maximal capacity of the body to use oxygen. A high CRF is closely linked with health and the ability to enjoy lifelong activities, while a low CRF is related to an increased risk for heart disease. Other terms used to reflect CRF that have synonymous meaning include aerobic capacity, maximal CRF, **maximal oxygen uptake**, or **VO$_2$ max**.

To ensure appropriate exercise program development, especially for sedentary clientele, it is important to evaluate CRF. Accordingly, when persons engage in regular aerobic activities, improvements in CRF occur, such as cardio (heart), vascular (blood vessels), respiratory (lung function) and aerobic (use of oxygen while exercising) components. It is not surprising that an increase in CRF can be observed with aerobic training programs, as the ability of the heart to pump blood and of muscular tissue to use oxygen are increased.

CRF Assessment: Variables Measured

The basic lab and **field tests** explained in this chapter require the monitoring of heart

Table 6.1

PURPOSES OF COMPREHENSIVE FITNESS TESTING

To develop a safe and effective individualized exercise program

To provide a baseline from which progress can be assessed

To identify attainable fitness and health goals that may enhance client motivation

To identify potential health/injury risk and offer appropriate referral

To enhance awareness of individual fitness status, along with education about fitness concept

rate. This important physiological measurement provides important information regarding how well the cardiovascular system functions. Heart rate should be obtained before, during and after exercise. During CRF assessment, it is also important to obtain subjective information from the client regarding how hard the work is perceived. Therefore, aerobics instructors should obtain a **rating of perceived exertion** (RPE) of the client during the fitness test to aid in effective exercise program development.

Heart Rate. **Heart rate,** or **pulse rate**, is a CRF indicator at rest and during submaximal levels of work, while maximal heart rate is commonly used when determining an appropriate target heart rate for aerobic workouts. **Resting heart rate** is usually determined while in bed after waking in the morning and is best reflected by an average of three to four separate early morning recordings. Because pulse rate is recorded in beats per minute (bpm), resting heart rate is most accurately measured for either a full minute or 30 seconds and multiplied by 2.

The measurement of resting or exercise pulse rate is most accurately obtained from **electrocardiogram** (ECG) recordings, but most fitness facilities are not equipped

Table 6.2

CRITERIA USED TO SELECT FITNESS TESTS

Validity of test	Does the test measure what it is supposed to measure? The test should accurately measure the fitness component (e.g., muscular endurance, muscular strength, flexibility, body composition). How accurate are the various tests that are used to measure health-related fitness components?
Reliability of test	Can the instructor repeatedly or consistently measure a given element? If the instructor measures a person's fitness level on separate days, he or she should get very similar results. The effort/motivation put forth by the client (e.g., muscle strength/endurance), the accuracy of the equipment used, as well as the skill of the person taking measures may influence reliability.
Norms for test	Can client scores be compared to a group of scores for persons with similar age, sex and/or activity level? Norms allow the aerobics instructor to accurately interpret and evaluate test results on an individual basis.
Economy of test	Can administration of test be easily performed, without expensive equipment, in a brief time period, and offer ease of interpretation by different persons?

with such costly equipment. Moreover, resting pulse rate can be accurately determined through the use of **palpation** techniques, while other methods of pulse measurement (e.g., stethoscope or commercial monitors) are most useful during the actual fitness tests.

Usually, resting heart rate for men averages 70 to 75 bpm and for women averages 75 to 80 bpm, while normal resting heart rate for adults can range between 40 to 100 bpm. Consequently, interpretation of resting heart rate is extremely difficult, especially for new clientele, as both genetics and fitness level influence the pulse rate at rest. Because resting heart rate usually decreases with aerobic exercise training, measurement of resting heart rate on follow-up assessments can be an indicator of improved cardiorespiratory fitness.

Perceived Exertion. Rating of perceived exertion (RPE) can be used by aerobics instructors to obtain subjective information from clients during fitness testing or exercise bouts (how does the client feel, or how hard the work seems to the client). The use of RPE as an indicator of exercise intensity during submaximal fitness testing aids the

aerobics instructor in identifying signs of exertional intolerance, undue fatigue or other abnormal responses (exercise intensity monitoring and use of RPE will be discussed later in the chapter). Borg (1982) has developed two RPE scales that are used for clients to subjectively gauge the intensity of perceived work (Table 6.3).

The 6 to 20 RPE scale has been frequently used in fitness testing, while the revised 10-point RPE scale may be easier for fitness professionals to explain to clients and for clients to understand. Regardless, either RPE scale can be used when assessing perceived exertion. When assessing RPE, it is important to explain to the client to pay close attention to the level of work and gauge the perceived effort by identifying a number that is verbally described (an RPE of 15 corresponds to an exercise intensity of "hard"). Care must also be taken by the test administrator to assess whether or not the test subject is misperceiving their level of exertion. This misperception can be either too high or too low.

Also, it should be emphasized that the client be as accurate as possible. In addition, when using this type of scale, a small percentage (5 to 14 percent) of clients underestimate RPE during early and middle phases of testing protocols.

CRF Assessment: Tests and Protocols

Different tests can be administered by aerobics instructors to assess maximal CRF. Regardless of the test protocol, the end-result of any CRF assessment is to determine a person's maximal ability to use oxygen during aerobic activity through direct or indirect measures. Such testing reflects the body's ability to use oxygen, which requires a fine-tuned integration in the function of the heart, lungs and muscles of the body when exercising.

Commonly, maximal oxygen uptake is expressed in milliliters of oxygen uptake per kilogram of body weight per minute ($mlO_2/kgBW/min$). By expressing maximal oxygen uptake relative to body weight, comparison of a client's value to other persons of similar age, sex and activity level can be made.

Maximal CRF Assessment

Maximal graded exercise tests, or stress tests, are the "gold standards" by which maximal oxygen uptake is determined. A graded exercise test to voluntary exhaustion using a treadmill or bicycle is an example of maximal testing. The obvious advantage of maximal testing is its accuracy, along with the ability of this test to diagnose heart disease through electrocardiographic and blood pressure monitoring.

However, maximal CRF assessment is usually reserved for laboratory or clinical settings, and requires a motivated client, close medical supervision, controlled conditions and special monitoring equipment. In addition, the need for extensive laboratory equipment, trained personnel and exercising to voluntary exhaustion often make maximal testing unlikely in fitness facilities.

Table 6.3

RATING INTENSITY USING PERCEIVED EXERTION (RPE)

6–20 RPE Scale	1–10 RPE Scale
6	0 Nothing at all
7 Very, Very Light	0.5 Very, Very Weak
8	1 Very Weak
9 Very Light	2 Weak
10	3 Moderate
11 Fairly Light	4 Somewhat Strong
12	5 Strong
13 Somewhat Hard	6
14	7 Very Strong
15 Hard	8
16	9
17 Very Hard	10 Very, Very Strong
18	• Maximal
19 Very, Very Hard	
20	

Source: Borg (1982).

Although not as accurate as maximal tests, many submaximal test protocols have been developed that are reasonably accurate and permit estimation of maximal CRF. Such tests require that clients exercise up to 70 to 85 percent of maximal capacity for a specified period of time, with test termination occurring well before exhaustion. Because of the lower exercise intensity, accuracy of the test, reliability of **submaximal exercise tests** and ease of administration, these alternate protocols are more desirable for aerobics instructors to indirectly assess maximal CRF.

A variety of submaximal tests have been developed; aerobics instructors can learn and administer selected field and laboratory submaximal protocols described below.

Submaximal CRF Assessment

A number of submaximal tests accurately and reliably estimate maximal CRF, maximal oxygen uptake or aerobic capacity.

Submaximal tests require either heart rate measurement during or after exercise (e.g., heart rate during bicycle test), or time to complete a specified distance (e.g., mile walk for time). Regardless of whether a heart rate is measured or a time recorded, the basic premise of submaximal CRF testing is that a highly fit person can do more work than a lesser fit person. Therefore, when measuring heart rate it is expected that a higher CRF level will yield a lower heart rate compared to a lower CRF person. Moreover, a specified distance can be completed by a fit person faster than an unfit person.

The use of any submaximal test to estimate aerobic capacity, or maximal oxygen uptake, is based on one or more of the following assumptions:

1. A linear relationship exists between heart rate, oxygen uptake and work load from submaximal to maximal levels;

2. Mechanical efficiency for all persons (oxygen uptake at a given work load) is uniform;

3. Age-adjusted maximal heart rate (MHR) assumes the same heart rate for all persons of the same age—error of this MHR is ± 12 bpm;

4. The subject is not taking heart rate-altering medications;

5. The subject is highly motivated and experienced in pacing him/herself for a specified distance or period of time.

A clarification of such assumptions is warranted. To begin with, assuming a linear relationship between heart rate and work may be inaccurate and may actually lead to an error of 10 to 20 percent when estimating maximal oxygen uptake. In some submaximal tests, heart rates are obtained during the workout and plotted at each work load. Assuming that heart rate and submaximal oxygen uptake are linear, an extrapolation of oxygen uptake is deter-

mined to maximal heart rate which is age-adjusted (Fig. 6.2). Although heart rate is related to oxygen uptake and work load during submaximal exercise to maximal exercise, substantial error can occur when using such extrapolations. Moreover, at any submaximal work load, oxygen uptake can vary by as much as 15 percent between clients, depending upon efficiency of movement.

When using submaximal tests to estimate maximal CRF, an assumption that maximal heart rate declines with age the same for all persons is made: **Age-predicted Maximal Heart Rate** = 220 - Age (years).

But age-adjusted maximal heart rate can vary by as much as 24 bpm (two thirds of the population varies an average of ± 12 bpm from the age-adjusted value) for any given age. The remaining one third of the population will vary by even more. As such, this formula can over- or under-estimate actual maximal heart rate, which similarly affects the accuracy of the estimated maximal oxygen uptake value.

For example, a person 40 years of age would be expected to have an age-adjusted maximal heart rate of 180 bpm; however, if actual maximal heart rate were determined from a stress test, the normal response of maximal heart rates could range from as low as 168 to 192 bpm because of the inherent error when using this formula.

Since submaximal protocols require measurement of heart rate response to work, these estimations of maximal CRF are valid only for persons who are not prescribed medications that alter heart rate (e.g., beta blockers, certain calcium channel blockers and certain vasodilators). Many clients who are treated for heart disease or mild to moderate hypertension may be prescribed these types of drugs. As a general rule, identify current medications and their effect on heart rate before

Cardiorespiratory
fitness assessment

administering any CRF test.

Finally, most field tests require that the person be familiar with exercising for a specific period of time or distance to make the test a valid estimation of maximal oxygen uptake. Although most field tests are less than maximal, these tests require the client be motivated and well-aware of the testing procedures. Knowing the limitations and assumptions of CRF tests aids the aerobics instructor in more appropriate administration and interpretation of the test.

Heart rate determination at submaximal work loads is very accurate and reproducible. With aerobic training and subsequent follow-up testing, changes in heart rate at similar work loads, or after performing a specific task (e.g., 1 mile walk), provide a relative marker for improvements in CRF, or aerobic fitness. Despite the possibility of error in estimating maximal oxygen uptake from submaximal tests, such tests are reliable indicators of maximal CRF and can be used to gauge CRF improvement as aerobic training progresses.

The recommended submaximal CRF test protocols do not require an expensive treadmill, electrocardiograph (ECG) and blood pressure monitoring during exer-

cise, and are not used for diagnostic purposes. Such submaximal test protocols are generally used in fitness facilities and include field testing (1 mile walk) and laboratory testing (3 minute **step test**).

The basic difference between field tests and laboratory tests is the degree of control over the variables that can affect the outcome of the test. In field testing, there is little control over how hard a person performs a given exercise, while laboratory tests require a greater degree of control over how much work a person performs. Although field and laboratory tests are reliable and reasonably accurate in estimating maximal oxygen uptake, field tests can accommodate mass testing, if needed. Also, field tests typically evaluate performance in normal activities, while laboratory tests measure certain parameters (e.g., heart rate) in response to a known amount of work. Depending upon the facilities, equipment and space, the field tests or laboratory testing protocols presented are adequate for CRF assessment.

Field Test: 1-mile Walk Test

The Rockport Walking Institute™ has developed a 1 mile walk test to estimate maximal oxygen uptake for persons between the ages of 30 and 69 years (Kline et al., 1987). This test is highly desirable for fitness professionals to use because it not only can estimate maximal oxygen uptake ($mlO_2/kgBW/min$) on a consistent basis for persons in this age range, but also can be used for mass testing of participants.

The intent of this test is to determine how fast each person can walk 1 mile. A well-orchestrated plan for administering this 1 mile test can yield excellent results. The following are the recommended procedures for administering the 1 mile walk test:

Required items:

• One-mile flat surface that is marke

Figure 6.2

Extrapolating Submaximal Heart Rates to Age-Adjusted Maximal Heart Rate to Estimate Aerobic Capacity. Note that this example, a 25-year-old has heart rates plotted and extrapolated on two different occasions, which result in a 12% error.

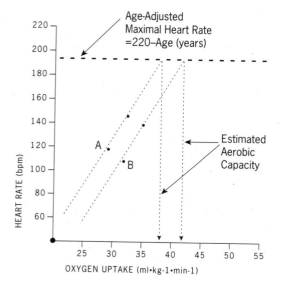

off (an oval track);

• A person to start and read performance time from a stopwatch;

• A partner with a watch (digital or second hand needed) for each walker, or a large clock with a sweep hand;

• Recording sheet, with name of each person and space for recording immediate exercise heart rate, body weight (pounds) and RPE of each walker.

Preparation before test day:

• Explain the purpose of the test to all participants (to determine how fast 1 mile can be walked to reflect maximal CRF);

• Identify that only walking is to be performed and to cover the distance as quickly as possible;

• Review the start and finish marks (prefer to use an oval track);

• Ensure that all persons have been walking the required distance and that previously sedentary persons have had a few weeks of activity before administering the test;

• Inform all clients of proper footwear for walking and appropriate clothing for the walking test.

Administration:

• Obtain body weight (pounds) of each participant before the walk test;

• Require all persons to warm up with slow walking and joint range-of-motion (stretching) activities;

• Each person should have a partner and each "couple" should have a stopwatch with a second hand (or a large clock with a sweep hand should be available);

• Review the purpose and procedures of the test;

• Determine which partner will walk, as larger numbers of persons can perform this test simultaneously;

• Administrator/timer readies the walkers and begins the timing after giving directions: "Ready, Set, GO!" All walkers begin at the same time;

• At each lap the administrator calls outs the elapsed time, while the partner counts the laps completed and indicates the number of laps remaining;

• Immediately upon completing the 1 mile distance, a 10- or 15-second heart rate should be obtained (by the walker or test assistant), which is multiplied by 6 or 4, respectively, to determine the heart rate in beats per minute;

• Each partner should record his or her heart rate and RPE during the last lap with the administrator;

• Walkers should actively cool down for 3 to 5 minutes.

Administration of the 1 mile walk test should closely follow the procedures above. It is imperative that all clients know the purpose of performing the test and are provided explicit instructions regarding test requirements; the instructor should recommend appropriate clothing and footwear, emphasize that only walking is to be performed, and caution that no person should partake in this test if previously sedentary. In addition, each person should be able to complete the distance and have been active for several weeks before participating in this test. Identifying prudent restrictions on client participation can eliminate unnecessary fatigue and possible injury.

The most important aspect of test administration for the 1 mile walk test is determining each client's time accurately. As indicated above, the critical task of obtaining a fairly accurate measure of the time to complete 1 mile can be performed by the test administrator or by pairing the clients with one another, especially when a large number of clients are being tested. After completion of the 1 mile walk test, maximal oxygen uptake can be estimated by using the tables in Appendix C.

The following example illustrates the use of the Appendix C tables to determine maximal oxygen uptake:

What is the estimated maximal oxygen uptake of a 28-year-old woman (Jane Fast) who walked 1 mile in 18 minutes and 15 seconds and has a heart rate (immediately after exercising) of 134 bpm?

To understand the estimated maximal oxygen uptake tables, first note that the tables are specific for the age and sex of participants, and that the heart rates (bpm) obtained immediately after finishing the 1 mile walk are placed along the far left-hand column, while the time to complete the distance (minutes/mile) is listed across the top of the table.

By referring to the estimated oxygen uptake table for 20- to 29-year-olds, one can ascertain Fast's estimated maximal oxygen uptake. First, locate the heart rate column on the far left side of the table and follow directly below to 130, which is closest to the heart rate obtained on Fast after completing the 1 mile walk. Second, using the 130 "row" as a guide, follow across the table to 18 minutes per mile, as Fast's completion time of 18 minutes and 15 seconds should be rounded off to the nearest minute per mile. As shown in the table, Fast's estimated maximal oxygen

uptake is 34.4 mlO_2/kgBW/min.

Remember that the estimated maximal oxygen uptake from the 1 mile walk test was developed with the assumption that the reference weight was 170 pounds for men and 125 pounds for women. Consequently, this test may slightly underestimate or overestimate maximal CRF depending on whether body weight is substantially more or less, respectively, than the reference weight for men and women. The maximal oxygen uptake may be corrected for weight differences by adding 1 milliliter to the maximal oxygen uptake for every 15 pounds less than 125 pounds or 170 pounds for men. Conversely, subtract 1 milliliter from the maximal oxygen uptake for every 15 pounds greater than the 125 pounds and 170 pounds for women and men, respectively. Also, since each walker must work as hard as he or she can, a lack of motivation will negatively influence the estimated value and underestimate maximal oxygen uptake.

In Table 6.4 classification of this client's CRF value can be examined. For Fast, her maximal oxygen uptake value of 34.4 mlO_2/kgBW/min for a 28-year-old woman is classified as "below average," ac-

Table 6.4

FITNESS CLASSIFICATION BASED ON MAXIMAL OXYGEN UPTAKE VALUES (mlO_2/kgBw/min)

Classification	20–30 years	31–40 years	41–50 years	51–60+ years
Above Average				
Men	>50	>47	>43	>40
Women	>47	>43	>40	>37
Average				
Men	42-49	39-46	36-42	32-39
Women	40-46	37-42	33-39	29-36
Below Average				
Men	36-41	32-38	30-35	27-31
Women	33-39	30-36	27-32	23-28
Needs Work				
Men	<36	<32	<30	<27
Women	<33	<30	<27	<23

cording to age and sex. From this information, it is apparent that Fast needs guidance in developing an appropriate exercise program to improve her CRF. Essentially, most sedentary persons will fall into either the "needs work" or "below average" categories of fitness.

Lab Test: 3-minute Step Test

The 3 minute step test, developed by Dr. Fred Kasch of San Diego State University, is currently used by YMCAs for mass testing of participants. Thanks to its relative ease of administration and minimal equipment requirement, this is a desirable test. Clients are given simple instructions to step up and down to a standardized cadence for 3 minutes. Immediately following the stepping, **recovery heart rate** is determined for a full minute.

The underlying premise for this test was that fitness level influences the rate of recovery heart rate; more fit persons recover more quickly than lesser fit persons following an equivalent bout of exercise.

Although norms are available for this test and it is economical, the weakness in this test lies in situational factors that can influence the accuracy and reliability of recovery heart rate, including prior exercise, tiredness, miscounting recovery heart rate, room temperature, coffee and smoking.

Procedures for Administering the 3 minute Step Test. Successful administration requires proper planning but can yield fairly good results.

Required items:
• 12-inch (30.5 centimeters) bench step—secure a sturdy bench;
• Metronome for accurate pacing—to be set at 96 bpm;
• Timing clock and test administrator;
• Stethoscope for measuring heart rate (optional);
• Recording sheet, with name of each person, sex and space for recording 1 minute recovery heart rate.

Preparation before test day:
• Explain the purpose of the test to all participants (to determine a 1 minute

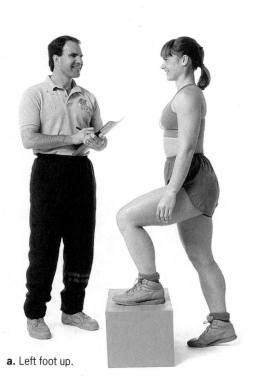

Figure 6.3
Step test.

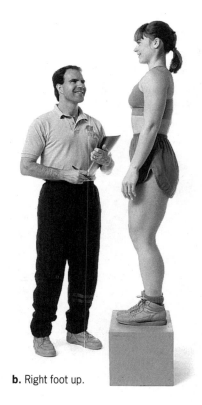

a. Left foot up.

b. Right foot up.

recovery heart rate after 3 minutes of stepping to reflect maximal CRF);

• Review and demonstrate proper cadence and procedure (e.g., step #1 - left foot up; step #2 - right foot up; step #3 - left foot down; step #4 - right foot down); either foot can lead;

• Inform all clients of proper footwear and appropriate clothing for the step test;

• Inform clients to refrain from coffee, smoking and exercise prior to this test, as the heart rate can be falsely elevated;

• Ensure all clients can accurately measure heart rate.

Administration:

• Allow a warm-up and practice of stepping at the desired rate of 96 bpm before test;

• Inform all clients to stop stepping if they experience lightheadedness or dizziness, excessive shortness of breath, nausea or if they feel they need to stop;

• Remind clients that the test is for 3 minutes and they are expected to sit down immediately afterward for a 1 minute pulse count;

• With clients facing the bench, begin the metronome, set at 96 bpm, and the test;

• Begin the clock when the clients begin stepping;

• Ensure the 4 beat cycle (up, up, down, down) is performed to cadence;

• Announce when 1 minute and 2 minutes have elapsed;

• When 20 seconds remain, remind the clients to be seated immediately after stepping;

• Obtain **radial** or **carotid pulse** within 5 seconds after sitting and count for 60 seconds;

• Record the post-stepping recovery heart rate in beats per minute;

• After pulse rate is determined, have client either remain sitting, or engage in an active cool-down.

Administration of the step test should closely follow the above procedures. To review essential points, it is important to inform the clients of the standardized cadence required while stepping (Fig. 6.3).

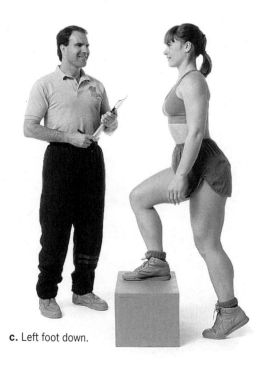

c. Left foot down.

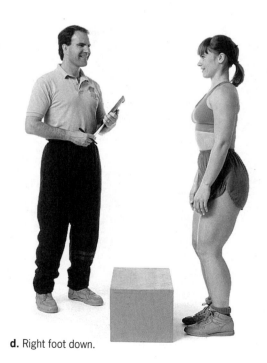

d. Right foot down.

Although a sequence is illustrated, either foot may lead during the 3 minute period. Both feet must contact the top of the bench on the "up" portion of the cycle, and both feet must contact the floor on the "down" portion of the cycle.

The client is expected to step up and down on the 12-inch bench at the rate of 24 stepping cycles per minute throughout the 3 minute test. With the metronome set at 96 bpm, each 4 beat cycle represents a complete step:

beat #1/ step #1 → right foot up (or left foot up)

beat #2/step #2 → left foot up (or right foot up)

beat #3/step #3 → right foot down (or left foot down)

beat #4/step #4 → left foot down (or right foot down)

Most importantly, clients should be well-aware of sitting immediately and beginning the recovery pulse count within 5 seconds after the 3 minute stepping period. A full-minute recovery heart rate is counted either by palpating the radial or carotid artery, or by stethoscope (the preferred method) and is recorded in beats per minute. Clients should carefully count

the recovery heart rate, since the rhythm during recovery can change quickly. The full-minute pulse rate reflects the heart rate at the end of stepping and the rate of recovery from the stepping.

Once recorded, the recovery heart rate can easily be compared to norms for both men and women of different ages. (Tables 6.5 & 6.6). For example, a 36-year-old man performs the step test and records 110 bpm for a recovery heart rate. Referring to Table 6.5, a fitness classification for a man who is 36- to 45-years-old with a recovery heart rate of 110 bpm is identified as "average." Be careful to use the appropriate reference norms for men and women, since the norms are sex-specific.

BODY COMPOSITION ASSESSMENT

Obesity accounts for about 15 to 20 percent of the annual mortality rate in the United States. It is linked with hypertension, diabetes mellitus (type II), coronary heart disease and high blood cholesterol. Other conditions commonly associated with obesity are cancer (colon, rectum, breast, gallbladder and prostate), gout, gallstones and respiratory insufficiency.

Table 6.5

NORMS FOR 3 MINUTE STEP TEST — MEN

Fitness Category	Age (Years) 18–25	26 -35	36 - 45	46 -55	56 -65	65+
Excellent	<79	<81	<83	<87	<86	<88
Good	79-89	81-89	83-96	87-97	86-97	88-96
Above Average	90-99	90-99	97-103	98-105	98-103	97-103
Average	100-105	100-107	104-112	106-116	104-112	104-113
Below Average	106-116	108-117	113-119	117-122	113-120	114-120
Poor	117-128	118-128	120-130	123-132	121-129	121-130
Very Poor	>128	>128	>130	>132	>129	>130

Source: Adapted from Golding et al. (1989). Reprinted with permission.

Table 6.6

NORMS FOR 3 MINUTE STEP TEST — WOMEN

Fitness Category	Age (Years) 18–25	26 -35	36 - 45	46 -55	56 -65	65+
Excellent	<85	<88	<90	<94	<95	<90
Good	85-98	88-99	90-102	94-104	95-104	90-102
Above Average	99-108	100-111	103-110	105-115	105-112	103-115
Average	109-117	112-119	111-118	116-120	113-118	116-122
Below Average	118-126	120-126	119-128	121-126	119-128	123-128
Poor	127-140	127-138	129-140	127-135	129-139	129-134
Very Poor	>140	>138	>140	>135	>139	>134

Source: Adapted from Golding et al. (1989). Reprinted with permission.

Americans spend tens of billions of dollars attempting to lose weight either through weight-reduction centers or diets. Considering that an American adult will have gained an average of 15 pounds since the early 1980s, it is little wonder that people have focused so much on weight reduction in this country. Despite such weight reducing options available, a more important public health concern is the body composition of individuals, not body weight. Accordingly, **body composition assessment** skills are essential for most fitness professionals in order to examine this important element of health-related fitness.

Definitions

Body composition assessment refers to identifying the fat and nonfat elements of body weight. Typically, assessment of body composition is based upon a two-compartment model; **fat mass** is determined from body weight and the remainder of body weight is referred to as fat-free mass, or **lean body mass**. In a two-compartment model, lean body mass is predominantly comprised of muscle and bone, while fat mass is strictly related to total body fat stores, including adipose tissue. Whenever body composition is discussed, the terms overweight and obese or overfat are commonly used. However, a clear distinction between these terms is necessary.

Overweight refers to excess weight (usually greater than 10 percent above ideal body weight) relative to a specific height according to established reference tables. **Obese** or overfat are synonymous terms referring to excess accumulation of body fat stores, which adversely affects health and is discussed below. Moreover, obesity is commonly identified when a person becomes more than 20 percent over ideal body weight, or at least twice what it is to be merely overweight.

Although body fat is commonly viewed as unimportant for normal human functions, it should be noted that total body fat is classified into two types: essential and storage fat. **Essential body fat** is necessary for normal physiological function; it insulates nerves and protects vital organs, and if eliminated, human health and function deteriorates. Normally, essential body fat constitutes about 3 percent of the total body fat in men and about 12 percent in women. The reason for such a difference between sexes in essential fat is that there is sex-specific fat, such as breast tissue, found in women only.

Storage fat is commonly associated with overweight or overfat persons. Storage fat refers to adipose tissue depots. This type of fat surrounds internal body organs for protection, and at least 50 percent of storage fat is found just under the skin and is called **subcutaneous fat.** Subcutaneous fat can be separated by connective tissue, which gives a dimpled look to the skin, commonly referred to as cellulite.

Cellulite is storage fat that contains proteins that attract water and tends to have a lattice-like indentation appearance. Although men and women usually possess excess storage fat, there is not much difference between sexes in the amount of storage fat, except that men tend to preferentially store body fat around the waist and women tend to accumulate body fat in the hips and thighs.

Knowing that many clients join a health club or fitness center to lose body weight or body fat, the fitness professional should evaluate body composition as a routine part of the overall fitness testing and evaluation. Proper guidance regarding weight loss, as well as periodic follow-up evaluations of body composition, can be easily performed and provide motivation to all clients, especially those attempting to lose weight. Moreover, fitness professionals can recommend a reasonable ideal body weight and develop a sound exercise program for those who desire to lose weight based on accurate, current body composition assessment. However, fitness professionals must exercise care with those clients who are obese and should be referred to appropriate weight-control specialists.

Measurement Techniques

There are several ways to indirectly measure body composition. Technological advances have been developed to permit accurate assessment of body composition, such as near-infrared interactance, magnetic resonance imaging, dual energy x-ray absorptiometry, and computed tomography. Despite their accuracy, these assessment methods are very expensive and are impractical for the fitness setting.

In such a venue, the more popular methods used to assess body fat and lean body mass include hydrostatic, or underwater weighing, bioelectric analysis and anthropometric measures.

Hydrostatic Weighing. **Hydrostatic**, or underwater weighing, is commonly referred to as the "gold standard" for body composition analysis. The premise of this technique is that body fat is less dense than water, while fat-free mass (bone and muscle tissue) is more dense. Consequently, fat will tend to float and weigh less in water than a corresponding amount of bone and muscle tissue.

When a person is weighed hydrostatically, complete submersion under water and maximal exhalation are required. Even though a maximal exhalation is performed, a small amount of air remains in the lungs. This **residual lung volume** should be measured; however, it can be estimated using a formula, but this may compromise the accuracy of body fat assessment.

Body density is determined from the relationship of body weight in air to underwater weight (corrected for residual lung volume). From body density, body fat is calculated and expressed relative to body weight. Although hydrostatic weighing is accurate, it is time-consuming to perform, requires expensive equipment and specially trained personnel, and is impractical for most fitness settings.

Bioelectric Impedance Analysis. A more recently developed technique used to assess body composition is **bioelectric impedance**

analysis (BIA). The premise of BIA is that lean body mass is composed of water and has a high electrolyte content, which allows for an electrical conductivity much higher than fat mass, while a higher fat mass tends to impede electrical conductivity. By placing four electrodes on the skin of the body in the supine position, conductance of a weak and imperceptible electrical current is measured. A greater electrical conductance suggests little impedance and is associated with higher lean body mass, or body density, while a lesser electrical conductance suggests impedance of the electric current and is related to a higher body fat mass.

Early research suggested that BIA was not very accurate, but recent research has refined this technique to be more applicable to the average person. To reliably or consistently measure body composition via BIA, each client must be well-hydrated, as this test is affected by dehydration, and no exercise should be performed within 4 to 6 hours of measurement.

BIA is a very quick and easy-to-administer technique; however, the measuring device can cost between $550 and $3,500, depending on its computerized capabilities. Despite its potential utility, BIA cannot yet be accurately used on all clientele, especially the very obese or lean, and the elderly. For persons who are at the extremes of the body fat continuum (either very lean or very fat), BIA is not very accurate, as lean body mass is overestimated in obese and underestimated in lean athletes. For the elderly, there is little research to indicate the relative accuracy of this method on persons over 65 years of age. Thus, caution should be taken before BIA is used.

Anthropometric Measurements. **Anthropometric measurements** are commonly used in the fitness industry to assess body composition. Anthropometric techniques are relatively easy to administer because they involve the measurement of varied combinations of skinfolds, girths and body weight.

Skinfold assessment is one of the most popular measures used to estimate body fat. Measurement of skinfolds affords fitness professionals an accurate, reliable and inexpensive method to assess body composition. The skinfold technique is designed to measure subcutaneous fat deposits, since approximately 50 percent of body fat stores is located just beneath the skin. With a relationship existing between subcutaneous fat and overall body density, measurements of skinfolds can be used to evaluate body composition.

Skinfold calipers measure the thickness of skinfolds in millimeters (mm). When skinfold measures are properly taken from a variety of sites, a higher value indicates a greater amount of fat stored beneath the skin and therefore a lower body density, and vice versa. The values obtained are applied to an appropriate formula to calculate body fat and fat-free percentages.

The recommended procedures for measuring skinfold thickness are:
• Standardize the measurement of all skinfolds by using the right side of the body;
• Identify the anatomical location of skinfold;
• Grasp the skinfold using the thumb and forefinger(s) of the left hand;
• Hold the calipers perpendicular to the skinfold and place the caliper pads on the anatomical skinfold site, while maintaining grasp of the skinfold;
• Within 2 to 3 seconds of releasing the caliper trigger, read the dial to the nearest 0.5 mm;
• A minimum of two repeat measures should be taken at each skinfold site to ensure accuracy; repeat measures should follow techniques for measurement;
• Measurements should be taken at

least 15 seconds apart to allow skinfold site to return to normal;

• Repeat measures of skinfold site thickness should be within ± 1mm.

The accurate prediction of body fat based on skinfold thickness is dependent upon a number of factors, including proper anatomical site location, tester's experience in skinfold assessment and use of appropriate formulas for predicting body fat. In addition, skinfold assessment should not be performed when the skin is moist, nor on clients who just finished an exercise workout, as a shift in body fluids toward the skin causes overestimation of skinfold thickness. Fitness professionals measuring skinfolds should be trained in proper measurement technique by an experienced associate who is familiar with anatomical landmarks and proper skinfold measurement techniques.

There are many equations for estimating body composition on the basis of skinfold measurements. Most are population-specific; that is, they are based on norms established for subjects of a certain age, sex and/or sport. Because fitness professionals come into contact with clientele of all ages and backgrounds, it is appropriate to utilize equations that are relatively quick, easy and generalizable to the population at large.

Two equations developed by Jackson and Pollock (1985) are intended for use in the general population. Each of these equations is based on the sum of three skinfold site measures. For women, skinfold measures are taken at the following sites:

1. Triceps (Fig. 6.4): A vertical skinfold taken on the back of the upper arm, halfway between the acromial (shoulder) and olecranon (elbow) processes;

2. Suprailium (Fig. 6.5): A diagonal skinfold taken above the crest of the ilium at the intersection of an imaginary anterior

axillary line;

3. Thigh (Fig. 6.6): A vertical skinfold taken midway between the hip and knee joints on front of the thigh.

For men, skinfold measures are taken at the following sites:

1. Chest (Fig. 6.7): A diagonal skinfold taken halfway between the anterior axillary line (crease of the underarm) and nipple;

2. Abdomen (Fig. 6.8): A vertical skinfold taken about 1 inch lateral to the umbilicus;

3. Thigh (Fig. 6.9): A vertical skinfold taken midway between the hip and knee joints on front of the thigh.

Once accurate measures are obtained for each site, add the three values, and refer to Table 6.7 for women or Table 6.8 for men to obtain an estimate of body fat percentage.

For example, Jane, a 48-year-old woman with skinfold measurements of 28 mm for thigh, 15 mm for triceps, and 22 mm for suprailium, has a value of 65 mm for the sum of three skinfolds. By referring to Table 6.7, a woman of 48 years with a sum of skinfolds of 65 mm has a body fat equivalent to 27.2 percent.

Because these tables were developed on men and women between 18 and 61 years, it is recommended that their use be restricted to persons of this age range. Also, because these tables can be generalized to a large population, the standard error of the body fat estimate is about ± 3.6 percent and ± 3.9 percent for men and women, respectively. Thus, in the above example, women who are estimated to have a body fat of 27.2 percent could normally range between 31.1 percent and 23.3 percent. Hence, it important to acknowledge the inherent error when using such body fat estimations.

How is the body fat percentage interpreted? General guidelines assist fitness

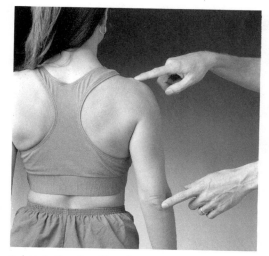

a. Locate the site midway between the acromial (shoulder) and olecranon (elbow) processes.

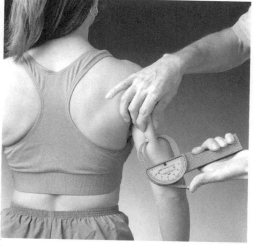

b. Grasp a vertical fold on the posterior midline of the upper arm.

Figure 6.4
Tricep measurement for women.

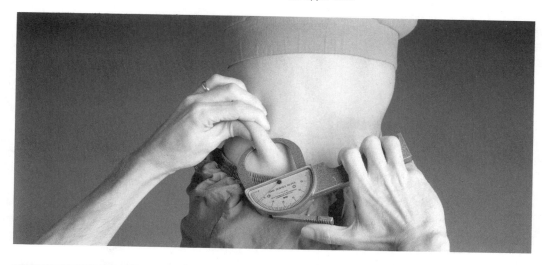

Figure 6.5
Suprailium measurement for women: Grasp a diagonal skinfold just above the crest of the Ilium, where an imaginary anterior axillary line intersects.

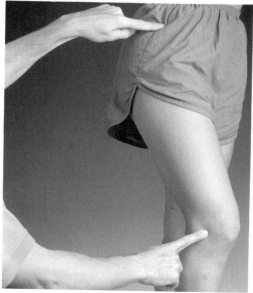

a. Locate the hip and the knee joints and find the midpoint on the anterior (top) of the thigh.

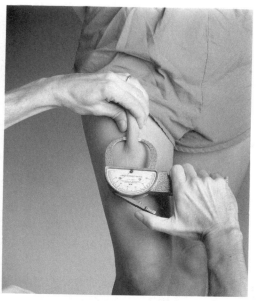

b. Grasp a vertical skinfold with the thumb and forefinger and pull it away from the body.

Figure 6.6
Thigh measurement for women.

professionals with interpreting body fat percentages. By referring to norms in Table 6.9, clientele can be classified on the continuum of health and fitness. In this table, there is no reference to age; creeping obesity is known to have ill effects on health and it is suggested to not allow for increased body fat with increasing age. It is highly recommended that men and women strive to attain a body fat that can be maintained and is associated with a low health risk, such as "healthy" body fat.

It is not precisely known what optimal body weight or percent body fat is necessary for health or physical performance for all persons. Once the percent body fat calculation is known, fitness professionals can help to develop realistic goals for clients, use a formula to calculate upper and lower desirable body weights, and monitor progress. To calculate desirable body weight, lean body weight must be determined. Lean body weight is derived by subtracting the body fat percentage from 100 percent, then multiplying this percentage by total body weight. Once lean body weight is derived, desirable

Table 6.7

PERCENT BODY FAT ESTIMATIONS FOR WOMEN

Sum of Skinfolds (mm)	Age Groups Under 22	23–27	28–32	33–37	38–42	43–47	48–52	53–57	Over 57
23–25	9.7	9.9	10.2	10.4	10.7	10.9	11.2	11.4	11.7
26–28	11.0	11.2	11.5	11.7	12.0	12.3	12.5	12.7	13.0
29–31	12.3	12.5	12.8	13.0	13.3	13.5	13.8	14.0	14.3
32–34	13.6	13.8	14.0	14.3	14.5	14.8	15.0	15.3	15.5
35–37	14.8	15.0	15.3	15.5	15.8	16.0	16.3	16.5	16.8
38–40	16.0	16.3	16.5	16.7	17.0	17.2	17.5	17.7	18.0
41–43	17.2	17.4	17.7	17.9	18.2	18.4	18.7	18.9	19.2
44–46	18.3	18.6	18.8	19.1	19.3	19.6	19.8	20.1	20.3
47–49	19.5	19.7	20.0	20.2	20.5	20.7	21.0	21.2	21.5
50–52	20.6	20.8	21.1	21.3	21.6	21.8	22.1	22.3	22.6
53–55	21.7	21.9	22.1	22.4	22.6	22.9	23.1	23.4	23.6
56–58	22.7	23.0	23.2	23.4	23.7	23.9	24.2	24.4	24.7
59–61	23.7	24.0	24.2	24.5	24.7	25.0	25.2	25.5	25.7
62–64	24.7	25.0	25.2	25.5	25.7	26.0	26.7	26.4	26.7
65–67	25.7	25.9	26.2	26.4	26.7	26.9	27.2	27.4	27.7
68–70	26.6	26.9	27.1	27.4	27.6	27.9	28.1	28.4	28.6
71–73	27.5	27.8	28.0	28.3	28.5	28.8	29.0	29.3	29.5
74–76	28.4	28.7	28.9	29.2	29.4	29.7	29.9	30.2	30.4
77–79	29.3	29.5	29.8	30.0	30.3	30.5	30.8	31.0	31.3
80–82	30.1	30.4	30.6	30.9	31.1	31.4	31.6	31.9	32.1
83–85	30.9	31.2	31.4	31.7	31.9	32.2	32.4	32.7	32.9
86–88	31.7	32.0	32.2	32.5	32.7	32.9	33.2	33.4	33.7
89–91	32.5	32.7	33.0	33.2	33.5	33.7	33.9	34.2	34.4
92–94	33.2	33.4	33.7	33.9	34.2	34.4	34.7	34.9	35.2
95–97	33.9	34.1	34.4	34.6	34.9	35.1	35.4	35.6	35.9
98–100	34.6	34.8	35.1	35.3	35.5	35.8	36.0	36.3	36.5
101–103	35.3	35.4	35.7	35.9	36.2	36.4	36.7	36.9	37.2
104–106	35.8	36.1	36.3	36.6	36.8	37.1	37.3	37.5	37.8
107–109	36.4	36.7	36.9	37.1	37.4	37.6	37.9	38.1	38.4
110–112	37.0	37.2	37.5	37.7	38.0	38.2	38.5	38.7	38.9
113–115	37.5	37.8	38.0	38.2	38.5	38.7	39.0	39.2	39.5
116–118	38.0	38.3	38.5	38.8	39.0	39.3	39.5	39.7	40.0
119–121	38.5	38.7	39.0	39.2	39.5	39.7	40.0	40.2	40.5
122–124	39.0	39.2	39.4	39.7	39.9	40.2	40.4	40.7	40.9
125–127	39.4	39.6	39.9	40.1	40.4	40.6	40.9	41.1	41.4
128–130	39.8	40.0	40.3	40.5	40.8	41.0	41.3	41.5	41.8

Source: Jackson, A.S. & Pollock, M.L.: Practical Assessment of Body Composition. (May 1985). Reprinted with permission of McGraw-Hill.

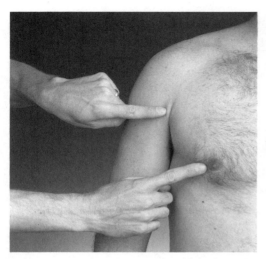

a. Locate the site midway between the anterior axillary line and nipple.

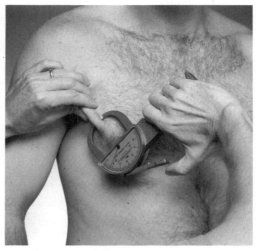

b. Grasp a diagonal fold.

Figure 6.7

Chest skinfold measurement for men.

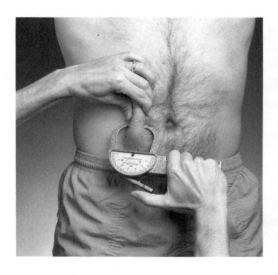

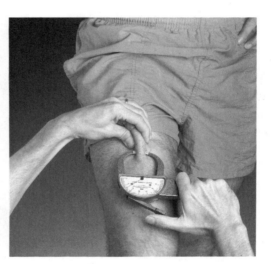

Figure 6.8 (left)

Abdominal skinfold measurement for men. Grasp vertical skinfold 2- 2.5 centimeters lateral (left) of the umbilicus.

Figure 6.9 (right)

Thigh skinfold measurement for men. Grasp a vertical skinfold with the thumb and forefinger and pull it away from the body (use Fig. 6.6a to determine location).

body weight is determined.

The formulas for determining lean body weight and desirable body weight are:

Lean body weight = (1.00 - percent fat) x body weight

Desirable body weight = lean body weight/(1.00 - percent fat desired)

For example, if a man weighs 220 pounds and is measured at 25 percent fat, and would like to be 20 percent fat, the desirable body weight can be calculated as follows:

Lean body weight = (1.00 - percent fat) x body weight

Step 1: Place all values into the lean body weight formula (body fat is expressed as a decimal):

Lean body weight = (1.00 - .25) x 220 lbs

Step 2: Subtract numbers within parentheses and multiply by weight to derive lean body weight:

Lean body weight = (.75) x 220 lbs

Lean body weight = 165 lbs

Step 3: Place values into the desirable body weight formula:

Desirable body weight = Lean body weight/(1.00 - percent fat desired)

Desirable body weight = 165 lbs/ (1.00 - .20)

Step 4: Subtract numbers within parentheses and divide lean body weight by desirable lean percentage:

Desirable body weight = 165 lbs/.80, or Desirable body weight = 206.3 lbs

Thus, if this man continues to exercise and does not change his eating habits significantly as he loses about 14 pounds, his body fat will decrease from an estimated 25 percent to an estimated 20 percent. Although a desirable body fat percentage can be difficult to achieve, it is recommended that the fitness professional establish a range of desirable body fat percentages to assist clients is achieving realistic goals.

The range should provide an upper and lower limit so that a desirable body weight range can be calculated.

Other Methods of Anthropometric Evaluation

Traditionally, recommended weight or ideal body weight has been determined through standardized height-weight tables based on age and frame size. Clinical settings regularly utilize such tables to recommend appropriate weight for clients

Table 6.8

PERCENT BODY FAT ESTIMATIONS FOR MEN

Sum of Skinfolds(mm)	Age Groups Under 22	23–27	28–32	33–37	38–42	43–47	48–52	53–57	Over 57
8–10	1.3	1.8	2.3	2.9	3.4	3.9	4.5	5.0	5.5
11–13	2.2	2.8	3.3	3.9	4.4	4.9	5.5	6.0	6.5
14–16	3.2	3.8	4.3	4.8	5.4	5.9	6.4	7.0	7.5
17–19	4.2	4.7	5.3	5.8	6.3	6.9	7.4	8.0	8.5
20–22	5.1	5.7	6.2	6.8	7.3	7.9	8.4	8.9	9.5
23–25	6.1	6.6	7.2	7.7	8.3	8.8	9.4	9.9	10.5
26–28	7.0	7.6	8.1	8.7	9.2	9.8	10.3	10.9	11.4
29–31	8.0	8.5	9.1	9.6	10.2	10.7	11.3	11.8	12.4
32–34	8.9	9.4	10.0	10.5	11.1	11.6	12.2	12.8	13.3
35–37	9.8	10.4	10.9	11.5	12.0	12.6	13.1	13.7	14.3
38–40	10.7	11.3	11.8	12.4	12.9	13.5	14.1	14.6	15.2
41–43	11.6	12.2	12.7	13.3	13.8	14.4	15.0	15.5	16.1
44–46	12.5	13.1	13.6	14.2	14.7	15.3	15.9	16.4	17.0
47–49	13.4	13.9	14.5	15.1	15.6	16.2	16.8	17.3	17.9
50–52	14.3	14.8	15.4	15.9	16.5	17.1	17.6	18.2	18.8
53–55	15.1	15.7	16.2	16.8	17.4	17.9	18.5	19.1	19.7
56–58	16.0	16.5	17.1	17.7	18.2	18.8	19.4	20.0	20.5
59–61	16.9	17.4	17.9	18.5	19.1	19.7	20.2	20.8	21.4
62–64	17.6	18.2	18.8	19.4	19.9	20.5	21.1	21.7	22.2
65–67	18.5	19.0	19.6	20.2	20.8	21.3	21.9	22.5	23.1
68–70	19.3	19.9	20.4	21.0	21.6	22.2	22.7	23.3	23.9
71–73	20.1	20.7	21.2	21.8	22.4	23.0	23.6	24.1	24.7
74–76	20.9	21.5	22.0	22.6	23.2	23.8	24.4	25.0	25.5
77–79	21.7	22.2	22.8	23.4	24.0	24.6	25.2	25.8	26.3
80–82	22.4	23.0	23.6	24.2	24.8	25.4	25.9	26.5	27.1
83–85	23.2	23.8	24.4	25.0	25.5	26.1	26.7	27.3	27.9
86–88	24.0	24.5	25.1	25.7	26.3	26.9	27.5	28.1	28.7
89–91	24.7	25.3	25.9	26.5	27.1	27.6	28.2	28.8	29.4
92–94	25.4	26.0	26.6	27.2	27.8	28.4	29.0	29.6	30.2
95–97	26.1	26.7	27.3	27.9	28.5	29.1	29.7	30.3	30.9
98–100	26.9	27.4	28.0	28.6	29.2	29.8	30.4	31.0	31.6
101–103	27.5	28.1	28.7	29.3	29.9	30.5	31.1	31.7	32.3
104–106	28.2	28.8	29.4	30.0	30.6	31.2	31.8	32.4	33.0
107–109	28.9	29.5	30.1	30.7	31.3	31.9	32.5	33.1	33.7
110–112	29.6	30.2	30.8	31.4	32.0	32.6	33.2	33.8	34.4
113–115	30.2	30.8	31.4	32.0	32.6	33.2	33.8	34.5	35.1
116–118	30.9	31.5	32.1	32.7	33.3	33.9	34.5	35.1	35.7
119–121	31.5	32.1	32.7	33.3	33.9	34.5	35.1	35.7	36.4
122–124	32.1	32.7	33.3	33.9	34.5	35.1	35.8	36.4	37.0
125–127	32.7	33.3	33.9	34.5	35.1	35.8	36.4	37.0	37.6

Source: Jackson, A.S. & Pollock, M.L.: Practical Assessment of Body Composition. (May 1985). Reprinted with permission of McGraw-Hill.

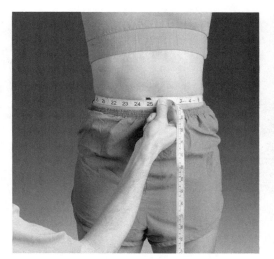

a. Waist measurement.

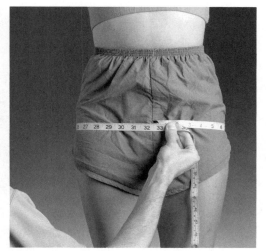

b. Hip measurement.

Figure 6.10
Waist and hip
measurements.

because of the relationship with mortality rates, as well as their simplicity of measurement and calculation, and low cost. Although such tables reflect the degree of excess weight and are easy to administer, body composition is not evaluated. Moreover, the derivation of height-weight tables is based upon a selected population (insurance policyholders) that is predominantly represented by young Caucasians. Thus, the reference of such tables to the average American may not be appropriate. Additionally, there is some controversy regarding an appropriate definition of ideal body weight (What is ideal body weight in reference to health, physical appearance or performance?).

The ability of height-weight tables to identify appropriate body weight is not very accurate, especially in younger adults. For example, young men and women who engage in strength-training regimes can tend to have a significant amount of muscle mass. Because the standardized tables address appropriate weight for a given height without consideration for composition, many persons who possess augmented muscle mass will be identified as overweight for their height, even though they are relatively lean and don't have much body fat.

Accordingly, the use of height-weight tables to determine appropriate body weight, let alone identify body composition, should be viewed with extreme caution because of the limitations cited above.

When assessing persons who are slightly overfat or obese, it is recommended to examine regional fat distribution, since the development of obesity has been linked to both genetics and environment. Recent research suggests that persons who tend to preferentially store body fat in the abdominal area (apple-shaped) are at higher risk for cardiorespiratory disease and type II diabetes, than those who have a similar amount of total body fat and tend to accumulate body fat in the hips and thighs (pear-shaped). Consequently, the terms pear-shaped versus apple-shaped have assumed far greater meaning when dealing with overweight persons.

Waist-to-hip Ratio. One means of addressing regional fat distribution in overweight clientele is to assess and compare circumferences of the waist and hip, referred to as the waist-to-hip ratio (WHR). To determine this ratio, the accurate measurement of both waist and hip circumferences is essential (Fig. 6.10).

Such measurements should be taken

Table 6.9

NORMS FOR BODY FAT PERCENTAGE OF ADULTS

Classification		% Fat Women	% Fat Men
Essential Fat		11.0–14.0	3.0–5.0
Storage Fat	Lean	<12	<7
	Healthy	13–20	8–15
	Slightly	21–25	16–20
Overfat	Fat	26–32	21–24
	Obese	>32	≥25

according to the procedures indicated:

• Use a nonelastic measuring tape;

• Record circumference in inches or centimeters;

• Have client wear minimal clothing (e.g., swimsuit) for accurate measurement;

• Waist circumference (most narrow abdominal girth at the umbilicus level);

• Hip circumference (largest girth of the buttocks)

The waist and hip measurements can then be expressed as a ratio according to this formula:

WHR = Waist circumference/Hip circumference

The use of this formula is very simple. For example, a woman's circumference measurements for waist and hip are 38 inches and 47 inches, respectively; these can be applied to the WHR formula as illustrated:

Step 1: Divide waist by hip measurement

WHR = 38 in./47 in.

WHR = 0.81

The value obtained—0.81—is the ratio of waist-to-hip for this woman. In general, a WHR above 0.95 for men and 0.85 for women place clients at increased risk of heart disease. Thus, fitness professionals can easily identify clients at risk and make appropriate physician referral.

Body Mass Index. The use of Quetelet's Index, or **body mass index** (BMI), is a unique

expression of height-to-weight and is more closely related to body fatness, as determined through hydrostatic weighing than are standardized height-weight tables. From this index, a high BMI is positively associated with hypertension, high blood cholesterol levels and cardiorespiratory disease.

As with height-weight tables, using BMI is very inexpensive and is easy to administer. Simple body weight scales that are reasonably accurate and calibrated, along with a stadiometer to measure height (a vertical ruler with right-angle measuring device) can be purchased at low cost. Most importantly, measurement of body weight and height should be standardized.

Body weight should be measured with minimal clothing, no shoes, and at similar times of the day on follow-up measures. Body height should be measured without shoes, heels together, person standing at attention with his or her back, buttocks, shoulders and head touching the wall after inhaling fully.

Height-to-weight expressed as BMI is characterized in the following formula:

BMI (kg/m^2) = Body Weight (kg)/ Height (m^2)

To use this formula, body weight must be expressed in kilograms (kg) (divide pounds by 2.2), as presented earlier. Also, height must be expressed in meters

AMERICAN COUNCIL ON EXERCISE

Body composition
assessment/
Musculoskeletal
fitness assessment

179

squared (m^2). Deriving the BMI for a man weighing 195 pounds and 5-feet-6-inches tall is illustrated below.

Step 1: Convert body weight from pounds to kilograms:

195 lbs/2.2 = 88.64 kg

Step 2: Normally body height is measured in inches; thus, record body height to the nearest one fourth of an inch and convert to inches:

5 feet 6 inches is easily converted to 66 inches

Step 3: Convert inches into centimeters (cm) by multiplying inches by 2.54:

cm = 66 inches x 2.54 cm per 1 inch
cm = 167.6

Step 4: Convert centimeters into meters (m) by dividing cm by 100:

m = 167.6/100
m = 1.676

Step 5: Square meters to convert to m^2:
m^2 = 2.81

Step 6: Place values into formula:
BMI = 88.64 (kg)/2.81 (m^2)
BMI (kg/m^2) = 31.54

From this example, this man exhibits a BMI value of 31.54 kg/m^2. This is evaluated by referring to general guidelines established when using the BMI; those clients requiring special weight-loss counseling can be easily identified (Table 6.10).

In evaluating the BMI for all clients, note that men are classified as obese with a BMI of 27.8 kg/m^2 or greater and that obese women have a BMI of 27.3 kg/m^2 or greater. Hence, using the BMI value is helpful to better address body fatness if other equipment is not available. Although more precise than typical height-weight tables, easy to administer at low cost and comparable across populations, the BMI is difficult to interpret to clients.

Consequently, the BMI may not be a useful tool to help a client determine the need to lose weight. In addition, it lacks the measurement sensitivity to reflect changes in body composition in follow-up visits.

MUSCULOSKELETAL FITNESS ASSESSMENT

In addition to evaluating CRF and body composition, fitness professionals should perform musculoskeletal fitness assessment (MSF). Because clients engage in activities that require varying levels of musculoskeletal fitness, assessing it can assist the fitness instructor in developing an individualized exercise program targeted toward comprehensive health-related fitness.

As previously shown in Fig. 6.1, MSF is comprised of three components, including muscular strength, muscular endurance and joint flexibility or range of motion.

Muscular Strength and Endurance Assessment

Adequate muscular strength and endurance are prerequisites for normal daily living activities and for engaging in varying levels of physical exercise.

In large part, muscular endurance depends upon muscular strength. Therefore, an important relationship exists between muscular strength and endurance. Muscular strength is defined as the maximum amount of force that a muscle can produce in a single effort. Muscular endurance is defined as the number of times a muscle

Table 6.10

BMI VALUES FOR ADULT MEN AND WOMEN

Desirable Range	20–25.0 kg/m²
Grade 1 Obesity	25–29.9 kg/m²
Grade 2 Obesity	30–40.0 kg/m²
Grade 3 Obesity (morbidly obese)	>40.0 kg/m²

Source: Jequier (1987).

repeatedly exerts a submaximal force or as the length of time a given muscular force can be sustained. Conceptually, when activities require a greater degree of one's muscular strength, then muscular endurance is shortened.

Given these two muscle functions, fitness tests have been developed to assess each of these as independent entities, or in combination. Usually, dynamic strength of major muscle groups is measured with a 1 repetition maximum test, commonly known as 1-RM. This involves the determination of the maximal amount of weight that can be lifted one time.

Short of conducting 1-RM testing, the measurement of muscular strength is difficult and requires well-trained professionals to supervise the testing session. Despite the validity of 1-RM testing, it is not practical for many settings and requires extensive equipment, such as barbells or multistation weight machines for assessment.

Measurement of muscular endurance or combined muscular strength and endurance performance can be assessed through easily administered fitness tests that don't require elaborate equipment, yet are valid and reliable and afford normative data for sex and age-related comparisons. Given that muscular strength and endurance are specific to each muscle group (triceps, hamstrings, biceps, quadriceps, pectorals), no single test is available to assess whole body muscular strength and endurance.

The following tests are recommended to evaluate muscular strength and endurance in fitness settings.

Push-up Test. The purpose of the push-up test is to evaluate muscular strength and endurance of the upper body, including triceps, anterior deltoid and pectoralis muscles. The standard push-up position is used for men, with only the hands and toes contacting the floor (Fig. 6.11a). The modified push-up position is used for women (Fig. 6.11b). Although the positions are different between sexes, the procedures for administering the test are similar, as described below.

Required items:

• Recording sheet, with name of client and space for recording push-ups completed

Preparation before test day:

• Explain the purpose of the test to each participant (to determine how many push-ups can be completed to reflect muscular strength and endurance);

• Review standard and bent-knee positions, and make sure that the hands are shoulder-width apart;

• Review the test counting: complete push-up is when the chest touches the fist of a partner and returns to the start position with arms fully extended;

• Allow clients to practice, if desired;

• Inform clients of proper breathing technique—to exhale on effort (when pushing away from the floor);

Figure 6.11

Push-up test.

a. Standard push-up position.

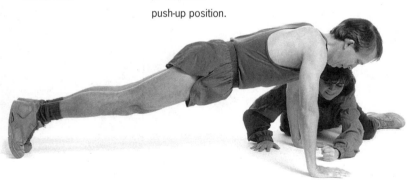

b. Modified push-up position.

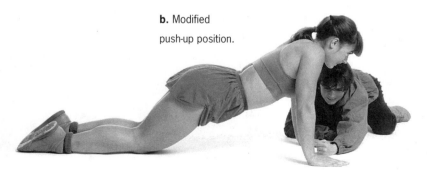

• Inform clients of proper clothing for the push-up test.

Administration:

• Have clients select a partner (or assign partners);

• Identify the exerciser and counter;

• Have exerciser assume the standard (for men) or bent-knee (for women) position, while the counter assumes a position in front of exerciser with fist below the chest;

• When ready, the exerciser can begin and the counter counts the total number of push-ups until exhaustion;

• Most importantly, rest is allowed in the UP position only!

• The score is the total number of push-ups performed.

From the push-up test, the fitness instructor can classify muscular strength and endurance for men and women by referring to Table 6.11. For example, a man of 52 years who performs 18 push-ups is classified as "above average" for his age.

Bent-knee Curl-up Test. The purpose of the bent-knee curl-up test is to evaluate abdominal muscle strength and endurance. Previous sit-up tests have been viewed with dissatisfaction because the hip flexor involvement during sit-up motion is potentially harmful to the low back, particularly when the feet are held motionless, as increased stress is created on the lumbar vertebrae. Even though modifications to the traditional sit-up have been instituted, including a bent-knee position, stress to the low back is still present during the sit-up movement. Consequently, the bent-knee curl-up test was recently modified to eliminate potential low-back problems and better assess abdominal muscle function. Moreover, the curl-up test remains inexpensive and easy to administer, is valid and reliable and affords standards for comparing men and women of similar ages.

The procedures for administering the bent-knee curl-up test are presented as follows:

Required items:

• Padded flooring or mat to conduct test;

• Metronome or cadence device set at 40 bpm;

• Recording sheet, with name of client and space to record number of curl-ups.

Preparation before test day:

• Explain the purpose of the test to each client (to determine how many curl-ups can be done to a set cadence without time constraints);

• Review and demonstrate the curl-up test, and allow client(s) to practice, if desired;

• Inform client(s) of proper clothing

Table 6.11

PUSH-UP NORMS FOR MEN AND WOMEN BY AGE GROUPS USING NUMBER COMPLETED

Age (Years) Gender	(15–19) M	F	(20–29) M	F	(30–39) M	F	(40–49) M	F	(50–59) M	F	(60–69) M	F
Excellent	≥39	≥33	≥36	≥30	≥30	≥27	≥22	≥24	≥21	≥21	≥18	≥17
Above Average	29–38	25–32	29–35	21–29	22–29	20–26	17–21	15–23	13–20	11–20	11–17	12–16
Average	23–28	18–24	22–28	15–20	17–21	13–19	13–16	11–14	10–12	7–10	8–10	5–11
Below Average	18–22	12–17	17–21	10–14	12–16	8–12	10–12	5–10	7–9	2–6	5–7	1–4
Poor	≤17	≤11	≤16	≤9	≤11	≤7	≤9	≤4	≤6	≤1	<4	≤1

Source: CSTF Operations Manual (Third Edition) Ottawa, Fitness and Amateur Sport, 1986. The Canadian Standardized Test of Fitness was developed by, and is reproduced with the permission of Fitness Canada, Government of Canada.

and footwear for the test.

Administration:

• For each client, two strips of tape should be placed parallel and 8 cm apart;

• Have client(s) actively warm-up before start of test;

• Pair-up clients if more than two for testing;

• Have client(s) assume a lying position with feet flat on the floor (knee bent about 90 degrees) and hands palm-down with the fingertips touching the first strip of tape, while the hands of the tester (partner) are placed behind the head;

• Begin the metronome cadence of 40 bpm—equal to 3 seconds per curl-up or 20 curl-ups per minute;

• When ready, the client slowly flattens the low back and curls the upper spine until the fingertips touch the second strip of tape (Fig. 6.12a);

• This is followed by a return to the orig-inal position with the back of head touching the tester's (partner's) hand (Fig. 6.12b);

• Every time the head touches the tester's hands one curl-up is counted;

• Clients perform as many curl-ups as possible without stopping, up to a maximum of 75;

• When cadence is broken, the test is terminated;

• Identify correct number of curl-ups performed and recorded.

By referring to Table 6.12, a classification of abdominal muscle strength and endurance for both men and women is obtained. For example, suppose a 41-year-old male performed 25 curl-ups during this test. According to the standards presented in the table, his score is considered to be "marginal" for his age. Interpretation of these results suggest that he needs to improve endurance of abdominal musculature.

FLEXIBILITY OR JOINT RANGE OF MOTION ASSESSMENT

Flexibility is the ability of a joint to move throughout its range of motion (ROM). Just as muscular strength and endurance are related to specific muscle groups, so is flexibility related to a specific joint ROM (hip, shoulder, knee, low back). Thus, no single flexibility test can be applied to total body flexibility. Although a variety of instruments measure ROM, many of the health-related fitness tests utilize centimeters or inches of movement, due to their ease of administration and simplicity, compared with more expensive and technically complicated measuring devices, such as goniometers or the Leighton flexometer.

The amount of joint movement is dependent upon age, physical activity, muscle temperature and soft tissue structures, including the joint capsule, muscles, tendons and ligaments. Physical activity usually

Figure 6.12

Curl-up test.

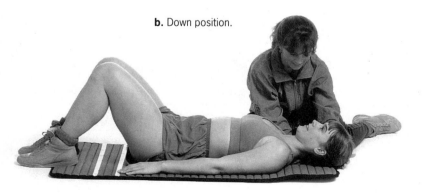

a. Up position.
Alternative tester hand position for added support.

b. Down position.

decreases with age, and this contributes to the reduced joint motion more than the aging process itself. Moreover, muscle temperature is critical for improving flexibility, which supports the rationale for stretching after a cardiovascular workout. Of the soft tissue structures, muscle is the most important modifiable joint structure for improving flexibility. Consequently, fitness professionals need to continue to stress the importance of stretching after each workout.

Fitness professionals have generally overlooked the importance of evaluating flexibility as a part of health-related fitness assessment. Improving and maintaining ROM of each joint is crucial to maintaining functional capabilities of daily living, as well as reducing the likelihood of muscular and joint injuries that directly impact upon quality of life. It has been suggested that good flexibility of the low back and hamstrings appear to be important elements in the treatment and prevention of low-back pain (LBP). Given that up to 80 percent of American adults will be afflicted with some type of LBP, it is imperative that fitness professionals make appropriate evaluation for such flexibility. Thus, tests which assess trunk flexion and back extension are highly recommended.

Canadian Sit-and-reach Test. The purpose of the sit-and-reach test is to assess forward trunk flexion. Administration of the sit-and-reach test is relatively quick, and its reliability is very good when adequate warm-up and joint readiness precedes the test, even though forward trunk flexion is affected by both low-back and posterior leg (hamstring) muscles. Given that limited forward trunk flexion is related to a greater likelihood of low-back problems, assessment of such flexibility is warranted for clientele of fitness programs.

The procedures for administering the sit-and-reach test include:

Required items:
• Sit-and-reach box with footline set to 26 cm (a step test box with a metric "yardstick" works quite well);
• Recording sheet, with name of client and space for recording forward flexion.

Preparation before test day:
• Explain the purpose of the test (to assess forward trunk flexion while seated on the floor and reaching forward as far as possible);
• Stress the importance of warm-up prior to performing this test;
• Review the procedure and have clients practice, if desired;
• Instruct clients on continued breathing while performing the test (don't hold breath);
• Instruct clients to wear clothing that won't restrict forward flexion movement.

Administration:
• Client should warm-up (a brisk walk or bicycle ergometer bout of 10 minutes) and perform sufficient static stretching exercises before administration;
• Have client remove shoes and sit facing the sit-and-reach box;
• Client assumes a position in which feet are flat (heels touching) against the foot box and about 4 to 6 inches apart, with knees fully extended;
• Client extends arms at shoulder level with hands on top of one another, finger-

Musculoskeletal fitness assessment/ Flexibility or joint range of motion assessment

Table 6.12

CURL-UP STANDARDS

Category	Men/Age			Women/Age		
	<35	35–44	>45	<35	35–44	>45
	Number Completed					
Excellent	60	50	40	50	40	30
Good	45	40	25	40	30	15
Marginal	30	25	15	25	15	10
Needs Work	15	10	5	10	6	4

Source: Faulkner et al. (1988).

tips even, and palms down;

• Client reaches forward with the arms and bends at the waist, as far as possible along the measuring scale and holds the position for 1 to 2 seconds, while the tester lightly touches the knees to ensure a straight leg position and records the maximal distance reached in centimeters (Fig. 6.13);

• Have client perform four trials, using the greatest forward flexion score.

The score from the sit-and-reach test can be compared to norms for both men and women, as presented in Table 6.13. For example, a woman of 45 years who has a maximal forward trunk flexion of 33 cm is classified as "average" for her age. Such information is important for the fitness instructor to obtain so that an exercise program can be individualized to the needs of the client without putting the client at risk for injury.

Back Extension Test. Imrie and Barbuto (1988) have developed a back extension test to assess ROM during slow and controlled spinal extension. In this test, the use of bony landmarks helps the fitness professional to measure consistently the amount of back extension.

Previously, back extension exercises have been discouraged by the fitness industry because of misconceptions regarding its usefulness and potential for causing injury to the low back. Certainly, spinal hyperextension is a contraindicated activity; however, spinal extension is a normal

function of the lowback. With physical inactivity, flexibility of most joints is reduced and muscles become stiff, including those muscles that allow for spinal extension. Consequently, the recommended back therapy exercises to help alleviate lowback pain have included both spinal flexion and extension.

The premise of this test is to determine how much back extension is present in clients who perform the movement in a slow and controlled manner, and without using the musculature of the low back. This is a "passive" test of extension, rather than an "active" test, and requires that the low-back musculature not be used.

Fitness professionals need to use such a test to assist in programming more appropriate activities to improve and maintain low-back ROM. The procedures for administering the back extension test are presented below.

Required items:

• Soft mat or flooring for conducting the test;

• Nonelastic measuring tape (preferably in centimeters);

• Recording sheet, with name of client and space to record amount of back extension.

Preparation before test day:

• Explain the purpose of the test (to assess spinal extension, which is a normal movement of the spine, and to compare the value to norms);

• Screen-out clients with a history of low-back pain;

• Stress the importance of warm-up prior to performing this test;

• Review the procedure of passive spinal extension, and have clients practice, if desired;

• Instruct clients to perform the spinal extension in a slow and controlled manner and to avoid using the back muscles to hyperextend;

Figure 6.13

Sit-and-reach

flexibility test.

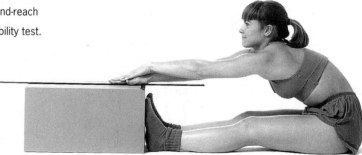

Table 6.13

SIT-AND-REACH NORMS FOR MEN AND WOMEN BY AGE GROUP USING FORWARD TRUNK FLEXION (CM)

Age (Years) Gender	(15–19) M	F	(20–29) M	F	(30–39) M	F	(40–49) M	F	(50–59) M	F	(60–69) M	F
Excellent	≥39	≥43	≥40	≥41	≥38	≥41	≥35	≥38	≥35	≥39	≥33	≥35
Above Average	34-38	38-42	34-39	37-40	33-37	36-40	29-34	34-37	28-34	33-38	25-32	31-34
Average	29-33	34-37	30-33	33-36	28-32	32-35	24-28	30-33	24-27	30-32	20-24	27-30
Below Average	24-28	29-33	25-29	28-32	23-27	27-31	18-23	25-29	16-23	25-29	15-19	23-26
Poor	≤23	≤28	≤24	≤27	≤22	≤26	≤17	≤24	≤15	≤24	≤14	≤23

Source: CSTF Operations Manual (Third Edition) Ottawa, Fitness and Amateur Sport, 1986. The Canadian Standardized Test of Fitness was developed by, and is reproduced with the permission of Fitness Canada, Government of Canada.

• Inform clients of proper clothing to be worn for the test.

Administration:

• Have client warm-up adequately prior to administering this test;

• Have client assume a front-supported position with hands under the shoulders, similar to a push-up position, front of thighs on the mat, and the pelvis in contact with the mat;

• Ensure that the client maintains contact with the mat throughout this test;

• Have the client slowly extend arms as straight as possible, while the pelvis remains on the mat;

• Locate the suprasternal notch and measure the distance from the floor to this anatomical landmark (Fig. 6.14);

• Record the distance of spinal extension in centimeters;

• Repeat this test two or three times for accuracy.

The back extension score obtained can be given a rating, according to Table 6.14. Note that the score is not age-dependent. For example, men of 53 years and 36 years who have a back extension score of 18 cm would be classified in the "marginal" category. This information is essential for fitness professionals to provide safe and effective

exercise programming for clientele.

After the health-related fitness testing is completed, an individualized exercise program can be developed.

EXERCISE PROGRAMMING

When developing an exercise program, fitness professionals must consider far more than just results from fitness tests. Although the majority of information to develop an exercise program will be derived from the health questionnaire, medical approval and health-related fitness evaluation, the process of developing a sound exercise program must address client-related interests and habits as well (Fig. 6.15). Personal interests and exercise habits of clients should be examined to increase the likelihood that the

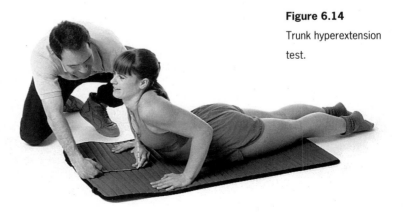

Figure 6.14

Trunk hyperextension test.

Table 6.14

STANDARDS FOR BACK-EXTENSION TEST

Rating	Back Extension (cm)
Excellent	≥30
Good	20-29
Marginal	10-19
Needs Work	≤9

Source: Adapted from Imrie & Barbuto (1988).

exercise regime will not only be safe and effective, but also will be adhered to regularly and established as a lifelong habit.

Although exercise programming should be based largely on the results of health-related fitness testing, the fitness professional must tailor the program to meet the desires, needs, goals and motivation level of the client. In some instances, clients may present physical or orthopedic limitations to specific exercises from either

a recent injury/surgical procedure or chronic condition. Consequently, modification of the exercise program must be made to meet individual needs. Moreover, fitness professionals must use established principles of exercise programming to develop an individualized regimen and educate clients about the benefits of their individualized exercise plan (see Chapter 10, "Adherence and Motivation").

The Conditioning Elements

The purpose of developing a well-rounded exercise program is to improve the health-related fitness of clientele through incorporation of both cardiorespiratory and musculoskeletal elements. Although cardiorespiratory fitness has been the cornerstone of most exercise programs, muscular strength, muscular endurance and flexibility are integral elements of health-related fitness and of a well-rounded conditioning program. Typically, a con-

Figure 6.15

Factors related to exercise program development.

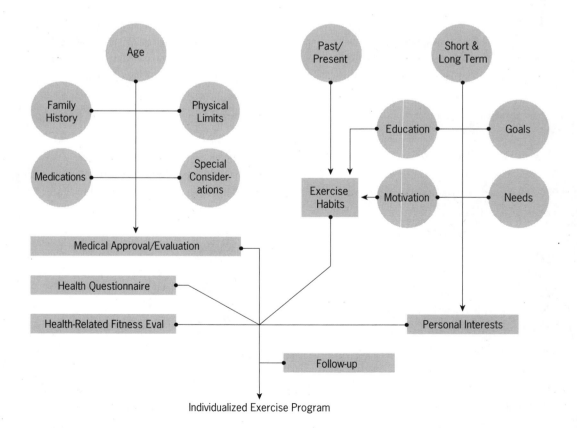

Table 6.15

ELEMENTS OF CONDITIONING PROGRAMS

Phase	Purpose
Warm-up	To gradually increase heart rate & body temperature
	To ensure joint readiness for activity
Aerobic Time	To elevate heart rate for 15-60 min
	55-90% HR max or
	40-85% HR reserve
	Three to five sessions per week
Cool Down	To allow slow, gradual recovery of heart rate
	To prevent pooling of blood in lower extremities
Muscular Time	15-20 minutes of strength/endurance training
	To increase strength & endurance of muscles not used in aerobic activity
	To enhance muscles used in daily living activities
Flexibility Time	15-20 minutes of stretching/flexibility activity
	To increase (maintain) ROM of all joints for activity and daily living activities
	To stretch musculotendinous junctions used during exercise

ditioning program has specific purposes related to each of its of five phases, including warm-up, aerobic time, cool-down, muscular time and flexibility time (Table 6.15) (see also the flexibility and strength training sections of Chapter 9, "Variations, From Step to Strength Training").

It is important that each of these phases be incorporated into the conditioning program and that clientele understand their importance. Health-related fitness assessment can help to identify areas in need of improvement and provides the basis of a well-constructed exercise plan.

Components of CRF Exercise Programs

The design of an exercise program must also incorporate four factors, including frequency of exercise (F), intensity of exercise (I), time or duration of exercise (T), and type or mode of exercise (T). Such factors are important for developing and maintaining cardiorespiratory and musculoskeletal fitness. The initials for each of these factors spell "FITT," an easy acronym to remember.

CRF Guidelines to Exercise Programming

The fitness professional can individualize CRF programs by using the **FITT principle.** Table 6.16 outlines the essential components for health enhancement and improvement in CRF, as recommended by the American College of Sports Medicine (ACSM).

For sedentary and unfit clients, it is recommended that the lower limits of the FITT principle be utilized, whereas most CRF programs tend to engage in exercise of moderate frequency (three to four times per week), intensity (60 to 70 percent heart

Table 6.16

RECOMMENDED COMPONENTS OF CRF EXERCISE PROGRAMS

Frequency *(How often to exercise)*	Three to five days per week
Intensity *(How hard to exercise)*	55-90% of maximal heart rate 40-85% of heart rate reserve or VO_2 max
Time (duration) *(How long to exercise)*	15-60 minutes (continuous)
Type (mode) *(What activity to engage in)*	Large muscle activity, rhythmic; biking/cycling, walking/hiking, jogging/running, aerobic dance (low impact), step aerobics, swimming, aquacize, rowing, stair-climbers

Source: ACSM (1991).

rate reserve), and duration (30 to 40 minutes). Fitness professionals must understand how each of these factors in the FITT principle interrelate and how to modify such elements in order to individualize the exercise program.

From the FITT principle, the most difficult, yet critical aspect of developing a proper exercise program identifies how hard a client should exercise. Typically, **exercise intensity** refers to the severity of the work being performed, such as the speed of walking/jogging, or the pace of music in step aerobics. In other words, intensity indicates how difficult the workout is.

For clients to derive cardiorespiratory benefits from an exercise program, it is imperative that the intensity be closely monitored, especially in newer clientele, so that exercise intensity is not too high. Monitoring and adjusting the exercise intensity is critical to safe and effective exercise programming.

ACSM (1991) recommends that exercise intensity be guided by developing **target heart rate** (THR) **ranges**. THR reflects a safe and effective exercise intensity and is derived by using a range between 55 to 90 percent of **maximal heart rate** (HR max), which corresponds to 40 to 85 percent of **heart rate reserve** (HR reserve) and maximal oxygen uptake, as shown in Fig. 6.16.

When using a percentage of HR max,

it is approximately 15 percent lower than a percentage of HR reserve. The percent of HR reserve most closely approximates maximal oxygen uptake percent during exercise, while percent of HR max reflects a work load that is about 15 percent less. A comparison between HR max and HR reserve for recommended exercise intensity levels is presented in Table 6.17.

Using the recommended HR max or HR reserve percentages, a THR "window" of 10 to 15 percent is developed for each client. For instance, one client may exercise between 55 to 70 percent of maximal heart rate, while another exercises between 70 to 80 percent of maximal heart rate. The rationale for establishing a 10 to 15 percent THR range is that the heart rate will naturally vary during the exercise session.

Although individual THR "windows" will vary among clientele, exercise intensity should remain within the recommended ranges of maximal heart rate or maximal heart rate reserve.

Fitness professionals should recognize the salient aspects of THR development. In essence, exercise intensities are based on the premise that health-related benefits are derived from low and moderate exercise intensities; however, CRF is more favorably altered with moderate exercise intensities, and performance training usually requires high exercise intensities.

Programmatic contrasts in exercise intensity among health-related physical activity, CRF exercise and performance training are presented in Fig. 6.17. Essentially, exercise intensity is the primary difference among these types of exercise programs. Older and more sedentary or unfit clients will commence their exercise program in health-related physical activity and may improve CRF at low intensities, depending upon their initial fitness level.

Usually, most clients will commence their exercising in the cardiorespiratory fitness category at about 60 to 75 percent of HR reserve and will improve CRF at this intensity. For the average fitness client, exercise intensity of performance training is too high, is linked to increased injury and yields no greater health benefits. Based upon client needs, goals, habits, fitness level and possible limitations, an appropriate THR range can be developed, using either HR max or HR reserve.

What exercise intensity is appropriate for beginning clients? To answer this question, the fitness level, prior activity and personal interests and goals must be addressed. In general, the range of intensities to consider for various clientele can be approximated by the following levels:

Previously sedentary = 40 to 55 percent of HR reserve, or 55 to 70 percent of HR max.

Currently active = 60 to 75 percent of HR reserve, or 70 to 85 percent of HR max.

Training = greater than 80 percent of HR reserve, or greater than 90 percent of HR max.

Knowing needs and goals of the client allows the development of a more appropriate exercise intensity. For example, many clients desire at least a modest amount of weight loss. When weight loss is a part of the exercise goal, the motivation and fitness level of the client must be care-

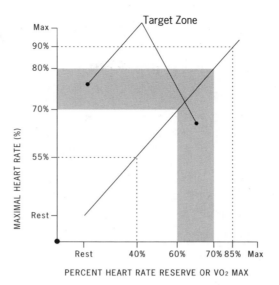

Figure 6.16

Exercise intensity: use of maximal heart rate and heart rate reserve.

fully considered. In the past, much of the advice related to exercise and weight control had been directed toward low-intensity (less than 70 percent HR reserve), long-duration exercise (30 to 60 minutes). While it is true that fat is preferentially burned with lower intensity exercise, the total amount of calories expended is really the primary factor (Ballor et al., 1989). For a given duration, an exerciser will burn more calories at a higher intensity. An instructor must also be aware that higher intensities also are accompanied by an increased risk for injuries, especially in an overweight population.

Estimation of Exercise Heart Rate. Accurate measurement of exercise heart rate is crucial to monitoring exercise intensity. Although digital heart rate monitors are available and are reasonably accurate, the use of palpation to measure pulse rate is a skill that clients are encouraged to perform.

Therefore, clients should be instructed on the proper pulse rate technique at the following sites:

Apical site. This pulse is taken at the apex of the heart and can sometimes be felt very clearly by placing the heel of the hand over the left side of the chest.

Carotid pulse site. This pulse is taken from the carotid artery just to the side of

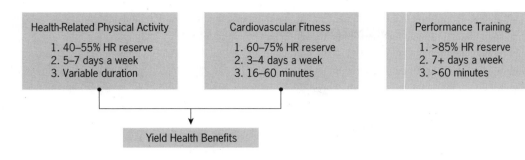

Figure 6.17

Contrast among physical activity, cardiovascular fitness and performance training.

the larynx using light pressure from the fingertips of the first two fingers, not the thumb (Fig. 6.18). Remember, never palpate both carotid arteries at the same time.

Radial pulse site. This pulse is taken from the radial artery at the wrist, in line with the thumb, using the fingertips of the first two fingers (Fig. 6.19).

Temporal pulse site. This pulse can sometimes be obtained from the left or right temple with light pressure from the fingertips of the first two fingers (Fig. 6.20).

Measuring heart rate immediately after exercising can provide a good estimate of the actual intensity of the workout. Knowing that a variety of factors (age, fitness level, and intensity and duration of exercise) influence the rate of recovery from an exercise bout, it is important to begin measuring the pulse rate within 5 seconds after stopping a given activity to closely

Table 6.17

COMPARISON BETWEEN PERCENT HR MAX AND PERCENT HR RESERVE DURING RECOMMENDED EXERCISE INTENSITIES

Percent HR Max	Percent HR Reserve
55	40
60	45
70	60
80	70
90	85
100	100

approximate the exercise heart rate. The pulse rate is counted for 10 or 15 seconds and multiplied by 6 (or 4) to determine beats per minute. The 10-second time period is preferred, since higher fit clients will recover rapidly, therefore allowing an adequate time frame to obtain a representative exercising heart rate.

The essence of counting pulse rate is to determine the number of cardiac cycles within a specified period of time. It is recommended that clients determine pulse rate by counting the first beat as one. In a group setting, the fitness instructor will not know what part of the cardiac cycle each member is in. Therefore, starting the count with zero may underestimate participants' heart rates.

Instructors should indicate in advance when the pulse is to be taken and should encourage clients to continue to move their feet while taking the pulse. Sudden cessation of activity may cause pooling of blood in the extremities and provoke light-headedness or dizziness, especially in clients who are either less fit or taking prescribed antihypertensive medication (beta blockers or vasodilators).

Clients should be encouraged to take their pulse routinely after a workout, while beginning exercisers should be instructed to take their pulse rate frequently—every 5 to 10 minutes of a 30-minute session—throughout the workout to familiarize themselves with the expected level of intensity. Once familiarized with one's bodily

Table 6.18

INTENSITY CLASSIFICATION OF PHYSICAL ACTIVITY

Intensity	Classification of HR max	HR reserve	VO$_2$ max or (6-20 Scale)	Rating of Perceived Exertion (RPE) (0-10 Scale)
Very Light (Weak)*	<35%	<30%	<10	≤2
Light (Moderate)*	35-59%	30-49%	10-11	3
Somewhat Hard (Strong)*	60-79%	50-74%	12-13	4-5
Hard (Very Strong)*	80-89%	75-84%	14-16	5-6
Very Hard (Very Strong)*	≥90%	≥85%	>16	>6

*Represents 0-10 RPE scale. Adapted from: Pollock & Wilmore (1990). Reprinted with permission.

responses to exercise, pulse rates can be taken less often, such as every 15 minutes.

Methods of Monitoring Cardiorespiratory Exercise Intensity

Fitness professionals must educate clients in the recommended ways to monitor exercise intensity for safe and effective programming. Several methods are used to monitor exercise intensity, and at least six such methods are recommended. The method selected will depend upon the fitness professional's expertise and access to testing data (stress test work load and heart rate), along with the client's exercise program, level of fitness and ability to perform certain monitoring techniques. It is important that the proper technique, precautions and limitations of each method be understood, so that fitness professionals can adapt or modify how clients gauge their exercise intensity. The following are methods recommended for monitoring exercise intensity:

Percent of Maximal Heart Rate. One very common and easy-to-calculate way of determining target heart rate method is the percentage of maximal heart rate method. To use this method of monitoring, HR max must first be determined from either a maximal stress test, or the age-adjusted maximal heart rate formula.

(Age-predicted Maximal Heart Rate = 220-Age [years]). The accuracy of THR is slightly compromised when using the age-adjusted maximal heart rate rather than a measured maximal heart rate. Also, if a client is taking medication which alters heart rate (e.g., beta blockers), then measured maximal heart rate must be used.

THR is calculated by taking a percentage of HR max. Adding 15 percent will approximate the same percent intensity of maximal oxygen uptake.

THR by HR max method:

THR = (HR max x percent intensity desired)

For example, a woman of 45 years who begins an exercise program at a desired intensity of 60 to 70 percent of HR max is calculated as follows:

THR = (HR max x percent intensity desired)

Step 1: Determine HR max—either measured from stress test or age-adjusted formula:

HR max = 220 - age

HR max = 220 - 45

HR max = 175 bpm

THR = (175 bpm x percent intensity desired)

Step 2: Convert the percentages of desired exercise intensities into decimal values by dividing by 100:

THR = (175 bpm x .60)
(lower intensity limit)
THR = (175 bpm x .70)
(upper intensity limit)

Step 3: Multiply HR max by upper and lower intensity limits:
THR = 105
(lower intensity limit)
THR = 122.5*
(upper intensity limit)
(*Note: round decimals to the nearest whole number)

By calculating her lower (60 percent) and upper (70 percent) intensity heart rates, a THR range of 105 to 123 bpm is identified.

Step 4: (Optional) Multiply heart rate by 1.15 to better reflect percent of aerobic capacity:
THR = 121 bpm (lower intensity limit)
THR = 141 bpm (upper intensity limit)

Percent of Heart Rate Reserve. Another method to determine THR range is to use a percentage of heart rate reserve, or commonly known as the Karvonen formula. The recommended percent of HR reserve (40 to 85 percent) corresponds to a similar percent of maximal oxygen uptake (40 to 85 percent). This method differs from the HR max method in that the resting heart rate is taken into account when determining THR. As in the HR max method, measured maximal heart rate must be used in this method when persons are taking prescribed medications that alter heart rate.

The key to this method is to take a percentage of the difference between maximal heart rate and resting heart rate, known as the reserve capacity of the heart, then add the resting heart rate to identify the THR. The reserve capacity of the heart reflects its ability to increase the rate of beating and cardiac output above resting level to maximal intensity.

THR is calculated using the HR reserve method:
THR = ([HR max - HR rest] x percent desired) + HR rest

For example, a 50-year-old man had a resting heart rate of 70 bpm and a maximal heart rate of 160 bpm during a stress test. What is his THR for an exercise intensity of 60 percent HR reserve?
THR = ([HR max - HR rest] x percent desired) + HR rest

Step 1: Determine reserve capacity of this client:
THR = ([160 bpm - 70 bpm] x percent desired) + HR rest
THR = (90 bpm x percent desired) + HR rest

Step 2: Convert intensity level to a decimal and place known intensity level and HR rest into formula:
THR = (90 bpm x .60) + 70 bpm

Step 3: Multiply desired intensity level by reserve capacity:
THR = (54) + 70 bpm

Step 4: Add resting heart rate to the percent reserve capacity:
THR = 124 bpm

From this example, it is important to remember that resting heart rate must be known and a THR range of upper and lower limits be recommended for each client. Knowing that heart rate can vary throughout an exercise session, it is important to establish a target zone of upper and lower heart rate limits for safe and effective programming. For this person, an upper limit of 75 percent is desired. By substituting 60 percent with 75 percent in the above formula, 75 percent of HR reserve is calculated as 138 bpm for the upper limit heart rate. Thus, a THR range of 124 to 138 bpm is desired for this 50-year-old man.

Rating of Perceived Exertion. Using the rating of perceived exertion is another common method of determining exercise intensity. Based on subjective perception steady-state work, using the 6 to 20 RPE scale or zero to ten RPE scale developed by Borg (1982). Interestingly, RPE is both valid and reliable, and is closely associated with increases in most cardiorespiratory parameters, including work, maximal oxygen uptake and heart rate.

In fitness settings, RPE can be used independent of, or in combination with, the heart rate to monitor relative exercise intensity of most clients. It must be understood that clients on medication that alters heart rate can use the RPE scale to monitor relative exercise intensity. Important when using either numerical RPE scale is the verbal description that reflects the intensity of work. Although clients should be instructed to gauge exercise intensity as closely as possible, some clients select inappropriate RPE values, and such persons should not use this method of monitoring exercise intensity.

To ensure that clients' perceived exertion corresponds to an appropriate relative exercise intensity, instructors should check the heart rate response. Although heart rate and RPE responses during a maximal stress test can identify an appropriate exercise intensity, such information is not usually available for most clients. By referring to Table 6.18, an approximate relative intensity classification for heart rate and RPE during exercise can be developed.

It is recommended that the RPE score reflect the recommended range of relative exercise intensities. When using the 6 to 20 RPE scale, clients should exercise between an RPE of 12 and 16 ("somewhat hard" to "hard") to reflect an approximate intensity of 50 to 85 percent of HR reserve, or 60 to 90 percent HR max, while an RPE of 4 to 6 ("somewhat hard" to "very strong") reflects similar intensities, using the 0 to 10 RPE scale.

Dyspnea Scale. **Dyspnea** refers to difficulty

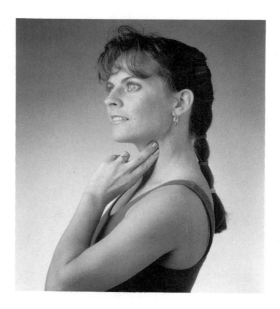

Figure 6.18
Carotid heart rate monitoring.

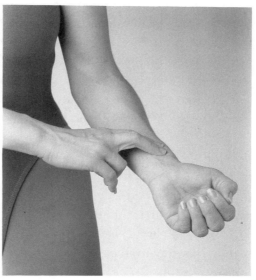

Figure 6.19
Radial heart rate monitoring.

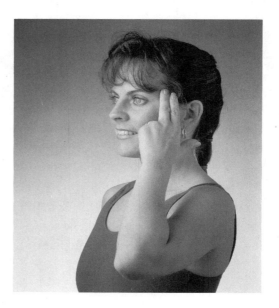

Figure 6.20
Temporal heart rate monitoring.

in breathing, or shortness of breath. The **Dyspnea scale** is a subjective score that reflects the relative difficulty of breathing as perceived by the client. Accordingly, this numerical scale can assist in monitoring exercise intensity:

+1 Mild, noticeable to client, but not to observer

+2 Mild, some difficulty that is noticeable to observer

+3 Moderate difficulty, client can continue to exercise

+4 Severe difficulty, client must stop exercising

The use of this scale is particularly helpful for those clients who have pulmonary conditions (asthma, emphysema) and those who feel limited due to breathlessness. Clients should be instructed to use the scale as a guide to their exercise intensity and in conjunction with the heart rate and RPE. Instructors should caution all clients who use this scale to reduce their intensity when breathing becomes labored (+3). If the severity of the pulmonary condition seems to worsen over time, instructors should consult with the client's physician and possibly recommend a more appropriate exercise setting for the client.

Talk Test. The **talk test** is another subjective method of gauging exercise intensity and can be used as an adjunct to heart rate and RPE. When clients exercise, it is highly recommended that breathing be rhythmical and comfortable. Particularly for newer clientele, talking while exercising can indicate whether an appropriate intensity is being performed. If the client is "winded" and needs to gasp for breath between words when conversing, then the exercise intensity is too high and should be reduced. As higher intensity activities are performed, it is expected that breathing rate will become faster and more shallow. For higher fitness levels, the use of the talk test may not be appropriate.

SUMMARY

The aerobics instructor must be aware of many aspects of exercise testing and programming for the wide variety of clientele being served. In order for aerobics instructors to be well-informed about the elements of comprehensive fitness testing, body composition, a thorough understanding of test limitations and applications is required. By using either the 3 minute step test or 1 mile walk test, aerobic fitness can be assessed. Body composition can be easily determined using skinfold assessment. To assess musculoskeletal fitness, it is important to evaluate muscular strength/endurance and joint flexibility using the tests described, which are easy to administer.

From health-related fitness assessment, clients are given an exercise program. It is important to develop the exercise plan, with goals and objectives, with both the health and needs of the client in mind. The recommended elements of exercise programming should include warm-up, aerobic time, cool-down, muscular time and flexibility time. When developing an exercise program, it is important that aerobic instructors design a well-balanced approach to exercise that not only focuses upon the health-related elements of fitness, but also meets the needs of the client. For CRF programming, instructors should identify the FITT principle of aerobic exercise programming for each client. Most importantly, clients should be instructed and regularly checked in their ability to monitor exercise intensity, through any of the six methods described in this chapter.

REFERENCES

American College of Sports Medicine (1992). *Health/Fitness Facility Standards and Guidelines*. (Sol, N. & C. Foster, eds). Philadelphia: Lea & Febiger.

American College of Sports Medicine (1991). *Guidelines for Exercise Testing and Prescription*. 4th ed. Philadelphia: Lea & Febiger.

American College of Sports Medicine (1990). Position Statement on the Recommended Quantity and Quality of Exercise for Developing and Maintaining Cardiorespiratory and Muscular Fitness in Healthy Adults. *Medicine and Science in Sports and Exercise*. 22: 265-274.

Ballor, D.L., J.P. McCarthy, E.J. Wilterdink, S.J. Hanson. (1989). Exercise intensity does not affect the composition of diet and exercise-induced body mass loss. *Medicine and Science in Sports and Exercise*, 21, (2): Supplement, #589.

Blair, S.F., H.W. Kohl, R.S. Paffenbarger, D.G. Clark, K.H. Cooper, and L.W. Gibbons (1989). Physical Fitness and All-cause Mortality: A Prospective Study of Healthy Men and Women. *Journal of the American Medical Association*. 262: 2395-2401.

Borg, G. (1982). Psychophysical Bases of Perceived Exertion. Medicine and Science in Sports and Exercise. 14:377-381.

Bray, G.A. & Gray, D.S. (1988). Obesity. Part I - Pathogenesis. *Western Journal of Medicine*. 149: 429-441.

Canadian Standardized Test of Fitness (CSTF) Operations Manual. 3rd ed. (1987). Published by authority of the Minister of State, Fitness and Amateur Sport Journal Tower(s), 365 Laurier Avenue West, Ottawa, Canada K1A0X6.

Faulkner, R.A., Springings, E.S., A. McQuarrie, & R.D. Bell, (1988). Partial Curl-up Research Project Final Report. Report Submitted to the Canadian Fitness and Lifestyle Research Institute.

Golding, L.A., Myers, C.R. & Sinning, W.E. (1989). *Y's Way to Physical Fitness*, 3rd ed. Champaign: Human Kinetics Publishers.

Howley, E.T. & Franks, B.D. (1992). *Health Fitness Instructor's Handbook*, 2nd ed. Champaign: Human Kinetics Publishers.

Hubert, H.B., Feinleib, M.N., McNamara, P.M. & Castelli, W.P. (1983). Obesity as an Independent Risk Factor for Cardiovascular Disease: A 26-Year Follow-up of Participants in the Framingham Heart Study. *Circulation*. 26: 968-977.

Imrie, D. & Barbuto, L. (1988). The Back-Power Program. In: *Resource Manual for Guidelines for Exercise Testing and Prescription* (Blair, S.N., P. Painter, R.R. Pate, L.K. Smith & C.B. Taylor, eds). Philadelphia: Lea & Febiger.

Jackson, A.S. & Pollock, M.L. (1985). Practical Assessment of Body Composition. *The Physician and Sports Medicine*, 5(May):76-90.

Jequier E. (1987). Energy, Obesity, and Weight Standards. *American Journal of Clinical Nutrition*, 45: 1035-1047.

Kline, G.M., Porcari, J.P., Hintermeister, R., Freedson, P.S., Ward, A., McCarron, R.F., Ross, J. & Rippe, J.M. (1987). Estimation of VO_2 max From a 1-Mile Track Walk, Gender, Age, and Body Weight. *Medicine and Science in Sports and Exercise*, 19: 253-259.

McArdle, W.D., Katch, F.I. & Katch, V.L. (1991). *Exercise Physiology: Energy, Nutrition, and Human Performance*, 3rd ed. Philadelphia: Lea & Febiger.

Pollock, M.L. & Wilmore, J.E. (1990). *Exercise in Health and Disease: Evaluation and Prescription for Prevention and Rehabilitation*, 2nd ed. Philadelphia: W.B. Saunders.

Sjostrand, T. (1947). Changes in Respiratory Organs of Workmen at an Ore Melting Works. *Acta Medica Scandinavica* (Suppl). 196: 687-695.

SUGGESTED READING

Cotton, R. (1991). Testing and Evaluation. In M. Sudy (Ed), *Personal Trainer Manual: The Resource for Fitness Instructors*, (pp. 155-192). San Diego: American Council on Exercise.

LaForge, R. (1991). Cardiorespiratory Fitness. In M. Sudy (Ed), *Personal Trainer Manual: The Resource for Fitness Instructors*. (pp. 195-233). San Diego: American Council on Exercise.

Wilmore, J.E. & Costill, D.L. (1988). *Training for Sport and Activity: The Physiological Basis of the Conditioning Process*. 3rd ed. Dubuque: Wm. C. Brown Publishers.

Chapter 7

Components

of an Aerobics Class

By Karen Clippinger-Robertson

An aerobics class is intended to enhance physical capacity so that overall health and quality of life improve. But to realize the potential gains from an exercise class, which include improved cardiovascular endurance, body composition, flexibility, muscular endurance and muscular strength, it is essential to design the class appropriately. Class design is probably the single most challenging task for the instructor. The challenge is to apply the scientific principles and exercise techniques presented elsewhere in this manual in a manner that will produce an effective, relatively

Karen Clippinger-Robertson, M.S.P.E., is a kinesiologist and a director of Seattle Sports Medicine Seminars, and of Pacific Northwest Ballet's Conditioning and Therapy Center. She has conducted fitness-instructor training programs for more than 15 years and has consulted for the U.S. Weight Lifting Federation, the U.S. Race Walking Team, and various dance companies, sports medicine clinics and fitness centers.

safe and highly motivating workout.

Table 7.1 outlines a sample design for an aerobics class. This design, based on principles discussed in this chapter, serves as a guide that may be varied to meet specific class objectives or the needs of a particular group of participants.

CLASS FORMAT

Typically, an aerobics class begins with a **warm-up**, which generally uses movements with a low to moderate speed and range of motion. These movements are designed to promote body awareness and to increase blood flow to the muscles. An aerobics or **calisthenics** component follows the warm-up. The aerobics component, which is aimed at improving cardiovascular endurance and body composition, uses large body movements performed continuously so that the heart rate remains elevated. Following the aerobic workout, a cool-down gradually reduces the heart rate toward resting levels and prevents excessive pooling of blood in the lower extremities. A calisthenics component includes exercises designed to increase muscular endurance or strength in specific muscles. The class ends with a further cool-down, which includes stretching and relaxation exercises designed to further lower the heart rate, help prevent muscle soreness, enhance flexibility and re-establish the body's equilibrium.

Emphasis

Although the four components—warm-up, aerobics, calisthenics and cooldown—are common to most exercise classes, the emphasis given to each will vary depending on the objective of a particular class, as well as the fitness level, age, health and physical skill of its participants. For example, a class for previously sedentary people may emphasize the calisthenics

portion while reducing the **duration** and **intensity** of the aerobics section. This approach could decrease the possibility of injury by increasing muscular strength and flexibility to prepare the body for the stresses of aerobics. The young or extremely fit may benefit from a 90-minute class that includes a 30- to 45-minute aerobics segment as well as a rigorous calisthenics section that uses resistance to enhance overload. With elderly or obese people, a longer slow cool-down is advisable.

Sequence

An area of continuing controversy in aerobics, about which there is little evidence at present, is whether it is better to place the calisthenics segment before or after the aerobics segment. The two sequences are outlined in Table 7.2. Proponents of calisthenics first (Cal-Aer) argue that calisthenics extend the warm-up, thus allowing the body to acclimate gradually to the increased work load of the aerobics segment (Gerson, 1985). They also argue that this sequence can alleviate the potential problem of postural hypotension. During exercise, there is a tremendous increase in blood flow to the working muscles. A change in position, especially raising the head above the heart by standing up after floor exercises can result in hypotension (a drop in blood pressure). The decreased blood flow to the brain can cause dizziness or faintness.

Some proponents of Cal-Aer also argue that fatigue after the aerobics segment could lead to poor technique and greater risk of injury during calisthenics. Others feel that because glycogen stores are used during calisthenics, the body will begin metabolizing fat sooner during aerobics. At this time, there is insufficient data to substantiate these arguments and more research is needed.

Table 7.1

SAMPLE AEROBICS CLASS DESIGN

Components		Examples of content
Warm-up (5-10 minutes)	Isolation exercises	Neck flexion, neck rotation side to side, shoulder circles, supported trunk flexion with pelvic tilts, hip isolations, knee flexion and extension, ankle circles, foot push-releases.
	Full body movements	Pliés, step-touches, step-touches with arm movements, small lunges, small lunges with increasing range arm movements.
	Flexibility exercises	Calf, hamstring and low-back standing stretches.
Aerobics (20-30 minutes)	Aerobic warm-up	Step-touches, touch-backs, heel-touches, knee lifts and light jogging with arms increasing in range of motion.
	Peak aerobics	Jogging with full arm movements, side leg-kicks, lunges with full arm movement, knee-lifts with hops, three-step kick with traveling.
	Aerobic cool-down	Same as aerobic warm-up (i.e., movements with less traveling, less range in leg and arm movements, less impact, slower tempo).
Cool-Down I (5-10 minutes)	Large, rhythmical movements	Rhythmical movements, such as walking or step-touches, decreasing range of motion to aid in returning blood to the heart, but at a low enough intensity to allow heart rate to gradually decrease toward a resting level.
Calisthenics (15-20 minutes)	Trunk exercises	Abdominal curl-ups, back extensions.
	Upper extremity exercises	Push-ups, posterior shoulder exercises.
	Lower extremity exercises	Hip flexor and quadriceps strengthening (front leg-lifts), hip abductor exercise (side leg-lifts), hip adductor exercise (side leg-pull), hip extensor exercise (back leg-lifts), tibialis anterior exercise, tibialis posterior exercise and peroneal exercise.
Cool-Down II (7-10 minutes)	Flexibility exercises	Flexibility routine, including stretches for the hamstrings, hip adductors, shoulder extensors, hip abductors, low back, quadriceps femoris, hip flexors, gastrocnemius and soleus.

Proponents of aerobics first (Aer-Cal) argue that calisthenics may fatigue the large muscles enough to increase the risk of injury during the faster pace of aerobics. In the author's experience, most group-exercise injuries result from overuse during aerobics rather than during calisthenics. Some proponents of Aer-Cal (Jones, 1985) believe that this sequence produces a slightly greater cardiovascular benefit and use of calories. When the heart rate has been ele-vated to the target zone by aerobic exercise, it may remain sufficiently elevated during part of the calisthenics to provide a greater aerobic benefit and caloric expenditure than would occur if the calisthenics were performed first. Individual class design might make the difference in this respect. For example, a calisthenics section that be-gan by using large muscle groups (such as hip, thigh or trunk) and emphasizing mus-cular endurance might be more likely to

Chapter 7
Components of an
Aerobics Class

provide these benefits than one that began with smaller muscle groups (ankles, arms) or one that emphasizes slow repetitions with holds. Further investigation is needed to see if these hypothesized benefits actually occur, and if so, if the gains they offer are large enough to have any practical significance.

Because so little scientific evidence is available to decide this issue of sequencing aerobics and calisthenics, instructors should stay abreast of new information, and in the meantime, carefully evaluate the alternatives for their own programs and participants. For purposes of illustration, this chapter will follow the Aer-Cal sequence.

In addition to appropriate sequencing of class components, it is important to design the movements within each component for safe and effective class development. An instructor who understands the purpose of each component and the physiological stress needed to produce desired changes can design movements that effectively produce these changes. See also Chapters 2 and 3 for illustrations and

descriptions of the muscles, joints and exercise techniques referred to in the following discussion.

WARM-UP

The purpose of the warm-up is to prepare the body for the more rigorous demands of the aerobics and calisthenics segments by raising the internal temperature. For each degree of temperature elevation, the metabolic rate of the cells increases by about 13 percent (Astrand & Rodahl, 1977). In addition, at higher body temperatures, blood flow to the working muscles increases, as does the release of oxygen to the muscles. Because these effects allow more efficient energy production to fuel muscle contraction, the goal of an effective warm-up should be to elevate internal temperatures one or two degrees, so that sweating occurs.

Increase in temperature has other effects that are beneficial for exercisers, as well. The potential physiological benefits of warm-up include:

Figure 7.1
Push-releases.

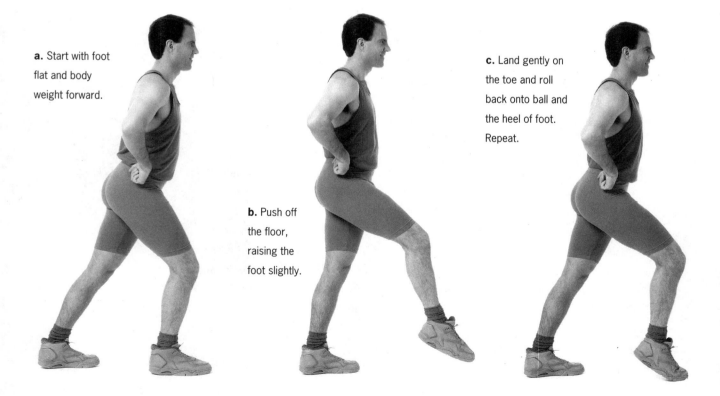

a. Start with foot flat and body weight forward.

b. Push off the floor, raising the foot slightly.

c. Land gently on the toe and roll back onto ball and the heel of foot. Repeat.

- higher metabolic rate
- increased blood flow to muscles
- higher rate of oxygen exchange between blood and muscles
- more oxygen released within muscles
- faster nerve impulse transmission
- decreased muscle relaxation time following contraction
- increased speed and force of muscle contraction
- increased muscle elasticity
- increased flexibility of tendons and ligaments
- rehearsal effect (the body practices muscular patterns to be used later)
- reduced risk of abnormal electro-cardiogram

Many of these physiological effects may reduce the risk of injury because they have the potential to increase neuromuscular coordination, delay fatigue and make the tissues less susceptible to damage (Astrand & Rodahl, 1977; Shellock, 1983; Lehmann & Koblanski, 1971; 1976).

Warm-up Exercise Selection Criteria

Considering time constraints, in a typical one-hour class, the warm-up should generally last 5 to 10 minutes. Movements should be selected that will help meet the goals of a warm-up—to prepare the body for more rigorous exercise and increase core temperature.

Specificity. Movements in the warm-up should specifically prepare the body for movements used in the aerobics routines. Specificity not only ensures that the appropriate muscles are warmed, but it also provides a **rehearsal effect.** That is, the neuro-muscular system has a chance to practice or rehearse muscular patterns similar to those used in later parts of the class. This rehearsal effect may enhance performance and reduce injury (DeVries, 1966). For example, the warm-up for a low-impact class

Table 7.2

CLASS SEQUENCING

Cal-aer class	Aer-cal class
Warm-up	Warm-up
Calisthenics	Aerobics
Aerobics	• Warm-up
• Warm-up	• Peak
• Peak	• Cool-Down*
• Cool-Down*	Cool-Down I**
Cool-Down I**	Calisthenics
Cool-Down II***	Cool-Down II***

*Reduce intensity to lower heart rate to low end of target heart rate zone.
**Rhythmic movements to lower heart rate to 120 beats per minute or less.
***Stretching and relaxation.

that uses a lot of arm patterns would include movements to prepare the shoulders and arms. In contrast, a high-impact class would include warm-up exercises for the ankles and feet, such as push-releases, which replicate the movements needed for jumping and landing. The push-release (Fig. 7.1) begins with the weight of the body forward, supported mostly by the foot in front. The exerciser forcefully pushes away from the floor while pointing the toe (ankle plantarflexion), so that the foot rises slightly off the floor. The exerciser then gradually lowers the body weight, using controlled movement, emphasizing eccentric use of the ankle plantarflexors and the intrinsic foot muscles.

Elevating Core Temperature. Although specificity is important, a common error in the warm-up is to over-emphasize body isolation exercises. Many classes begin with a series of isolation movements, such as forward head rolls (without forcing the head back into full hyperextension), shrugs, shoulder rolls and torso twists. Although these exercises are useful to begin with and to increase kinesthetic awareness, they should progress to movements that use more muscle mass so that internal body temperature is elevated. Remember that it

Figure 7.2

Shoulder shrugs and
shoulder rolls.

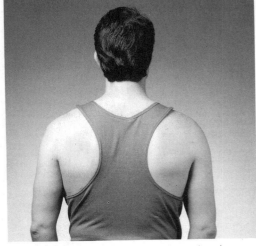

a. Begin with shoulders relaxed and arms hanging.

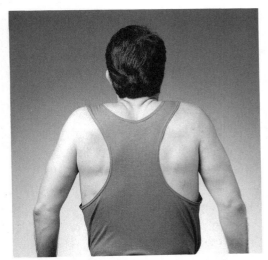

b. Shoulder shrugs: Bring shoulders up, elevating
shoulder blades, and then lower.

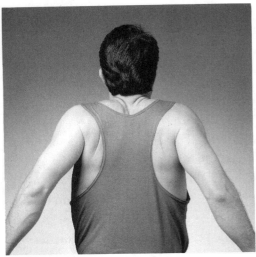

c. Shoulder rolls: Bring shoulders up. Pull the
shoulders back and down.

is this rise in core temperature that provides many of the benefits attributed to a warm-up.

Stretching. Studies have shown that the combination of warm-up and stretching enhances flexibility more than either used alone (Lehmann, 1970; Masock & Warren, 1970; Wiktorsson-Moller et al., 1983). This combination will allow a muscle to be stretched farther during activity before damage occurs. Hence, these stretches should specifically prepare the exerciser for the stresses and range of motion demanded by the following aerobic component.

Warm-up Format and Content

One way to meet the various criteria for the warm-up is to organize it into three phases. These phases will be termed Isolation Movements, Full Body Movements and Flexibility Exercises.

Isolation Movements. This first phase uses small, isolated movements intended primarily to increase kinesthetic awareness, or help participants shift from their previous activities and focus on their bodies. These movements, which also begin to increase blood flow to the contracting muscles, include side-to-side neck rotations, shoulder shrugs, shoulder rolls (Fig. 7.2), hip isolations, ankle circles and pelvic tilts. Pelvic tilts can provide practice for correct postural alignment throughout the rest of the class (Fig. 7.3). It is usually easier for participants to follow movements that flow in sequence, either from head to toe or from toe to head.

Full Body Movements. From the first phase, movements should progress to include more muscle groups simultaneously and thus, facilitate elevation of internal body temperature. During the second phase, include movements such as knee bends (pliés), side reaches, step-touches and heel-touches. This second phase, with movements that are slower and simpler than during peak aerobics, is a perfect time to emphasize correct alignment and technique. Because the body is not yet prepared to generate or absorb large forces, movements should be limited in impact and range of motion. Exercises such as deep lunges, high kicks, jumping jacks, or single-leg jumps are best saved for peak aerobics. As the warm-up proceeds, movements can build both in range of motion and complexity, always being carefully selected to prepare the body for the specific challenges of the particular class.

Range of Motion/Flexibility Exercises. A short series of full range-of-motion movements composes the third and last phase of the warm-up. These movements are designed to take each muscle group to the limits of its range of motion in a slow, controlled manner. The purpose is to prepare for more vigorous full range movement in the aerobic segment. They may be referred to as stretches, although they are often held less long than is optimal for flexibility training. The longer-held stretches desirable for long-term flexibility gains come at the end of the class. At this point, standing stretches (Figs. 7.4 & 7.5) work well, so that the class can see the positions and move easily into aerobics. The "stretches" the instructor chooses depends on the type of class he or she is teaching. Full range of motion for the low back, hip flexors, hamstrings and both calf muscles are especially important. With any standing stretch, the hands may be used to help support the upper body by placing them on the thighs or on a wall, chair or barre. For descriptions of specific standing stretch positions, refer to Chapter 3, (lumbar extensors, hamstrings, gastrocnemius, soleus).

Additional stretches may also be appropriate, depending on the specific format and content of the aerobic segment. For example, shoulder extensor range of motion is desirable for low-impact classes or other classes that use many full, overhead arm movements. A stretch for the hip flexors may also be desirable, particularly in bench classes or classes utilizing lunges (Fig. 7.5).

AEROBICS

The purpose of the aerobic segment of an exercise class is to improve cardiovascular endurance by challenging the heart and lungs. To achieve this desired effect, participants must maintain their heart rates within a target zone for an extended period. To maintain this elevated heart rate, aerobic exercise uses prolonged, continuous movement of large muscle groups. This type of exercise can also improve body composition by reducing body fat.

Duration

Although the American College of Sports Medicine (ACSM) (1991) recom-

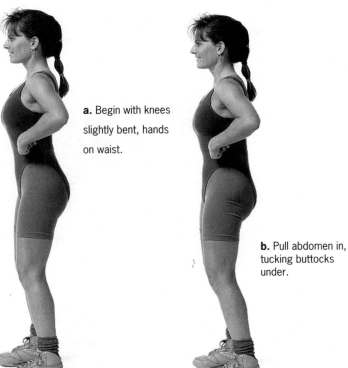

Figure 7.3

Standing pelvic tilt.

a. Begin with knees slightly bent, hands on waist.

b. Pull abdomen in, tucking buttocks under.

Chapter 7

Components of an
Aerobics Class

mends aerobic-exercise periods ranging from 20 to 60 minutes, within the constraints of a one-hour exercise class it usually works best to allow 20 to 30 minutes for the aerobics segment. At least 20 minutes is needed to burn enough calories and apply sufficient stimulus to improve body composition and cardiovascular fitness while working at a safe intensity. Usually a maximum of 30 minutes is recommended for the basic aerobics class. In that time, participants can achieve cardiovascular benefits (assuming they are working at appropriate intensities) while still keeping musculoskeletal risk low.

For some specialized classes the duration of the aerobics segment may be extended. For example, a longer duration—approximately 40 minutes—at a lower intensity would be appropriate for a class of overweight students with a primary goal of improving body composition. Some studios offer a 90-minute class for persons who are very healthy and fit, and in these cases, a longer aerobics segment of 40 to

50 minutes may also be appropriate. However, with these longer durations, careful medical screening, meticulous class design and gradual increase in intensity are essential to avoid musculoskeletal injury. One study found that musculoskeletal injuries to the lower body doubled when a 30-minute aerobics segment was increased to 45 minutes in walk-jog-run programs for beginners (Pollock et al., 1977).

Intensity

For effective but lower risk cardiovascular gains in adult fitness programs, exercising at an intensity of 60 to 80 percent of maximum heart rate reserve (Karvonen formula) or 70 to 85 percent of maximal heart rate (maximal heart rate formula) is commonly recommended (see Chapter 6, for a detailed discussion of target heart rate ranges). Although 60 percent, the threshold necessary for cardiovascular improvement, is a helpful guide, it is important to understand that fitness gains will be affected by the initial fitness of each partic-

Figure 7.4

Standing stretches.

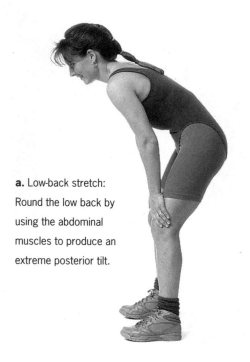

a. Low-back stretch: Round the low back by using the abdominal muscles to produce an extreme posterior tilt.

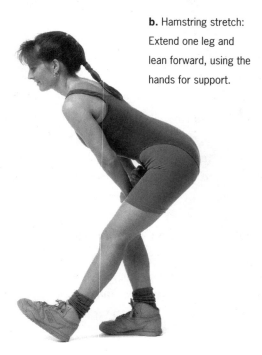

b. Hamstring stretch: Extend one leg and lean forward, using the hands for support.

ipant. Cardiovascular gains occur in unfit persons at exercise intensities lower than 60 percent, while the fit exerciser often has to work at higher intensities to show significant improvement (Pollock et al., 1984). However, as the upper range of the recommended intensities is approached or surpassed, risk increases for musculoskeletal injury and cardiovascular symptoms, while participant compliance decreases. Therefore, in a recreational aerobics class it is probably best to avoid the intensities higher than 85 percent of maximal heart rate. Pollock et al., (1984) recommend an intensity in the lower to middle range for beginning, asymptomatic adults, and the upper ranges are generally reserved for very fit and healthy individuals who have been exercising consistently.

Interaction of Intensity and Duration. It is important to remember that it is the total work load (energy expenditure) that determines cardiovascular improvement. Thus,

similar gains can result from either longer duration at lower intensity or shorter duration at higher intensity workouts. It is the combination of exercise intensity and duration that counts. Considering that medical histories are often incomplete and that it is difficult to individualize classes adequately, it seems prudent for an instructor to aim for a moderate combination of exercise duration and intensity in the aerobics class. Encouragingly, studies have found that exercise sessions of 30-minutes duration, at a moderate intensity, performed three to five times per week, can increase aerobic fitness and provide significant protection from heart disease (Cooper, 1982).

Monitoring Aerobic Intensity. Aerobic exercise must be of a high enough intensity to overload the cardiovascular-respiratory system but of low enough intensity that oxygen can be delivered fast enough to allow aerobic metabolism to predominate. Participants need to know what their appro-

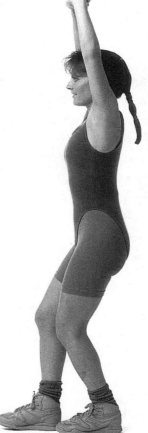

e. Shoulder extensor stretch: From soleus stretch position bring clasped arms overhead and back.

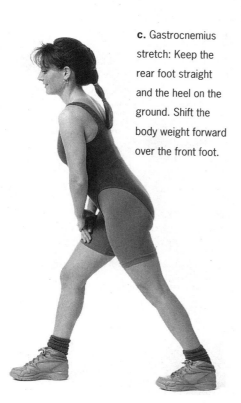

c. Gastrocnemius stretch: Keep the rear foot straight and the heel on the ground. Shift the body weight forward over the front foot.

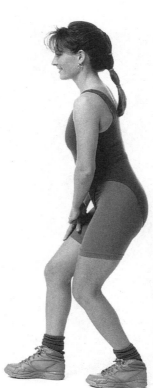

d. Soleus stretch: Shift the weight slightly to the back and bend the back knee.

priate target heart rate ranges are in order to optimize cardiovascular benefits while keeping risk low. They must also be trained to estimate their heart rates by monitoring their pulse or rating their perceived exertion. It is important to give the participants opportunities to monitor their exercise intensity. It is also important that the instructor receive feedback about the intensity. This enables the instructor to adjust the exercise intensity if necessary by altering exercise content, sequence and progression (for a detailed discussion of monitoring exercise intensity see Chapter 6).

Modification of Aerobics Intensity

To be able to provide appropriate individual modifications and to select appropriate intensity movements for a given class, it is important to understand what determines the intensity of movements. A simple way to think of intensity is how much body mass must be moved how far in what amount of time. This, in turn, will influence how much muscle mass must be

Figure 7.5

Hip flexor stretch: Standing in a lunge position, press the bottom of the pelvis forward until a stretch is felt across the front portion of the rear hip. Lift heel of rear foot slightly bending the knee.

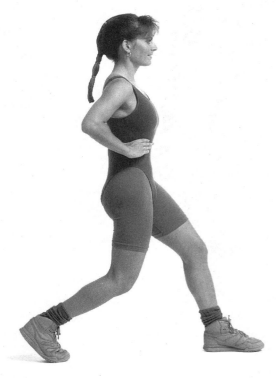

used and what the oxygen needs of that tissue will be. Some examples of applying these principles follow.

Raising and Lowering Center of Gravity. Movement of the human body as a whole is often described in reference to the center of gravity. The center of gravity can be defined as the point at which the mass of a body would be located if all of the mass were concentrated in an infinitely small volume (i.e., a point). It can be thought of as the center of mass in all directions (i.e., front/back, side/side, top/bottom). One way to increase intensity is to increase the movement of the center of gravity in a vertical dimension. For example, with low-impact movement this is often done by bending the knees and then straightening the knees (Fig. 7.6). This utilizes some of the large muscle groups of the lower body to affect the alternate lowering and raising of the center of gravity.

Adding Jumps. In high-impact aerobics, the emphasis is often on an upward vertical excursion of the center of gravity, as with hops or jumps. Intensity is significantly increased by recruiting enough large muscles and exerting enough force to propel the body through space. Large muscles are also recruited eccentrically to control the landing of the body.

Lifting Limb/Body Segment. Lifting a limb, such as an arm or leg, will also increase exercise intensity (Fig. 7.7). Muscular effort is required to lift the limb, and lifting a limb (mass) has an effect on the whole body of raising the center of gravity. For example, adding a knee-up to the basic step (Fig. 7.8) will slightly increase cardiovascular intensity (oxygen cost) and calories burned (metabolic cost). Adding lifting of a leg appears to be more effective than an arm. This is probably related to the larger muscle mass involved. One study with low-impact aerobics showed that there was no significant difference between performance of a routine with or without arm movements (Stanforth et al., 1988). This may be due to the tendency to make lower body movements smaller when arm movements are added. This conjecture is given support by the finding that addition of arms does increase intensity with bench-stepping during which lower body work is more standardized by step height.

Addition of Weights. Most studies have found that adding small hand weights to low-impact routines does not significantly increase the oxygen cost or calories burned. With step aerobics, no significant increases were found with 1-pound weights, while only slight increases were found with the addition of 2-pound weights. Also, risk of shoulder injury may increase significantly if hand weights are used improperly. This would not be the method of choice for effective elevation of intensity in most instances.

Traveling More. Traveling more through space emphasizes increasing the horizontal movement of the center of gravity. The traveling can be forward and back, side to side, on diagonals, in circles or any combination of these. Traveling is a very effective way to use a large amount of muscle mass and to increase intensity. Studies with both low-impact and step aerobics have shown marked increases in exercise intensity and metabolic cost with movements that include traveling. For example, one study found that by emphasizing continuous, very large traveling movement through space, low-impact movement could achieve the oxygen and metabolic cost associated with high-impact movements (Otto et al., 1988).

Faster Tempo. If the same full range of motion can be maintained, increasing the tempo of the music will increase the intensity of the workout. This can be explained by the fact that the body is performing the same work in a shorter period of time, resulting in more work per unit of time. Hence, the muscles involved will require

Aerobics

Figure 7.7

Increasing exercise intensity by adding a knee-up.

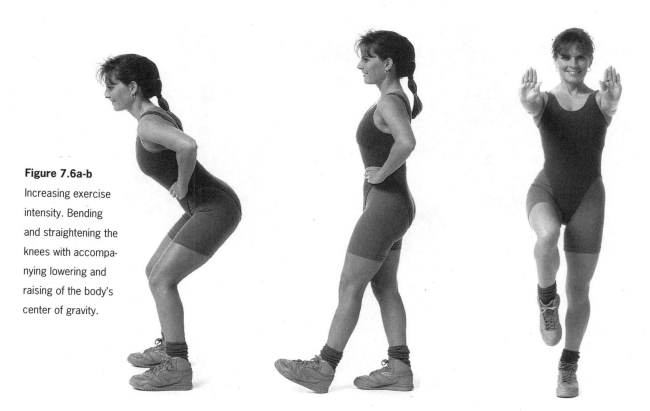

Figure 7.6a-b

Increasing exercise intensity. Bending and straightening the knees with accompanying lowering and raising of the body's center of gravity.

more oxygen. Again, this is most effective with the large muscle groups of the legs. However, as tempo increases too much, there is a tendency to decrease the range of motion which can diminish or even halt potential intensity increases. Furthermore, excessive **tempo** can increase injury risk, especially in the shoulders. Fast, full range of motion, of the shoulders with the elbows extended is not recommended.

When attempting to alter exercise intensity, these principles can be applied alone or in combination. For example, taking the movement phrase of three walks forward + kick, followed by three walks backward + lunge, intensity can be increased by: (1) rising up on the toe for the kick and bending the front knee farther to go lower in the lunge, (2) adding a jump with the kick or substituting jogs for the walks, (3) kicking the leg higher, (4) rigorously pushing up with the arms with the kick and pulling back with the arms with the lunge without diminishing lower body

movement, (5) traveling farther forward and back with the walks and lunge, or (6) performing the same movement range with a slightly faster music tempo.

Note that addition of weights was excluded. Because of the limited gains and relatively high musculoskeletal risk, the use of hand weights was excluded from this example. Weights are appropriate for an isolated, carefully choreographed routine with slower tempo music and good safety cueing (i.e., the last song of the aerobics segment or Cool-Down I). The primary purpose of the hand weight is to increase intensity locally for a particular muscle (potentially enhancing muscular endurance) or to add choreographic variety, rather than to increase overall cardiovascular intensity.

The same principles discussed above can also be applied in reverse to decrease intensity. When individual modifications are needed while still staying with the same movement phrase, the most effective means

Figure 7.8

Increasing exercise intensity.

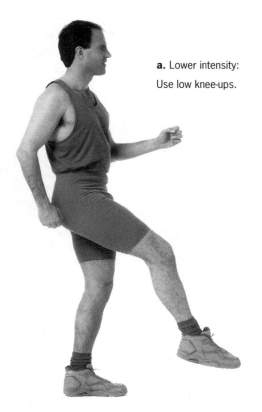

a. Lower intensity: Use low knee-ups.

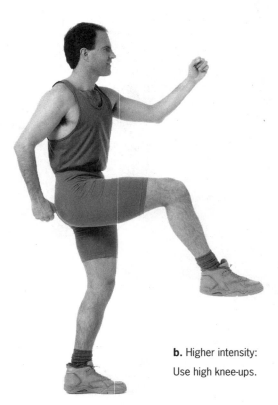

b. Higher intensity: Use high knee-ups.

is to decrease the movement of the body as a whole. So, participants can be cued to make their movements smaller with less traveling to decrease intensity. For example, with low-impact movements intensity can be reduced by lifting the knee less high; with high-impact movements the jump or hop can be lessened or removed; and with step choreography, arm movements can be made smaller or deleted. It is important to remember that arm movements do not necessarily contribute significantly to cardiovascular intensity with non-step aerobics, so deleting arm movements may not decrease overall intensity unless leg movements are also made smaller.

Aerobics Class Types

Since the origin of aerobics classes, many different types of classes have evolved to enhance various benefits or reduce various risks. It is important to understand the advantages and disadvantages of various class types so that appropriate choices can be made for working with different participants and populations.

High-impact. High-impact aerobics utilizes aerobic movements such as jumping, or hopping, in which there are moments when the body is projected into space and both feet lose contact with the ground. The primary advantages of high-impact movements are very good cardiovascular overload and metabolic benefits (i.e., kilocalories utilized per minute of exercise). High-impact classes also have a high fun and popularity factor, encouraging compliance. Thus, high-impact aerobics potentially offers very good fitness benefits for the appropriate participant. However, the disadvantage of high-impact aerobics is the relatively high reported injury incidence, particularly in the lower body. High-impact movements may be inappropriate for indi-

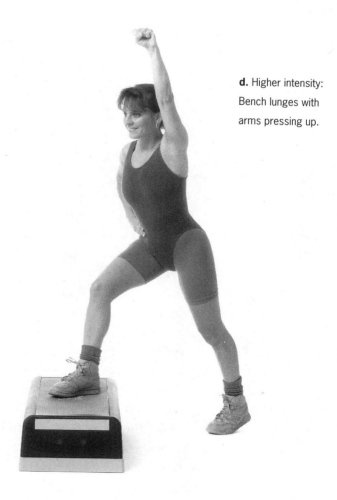

d. Higher intensity: Bench lunges with arms pressing up.

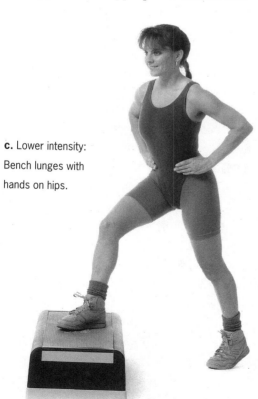

c. Lower intensity: Bench lunges with hands on hips.

viduals with biomechanical or other factors that predispose them to injury in the lower leg and foot regions. Some instructors attempt to accommodate such individuals by demonstrating both a high- and low-impact version of the same movements. The effectiveness of such an approach is highly dependent on the choreography and demonstrations used. Since most beginners will need to follow someone, it is important that the instructor or an assistant continuously or frequently model the low-impact variation.

Low-impact. Low-impact aerobics utilizes aerobics movements in which at least one foot contacts the ground at all times. Low-impact aerobics evolved to decrease the lower leg overuse injuries associated with high-impact classes. Low-impact aerobics offers lower impact-related musculoskeletal stress, particularly useful for individuals with a tendency toward stress fractures, shin splints and other lower extremity injuries. They are ideal for special populations, such as seniors, pregnant women and overweight individuals. However, with the reliance on the repetitive use of a flexed knee, some susceptible participants may complain of knee (particularly patellofemoral) problems.

The primary disadvantage of the low-impact class is achieving adequate intensity for the more fit individual. Early studies using traditional low-impact moves (more stationary and emphasizing arm movements) found markedly lower oxygen and metabolic costs than traditional high-impact classes. Furthermore, it was shown that the heart rate associated with a low-impact routine was often associated with a lower rate of oxygen consumption than the same heart rate accompanying a high-impact routine. Thus, having a heart rate in the desired target zone with low-impact aerobics would not necessarily yield the ex-

pected fitness benefits. This occurs if one relies on arm movement to elevate the heart rate. Arm movement causes a heart-rate increase without necessarily increasing oxygen demand. This type of low-impact aerobics could actually result in fitness losses for the more fit individual.

However, later studies suggest that certain low-impact movements have a place for the more fit individual. If low-impact movements emphasize continuous traveling through space, similar benefits to a high-impact class can probably be achieved. So to maximize the benefits of low-impact aerobics, emphasis should be on lower body movement and large movement of the whole body through space, rather than on more stationary routines emphasizing arm movement.

Non-impact. Non-impact aerobics is often erroneously used to describe low-impact classes. Even walking is associated with impact (about 1.2 x body weight). Non-impact aerobic activities would refer to non-weight-bearing activities, such as swimming laps or doing exercises in a chair.

Impact, however, is not necessarily bad; in fact, it is an important stimulus for maintaining or increasing bone density. Furthermore, the muscular effort associated with propelling the body or recovering the body is useful in creating adequate cardiovascular overload. Although in select cases of obesity or with certain musculoskeletal conditions impact must be deleted, most healthy individuals benefit from some impact. Simply vary the impact so that high-impact duration is limited to enhance fitness without injury.

Combination-impact. Combination-impact aerobics utilizes both low- and high-impact movements. The high-impact movements promote higher intensity while the low-impact movements vary the musculoskeletal stresses. High- and low-impact movements can be combined within a movement phrase (e.g., three low walks plus a hop), a routine (e.g., a low-impact phrase interspersed with a high-impact phrase), or a song (e.g., first song of aerobic segments uses low- followed by high-impact movements in the second song). The duration of high- and low-impact movements used and their particular formatting should be based on the profile of participants in a given class. When carefully choreographed, combination-impact classes offer the advantage of minimizing injury risks while maximizing the benefits of both low- and high-impact approaches.

Step Aerobics. Step aerobics utilizes stepping up and down from a platform. Step aerobics can offer a moderate- to high-intensity cardiovascular workout with low-impact stresses. Intensity can be easily individualized further by changing platform heights. However, the higher platform heights are associated with increased knee discomfort. This has led to attempts to increase intensity through other methods, such as faster music, more complex choreography, addition of jumps (higher impact) and addition of weights. Further research is needed to address the relative benefit and risk of these approaches. At this point it appears that careful selection and sequencing of higher intensity movements, such as repeaters and propulsions, can produce the desired high-intensity workout while still keeping risk low.

The disadvantage of platform-stepping is that the associated repetitive knee flexion can produce knee problems in susceptible exercisers. By adding movements performed on top of the platform, off the platform and around the platform, needed recovery time can be allowed for the knees—"combination bench." Similar to the combination-impact approach, this recovery can be allowed within a movement phrase, with-

in a routine or from song to song. The key is to alternate musculoskeletal stresses (see Chapter 9, "Variations: From Step to Strength Training").

Aerobic Format Options

In addition to selecting the type of class in terms of impact or bench, there are various options for formatting these movements. The most commonly used is the continuous format, but some other options may provide variety or be useful for specific populations or fitness goals.

Continuous. With the continuous format, an attempt is made to keep heart rate at the goal level (e.g., 75 percent of maximal heart rate) throughout the aerobics portion of the class. Choreography must be selected that uses large muscle mass and is of appropriate intensity to maintain fairly steady heart rates within the target heart rate range. Through choreography, cueing, and music tempo, an attempt is made to minimize intensity "ups and downs" during peak aerobics.

Interval. In contrast to the continuous format, the interval format uses alternating periods of higher and lower intensity movement. This approach was originally used with athletes with very high intensity work intervals (≥ 85 percent of maximal heart rate) designed to stress the anaerobic energy systems and upper limits of the aerobic energy systems. During active recovery, the exercise intensity is low enough to facilitate lactic acid removal. The advantage of interval training is that more work is done in the same amount of time, yielding better cardiovascular and metabolic benefits.

The disadvantages of the interval approach are greater cardiovascular and musculoskeletal injury risk and decreased compliance. Hence, it is commonly recommended that the traditional interval format be reserved for young, healthy athletes.

Chapter 7
Components of an
Aerobics Class

Modified for adult fitness programs, the work intervals are lower intensity, about 10 percent above the goal target heart rate to a maximum of 85 percent. The rest intervals are about 10 percent below the target heart rate. The duration of the work interval, the ratio of the work interval to the recovery interval, and the maximum and minimum heart rates used would be based on the fitness profiles of the specific participants (see Chapter 9, "Variations: From Step to Strength Training").

Circuit. The traditional circuit format uses resistance stations (using body weight, free weights, bands, weight apparatus) with aerobic movement interspersed between these stations to keep heart rate elevated (see Chapter 9 for detailed circuit formats appropriate for the aerobics classroom). The advantage of circuit training is the

multiple benefits of moderate improvements in muscular strength/endurance, cardiovascular endurance and body composition.

The disadvantage of circuit formats is that slightly better cardiovascular gains can be achieved by doing only aerobic movement and better strength gains can be achieved by using heavier overload with fewer repetitions. However, for individuals who do not have the time or interest to do supplemental strength training, this format enables some gains in strength and muscle mass, in addition to moderate cardiovascular benefits. Maintaining adequate muscle mass and strength is important for body composition, injury prevention and prevention of osteoporosis.

Selecting and Sequencing Aerobic Movements

Aerobics routines are built from basic locomotor movements, such as walks, runs (jogs), skips, hops and jumps. Figure 7.9

Figure 7.9

Aerobics routine using varied arm movements while jogging.

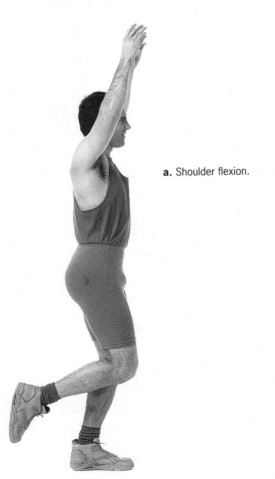

a. Shoulder flexion.

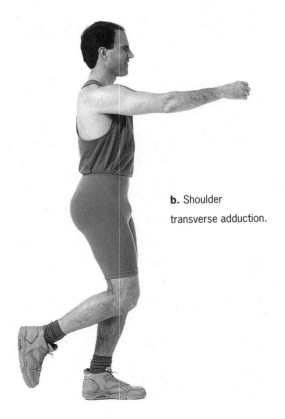

b. Shoulder transverse adduction.

presents variations of arm movements combined with jogging in place. Additional variety can come from adding traditional dance steps (Charleston, cha-cha, hustle, swing, polka, pony), movements from other dance forms (ballet, jazz, funk, hip-hop) and sports-related movements (karate, boxing, tennis, skiing). Movement selection and sequence are very important for overall exercise effectiveness and safety. Some important considerations for selection and sequencing are described below.

Cardiovascular Considerations. Exercises should be selected to produce the desired intensity. For example, when selecting movements for peak aerobics, use moderate- to high-intensity variations to keep heart rates elevated. In contrast, during the aerobic warm-up, sequence a moderate-intensity movement between two low-intensity movements, changing the proportion as the warm-up progresses. The class profile (i.e., advanced, beginning, special populations) influences the relative inten-

sity of movements. Also, remember that for cardiovascular safety, it is advisable to use an upper limit of 85 percent of maximal heart rate. A majority of cardiovascular problems, some of which can be life threatening, occur at higher intensities.

Musculoskeletal Considerations. In many cases the limiting factors for exercise progression are musculoskeletal. That is, as exercise intensity, duration or frequency are increased, the cardiovascular system adapts but the musculoskeletal system does not, and injury occurs. Hence, altering impact and stresses to specific body parts through selection and sequencing of movements is very important for long-term program effectiveness and safety.

To lessen musculoskeletal risk, it is important to build routines that use a balance of muscle groups, including movements to the front, back, sides and on various diagonals. The primary joints of the arms and legs should be worked in all possible directions; for example, flexion, exten-

Aerobics

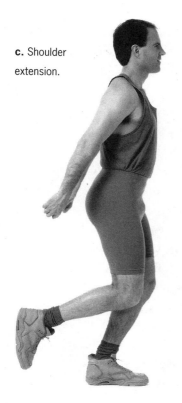

c. Shoulder extension.

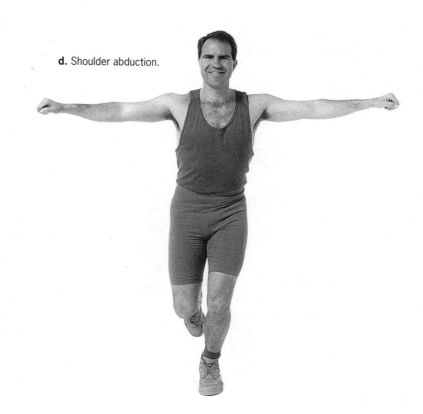

d. Shoulder abduction.

sion, abduction, adduction, circumduction and rotation at the hip and shoulder. In designing hip movements, many instructors have a tendency to emphasize the hip flexors with exercises such as front knee-lifts (Fig. 7.10), and to forget the importance of movements such as side kicks (Fig. 7.11) that work the hip abductors, and back knee curls (Fig. 7.12) that work the hamstrings. With the arms there is a similar tendency to use front and overhead movements excessively. It is important to work the arms backward (Fig. 7.9c) and to rotate them as well. Including movements on diagonal planes will also incorporate varied muscle groups. Incorporating movements of the scapular muscles is particularly necessary.

To lessen musculoskeletal risk, it is also helpful to evaluate movements in terms of their primary site of stress, the magnitude of stress and the repetitive nature of the stress. For example, the primary area of stress for many high-impact movements is the lower leg/foot and the magnitude is greater for movements landing on one leg versus two. In contrast, with many low-impact and step movements, the primary stress area is the knee (particularly the patellofemoral joint) and the magnitude is greater with movements involving more forceful quadriceps contraction and greater degrees of flexion. In the latter case, the relative magnitude of force is still not that high (i.e., as compared to jumping) but it is the repetitive nature that is of concern.

The absolute magnitude of force is better kept low when selecting movements for seniors or pregnant women. For these populations, low-impact movements are ideal. However, in a regular aerobics class higher forces can be carefully included with the following precautions: (1) limit the number of consecutive repetitions, (2) cue participants to limit the absolute magnitude of force if necessary (i.e., by limiting height of jump or depth of knee flexion), and (3) sequence higher risk movements so that musculoskeletal stress can be alternated (Fig. 7.13). With a step platform routine, a lunge series could be sequenced with something performed on top of the platform or on the floor to allow recovery to the knee area. Careful sequencing allows the use of a wider diversity of movements with a lower injury risk.

Choreographic Considerations. In addition to safety and effectiveness considerations, movement selection and sequencing must address choreographic needs. Choreographic factors, such as flow, transitions, variety, use of different rhythmic patterns, use of different planes and levers and use of different directions and spatial arrangements, should be taken into account. To enhance learning, successful performance, and maintain a safe and effective exercise intensity, it is important that each movement sequence lead smoothly into the next.

Figure 7.10

Front knee-lifts work the hip flexors.

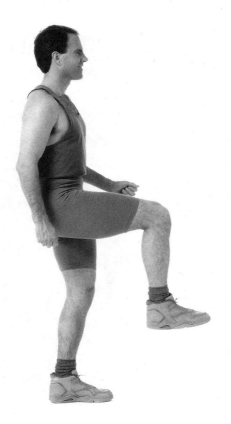

If dance steps are selected, break each one down to its simplest component, then gradually add or change one element (plane, lever, direction, rhythm) at a time until everyone is performing the dance step. For example, a cha-cha: Base movement: walk in place 8 counts. Change rhythm: 1-2, quick 3-and-4, 1-2, quick 3-and-4. Add direction: Step front with right, 2, quick 3-and-4; step front with left, 2, quick 3-and-4. Change direction: Cross right over left, 2, quick 3-and-4; cross left over right, 2, quick 3-and-4. Now the whole cha-cha step is established.

At this point different arm combinations could be added, or another directional change could occur by doing a cha-cha set facing the front wall, side wall, back wall and side wall. Intensity could change by substituting a lunge for the crossover step, and by performing the quick 3-and-4 on the balls of the feet. The advantage of building choreographic patterns is that everyone stays together, intensity is main-tained and variety can be introduced gradually increasing complexity. The degree to which a movement pattern is broken down and how quickly variations are built will depend on the fitness and skill level of the class. Another important aspect of these choreographic concerns is that the movement sequences are fun, motivating and encourage compliance.

A Three-phase Approach

When selecting and sequencing aerobic movements it is helpful to think of the aerobic segment in phases. Like the class warm-up, it may be thought of in three phases: the aerobic warm-up, peak aerobics and the aerobic cool-down.

Aerobic Warm-up. The aerobic warm-up allows the cardiovascular system to adjust gradually to the increasing exercise demands; it also prepares the musculoskeletal system. In contrast to the warm-up at the beginning of class, the aerobic warm-up avoids isolation movements and instead

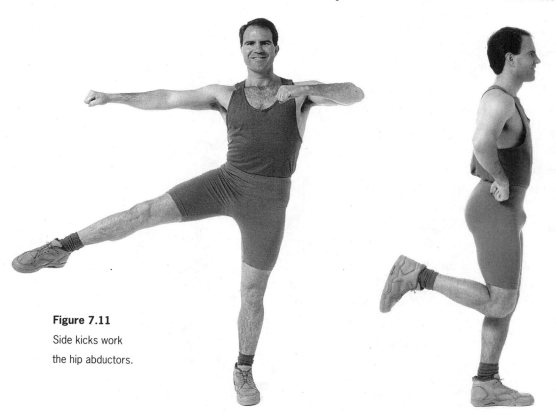

Figure 7.12

Back knee curls work the hamstring muscles.

Figure 7.11

Side kicks work the hip abductors.

emphasizes continuous movements that involve large muscle mass and that increase internal temperatures along with heart rate. Appropriate exercises include step-touch (Fig. 7.14a), touch-back (Fig. 7.14b), and heel-touch (Fig. 7.14c)—all with lower range-of-motion arm movements (i.e., shoulder range of motion 45 to 90 degrees in flexion and abduction). In all of these foot-touches, one foot is always on the ground, so that impact is low and range of motion is low to moderate.

Peak Aerobics. As the class continues into the aerobics segment, intensity and heart rates should gradually build. The instructor can use any of the techniques discussed earlier in choreographic considerations and building intensity (see "Modifying Aerobic Intensity"). However, three techniques that work particularly well for peak aerobics are traveling more, adding a jump or hop and lifting a limb higher (Fig. 7.15).

Aerobic Cool-down. Frequently short-changed in aerobics classes, the **aerobic cool-down** allows the cardiovascular system to gradually re-establish equilibrium at a lower intensity. The instructor can gradually reduce intensity by progressively reducing range of motion, traveling, impact and amount of muscle mass used. By the end of the aerobic cool-down, heart rate should be decreased to the lower end of the target heart rate range. The aerobic cool-down provides a smooth transition into the class cool-down. For the purpose of clarity, this chapter refers to the aerobic cool-down as Cool-Down I and the class cool-down as Cool-Down II.

Cool-down I

In the Aer-Cal sequence, the **cool-down** following the aerobics component is often incorporated into the beginning of the calisthenics component (Table 7.2). How-

ever, because cardiac complications most often occur with the cessation of exercise, this part of the workout is being addressed separately to emphasize its importance. When appropriately designed, the aerobic cool-down will continue to lower the heart rate to 120 beats per minute or below and will help to prevent excessive pooling of blood in the lower extremities, reduce muscle soreness and promote faster removal of metabolic wastes (Astrand & Rodahl, 1977; Pollock et al., 1984).

During this segment, the music is slower and the range of motion is smaller than in the aerobics component. Movements in which the head is lowered below the heart and then raised again should be avoided because these movements may cause dizziness. The aerobic cool-down is an appropriate time for upper-body strengthening, using surgical tubing or weights, while the legs make simple and small movements, such as walking or step-touches (Fig. 7.16). The rhythmic contractions of the legs act as an important muscle pump to help return blood from the

Figure 7.13
Alternate stresses by choosing movements that challenge different muscle groups and joints.

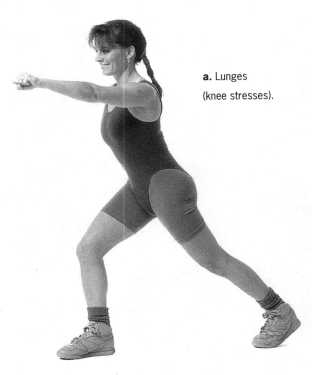

a. Lunges (knee stresses).

lower extremities to the heart.

Without such activity, blood pooling in the lower body can result in reduced blood pressure, dizziness and (in exceptional cases) cardiac arrhythmias. This pooling can be of particular concern with sustained isometric contractions of the legs because isometrics occlude blood flow. For example, some instructors direct students to hold a deep knee bend (isometric quadriceps work) for an extended period while performing upper-body exercises. Instead of maintaining this fixed position, exercisers should rhythmically flex and extend their legs and use other small, simple, rhythmic movements. Isometrics are better placed later in the class after sufficient cool-down has been achieved.

In the Aer-Cal sequence, the final cool-down period follows the calisthenics component. This cool-down (Cool-Down II) is composed of flexibility and relaxation exercises. In classes that follow the Cal-Aer sequence, Cool-Down I (lowering the heart rate) immediately precedes Cool-Down II (flexibility and relaxation).

CALISTHENICS

The purpose of the calisthenics component is to improve strength and endurance in major muscle groups. This section will address considerations for incorporating calisthenics into a standard aerobics class.

General Calisthenics Component Design

To design an effective calisthenics component with limited risk it is important to understand the difference between muscular strength and muscular endurance. Muscular strength is the maximum force

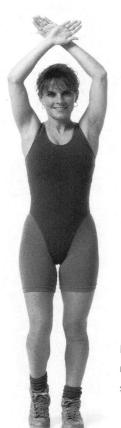

b. Vigorous overhead movements (shoulder stresses).

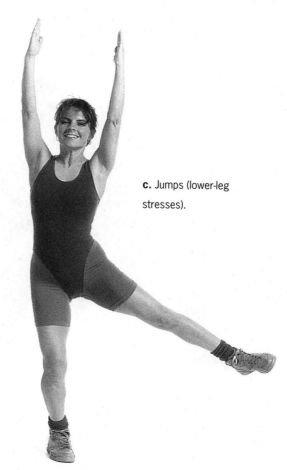

c. Jumps (lower-leg stresses).

Chapter 7
Components of an
Aerobics Class

a muscle can exert against a resistance in a single effort. In contrast, muscular endurance refers to the number of times a muscle can exert force against a given submaximal resistance or the ability to sustain an isometric contraction over time.

Training programs designed to maximize strength gains utilize higher resistance and lower repetitions while programs designed to maximize muscular endurance gains utilize lower resistance with higher repetitions (see Chapters 1, 3 and 9).

Maximizing Calisthenic Effectiveness. Muscular strength is important to prevent injuries, and several studies suggest that increases in strength will also produce moderate increases in muscular endurance (Anderson & Kearney, 1982; Fox, 1984). However, exercise regimens designed to increase muscular endurance do not appear to be as effective for improving strength. For example, performing many consecutive abdominal curls does not gen-

erally produce adequate gains in abdominal strength. Many athletes and aerobics instructors who perform hundreds of abdominal crunches daily still test out weak in their abdominal muscles (Clippinger-Robertson, 1986). Of 88 aerobics instructors recently tested, 89 percent scored inadequately on standard physical therapy strength tests for the abdominals (Kendall et al., 1971).

With the information currently available, it seems more time-efficient and effective to design the calisthenics routine to emphasize increasing muscular strength rather than muscular endurance. Although optimal strength gains occur with quite high resistance and low repetitions (for example, four to six sets of 2 to 6 repetitions of 90 percent of maximum resistance), such an approach is also associated with a higher injury risk. So, a more moderate approach of one to three sets of 8 to 12 repetitions at 70 to 80 percent of maxi-

Figure 7.14a-c
Aerobic warm-up movements.

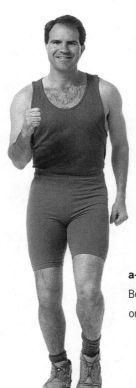

a-1. Step-touches: Begin with weight on right foot.

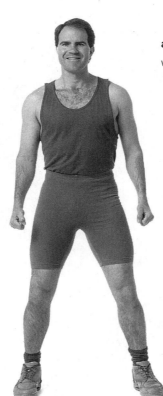

a-2. Step to side with left foot.

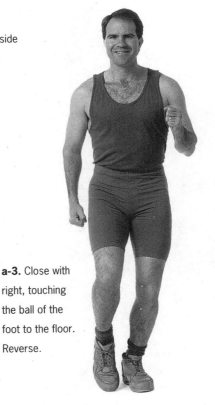

a-3. Close with right, touching the ball of the foot to the floor. Reverse.

mum resistance is commonly recommended for recreational athletes. This more moderate approach will lessen the risk of injury while still allowing good strength gains and some muscular endurance gains.

This recommended intensity can be easily achieved in traditional strength training in which external resistance, such as free weights, wall pulleys or weight apparatus, are used to effect sufficient overload. However, within the confines of an aerobics class, it is often difficult to achieve sufficient overload so that adequate fatigue is achieved by 12 repetitions. Care must be taken to select and modify exercises in an attempt to create adequate overload through techniques such as using slower repetitions, holds, a greater range of motion, changing body position to maximize gravity effects, or adding external resistance, such as light weights, surgical tubing or elastic bands.

Several of these techniques can be illustrated with abdominal curls. Many exercisers who routinely perform 100 curls can achieve better gains with fewer repetitions of harder variations. These individuals can often achieve adequate muscle fatigue in about 10 repetitions when they perform the curls slowly and increase the height, working up to about 30 degrees of spinal flexion. Keeping the lower waist on the floor will enhance safety but the trunk should be fully flexed, sequentially curling up against gravity (Fig. 7.17a). Initially the hands can be used on the thighs to flex the trunk slightly more. Stronger individuals can perform this same exercise with the hands behind the head or with a weight in the hands behind the head. Another way to increase difficulty is to add holds at one or more arcs (Fig. 7.17b). The exerciser can curl up to about 20 degrees, hold for 4 counts, gradually curl back down to the floor, and immediately curl up again, repeating the whole exercise five to ten

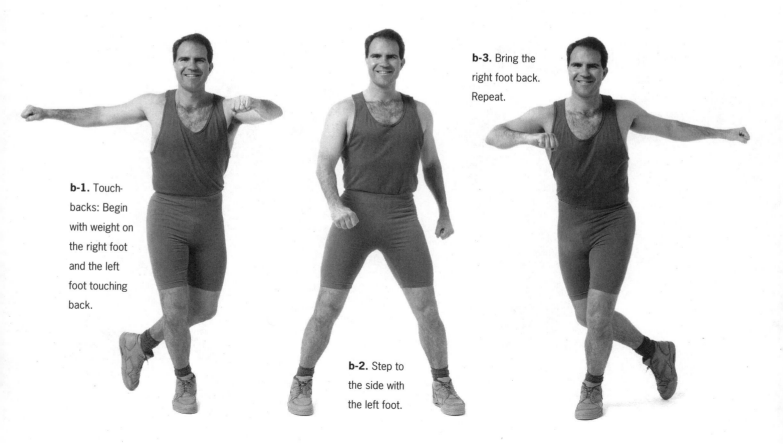

b-1. Touchbacks: Begin with weight on the right foot and the left foot touching back.

b-2. Step to the side with the left foot.

b-3. Bring the right foot back. Repeat.

times. Difficulty can be further increased by bringing the hands back behind the head during the 4-count hold.

Adding rotation also increases difficulty (Fig. 7.17c). The exerciser curls up to about 20 degrees and rotates to the side, keeping the pelvis stationary as the torso rotates. The opposite shoulder should come up and around to encourage use of abdominal instead of back muscles for rotation. After holding this rotated position for several counts, the exerciser rotates to the other side, rotates back to the center, and then lowers the trunk carefully to the floor.

Another factor for effective strength development is the amount of recovery allowed between sets of the same exercise or different exercises that target the same muscle group. If inadequate recovery is allowed, the training will foster muscular endurance versus strength. With heavy resistance training for strength and power, 2- to 3-minute rest periods are recom-

mended, while for muscular endurance rest periods of less than 1 minute are commonly used. In an aerobics class in which goals lie between these two extremes, a recovery of 1 to 3 minutes can be allowed. In the interest of time economy, one approach is to perform a sequence of exercises that target different regions and then return for a second set for key muscles.

For example, 8 reps of an abdominal exercise could be followed by a set of 8 reps for the right hip abductors, the left hip adductors and the back extensors, using bands for resistance. Then a second set of abdominal exercises could be performed followed by the left hip abductors and the right hip adductors. It is important to realize that just doing a different variation for the same muscle group (e.g., 8 straight curls followed by 8 curl-ups with rotation) does not allow adequate recovery and is similar to performing 16 reps in a row (emphasizing muscular endurance

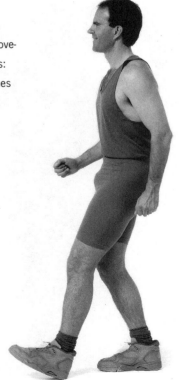

Figure 7.14c
Aerobic warm-up movements. Heel-touches: Alternate heel-touches in front of the body.

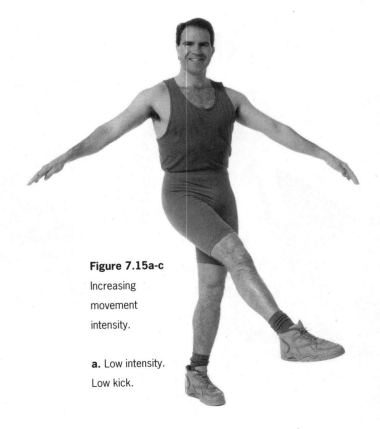

Figure 7.15a-c
Increasing movement intensity.

a. Low intensity. Low kick.

versus strength).

Better strength gains can be achieved by performing 8 reps of adequate difficulty to produce muscular fatigue followed by several other exercises so that the desired 1- to 3-minute recovery is allowed before doing a second set. It is also important to realize that if a single set can be done with sufficient intensity, it may not be necessary to do additional sets. Research suggests that about 70 percent or more of the strength gains associated with three sets can be achieved by doing one high intensity set (ACSM, 1990).

The ACSM recommends a minimum of one set of 8 to 12 repetitions performed a minimum of two times per week for adult fitness programs. Given the time constraints of an aerobics class, one approach is to perform just one set of most exercises with two or three sets for only key muscle groups, such as the abdominals.

Still another concern for maximizing strength effectiveness is the range of motion utilized by the given exercise. Strength gains are specific to the angle exercised and diminish the farther away one goes from the exercised angle or range (Graves et al., 1989). Exercising joints through their full range of motion is also important for maintaining or increasing flexibility. Hence, it is generally recommended that strength-training exercises be performed through a full range of motion for maximum benefits. Although this usually can be done easily with the use of weight apparatus, it is often difficult to do within the aerobics class. In many cases, gravity is serving a primary role of resistance and so requires a set position of the body that might not allow full range of motion.

For example, when performing pectoral flys (shoulder transverse adduction) with dumbbells, the exerciser must be supine to have the necessary relationship to gravity for effective overload. However,

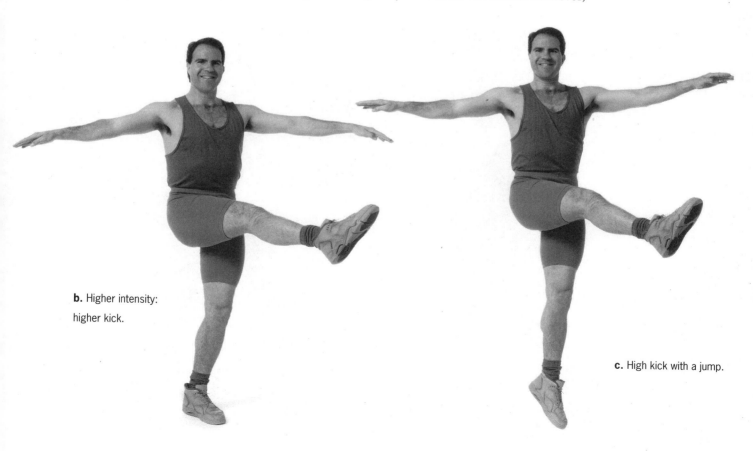

b. Higher intensity: higher kick.

c. High kick with a jump.

when performing this lying on the floor, the floor prevents the arms from going behind the body. Outside of class, this exercise would generally be performed supine or inclined on a bench to allow full range. In other cases, safety also dictates a less than full range of motion be utilized. For example, when doing hip extension supported on the hands and knees, unless adequate trunk stabilization is effected, full hip hyperextension will generally be accompanied by forceful arching of the low back. To lower risk, range is commonly limited to lifting the leg from the floor to a position in line with the trunk or just beyond.

When elastic resistance is used (bands or tubing), the range of motion is not usually as limited since the body does not have to be positioned in a set relationship to gravity. However, even though a larger range can theoretically be used, resistance is not equivalent throughout the range. Because of the nature of elastic resistance,

there is not much resistance at the beginning of the range and the resistance increases as the band or tube is stretched farther. A participant may not be able to complete the full range of motion due to an inability to overcome the resistance and resistance may be inadequate to overcome gains in the early part of the range. This shortcoming can be lessened by adjusting handgrip (how close the hands are to each other) and range so that adequate resistance occurs in the most functional portion of the range. Additionally, one could perform several sets with different handgrips and ranges to facilitate transfer to a fuller range of motion.

Enhancing Calisthenic Safety. In making the decision to emphasize muscular strength over muscular endurance, the safety and the specific needs of the class must be considered. For example, adding holds, with the associated elevation of blood pressure, may cause problems for seniors, pregnant women or exercisers

Figure 7.16

A Cool-Down I exercise.

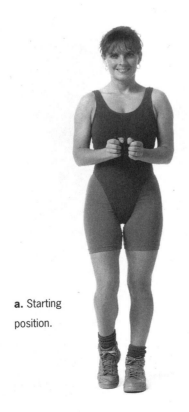

a. Starting position.

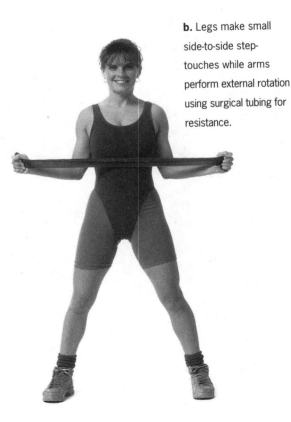

b. Legs make small side-to-side step-touches while arms perform external rotation using surgical tubing for resistance.

with heart disease. Adding weights may endanger pregnant women or students with arthritis. One approach is to use exercise at higher resistance only in intermediate or advanced, unrestricted classes. Another approach is to add higher resistance to exercises after a 6- to 10-week conditioning period that uses lower resistance.

However, the most common consideration is a class of unrestricted individuals at various levels of strength and endurance. As in aerobic choreography, it is important to begin with the easiest version of a movement, then add on or introduce more difficult variations, one change at a time. In this way, each participant can stay at an appropriate level. If an instructor starts with the most difficult or intense variation first, then demonstrates a lower level variation, the first segment will be poorly performed by the weaker class members. Participants are also often embarrassed and reluctant to drop down to a lower level; they will continue to try the more intense version using substitution patterns, poor technique, limited range of motion or will stop altogether. Instructors must sequence the exercises to encourage participants to work carefully at their individual fitness levels and with proper technique.

It is also important to give class members cues so that they know when and how to progress properly. For example, in abdominal work, begin with a series of pelvic tilts, then add an abdominal curl with arms on the floor beside the hips. Cue the participants that their goal is to lift their shoulder blades from the floor, bringing the trunk through full ROM. If they cannot, they should keep the arms on the floor. If they can, cross the arms on the chest. Continue the abdominal curls with the arms on the chest. If they can still clear their shoulder blades from the floor (achieve full range of motion), they can

change the arm position to hands behind the head. If not, continue with arms across the chest. Cue participants to continue to move at the waist through the full range of motion without pulling on the head or neck. As the abdominals fatigue, participants may perform additional repetitions in the full range of motion by changing the arms back to the chest or sides.

Alignment and Technique. Although certain exercises may be inherently too risky for an aerobics class (see "Enhancing Calisthenic Safety"), almost any exercise can be potentially dangerous if performed with poor alignment and technique. With most exercises, the manner in which they are performed is the most critical issue. If instructors understand the correct execution of exercises, anticipate common errors and

Figure 7.17
Increasing overload in curl-ups.

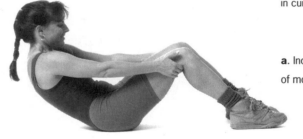

a. Increase the range of motion.

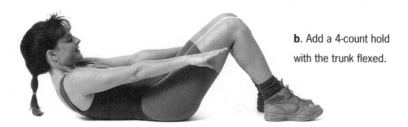

b. Add a 4-count hold with the trunk flexed.

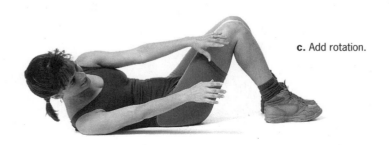

c. Add rotation.

Chapter 7

*Components of an
Aerobics Class*

cue effectively so that participants can achieve correct form, they considerably reduce the risk of injury in their classes as well as enhance exercise benefits (see Chapter 3, for details on cueing, correct exercise form and alignment).

One common source of error is the tendency to "cheat" by substituting other muscles as fatigue increases. The resulting musculoskeletal compensation can both cause injury and interfere with desired gains in muscular strength or endurance. To avoid this error, the exerciser must maintain trunk and pelvic stability as well as the movement pattern that uses the correct muscles. Trunk and pelvic stability can generally be achieved through contraction of the abdominal muscles, or in some cases, co-contraction of both the abdominals and the back extensors such that a neutral position of the spine is maintained. After attaining this pelvic and spinal alignment, the goal is to maintain it throughout the exercise without letting the pelvis exces-

sively tilt forward (arching the low back), tilt laterally or excessively rotate. A subtle change in position can have a dramatic effect on muscle use and body stresses.

For example, in exercises involving bringing the leg behind the body (hip extension) and exercises using overhead arm movements (Figs. 7.18a & 7.18b) there is a tendency to let the top of the pelvis tilt forward. Cueing for firm abdominal stabilization is important. Excessive lateral tilting of the pelvis is particularly prevalent in movements involving hip abduction or adduction. For example, a common error in performing standing or side-lying hip abduction exercises (side leg lifts) is to allow lateral tilting of the pelvis while the actual movement at the hip joint proper stays the same (Fig. 7.19). This technique error permits the lateral trunk flexors to assist with the movement, appearing to lift the leg higher. However, the load to the hip abductors is about the same and the stress to the low back is increased. Exces-

Figure 7.18
Maintaining correct
alignment.

a. Use the abdominals
to stabilize the trunk and
pelvis to avoid distortions such as arching
the low back. This
shows hip hyperextension with both correct
and incorrect alignment.

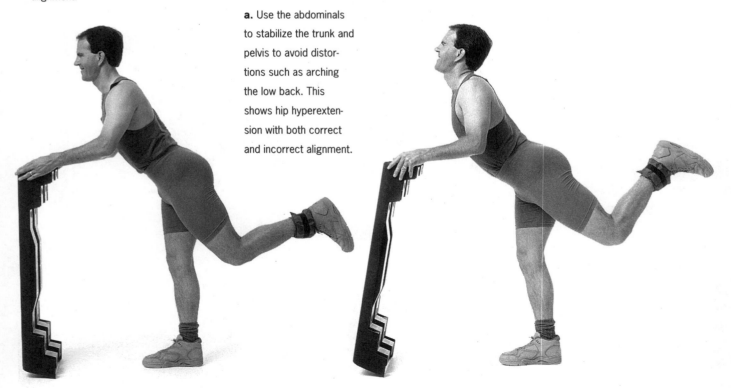

sive pelvic rotation can be linked with hip flexion, extension, abduction, adduction or rotation and commonly occurs toward the end of the range of motion. Instructors, therefore, must be familiar with the normal range of motion for each joint and be able to spot and correct class participants when they deviate from neutral alignment.

Correct technique often requires reducing the range of motion, the repetitions and the speed, so that the appropriate muscles can stabilize the pelvis and spine, preventing undesired movement. For example, with the donkey kick (Fig. 7.20a) or back leg lift, only about 10 to 15 degrees of hip hyperextension is possible in the average individual before the spine must arch and the pelvis tilt forward (Fig. 7.18a). Many exercisers will also attempt to achieve a greater range by allowing the

pelvis to rotate (Fig. 7.20b & c). Thus, the hip extension movement should use a small range and adequate abdominal stabilization to maintain correct alignment and prevent excessive hyperextension or rotation of the spine. To achieve sufficient overload, bands, tubing or weights can be added for resistance. Performing fewer repetitions or using a lower resistance in which proper form can be maintained is far safer and more effective than compromising correct technique.

Participants also need to be educated as to the expected range of motion of the working joint.

Selecting Specific Calisthenic Exercises

It is ideal to develop a balance between agonists and antagonists of a given movement by strengthening the prime movers, the muscles that assist with a movement

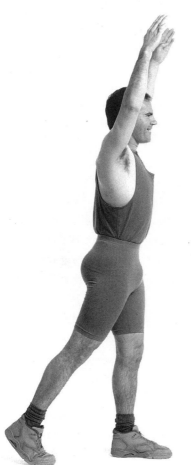

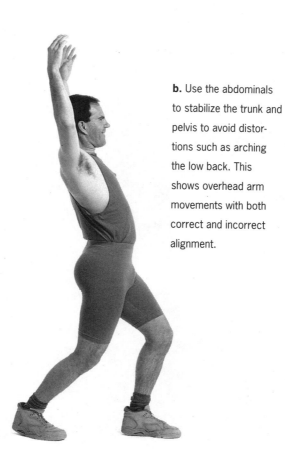

b. Use the abdominals to stabilize the trunk and pelvis to avoid distortions such as arching the low back. This shows overhead arm movements with both correct and incorrect alignment.

(synergists) and the muscles that have the opposite action (antagonists). Overdevelopment of one muscle group can actually be counterproductive, as evidenced in studies that find hamstring strains resulting from strength imbalances between the quadriceps and hamstrings (Burkett, 1970; Liemohn, 1978). However, in an aerobics class with only 15 to 20 minutes available for calisthenics, it is difficult to design routines that develop such a balance. One approach is to select some exercises, such as the push-up, that work several muscle groups at once. Another approach is to emphasize muscle groups that tend to be weak in most people and that are important for posture and for injury prevention. In addition, upper extremity muscles can be challenged during Cool-Down I with the use of bands, tubing or light weights, so that only trunk and lower-extremity muscles remain for the calisthenic portion of class.

Current ACSM recommendations are to include a minimum of eight to ten strengthening exercises that condition the major muscle groups in adult fitness programs. Certainly the challenge in a 15- to

20-minute segment is to effectively overload the chosen muscle groups progressively for various fitness levels so that everyone actually benefits from the time spent.

Several considerations are important for an instructor designing exercise sequences for calisthenics:

1. Position the body so that resistance is working to provide effective overload in accordance with a given participant's fitness level. When the weight of the body provides the primary resistance, this overload can be achieved by using antigravity positions that lift more of the body or in which the principles of leverage are applied such that a given body mass produces a greater resistance (torque). An example of the former is performing standing toe raises (ankle planterflexion) on one leg versus two. An example of the latter is performing abdominal curls with the hands behind the head versus down by the sides.

When free weights provide the primary resistance, select a body position in which the weight is moving directly against gravity in the up phase for as large a range of motion as possible. For example, pectoral flys with dumbbells (shoulder transverse adduction) should be performed supine versus standing.

Lastly, when bands or tubing are used for resistance, position the body so the band is in line to resist the desired motion as directly as possible. For example, standing in a lunge position with the right leg back works well to resist right shoulder flexion. When elastic resistance is used, the most important factor becomes the line of pull relative to the stable end of the band or tube rather than gravity.

2. Group exercises together that are best performed in the same or similar positions, or in positions that transition easily from one to another. When weights or the body itself provide the primary resistance,

Figure 7.19

Side leg lifts.

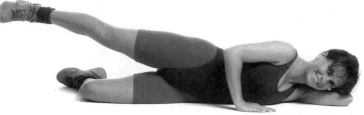

a. Correct: Proper pelvic-spinal alignment.

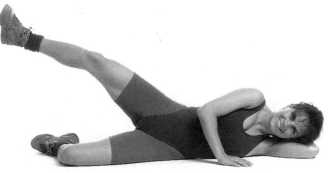

b. Incorrect: Excessive lateral tilting of the pelvis (a common compensation).

muscle groups that are antigravity in the same position can be sequenced together. However, particularly with standing combinations, it is often necessary to include some variety to allow recovery for the stabilizing muscles and joints. For example, standing in a lunge position with hand support on the forward thigh and a weight in the other hand, perform single back arm raises for the shoulder extensors and single arm rows (elbow-out position) for the scapular adductors. Then bring the front leg back next to the other leg to perform standing side leg raises for the hip abductors (with ankle weights), front arm raises for the shoulder flexors and external rotation for the shoulder rotator cuff. Also stretch the calf muscle of the back leg while performing single back arm raises and rows.

3. Use alternating sets of repetitions to give each muscle group an "active" rest (recovery). Depending on the number of repetitions and the speed of performance, two to five exercises can be grouped together such that 1 to 3 minutes of recovery is allowed a given muscle group before an additional set is performed. Continuing the example above, do a set of 8 back arm raises, 8 rows, 8 side leg raises, 8 front arm raises and 8 shoulder rotations. Then repeat the whole sequence (i.e., perform a second set) on the same side before changing sides. When time is limited, another option is to only perform a second set of the muscle groups that tend to be weaker. In this example, after performing the sequence once, only a set of back arm raises, rows and shoulder rotations would be repeated. If the repetitions are performed slowly, another option would be to group a smaller number of exercises together. For example, back arm raises, rows and side leg raises would be performed in sequence and then repeated before going onto the additional exercises. Time the exercise to decide how

many to link together so that appropriate recovery is allowed.

Abdominal Strength. Abdominal strengthening (Fig. 7.17) is important both to correct the common postural problem of lumbar lordosis and to prevent low-back injury. The oblique and transverse abdominal groups are particularly important in these functions because they generate intra-abdominal pressure (Clippinger-Robertson, 1986).

There is some evidence from studies of other muscle groups that performance of

Calisthenics

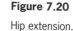
Figure 7.20
Hip extension.

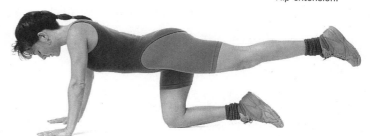
a. Correct alignment: Limited range and adequate abdominal stabilization.

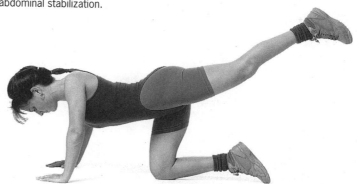
b. Incorrect alignment: Excessive range and inadequate abdominal stabilization.

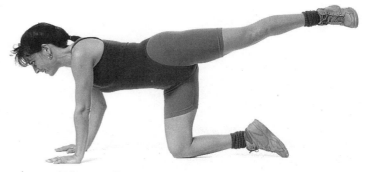
c. Incorrect alignment: Excessive rotation of the pelvis and spine.

different functions of the same muscle will slightly alter which motor units are recruited within the same muscle, and slightly different muscle soreness patterns are sometimes noted between "upper" and "lower" abdominal exercises. Since both functions of the abdominals (pulling the ribs down and posteriorly tilting the pelvis) are important for posture and movement, it appears advisable to include abdominal exercises that utilize both of these functions. This very controversial area requires additional research, but until more data are available, include a combination of abdominal exercises that emphasizes the following: bringing the ribs toward the pelvis, bringing the pubic bone toward the ribs, pulling the abdominal wall inward and rotating against resistance.

A possible combination to include would be: (1) a set of supine pelvic tilts with knees bent and feet flat on the floor, (2) a set of partial curl-ups (raising the ribs toward the pelvis), (3) a set of reverse abdominal curls (lifting the hips off the floor with knees pulled in toward the chest), (4) a set of "crunches" in which both the shoulders and hips lift from the floor, and

(5) a set of "oblique curls" in which a shoulder is raised toward the opposite hip. Incorporating isometric holds at various points in the range of motion, and emphasizing the concentric then the eccentric phase of the movement may help to recruit muscle fibers differently and contribute to the overall strength and endurance of the abdominals. Remember, in order to achieve the desired strength gains, these different abdominal variations would not be done consecutively, but rather with exercises for other muscle groups in-between so that 1- to 3-minutes recovery is allowed.

Back Strength. In the past, many instructors avoided back extensor strengthening and instead emphasized strengthening the anterior muscles (the abdominals). The theory was that excessive lumbar lordosis was due in part to a strength imbalance between the abdominal muscles and the back extensors. However, increasing evidence shows many individuals are weak in their back extensors as well as their abdominals. Back extensor weakness as well as abdominal weakness seems to be a risk factor for low-back problems. Several studies have shown that individuals with good back extensor endurance and better general conditioning have a lower incidence of back problems than deconditioned individuals.

It appears prudent, then, to strengthen back extensors as well as abdominals. However, back extensor exercises should be done carefully, progressing gradually, without ballistic movements of the lumbar spine. If students experience back pain or discomfort when performing these exercises, they should immediately stop and see their attending physician before attempting them again. In some cases, the physician may recommend modification or even deletion of some back extensor exercises for their patient.

Shoulder Strength. Most people use their

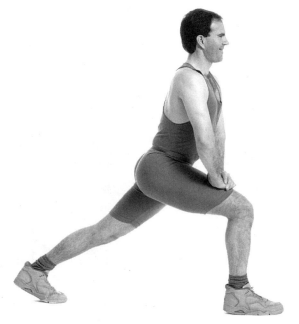

Figure 7.21

Limit knee flexion in lunges to lower risk.

arms in front of them to lift, carry and reach, thus developing stronger and shorter shoulder muscles in front (anterior) than in the back (posterior). Hours of sitting in sedentary jobs, often with slumping posture, further aggravate this tendency by weakening and stretching posterior shoulder and upper-back muscles. This common imbalance between posterior and anterior shoulder muscles can produce the postural problem of rounded shoulders. Rounded shoulders generally involves weak, long scapular adductors, with tight humeral internal rotators (pectoralis major, latissimus dorsi, and anterior deltoid). Correction of this problem involves strengthening the upper back and posterior shoulder region (scapular adductors, thoracic spinal extensors, and humeral external rotators) and stretching the shoulder transverse adductors (pectorals). Correction of rounded shoulders is important, not only for aesthetic reasons, but because the condition can cause improper shoulder mechanics that can lead to problems such as tendinitis.

If the class has time for additional shoulder strengthening, a well-rounded program would include shoulder extension exercises and the more commonly used flexion and abduction exercises see Chapter 3, for specific exercises and technique.

Hip and Knee Strength. Strengthening the quadriceps is important to protect the knee and prevent problems with the kneecap, such as chondromalacia patella (Clippinger-Robertson et al., 1986). To prevent muscle strains, however, balanced strength between the quadriceps and hamstrings is necessary; thus, the hamstrings need to be strengthened along with the quadriceps. Remember that the hamstrings and the rectus femoris are biarticulate (cross two joints), and exercises that combine actions at both hip and knee are an effective means of strengthening these muscles.

A possible sequence for these muscle groups would include 8 stationary lunges with right foot forward, 8 left hip extensions with the knee straight, 8 right knee extensions, and 8 right hamstring curls with the right hip held in slight hyperextension and pelvis stabilized with the abdominals. Repeat with a left lunge-right hip extension-left knee extension-left hamstring curl

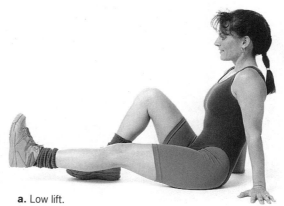

Figure 7.22
Increasing intensity of front leg lifts.

a. Low lift.

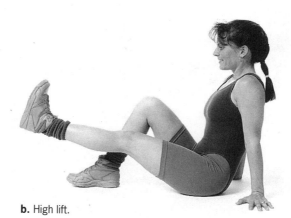

b. High lift.

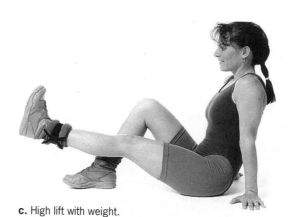

c. High lift with weight.

Figure 7.23

Leverage principles applied to curl-ups. By modifying arm positions, curl-ups are made progressively more difficult.

series. To achieve adequate overload by 8 reps, most individuals would have to perform these latter exercises with ankle weights or looped bands for resistance. The lunges could be performed as a warm-up, or to achieve adequate overload, add weights in the hands or substitute wall squats. If there is inadequate time to perform the whole series, hip extension can be combined with knee flexion in one exercise and balanced by performing knee exten-

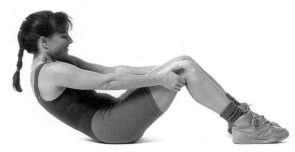

a. Least difficult: Curl-up with arms reaching forward.

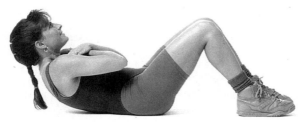

b. More difficult: Curl-up with arms crossing at chest.

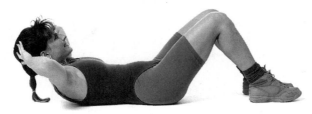

c. More difficult: Curl-up with hands behind head.

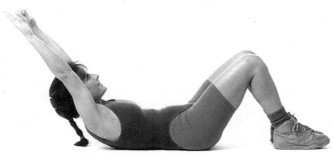

d. Most difficult: Curl-up with arms overhead.

sion with bands or weights for resistance.

In addition to the hip flexors and extensors, it is desirable to strengthen the hip abductors and adductors, which help to stabilize the gait and assist with other movements such as flexion, extension and rotation. The abductors may be exercised with a side-lying leg lift, or the standing side lift with bands or weights for resistance. Adductors are probably best strengthened side-lying.

Ankle and Shin Strength. Another area that needs strengthening for injury prevention is the shin and lower leg, the most commonly injured areas in high-impact aerobics classes. Although many people believe that jumping strengthens the shins, it actually primarily strengthens the calf muscles (plantarflexors), which work concentrically on the takeoff and eccentrically on the landing. It is particularly important to strengthen the tibialis anterior, the tibialis posterior and the peroneals. Although some of these muscles aid with plantarflexion, they can be overloaded more effectively when inversion and eversion, respectively, are added. It is also very important to warm these muscle groups prior to impact activities.

In some classes and with some populations it may also be desirable to include calf strengthening exercises. For example, with older adults calf weakness is prevalent and a low-impact aerobics segment may not provide sufficient overload in itself. In a 15-minute calisthenic segment in a regular aerobics class, however, this muscle group need not necessarily be emphasized as it is overloaded with the jumps and hops of aerobics. Most people would benefit, however, from stretching this area.

Calisthenic Exercise Modification

As in the aerobics component, the goal of the calisthenics component is to provide appropriate exercises so that muscular strength and endurance improve while injuries are avoided. Because it is common to find wide variation in strength among class members and even among joints and muscles in the same person, the instructor must provide options for modifying exercises. Participants should be warned that if their joints hurt or if they cannot maintain correct form, they are working too hard and should substitute easier versions of the exercises.

Modifying Calisthenic Safety. Some exercises are probably better to avoid in the aerobics class after assessing their risk and benefit. Chapter 3 lists several higher risk exercises with suggested substitutions. However, most exercises can simply be modified to enhance safety (Clippinger-Robertson, 1988). With strengthening exercises, one of the most common methods of modifying is to limit range of motion. For example, when bending the knees, the stress on the knees (patellofemoral compression force) dramatically increases with greater degrees of flexion. Although some athletes may need to use a fuller range of motion, in the aerobics class it is commonly recommended that knee flexion be limited to about 90 degrees in strengthening movements such as squats and lunges so that risk is lowered (Fig. 7.21). Another previously discussed example is limiting range in hip extension exercises (Fig. 7.20) so that excessive arching of the back is avoided and proper technique is maintained. Additional recommendations for modification of strengthening exercises are provided in Table 7.3.

Modifying Calisthenic Intensity. Three convenient ways to modify the difficulty of an exercise are to vary the repetitions, the distance a body part is lifted, or the resistance. Increasing these variables will increase difficulty. For example, with straight-leg raises, difficulty may be increased by performing 12 instead of 8 reps, lifting the leg higher (Fig. 7.22a & b) or adding ankle weights (Fig. 7.22c). Resistance may also be in-

creased by changing the configuration of body parts, a technique commonly used in curl-ups and push-ups in which altering the relationship of body parts to the axis of rotation significantly affects the difficulty of the exercise. Curl-ups, for instance, become progressively more difficult as the arms move farther away from the lumbar spine (Fig. 7.23a-d). A participant who has difficulty performing a series of curl-ups can modify the exercise by changing the arm position, by curling to a lower arc, or by performing fewer repetitions interspersed with rests; for example, a sequence of 4 curls, brief rest, 4 curls.

Calisthenic Transitions

When combining exercises into a sequence, it is important that smooth transitions occur between movements. When

Figure 7.24a-b
Strengthening the hip abductor and adductor.

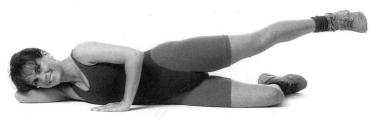

a. Lift top leg toward ceiling and lower slowly to the floor.

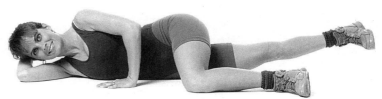

b. Lift bottom leg and lower slowly to the floor.

Figure 7.25
Modified side-ups.

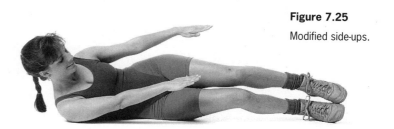

Table 7.3

BASIS OF EXERCISE RISK ASSESSMENT AND MODIFICATION

Region	Common Injury Mechanism/Joint Vulnerability	Potential Structures at Risk	Example of Exercise	Degree of Controversy	Recommended Modifications
Spine *Cervical*	Percussive hyperextension	Muscles, ligaments	Fast head forward-back in warm-up	Moderate	Delete or limit range and speed (slowly, look up without letting head drop back). Change position to work against gravity.
	Momentum	Muscles, ligaments	Fast head circles	Moderate	Perform slowly, with control & limit range to back.
	Percussive or loaded extreme flexion	Cervical compression Low back/sciatic nerve	Plough	Moderate	Substitute gentle stretch using hand to pull head forward for neck; supine double-knee-to-chest for low back.
Lumbar & Sacroiliac Joints	Percussive hyperextension	Vertebrae, disc, muscles, ligaments	Donkey kicks Hamstring leg-lifts	Moderate	Limit height of leg lifted so that back does not arch.
			Roman chair extension	High	Limit degree of spinal hyperextension and preceding flexion.
	Percussive or weighted extreme flexion	Ligaments, disc, muscles facet joints	Standing toe-touches	Moderate	Substitute sustained, supported stretch
			Stiff-legged dead lifts	High	Delete for non-power-lifters.
	Addition of rotation to percussive hyperextension or extreme flexion	Disc, ligaments, muscles	Windmills	Low	Substitute sustained, controlled stretch.
	Sustained extreme flexion	Disc, ligaments	Many standing hamstring stretches	High	Use hands on thigh, wall or floor for support.
			Ballet barre stretches		Reserve for dancers.
			Sit and reach stretch		Use selectively for appropriate populations.
	Hip flexor traction on lumbar spine	Disc, muscles, ligaments	Double leg-lifts Full sit-ups	Low Moderate	Substitute ab curls. Substitute ab curls.
	Long lever arm relative to lumbosacral an sacroiliac joints	Muscle, ligaments, disc	Flat back bounces	Low	Delete.
			Good Morning	High	Substitute prone back extension.
			Hip horizontal abduction	High	Perform with bent knee or lower leg to 45° hip flexion or below.

Table 7.3 (Continued)

BASIS OF EXERCISE RISK ASSESSMENT AND MODIFICATION

Region	Common Injury Mechanism/Joint Vulnerability	Potential Structures at Risk	Example of Exercise	Degree of Controversy	Recommended Modifications
Lumbar & Sacroiliac Joints	Compression	Disc	Overhead press	High	First develop adequate strength in trunk stabilization muscles and proper technique.
Shoulder	Impingement	Supraspinatus	Excessive overhead arm movements with poor mechanics	Low	Encourage correct shoulder mechanics, limit consecutive reps.
	Excessive deceleration and momentum	Rotator cuff	Jumping jack arms with too fast a tempo	Low	Use appropriate tempo music or decrease range of arms.
		Pectoralis major strain Shoulder strain/ dislocation	Supine flys Stiff arm pullovers	Low	Use appropriate weight, good control and gradually develop ROM.
Hip	Excessive range of motion/momentum	Muscle strains, lumbosacral joint	Bounce lunge stretch Straddle stretch	Low High	Adequate warm-up, substitute static techniques, alternative positions for less flexible.
			Scissors exercise	High	Substitute side-lying, adductor strengthening exercises.
Knee	Extreme flexion	Menisci, ligaments, patellofemoral joint	Duck walks Deep lunges Grand pliés	Low	Delete. Limit range to about 90°.
			Full squats	High	Limit use to training athletes with qualified instruction.
	Twisting of tibia relative to femur	Menisci, ligaments, patellofemoral joint	Lotus position	Low	Substitute adductor stretch with soles of feet together.
			Hurdler's stretch Poor technique in half-squats, lunges	High	Change knee position. Encourage correct alignment with mid-kneecap over 2nd toe.
Ankle/foot	High impact	Ankle/foot structures, patellofemoral joint, spine	Large jumps landing on one foot	High	Careful sequencing with lower impact moves, correct technique, showing low-impact modification.
	Excessive pronation	Ankle/foot structures	Poor technique with jumps	Moderate	Encourage correct technique.

the routine includes several sets, working alternate muscle groups in a similar body position helps keep a smooth flow. For example, a set of 10 right side leg-lifts (Fig. 7.19a) may be followed by a set of 10 left side leg-pulls (Fig. 7.24) and a set of side-lying abdominal curls (Fig. 7.25). This alternation may be repeated several times with variations in leg position or counts, if desired. If a single set is being performed, this series could easily sequence to an exercise performed on the back or stomach before repeating the original series on the other side. An instructor who knows several strengthening exercises for each major muscle group will find it easier to design a sequence that flows well.

Including a few calisthenics in preceding and following segments can also sometimes enhance smooth transitions and effective use of limited class time. Shoulder and upper-back exercises can easily fit into Cool-Down I while the legs perform simple rhythmic movements. These movements can make a smooth transition into floor

work for the abdominals, hip and knee, or into standing leg work such as front, side, or back leg-lifts, knee extension and knee flexion. In a similar manner, exercises for strengthening the shins fit well with simple stretches during Cool-Down II.

Cool-down II (Flexibility)

The primary purpose of Cool-Down II is to enhance flexibility. Adequate flexibility is important for injury prevention, optimal joint biomechanics and for enhanced performance. Current evidence indicates that stretching muscles when they are warm tends to reduce tissue damage and increases the amount of muscle elongation that persists after the stretch is removed (Taylor et al., 1990). Therefore, placing flexibility exercises at the end of class during this final cool-down works well, even though some specific stretches may be used after working particular muscle groups during calisthenics.

As in other segments of the class, a smooth flow between exercises is desir-

Figure 7.26

Stretching the hip flexors.

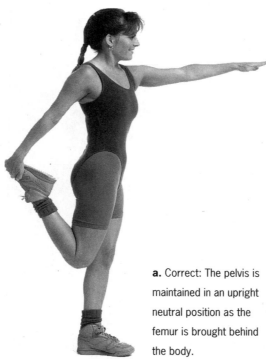

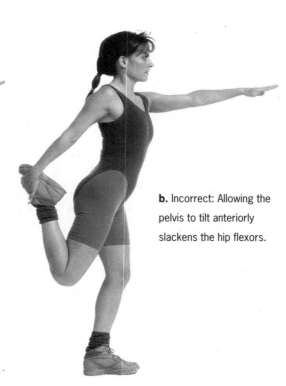

a. Correct: The pelvis is maintained in an upright neutral position as the femur is brought behind the body.

b. Incorrect: Allowing the pelvis to tilt anteriorly slackens the hip flexors.

able. Instructors should group flexibility exercises to avoid awkward transitions and minimize the number of changes in body position.

General Flexibility Component Design

Cool-Down II is composed of a series of stretches to maintain or increase range of motion at key body joints. How a stretch is applied in terms of intensity and duration will have an important effect both on effectiveness and safety.

Maximizing Stretching Effectiveness. To maximize flexibility gains and lessen the risk of injury, a stretch should ideally be of a slow, lower-force, longer-duration nature (Sapega et al., 1981).

Enhancing Stretching Safety. Because there is a fine distinction between the deformation of connective tissue associated with increasing flexibility and the deformation that will cause injury, control of stretching intensity and the speed of stretch application is very important for injury prevention. Ballistic exercises that utilize a rapid application of stretch and a relatively high magnitude of stretch should be modified or avoided. Stretches that are selected should allow a sufficiently low magnitude of stretch with a slow, controlled application.

Alignment and Technique. An instructor who understands which muscles are the focus of each stretch and which position of the joints is necessary will be able to help participants stretch more effectively and more safely. For example, in stretching the hip flexors the exerciser should bring the hip into extension while the pelvis maintains a neutral position—straight up and down (Fig. 7.26a). A common error is to allow the pelvis to tilt forward as the hip is brought into extension (Fig. 7.26b). This error slackens the muscles that the exerciser intends to stretch. Careful attention to technique and use of the abdominals to stabi-

lize the trunk will enhance flexibility gains while lessening risk to surrounding joints.

Selecting Specific Flexibility Exercises

This final flexibility routine should ideally include a balance of stretches for key muscles groups with an emphasis on areas that are commonly tight and that are important for injury prevention. Adequate flexibility is especially important for injury prevention in general populations in the anterior shoulder, hip flexors, low back, hamstrings and calf muscles. Inadequate shoulder flexibility frequently leads to round shoulders and compensatory arching of the low back in positions in which the arms are overhead (Fig. 7.27). Tight low-back muscles, hip flexors and hamstrings can disrupt optimal spinal mechanics and increase the risk for low-back injury. Tight calf muscles (gastrocnemius-soleus complex) limit needed dorsiflexion at the ankle during typical

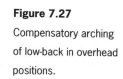

Figure 7.27

Compensatory arching of low-back in overhead positions.

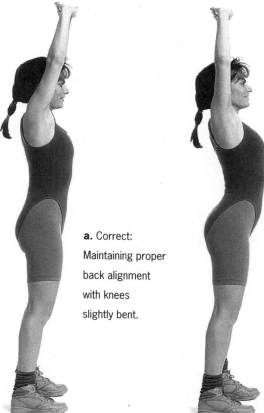

a. Correct: Maintaining proper back alignment with knees slightly bent.

b. Incorrect: Tight shoulder extensors can limit shoulder flexion so that compensatory hyperextension of the lumbar spine is necessary to reach overhead.

Chapter 7
Components of an
Aerobics Class

locomotor movements. This can interfere with needed shock absorbency and often leads to compensatory foot pronation to achieve greater dorsiflexion at the ankle. Excessive pronation contributes to many lower extremity injuries, including shin splints, Achilles tendinitis and plantar fasciitis. Flexibility exercises for the anterior shoulder, low back, hamstrings and calf that should be included in all classes are described in Chapter 3.

Additional flexibility exercises may be chosen to fit the needs of a specific class. Generally, stretches should also be included for the quadriceps femoris, hip abductors and hip adductors.

Flexibility Exercise Modification

Like strength, flexibility varies widely among people and among joints and muscles within the same person. An individual may be fit from both cardiovascular and muscular strength perspectives and yet inflexible in certain muscle groups. Some stretch positions are particularly rigorous and can produce discomfort or even injury, particularly in less flexible people or special populations, such as overweight, pregnant or senior participants. If participants show discomfort or are unable to achieve the desired position for effective stretching, the instructor should modify exercises or substitute less advanced or lower-risk variations.

Modifying for Stretching Safety. To select flexibility exercises that yield effective gains without endangering the spine or other joints, the instructor needs a basic understanding of joint biomechanics, and a knowledge of the fitness levels and musculoskeletal health of his or her students. Some high-risk stretches and alternatives are described in Table 7.3.

Modifying for Flexibility Level. For less flexible participants, stretch positions are often safer and more effective if they isolate the stretch to a single muscle group so as not to require marked flexibility at other joints, if they have a built-in mechanism to allow variation in intensity with an adequately low minimum, and if balance can be easily maintained.

In the supine hamstring stretch for example, balance is easy because the back provides a wide base of support on the floor. This position with the back flat and supported also limits involvement of the low back in the stretch and helps isolate stretching to the hamstring muscle group. Furthermore, the exerciser's ability to bend the knee, which slackens the hamstring, and to vary the angle of the leg as it is brought toward the chest allows even a very tight individual to achieve the position and to easily control stretch intensity. In

Figure 7.28

Enhancing safety while stretching the hamstrings.

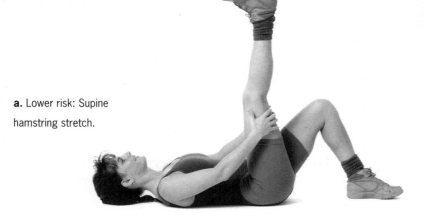

a. Lower risk: Supine hamstring stretch.

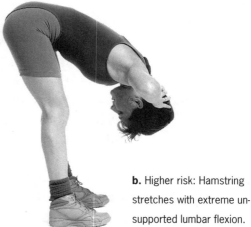

b. Higher risk: Hamstring stretches with extreme unsupported lumbar flexion.

contrast, hamstring stretches that use forward trunk flexion (Fig. 7.28) place the stretch on several muscle groups, including the calf and low back. The weight of the whole upper body produces the force elongating the hamstrings, making the stretch intensity high and difficult to control for the less flexible individual. That is, people with tight hamstrings and low-back muscles cannot bring the trunk close to the legs, and so the force stretching the hamstrings actually increases in less flexible persons. Furthermore, they often cannot reach the floor and so cannot use hand support on the floor to reduce stress to the low back. Finally, this position is often awkward and requires tricky balance for less flexible exercisers who often resort to undesirable compensations to achieve stability, such as shifting the weight back on the feet and hyperextending the knees.

Designing stretches for less flexible participants, especially beginners, makes it important to choose positions carefully. Two effective ways of modifying stretches are to change the relationship of the body to gravity or to simplify the movement to involve fewer muscle groups. For example, the straddle stretch (Fig. 7.29) is frequently uncomfortable for beginners. Although this stretch is intended to increase flexibility in the hamstrings and hip adductors, the proper position to achieve this stretch— with upper-body weight in front of the hip sockets—requires more low-back and hamstring flexibility than many participants possess. The straddle stretch may be modified by simplifying it into stretches for single

Figure 7.29
Modifications of straddle stretch. (See Figure 7.28a for supine hamstring stretch)

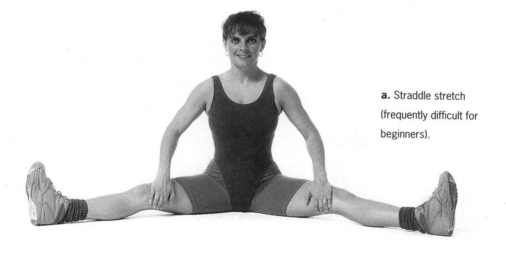

a. Straddle stretch (frequently difficult for beginners).

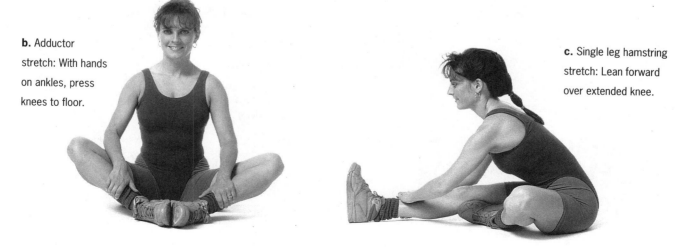

b. Adductor stretch: With hands on ankles, press knees to floor.

c. Single leg hamstring stretch: Lean forward over extended knee.

Table 7.4

CLASS EVALUATION

Class Warm-Up	Movement selection	Completeness, balance, appropriateness, specificity for class demands.
	Sequencing	Progressive increase in range of motion, complexity, muscle use.
	Rhythmical flow	Appropriate ordering and transitions.
Aerobics Component	Movement selection	Safety and effectiveness for class positioning and participants.
	Intensity	Gradual increase at beginning and decrease at end.
	Modifications	Modifications clearly demonstrated for intensity and impact.
	Choreography	Variety and interest.
	Muscle balance	With arm and leg movement.
	Stressful movements	Limited consecutive repetitions with modifications where appropriate.
	Stress alternation	Between different regions of body (i.e., shins, knees, hips).
	Impact	Appropriate use for class level and participants' fitness/health history.
	Sequence/progression	Logical building (i.e., intensity, impact, complexity).
	Transitions	Smooth, easy-to-follow.
	Cueing	Clear, concise, appropriate timing, safety emphasis.
	Heart rate monitoring	Quick and accurate with appropriate feedback given.
Class Cool-Down I	Movement selection	Rhythmic leg movements, no isometrics, avoid lowering head below heart.
	Intensity	Gradually decreasing.
	Heart rate monitoring	Accurate with instructions on modification if too high.
Calisthenics/Muscle Conditioning	Exercise selection	Safety, effectiveness, relevance to participants.
	Muscle balance	Key muscles, antagonist pairs or weak partner in pair.
	Technique	Emphasis on technique rather than just repetitions.
	Cueing	Clear, concise, whys, safety emphasis.
	Demonstration	Correct technique, clear, do's and don'ts.
Cool-Down II (Flexibility Exercises/ Relaxation)	Exercise Selection	Safety, effectiveness, relevance to participants' modifications.
	Muscle balance	Key muscles for class, posture and injury prevention.
	Technique	Emphasis on technique and where stretch should be experienced.
	Cueing	Clear, consider, whys, safety emphasis.
	Demonstration	Correct technique, clear, do's and don'ts.
Instructional/Leadership Techniques	Persona	Motivating, enthusiastic, caring, diplomatic when handling problem students.
	Professionalism	Attitude, presence, dress, educator vs. just performer.
	Movement skills	Defined, coordinated, articulate, easily followed, proper alignment.
	Verbal cueing	Clarity of voice, projection, pitch, voice modulation, conciseness.

Table 7.4 (Continued)

CLASS EVALUATION

Instructional/Leadership Techniques	Verbal cueing variety	Footwork, directional, rhythmic, numerical, step.
	Nonverbal cueing	Visual cueing, eye contact, mirroring, overexaggeration, hand signs, different facings.
	Choreography	Appropriate movement selection, freestyle vs. choreographed or structured, add-ons, progressions, part-whole, simple-complex.
	Corrections/modifications	Nutrition, benefits of exercise, injury prevention.
Safety/Injury Prevention	Contraindicated exercises	Avoidance of or modification of.
	Safe transitions	To and from floor, from full knee flexion, with spinal flexion.
	Technique	Proper alignment, controlled movement, appropriate tempo music.
	Encouragement for self-monitoring	Heart rate, RPE, talk test.
	Encouragement to work at own level	Avoid encouraging competition with instructor or other students. Emphasize self-improvement.
	Heart rate monitoring	Appropriate placement in class, accurate procedures, adequate feedback.
Overall Impressions	Program content	Effectiveness/safety for participant level.
	Overall class flow and organization	Well-organized and balanced, instructor knows music.
	Safety precautions and techniques	Floor transitions, class transitions such as cool-down, potential higher-risk exercises, modifications, awareness of warning signs of exercise, use of resistance, platforms and props.
	Music	Tempo (according to ACE's manual): <100 bpm — stretching 100-120 — warm-up and cool-down 130-170 — aerobic routines 110-130 — floor exercises Interest, variety appropriateness for participants.
	Staying power/interest	Challenging but reachable, fun, creative.
	Variety	Movement, music, cueing.
	Motivational qualities	Appropriate goal-setting and evaluation (heighten awareness and importance of subtle improvements). Minimizing perfectionism (emphasize improvement vs. absolute performance). Quantitative measures (sit-reach, ab-curl). Individualization, recognition, social contacts.

muscle groups, the hamstrings and hip adductors. Other modifications include bending the knees to slacken the hamstrings or bringing the legs closer together to slacken the adductors. People who are too tight to sit with the trunk leaning forward can keep the outstretched knee or knees bent slightly, allowing the bottom of the pelvis to move back to the proper position. For the hamstrings, they may use a supine position with the outstretched knee slightly bent.

As flexibility increases, stretches can progress to include more muscle groups and more complex positions. However, it is still important to keep participants focused on technique and relaxing their muscles, not on keeping their balance. It is always important not to jeopardize the back or other joints. Many simple "beginning" stretches are effective enough to be carried over into advanced classes. Unlike strength exercises, in which positions must often be altered to ensure adequate overload as participants' strength improves, most stretches may progress simply by further approximating the appropriate body segments. For example, leaning farther forward with the trunk in the butterfly stretch (Fig. 7.29) or bringing the leg farther toward the chest in the supine hamstring stretch will increase stretch intensity.

Stress Reduction

Stretching may also offer benefits in regard to muscle relaxation and stress reduction. Excessive stress is thought to play a role in many of the health problems of today and stress reduction is one of the commonly reported reasons that individuals choose to take aerobics classes. When used for stress reduction, stretching is commonly performed very slowly, with concentration on slow breathing, and in

a darkened room with quiet or relaxing music. It can also be combined with other relaxation techniques.

SUMMARY

Safe and effective class design requires a specific structuring of exercises so that the appropriate overload is provided to help achieve the desired gains (Table 7.4). Instructors should balance each segment of the class—warm-up, aerobics, calisthenics, flexibility—in terms of muscles used and in terms of maximizing benefits while minimizing risks. Application of basic scientific principles from kinesiology and exercise physiology is necessary for appropriate exercise selection, to anticipate problems, to know how to cue exercises and to design effective routines. If instructors frequently explain and demonstrate modifications of exercises, participants can work at the appropriate intensity for their level of fitness with reduced injury risk. Instructors should move beyond emphasizing just quantity toward the fitness gains that come from emphasizing specificity and performance quality.

REFERENCES

American College of Sports Medicine. (1991). *Guidelines for Exercise Testing and Prescription*. Philadelphia: Lea and Febiger.

American College of Sports Medicine. (1990). Position Stand: The Recommended Quantity and Quality of Exercise for Developing and Maintaining Cardiorespiratory and Muscular Fitness in Healthy Adults. *Medicine and Science in Sports and Exercise*, 21, 265-274.

Anderson, T., & Kearney, J. (1982). Effects of Three Resistance Training Programs on Muscular Strength and Absolute and Relative Endurance. *Research Quarterly in Exercise and Sport*. 53, 1-7.

Astrand, P., & Rodahl, K. (1977). *Textbook of Work Physiology*. New York: McGraw-Hill,

Burkett, L. (1970). Causative Factors in Hamstring Strains. *Medicine and Science in Sports* 2, 39-42.

Clippinger-Robertson, K. (1988). Understanding Contraindicated Exercises. *Dance Exercise Today*, January/February, 57-60.

Clippinger-Robertson, K.; Hutton, R., Miller D., & Nicholas, D. (1986). Mechanical and Anatomical Factors Relating to the Incidence and Etiology of Patellofemoral Pain in Dancers. *In The Dancer as Athlete*, ed. C. Shell. Champaign, Il: Human Kinetics Publishers.

Cooper, K. (1982). *The Aerobics Program for Total Well-Being*. New York: Evans.

DeVries, H. (1966). *Physiology of Exercise*. Dubuque, Iowa: Brown.

Fox, E. (1984). *Sports Physiology*. Philadelphia: W.B. Saunders.

Gerson, R. (1985). Point-Counterpoint: Calisthenics Before Aerobics. *Dance Exercise Today*, May/June, 26-28.

Gettman, L., Ward, P., & Hagan, R. (1982). A Comparison of Combined Running and Weight Training with Circuit Weight Training. *Medicine and Science in Sports*, 14, 229-234.

Graves, J., Pollock, M. Jones, A. Colvin, A., & Leggett, S. (1989). Specificity of Limited Range of Motion Variable Resistance Training. *Medicine and Science in Sports*, 21, 84-89.

Jacobson, E. (1938). *Progressive Relaxation*. Chicago: University of Chicago Press.

Jones, A. (1985). Point-Counterpoint: Calisthenics Before Aerobics. *Dance Exercise Today*, May/June, 27-28.

Kendall, H., Kendall, F., & Wadsworth, P. (1971). *Muscle Testing and Function*. Baltimore: Williams and Wilkins.

Lehmann, J., Masock, A., & Warren, C. (1970). Effect of Therapeutic Temperatures on Tendon Extensibility. *Archives of Physical Medicine and Rehabilitation*, 51, 481-487.

Liemohn, W. (1978). Factors Related to Hamstring Strains. *American Journal of Sports Medicine*, 18, 71-76.

Otto, R., Yoke, M., Wygand R., & Kamimukai, C. (1988). The Metabolic Cost of Two Differing Low Impact Aerobic Dance Exercise Modes. *Medicine and Science in Sports and Exercise*, 20-2 (abstract), 525.

Pollock, M., Gettman, L., Mileses, C., Bah, M., Durstine, J., & Johnson, R. (1977). Effects of Frequency and Duration of Training on Attrition and Incidence of Injury. *Medicine and Science in Sports*, 9, 31-36.

Sapega, A., Quedenfeld, T., Moyer, R., & Butler, R. (1981). Biophysical Factors in Range-of-Motion Exercise. *Physician and Sportsmedicine*, 9, 57-65.

Shellock, F. (1983). Physiological Benefits of Warm-Up. *Physician and Sportsmedicine*, 11, 134-139.

Stanforth, D., Hamman, & Senechal, C. (1988). Relationship of Heart Rate and Oxygen Consumption During Low Impact Aerobic Movements. *Medicine and Science in Sports*, 20-2 (abstract), S88.

Taylor, D., Dalton, J. Seaber, A. & Garrett, W. (1990). Viscoelastic Properties of Muscle-tendon Units: The Biomechanical Effects of Stretching. *American Journal of Sports Medicine*, 18-3, 300-309.

Warren, C., Lehmann, J., & Koblanski, J. (1976). Heat and Stretch Procedures: An Evaluation Using Rat Tail Tendon. *Archives of Physical Medicine and Rehabilitation*, 57, 122-126.

Warren, C., Lehmann, J., & Koblanski, J. (1971). Elongation of Rat Tail Tendon: Effect of Load and Temperature. *Archives of Physical Medicine and Rehabilitation*, 52, 465-474.

Wiktorsson-Moller, M., Oberg, B., Ekstrand, J., & Gillquist, J. (1983). Effects of Warming Up, Massage and Stretching on Range of Motion and Muscle Strength in the Lower Extremity. *American Journal of Sports Medicine*, 11-4, 249-252.

SUGGESTED READING

American College of Sports Medicine. (1991). *Guidelines for Exercise Testing and Prescription*. Philadelphia: Lea and Febiger.

American College of Sports Medicine. (1990). Position Stand: The Recommended Quantity and Quality of Exercise for Developing and Maintaining Cardiorespiratory and Muscular Fitness in Healthy Adults. *Medicine and Science in Sports*, 21, 265-274.

Clippinger-Robertson, K. (1988). Understanding Contraindicated Exercises. *Dance Exercise Today*, January/February, 57-60.

Graves, J., Welsch, M., & Pollock, M. (1991). Exercise Training for Muscular Strength and Endurance. *IDEA Today*, July/August, 33-40.

Pollock, M., Wilmore, J., & Fox, S. (1984). *Exercise in Health and Disease*. Philadelphia: W. B. Saunders.

Sapega, A., Quedenfeld, T., Moyer, R., & Butler, R. (1981). Biophysical Factors in Range-of-Motion Exercise. *Physician and Sportsmedicine*, 9, 57-65.

Taylor, D., Dalton, J., Seaber, A., & Garrett, W. (1990). Viscoelastic Properties of Muscle-tendon Units: The Biomechanical Effects of Stretching. *American Journal of Sports Medicine*, 18-3, 300-309.

Wescott, W. (1989). *Strength Fitness: Physiological Principles and Training Techniques*. Dubuque, IA: Wm. C. Brown.

Chapter 8

Teaching an Aerobics Class

By Lorna L. Francis

The learning process

- Stages of learning
- Teaching approaches

Teaching strategies

- Selecting appropriate exercises
- Exercise skill analysis and modifications
- Feedback and knowledge of results

Designing instruction

- Goal setting
- Lesson planning
- Teaching styles
- Evaluating performance

Preparing and teaching class activities

- Selecting music
- Choreography
- Cueing

A safe and successful aerobics program depends on the instructor's ability to apply sound instructional principles and practices. In fact, effective teaching may well be the most important aspect of the aerobics instructor's role. Inadequate leadership is often cited by participants as a reason for dropping out of formal exercise programs. Unfortunately, many people believe that teaching is intuitive and spontaneous. Without proper training, however, an intuitive and spontaneous approach to teaching often results in ineffective leadership. Over the years, researchers have provided

Lorna Francis, Ph.D., a physical education professor at San Diego State University, and an internationally recognized speaker, is the author of several fitness books. Dr. Francis serves on the board of directors of ACE and is a member of the development team for Step Reebok and Bodywalk. An ACE-certified instructor, Dr. Francis was co-recipient of the 1989 IDEA Lifetime Achievement Award.

invaluable information to help instructors effectively plan and implement their programs. Scientific investigation of teaching techniques has led to an understanding of the phenomenon of teaching and its impact on **learning** behavior. A theoretical approach to teaching has provided a way to identify role expectations for teachers and students. More importantly, a scientific approach has helped determine whether a teacher's actions result in the intended outcome. The purpose of this chapter is to provide exercise leaders with a sound teaching foundation by exploring the elements of effective teaching and how they apply to an aerobics setting.

THE LEARNING PROCESS

Many instructors do not appreciate the complexity of the process required to learn a new exercise or movement pattern. In a matter of seconds, the student must perceive and react to the proper cues, must remember similar situations and instruction on what to do, must determine the proper strategy and make the correct response, and finally, through feedback, must determine whether he or she performed the exercise correctly. This section examines the learning process and describes learning strategies that will facilitate the teaching of motor skills.

Magill (1980) defines learning as an "internal change in the individual that is inferred from a relatively permanent improvement in performance of the individual as a result of practice." Instructors can therefore infer that learning has occurred when a person's performance shows less variability over time.

Learning takes place in three domains of human behavior: cognitive, affective and motor. All three domains are important within the aerobics field.

The **cognitive domain** describes intellec-

tual activities and involves gaining knowledge. Studies have shown that education within an exercise program positively affects motivation and exercise compliance. Therefore, competent instructors should remain up-to-date on the latest research in exercise and related fields in an effort to inform their students and to respond intelligently to their questions or concerns.

The **affective domain** describes emotional behaviors. Motivation to exercise depends on a person's feelings toward exercise. Instructors are therefore instrumental in helping participants develop positive attitudes about exercise.

Finally, the **motor domain** refers to those activities requiring movement. Learning motor skills is the foundation of exercise classes.

Within the aerobics profession, the motor domain has been heavily emphasized, and limited attention has been given to the affective and cognitive domains. However, research has shown that teaching within all three domains is critical to exercise compliance.

Stages of Learning

To teach effectively, an instructor must be aware of the various stages of learning. One of the most commonly cited learning models was developed by Fitts and Posner (1967), who theorized that there are three stages of learning for a motor skill: cognitive, associative and autonomous. Within the first or **cognitive stage** of learning, learners make many errors and have highly variable performances. They know they are doing something wrong, but they do not know how to improve their performance. At this stage, participants seem terribly uncoordinated and consistently perform exercises incorrectly. Learners in the second or **associative stage** have learned the basic fundamentals or mechanics of the skill. Their errors tend to be less gross in nature and they can now concentrate on refining their skills. During this stage, exercise participants are able to detect some errors and the instructor needs to make only occasional corrections. During the third or **autonomous stage** the skill becomes automatic or habitual. Learners can now perform without thinking and can detect their own errors. Highly skilled participants, for example, do not think about individual steps in a routine, but instead concentrate on the more difficult aspects of the choreography.

The kind and amount of information that exercise participants can understand depends on the stage of the learning process they are in. For example, beginning aerobic exercisers see a choreographed routine as composed of many steps, each step demanding their full attention. However, advanced aerobic exercisers see only a few steps as crucial, perhaps where the tempo changes or at the beginning of a difficult part of the routine. Because beginners are less skilled at determining what information they must attend to, the exercise instructor must provide them with specific information about what is important. For example, since maintaining appropriate posture is necessary to properly execute many exercises and movement patterns, instructors must constantly remind beginners to maintain correct exercise posture. To employ appropriate teaching strategies, instructors need to be aware of each participant's stage of learning.

Teaching Approaches

When teaching an exercise or movement pattern, instructors should determine which teaching approach will be most effective. They can use either a **part approach** in which the skill is broken down into its component parts and each part is practiced, or a **whole approach** in which the skill is practiced in its entirety. The most efficient teaching approach depends on the task complexity and the task organization of the skill (Magill, 1980). **Task complexity** refers to the number of parts or components within a task and the level of information processing required to complete the task. A highly complex task has many components and requires much attention. Aerobic combinations with intricate footwork and arm movements, for example, can be highly complex. Low complexity tasks have few components and relatively limited attention demands. Many floor exercises are low in complexity. **Task organization** refers to the number of parts of the task that are interrelated. A task high in organization is composed of closely related components, such as the parts of a specific floor exercise. A task low in organization is composed of independent parts, such as the individual steps making up an aerobics routine.

Tasks or skills that are high in complexity and low in organization should be taught by practicing the parts. The part approach to teaching is therefore appropriate for aerobics routines. Instructors should teach each step in its simplest form. Once participants have mastered the steps, they can be placed in the proper sequence. Tasks or skills that are low in complexity but high in organization should be practiced in their entirety. When teaching a floor exercise, instructors should explain the entire exercise in terms of the correct execution and then ask their students to perform the activity.

TEACHING STRATEGIES

To become proficient at teaching aerobics, instructors must be familiar with methods for selecting appropriate exercises and movement patterns, analyzing exercise skills, and modifying exercise for various fitness levels and special populations. They must also be knowledgeable concerning techniques for increasing participant motivation and exercise adherence (see Chapter 10, "Adherence and Motivation"). The following section addresses these important teaching strategies.

Selecting Appropriate Exercises

An effective aerobics instructor must develop skills to determine which exercises and movement patterns are effective and safe to use within the exercise class. A thorough knowledge of exercise science is essential in this decision-making process. Each exercise or movement pattern should be evaluated according to its effectiveness and safety. To determine exercise effectiveness, instructors must ask themselves, "Does this particular exercise do what it is suppose to do?" In other words, what is the purpose of the exercise and does it meet the intended objective? When considering stretching exercises, the instructor must ask, "Does this particular exercise effectively stretch the muscle(s) it is suppose to stretch?"

For example, while it is possible to stretch the erector spinae and hamstrings using a straight-legged sitting toe-touch exercise, class participants with tight erector spinae or tight hamstrings may be unable to put sufficient stretch on the targeted muscles. Compound stretches, where several major muscle groups are being stretched at the same time are not as effective as stretches that isolate a specific muscle or muscle group. Therefore, it might be more effective to use two different stretches, one that targets the hamstrings and one that targets the erector spinae.

When considering the effectiveness of strength exercises, the instructor must ask, "Does this exercise strengthen the intended muscle(s)?" Some fitness leaders are con-

fused about the direction in which the resistance is being applied when evaluating certain strength exercises and consequently tend to teach exercises that do not target the intended muscle group. For example, holding a rubber band in the right hand above the head while pulling the band down toward the hips with the left hand, will help to strengthen latissimus dorsi (lat pull-down). However, performing this same movement with a hand-held weight will strengthen the deltoids. Knowledge of muscles and their actions and an understanding of the direction in which the resistance is being exerted is invaluable in helping instructors select effective strength exercises.

If an exercise does not fulfill the instructor's objective, it should not be selected for inclusion in the aerobics class. If an exercise is determined to be effective, the instructor must then decide if it is safe. Instructors must ask, "Does the selected exercise cause pain in the joints or does it put unnecessary stress on other vulnerable parts of the body?" For example, while unsupported, sustained forward flexion in a standing position is often used to stretch the hamstrings, this particular position is hazardous to the lumber spine. Therefore, a safer alternative for stretching the hamstrings should be considered. While in many instances an instructor will probably choose to reject an exercise that is determined to be unsafe or contraindicated, there are times when the benefits of an exercise can outweigh the risks. For example, to effectively stretch the quadriceps it is necessary to apply an external force to move the heel of the foot toward the buttocks. This position can be mechanically stressful to vulnerable structures of the knee. However, if the exercise is performed with care, the benefits often outweigh the risk for participants with healthy knees.

An instructor's ability to evaluate the

effectiveness and safety of exercises will improve as he or she learns more about the functional anatomy of the human body and the many factors that can affect efficient human movement.

Exercise Skill Analysis and Modifications

An important role of the exercise instructor is to effectively analyze the movement skills of class participants. An exercise that is performed incorrectly will not achieve the desired goal, but more importantly, improper exercise execution could result in injury. Body alignment is crucial to proper exercise execution. Instructors must therefore have a thorough knowledge of appropriate body alignment.

Most exercises require class participants to maintain a neutral pelvis. The neutral position of the lumbar spine is found by alternately performing an anterior (forward) pelvic tilt and a posterior (rearward) pelvic tilt. The midpoint between these two extreme positions of the pelvis is the neutral position. The neutral position of the cervical spine is also important. The head should be comfortably balanced with a minimum of activity of the muscles of the neck. Class participants should be frequently reminded of mechanically sound posture—neutral head, shoulders back, chest up, neutral pelvis and relaxed knees (standing posture). For more information on proper body alignment see Chapter 3, "Biomechanics and Applied Kinesiology".

Instructors must also be familiar with the specific mechanics of each exercise. For example, when using rubber bands, there is a natural tendency to hyperextend the wrist joints when flexing and extending the elbow joint (this gives the exerciser a mechanical advantage). Since wrist hyperextension puts considerable stress on the tendons that cross the wrist joint, class participants must be frequently reminded to maintain a neutral wrist position. Shoulder impingement is a growing problem in aerobics classes. This condition can occur when class participants repeatedly use lateral movements of the arms above shoulder level with the palms facing downward (with or without weights). Students must be encouraged to turn the palms upward as the arms are raised above shoulder level. When performing lunging or squatting exercises, it is advisable that the load-bearing knees are not flexed deeper than 90 degrees. Squatting beyond 90 degrees places high levels of compression stress on the back of the kneecaps.

These are but a few examples of common technique errors performed by class participants. To effectively teach and correct exercises, instructors must have a good understanding of sound mechanics for every exercise they select.

When teaching exercises, instructors must communicate important alignment and execution cues. It is also recommended that instructors walk around the room as much as possible to make appropriate corrections. This is particularly important during the floor work and poststretch phase of the exercise class. Unless the instructor provides appropriate feedback, few participants, especially beginners, will have any idea that they are not performing an exercise properly.

Instructors must be very cautious with hands-on corrections. Pushing a participant's limb into proper position during a stretch could result in a serious injury for the exerciser, especially if he or she is inflexible. As a rule of thumb, instructors should not perform hands-on corrections for exercises that require the manipulation of a muscle being stretched. Instead, the instructor can demonstrate proper execution of the exercise and offer verbal corrections.

However, if a participant is hyperextending a joint, for example, it might be beneficial for the instructor to lightly touch the exerciser's knees or elbows as a reminder to soften them. Common sense must always be applied by instructors when making decisions about whether to physically correct an inappropriate exercise position.

Many aerobics classes are composed of participants with varying levels of fitness and skill. In smaller communities, special populations, such as pregnant, obese or handicapped individuals, are mainstreamed into regular aerobics classes. This state of affairs presents a challenging teaching environment for instructors. To effectively provide appropriate modifications, it is important that instructors be familiar with the health history and fitness level of each class participant. Knowing this information will help instructors reduce a participant's risk of developing health complications during exercise. For example, participants with a history of high blood pressure should be reminded by the instructor not to perform static strength exercises and to avoid holding the arms at or above shoulder level for an extended period of time. A pregnant woman should be advised by her teacher not to perform exercises on her back after the fourth month of pregnancy. Mainstreaming special populations can be done as long as these individuals are appraised of specific exercise modifications and are periodically reminded of those modifications throughout the class session. For more information on modifying exercise for special populations see Chapter 11, "Special Populations and Health Concerns."

The most common modification that needs to be addressed by aerobics instructors is that of modifying exercise intensity to provide safe and effective activity for all fitness levels. Factors that affect exercise intensity include music tempo and the size of arm and leg movements. In a multilevel program, the speed of music must be selected to accommodate the less-fit individuals in the class. It is hazardous for individuals with a poor level of fitness to exercise to fast music. However, the person with a higher level of fitness can manipulate the choreography by performing larger leg and arm movements to increase exercise intensity. Instructors can assist this process by demonstrating movement modifications for each of two or three intensity levels.

For example, a level-one march with arm curls (elbow flexion and extension) can be modified to a level-two jog with arm curls to a level-three jog with overhead presses (shoulder abduction/adduction and elbow extension/flexion). It should be noted that overarm movements are not necessarily more intense aerobically than arm movements below shoulder level. While it is true that an overhead press is more intense than an arm curl, this is because the arm curl is performed with a shorter lever and therefore requires less energy expenditure to perform than an overhead press which moves from a short lever to a long lever. However, side laterals (a long-lever exercise that involves shoulder abducting to shoulder height with the elbows extended) would require about the same energy expenditure as an overhead press, even though side laterals are performed at a lower level than overhead presses.

Teaching to two or three levels requires some skill on the part of the instructor. The instructor needs to demonstrate each of the levels every time a new movement is introduced. While it is tempting for the instructor to spend most of his or her time demonstrating the more intense version of a movement, it is probably the least-fit or beginner student that requires constant visual cues. It is not surprising that deconditioned individuals (who, more often than not, are also less skilled at movement performance) emulate the more intense choreography being demonstrated by the instructor, even when the instructor tells participants to move at their own pace. Unfortunately, beginning-level participants are not skilled enough to perform movements without visual cues. After intensity levels one, two and three have been demonstrated, the instructor should come back to performing level one. Instructors must not forget that their primary objective as an exercise leader should be to teach rather than to perform.

It is the responsibility of both the instructor and the participant to monitor exercise intensity. The instructor controls intensity according to the music tempo selected and the types of movements demonstrated. The participant manipulates the exercise intensity by controlling the size of the movements performed. Instructors should encourage beginners to take their heart rates frequently and they should also be aware of the progress participants are making. One approach is to ask for a show of hands for those above, below and within their target heart-rate range. Instructors should advise those participants who are above their target zone to keep their feet closer to the ground and reduce the size of their arm movements. Those students exercising below their target zone should be encouraged to take larger steps and increase the size of their arm movements if they are ready to do so.

Instructors must make sure that exercise heart rates can be reported in a non-threatening and noncompetitive environment to ensure honesty. Accurate reporting is particularly important for participants who must maintain strict exercise heart rates due to specific medical conditions.

To avoid injury, it is extremely impor-tant that participants adjust the intensity of their movements to their cardiorespiratory fitness level. Within a multilevel class, beginners should be encouraged to progress slowly in both the intensity and duration of exercise. After deconditioned exercisers have reached their aerobic goal for the day, instructors should request that these individuals lower the intensity by "walking" through the rest the movements while more experienced participants continue to exercise at a higher intensity. Instructors should be very careful not to give conflicting messages to participants. If everyone is expected to work at his or her own intensity level, instructors must avoid general phrases such as "Get your feet up higher," "Push through it," or "Just do one more routine." Participants will feel compelled to work at higher intensities regardless of whether they are ready to do so.

Feedback and Knowledge of Results

A very important part of learning is feedback and knowledge of results. **Feedback** is an internal response within a learner. During information processing, the correctness or incorrectness of a response is stored in memory to be used for future reference. The instructor has little influence on this type of feedback. **Knowledge of results**, or KR, is feedback from external sources such as the instructor (Magill, 1980). By providing KR, exercise leaders can greatly influence a participant's performance. KR serves three important functions in learning: it provides information about performance, it serves as a motivator for further performances, and it reinforces or strengthens correct responses. An instructor must determine the critical elements of a skill in order to know which aspects of the skill to evaluate. For example, if the primary objective of the class is to achieve target heart rate, the instructor should give KR that is specific to the intensity of movement.

Three types of statements can be used when giving KR: corrective statements, value statements and neutral statements (Mosston, 1981). **Corrective statements** are used when a learner's response is incorrect. The statement identifies the error and tells the learner how to correct it. For example, "You are raising your back too far off the floor during your curl-up; keep the lower back on the floor at all times." Corrective statements are the most effective type of KR for ensuring immediate improvement in performance. A **value statement** projects a feeling about a performance, using such words as "good" or "well done." This type of statement can motivate or encourage a participant whose performance is still not altogether correct but is improving. For example, "Good, Mary, you are getting better." Finally, a **neutral statement** acknowledges the performance but does not judge or correct it. "I see you did 30 curl-ups" is an example of a neutral statement. All three statements have a place in the teaching environment, however, beginning instructors who have not yet developed effective skill analysis techniques often find themselves relying on value statements.

An instructor relies on kinesiological principles, past experience and aesthetic standards to determine the correctness of a performance (Mosston, 1981). Kinesiological principals are used to determine which postures and movements are mechanically correct. For example, curl-ups are performed with the knees bent to reduce stress on the lower back and to isolate the abdominal musculature. Past experience is often used to correct a movement based on subtleties accumulated from observing many exercisers perform the same movement. Experienced instructors can often find just the right word or phrase to

correct consistently inappropriate performances. Aesthetic standards are used to correct movements and postures determined to be culturally attractive. Aerobics movements are often corrected on the basis of aesthetic standards.

In the early stages of learning, performers cannot determine what they are doing wrong and therefore require a great deal of KR. On the other hand, proficient performers rely more on internal feedback and require little KR. Since beginners depend more heavily on visual cues than do experienced exercisers, instructors teaching multilevel classes should spend much of their time demonstrating exercises and movement patterns at the level appropriate for beginners while occasionally demonstrating exercises for more advanced participants.

A person can attend to only a few cues at any given moment. Therefore, when giving KR, instructors should limit the number of corrections offered at any one time. Positive reinforcement is very important in the early stages of learning. Instructors should use positive value statements when participants make a good attempt even if the performance is not yet correct. Appropriate feedback should always be given in a friendly manner. If several participants are performing a move incorrectly, the instructor can give feedback to the entire class. However, if one person consistently performs an exercise or movement incorrectly, the instructor should talk to that person privately, either when other class participants are working individually or after class.

DESIGNING INSTRUCTION

Effectively designing an aerobics routine involves setting goals, planning specific instructions or lessons for each component part of a class, including facility and equipment considerations, selecting the appropriate teaching style, and evaluating student performance.

Goal-setting

The effective use of goal-setting facilitates both learning and performance of motor skills. The competent exercise instructor establishes program goals and aids participants in developing their personal goals. Program goals should reflect what the instructor expects students to gain from the program. Examples of program goals might include the following:

1. The participant will increase or maintain adequate aerobic fitness to acquire cardiorespiratory health benefits.

2. The participant will increase or maintain adequate and specific joint range of motion to prevent muscle imbalances and to provide appropriate range of motion for aerobic- and floor-exercise movements.

3. The participant will increase or maintain adequate and specific muscular strength to prevent muscle imbalances and to provide adequate strength to effectively perform aerobic movements.

Once the program goals have been determined, instructors should establish class objectives and plan daily activities that will result in the achievement and maintenance of program goals. For a more complete discussion related to motivations and goals refer to Chapter 10, "Adherence and Motivation."

Lesson-planning

Planning and class preparation result in the efficient use of time, smooth progression of activities and greater program variety. Often instructors who do not plan their lessons present the same music, exercises and movement patterns day in and day out. Participants and instructors alike become bored with this daily routine.

It is particularly important that inexpe-

rienced instructors write out their daily class activities. While experienced instructors may no longer need to write a daily lesson plan, they should at least spend time before each class mentally preparing class activities. A daily lesson plan should consist of class objectives, planned activities and the time allotted for each activity, necessary equipment and patterns of class organization. Figure 8.1 contains a sample lesson plan that can be modified to meet the needs of individual instructors and the objectives of specific classes.

Class Objectives. Just as exercise instructors need to establish program goals, they also need to develop more specific objectives for each class meeting. Class objectives state what instructors expect their participants to accomplish during each exercise session. The following are examples of class objectives:

1. The participant will maintain or increase cardiorespiratory fitness by exercising aerobically for 15 to 30 minutes at an intensity of 50 to 75 percent maximal heart-rate reserve.

2. The participant will increase or maintain adequate and specific flexibility by performing the following stretching exercises to their fullest range of motion: hamstrings, quadriceps, (and so on).

3. The participant will increase or maintain adequate and specific strength and endurance by performing 8 to 12 repetitions of the following exercises: curl-ups, prone shoulder and hip extensions, (and so on).

Objectives help instructors focus on the purpose of each selected exercise and activity. In fact, novice instructors should list the purpose of each strength and flexibility exercise used in their classes. Knowing the purpose and benefits of each exercise will help instructors select appropriate class activities.

Class Activities and Time Allocations. Class activities are planned to meet the objectives of each component part of an aerobics class. Component parts of a class include:

1. Warm-up and prestretch.
2. Aerobic conditioning.
3. Aerobic cool-down.
4. Resistance training.
5. Poststretch.

An important but often overlooked activity is a regularly planned educational mini-lecture that focuses on pertinent

Figure 8.1

SAMPLE LESSON PLAN

Class: Aerobic Exercise   **Date:** December 31, 1993   **Time:** 9–10:15 a.m.

Class Objectives:

1. Participants will improve or maintain cardiorespiratory fitness by performing aerobics movements for 15 to 25 minutes at 50 to 75 percent heart-rate reserve.

2. Participants will improve or maintain flexibility by performing specific stretching exercises, holding for 10 seconds at maximum range of motion.

3. Participants will improve or maintain strength by performing specific strength exercises for three sets of 12 repetitions.

Activities	Time (minutes)	Patterns of Class Org.	Equipment	Music	Comments
Discussion (Spot-reducing)	5	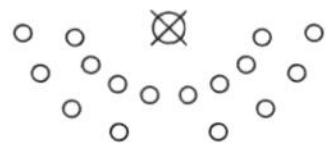			
Warm-up	5	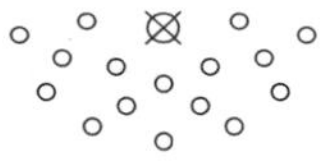		Will vary according to season, age group and participant interest	Nice and easy
Preaerobic Stretch (Pectoralis Major, Hamstrings, hip flexors, Erector Spinae, Quads, Gastrocnemius)	5	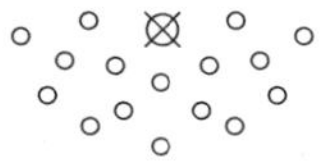		(same as above)	Stretch to point of tightness not pain
Aerobic Exercise (Freestyle technique using a linear progression)	25	(same as above)		(same as above)	Take ExHR. Check ExHRs with a show of hands
Cool-down	4	(same as above)		(same as above)	Take recovery HR
Floor Exercise (Curl-ups, Toe-raises, Prone hip extension, Tricep extension, Scapulae adduction)	20	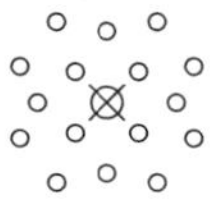	Mats, rubber bands	(same as above)	Slow and controlled; breathe on exertion
Postaerobic Stretch (Same muscle groups as preaerobic stretch)	10	(same as above)	Towels	(same as above)	Perform exercises on the floor
Record Progress	1		Card file		Give praise/ encouragement

physiological, kinesiological or nutritional information. These discussions, which should be concise and brief (5 minutes) can include such topics as exercise myths and misconceptions, the latest findings on fat utilization during exercise, and methods of reducing low-back pain. The instructor can offer additional educational information during the workout by discussing the purpose of a particular segment or exercise while it is being performed. Educational handouts are also extremely valuable to participants and can serve as a motivator for continued attendance.

Strength and flexibility exercises should be carefully planned. Specific stretching and resistance training exercises are discussed in Chapters 3, "Biomechanics and Applied Kinesiology" and 9, "Variations: From Step to Strength Training". The selection of music and movement patterns for the warm-up, aerobic conditioning and cool-down segments of the class are one of the instructor's most challenging tasks. These two very important activities are addressed in greater detail later in this chapter.

The time allotted for each activity varies according to the total class time available and according to the specific nature of the activity. Some activities will naturally require more time than others. Minimum and maximum time requirements for the warm-up, aerobics and cool-down segments are discussed in Chapter 7, "Components of an Aerobics Class". The time allotted for stretching and strengthening depends on the number of exercises to be performed.

Beginning and ending class on time is also important. Instructors who methodically plan their lessons will know the precise length of time for each activity. However, since unforeseen events, such as a tape deck malfunction, do occur, the competent instructor needs to be flexible and able to improvise at the last minute if necessary.

Patterns of Class Organization. Aerobics classes should be arranged to ensure the safety of participants and to enable everyone to hear the instructions and see the demonstrations. Patterns of class organization refer to the formations used by instructors to provide their students with maximum opportunities for learning and performing. In a typical aerobics class formation, the instructor stands at the front of the room and participants face him or her. While this formation can be effective, there is one major disadvantage. Usually the enthusiastic, experienced participants stand in the front of the room while the less experienced stay in the back. The result is a potentially unsafe situation, because it is difficult for an instructor to observe those in the back of the room. To resolve this problem, instructors can periodically move from the front to the sides and to the back of the class, asking participants to turn and face them in each new position. A circle formation can be used occasionally for variety. Instructors stand in the center of the room and have participants form a single or double circle around them. Exercise leaders using this formation should change their point of focus by rotating a quarter turn from time to time.

Facility and Equipment Considerations. Not all instructors can choose the facility in which they teach. Ideally the exercise facility should have the following:

1. Good ventilation, with a temperature range of 60 to 70 degrees Fahrenheit.

2. A floor that will effectively absorb shock and will control undesirable medial-lateral motions of the foot. A hardwood sprung floor is ideal.

3. Sufficient space for each student to move comfortably (with arms outspread, each participant should be able to take two large steps in any direction without touching another student).

4. Mirrors for participants to observe their own exercise positions and postures.

5. In large classes, a raised platform for the instructor.

Equipment needs will include music tapes, tape deck and speakers, microphone, mats and some form of resistance training equipment, such as weights, tubes or rubber bands. Equipment for additional activities, such as circuit training, might include balls, hoops, jump ropes and steps.

Instructors should always arrive early to check that all equipment is in working order before class begins. Class time should never be spent cueing tapes or searching for equipment.

One of the most important pieces of aerobics equipment is the sound system. Although instructors rarely have the opportunity to select the sound system, they should be familiar with the basic features of the equipment they are using. Before instructors begin their classes they should always check the proper setting of the volume, bass, treble and pitch controls. According to Price (1990), audiologists recommend that exercise instructors keep their music volume under 85 decibels (Normal conversation ranges from 60 to 70 decibels, an alarm clock ringing two feet away is about 80, a chainsaw is 100, while a jet plane takeoff is around 120). The Occupational Safety and Health Administration (OSHA), which regulates noise standards for workers, states that ear protection must be provided for workers if noise level on the job averages 90 decibels over an 8-hour period. Extended exposure to sound levels at 85 to 90 decibels and above can eventually damage a person's hearing. Instructors who use loud music are not only at risk of damaging their hearing and that of their participants but they are much more likely to suffer from voice injury as they find themselves having to

shout over loud music.

In addition to keeping the music volume at an appropriate level to protect the hearing of class participants, audiologists recommend that instructors turn up the bass and lower the treble since high frequencies can be more damaging than low frequencies (Price, 1990). A higher base setting can also be beneficial for class participants who have difficulty hearing the underlying beat. If a tape deck has pitch control (a feature that allows an instructor to speed up or slow down the music tempo), it should be checked for proper positioning before class begins (the center position usually indicates normal speed). Nothing is more frustrating for an instructor than to begin a class and find that the music is much slower or faster than anticipated. Instructors should attempt to minimize the use of the pitch control as extreme changes in the speed of the music distort the sound. If instructors find themselves constantly pitching the music speed up, they might want to consider selecting music that is performed at a faster tempo.

Teaching Styles

The teaching style chosen is an important factor in determining the instructor's success in effectively presenting class activities. Instructors should be familiar with a variety of teaching styles. Mosston (1981) has identified eight specific teaching styles. Each accomplishes a different set of objectives, and it is both possible and desirable to use several styles in an aerobics class. The five styles directly applicable to an exercise class include command, practice, reciprocal, self-check and inclusion. Each style is described and discussed in terms of its practical application to aerobic exercise.

An instructor using the **command style** of teaching makes all decisions about posture, rhythm and duration, while participants

Figure 8.2

SAMPLE CRITERIA CARD

Name_____

Test	Passing Criteria	Performance Level		
		1	2	3
	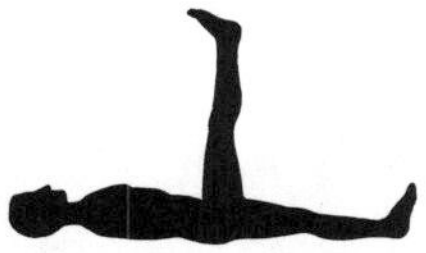 Date:	_____	_____	_____
Flexibility *Hamstrings* *	Leg raised to vertical	_____	_____	_____
Quads *	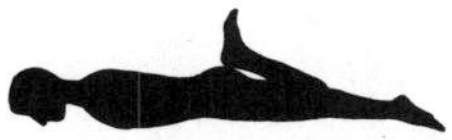 Heel touching buttocks	_____	_____	_____
Strength *Sit-ups (1 min)*	Males Age < 35 35-44 > 45 45+ 40+ 25+	_____	_____	_____
	Females Age <35 35-44 >45 40+ 30+ 15+	_____	_____	_____
Cardiovascular *3-min. step test HR*	Males Females < 105 < 116	_____	_____	_____
Body Composition *Percentage body fat*	Males Females < 19% < 26%	_____	_____	_____

*Draw the leg position of the exerciser being tested.

follow his or her directions and movements. This style is most appropriate when instructors want to achieve the following objectives:

- immediate participant response
- participant emulation of instructor as role model
- participant control
- safety
- avoidance of alternatives and choices
- efficient use of time
- perpetuation of aesthetic standards

The command style has been perhaps the most commonly used style in aerobics classes. While this style is particularly suited to warming up, cooling down and learning new routines and exercises, it leaves no room for individualization. The participant has little say in decisions about personal physical development and few opportunities exist for social interaction. To achieve these objectives, an instructor must rely on other teaching styles.

The **practice style** of teaching provides opportunities for individualization and includes practice time and private instructor feedback for each participant. While all exercisers are working on the same task, individual participants can choose his or her own pace and rhythm. The practice

Figure 8.3

SAMPLE RECORD CARD

Name _____   Date _____

Resting Heart Rate _____   Target Heart-Rate Zone _____ to _____

Activity	
Aerobic exercise HR	158
Aerobic exercise recovery HR	118
Curl-ups	20-20-20
(Body weight)	(3 sets of 20 reps)
Leg lifts (5lbs)	12-12-10
Shins (rubber bands)	12-10-10

style is particularly suited for floor exercises in classes where the fitness level of participants varies greatly. Using this style, instructors can encourage students to perform the maximum repetitions suitable to their skill or fitness level. The real key is that once instructors determine the task, such as curl-ups, they are free to move around and give individual feedback where necessary. A disadvantage to this style is that not all participants are sufficiently motivated to achieve their maximum potential.

The **reciprocal style** of teaching involves the use of an observer or a partner to provide feedback to each participant. This style enables everyone to receive individual feedback, an often impossible task for the instructor. The reciprocal style can best be used for fitness assessment. For example, tests evaluating posture, girth measurements, strength and flexibility can be quickly administered by partners. Using a criteria card that describes the test, the criteria for passing, and the performance level achieved will allow students to monitor their own progress. A sample criteria card is presented in Fig. 8.2. Aside from providing the participant with important feedback, the reciprocal style encourages

social interaction, which is one reason people choose to participate in organized exercise programs. One major disadvantage of this style is that the observer or partner may not provide appropriate KR.

The **self-check style** of teaching relies on participants to provide their own feedback. Participants perform a given task and then record the results, comparing their performance against given criteria or past performances. This style lends itself nicely to the recording of target heart rate, recovery heart rate and number of floor-exercise repetitions. Instructors will need to provide a record card for each individual participant. A sample record card is presented in Figure 8.3. Because a key component of motivation and exercise compliance is self-monitoring of progress, it is desirable to incorporate the self-check style into every exercise program.

The **inclusion style** of teaching enables multiple levels of performance to be taught within the same activity. Perhaps one of the most significant problems facing the aerobics industry is teaching multiple skill and fitness levels within one class. Skill and fitness level can vary in each segment of the exercise class, including stretching, strengthening and aerobic work. Because most people tend to overestimate their ability, instructors should first administer tests to determine the skill and fitness levels of individual participants. Then the class should be designed to incorporate all levels so that each person can achieve maximum success. During the stretching and strengthening segments of the program, the instructor can offer alternate positions for the different levels. For example, during the abdominal work the participant with weak abdominal muscles can choose to do pelvic tilts, while the person with stronger abdominals can perform curl-ups. The instructor can also offer different levels of difficulty during the aerobic segment. For example, beginners can perform marches with claps while the more advanced students jog with overhead presses. Instructors periodically need to demonstrate each level of movement, spending more time on the patterns for beginners.

Evaluating Performance

The effective exercise leader monitors participants' progress toward personal goals through periodic testing. Each aerobic exerciser should be evaluated initially to establish a baseline by which to measure progress. Physiological measures such as cardiorespiratory fitness, body composition, strength and flexibility are described in Chapter 6, "Fitness Testing and Aerobic Programming."

Instructors should attempt to use valid tests that can be easily administered either by partners or by the participants themselves. Providing criteria cards that indicate test directions, criteria for passing, and performance level achieved by exercisers saves valuable class time and can serve as a motivational tool for participants (Fig. 8.2).

In addition to periodic testing, instructors should encourage participants to monitor their daily accomplishments. A record card can be used to keep track of daily progress (Fig. 8.3). Items such as heart rate (resting, exercise and recovery) and the number of floor-exercise repetitions can be regularly monitored and recorded by participants themselves. Criteria and record cards should be stored in an alphabetized file that is available to participants at each class meeting. Instructors can remind participants to pick up their cards, record the appropriate information, and refile them before leaving class.

It is important that instructors be aware of their students' progress toward their goals. They can become so by periodically examining participants' record cards and through one-on-one interaction with participants either before, during or after class. If a participant is not showing progress, it is the instructor's responsibility to help determine the problem. It may be that unrealistic goals have been set or there has been an attendance problem. Showing genuine concern for students encourages long-term participation in a formal exercise program.

PREPARING AND TEACHING CLASS ACTIVITIES

The majority of an aerobics instructor's time is spent selecting music and developing movement patterns. The purpose of this section is to explain music selection, to explore different choreographic techniques and to become familiar with successful cueing skills.

Selecting Music

Music not only provides the timing for exercise movements, it also makes a class enjoyable and it helps to motivate participants. Because music is the basis of aerobics programs, instructors should be familiar with its fundamental elements.

The music **beat** is the regular pulsations that have an even rhythm and occur in a continuous pattern of strong and weak pulsations. Strong pulsations are called the **downbeat** while weaker pulsations are called the **upbeat**. A series of beats form the underlying rhythm of a song. The **rhythm** is the regular pattern of sound that is heard when listening to music. A **meter** organizes beats into musical patterns or measures, such as four beats per measure. A **measure** is a group of beats formed by the regular occurrence of a heavy **accent** on the first beat or downbeat of each group. Most aerobics routines use music with a meter of 4/4 time (the first four indicates 4 beats per measure while the second four shows that the quarter note gets the beat).

To successfully choreograph movement patterns, instructors must be familiar with their music. Determining music tempo is the first requirement. The **tempo** or speed of the music determines the progression as well as the intensity of exercise. The beats per minute (bpm) or tempo for a song can be determined by counting each beat for one minute. Using experience and common sense, instructors have adopted general guidelines for selecting the appropriate music tempo for the various component parts of an aerobics program. Slow tempos under 100 bpm and without a strong underlying beat are generally used for poststretching, while tempos from 120 to 140 bpm are frequently used for warm-ups, prestretch and cool-downs. Floor exercises are often performed to tempos of 110 to 130 bpm. The tempo for floor exercises should be slow enough for participants to control their movements. Aerobic activities are generally performed at a tempo of 130 to 160 bpm. Instructors must be cautious when choosing music speeds over 150 bpm because participants need to move quickly at higher tempos.

Encouraging students to perform smaller movements will help them preserve the control necessary for safety when using high music speeds. Beginners should never be expected to move at fast speeds because they are not yet proficient enough to perform quick movements under control. Another consideration with fast-paced music is that participants with long arms and legs need more time to cover the same spatial area as participants with shorter limbs. For example, people with short arms can bring their arms above their heads more quickly than can people with long arms. Consequently, participants with long arms often appear to be uncoordinated unless they bend their elbows to keep in time with the instructor and the music.

After determining the tempo, it is useful for instructors to break down the music into musical phrases. According to Bricker (1991), "as letters of the alphabet combine to form sentences, so beats of music combine to form measures, and measures combine to form phrases. A **phrase** is composed of at least two measures of music. To learn to recognize musical phrases, imagine where you would pause for breath if you were singing a song." Shyba (1990) likes to think of a musical "sentence" as a group of four phrases (usually 32 counts). Shyba recommends that instructors indicate on a piece of paper each musical phrase with a pen stroke crossing the set out with the last phrase in the sentence (卅). Therefore, if an instructor were listening to 32 measures (4 beats per measure) making up 16 musical phrases (8beats per phrase) or four musical sentences (32 beats per sentence), there would be four sets of three vertical pen strokes crossed by one diagonal pen stroke (each pen stroke representing an 8-count phrase: 卅 卅 卅 卅). Musical phrasing is ideal when it groups into musical sentences of 32 counts. However, there are times when a phrase may be subdivided and it becomes awkward if the instructor is in the middle of a 32-count combination when the musical phrasing becomes inconsistent. Shyba (1990) recommends that instructors use phrasing inconsistencies to introduce a new step or to perform simple free-form footwork until the musical sentences re-establish themselves.

When choreographing movements to music, instructors should take care to begin the movement pattern on the downbeat of the measure (the first count of the measure). Combining 8-count movements, such as eight marches or four jumping jacks to make up a 32-count combination, will help participants anticipate movement changes on the downbeat, thus giving them a feeling of success.

While many movement patterns are performed on each beat of the music, it is possible to change the rhythm of the movement so that it is being performed double time to the basic beat (one and two and three and four and), half-time (2 counts per movement) or in **syncopation** where the accent is temporarily displaced from the naturally occurring accent in music (one AND two AND with the accent occurring on the AND rather than on one or two).

The rhythm of the music can often dictate the style of movement. Instructors will find it easiest to work with music that has a steady rhythm and a strong beat. The type of music selected will depend on the demographics of the exercise group and the creativity of the instructor. Staying open-minded is important. Instructors must not rely exclusively on their personal music preferences. The music style selected should reflect, in part, the interests of the age group. For example, young people may enjoy Top-40 pop, while an older group may prefer swing or big-band music. Age should not be the only criterion for

selecting music, however. In some parts of the country, gospel, folk and country music are more appealing than rock 'n' roll. Instructors may also want to consider the time of the year. At Christmas, for example, participants may be delighted to exercise to "Rudolph The Red-Nosed Reindeer." For further variety, instructors can select music for special "theme days"—square dance, clogging and polka music for a country music day or cha-cha, rumba and samba music for a Latin music day. The greater the variety of music, the more enjoyment most participants will receive from an aerobics program.

To keep participants interested, instructors should change music frequently. For instructors who have trouble staying current with music selections, there are national music organizations that manufacture music tapes for aerobics classes. In addition, instructors can ask regular participants for music suggestions.

Choreography

Once the music has been selected, instructors must choose appropriate movement patterns. The first consideration is whether the selected movement or the sequencing of movements is safe. Other chapters in this manual address contraindicated exercises, but for review purposes, instructors should keep in mind the following general guidelines when selecting choreography:

1. Avoid movements that result in hyperextension of any joint.

2. Avoid excessive repetitions on one weight-bearing leg. Alternate legs frequently.

3. Avoid flinging the limbs at any time.

4. Make sure lateral foot movements are well-controlled to avoid tripping or falling (especially on carpet).

5. Avoid contraindicated positions such as sustained and unsupported

forward flexion.

6. Avoid stretching muscles ballistically while performing movement patterns.

7. Avoid changing directions rapidly. Transitions between complex step patterns may require a movement sequence in place before changing directions.

8. Avoid continuous movement that requires participants to remain on the balls of their feet for extended periods.

9. Avoid holding the arms at or above shoulder level for an extended period of time. Frequently vary low-, mid- and high-range arm movements.

10. Balance routines so that the same movements are performed equally on both sides of the body.

Instructors teaching aerobics should be familiar with the basic foundations of movement. Four **basic locomotor steps** use the feet as the base of support:

Walk or Step—A transfer of weight from one foot to the other in which one foot remains in contact with the floor at all times.

Run or Leap—A transfer of weight from one foot to the other in which both feet momentarily lose contact with the floor.

Hop—Pushing the body upward off one foot and landing on that same foot.

Jump—Pushing the body upward off one foot or both feet and landing on both feet.

All other steps are either variations or combinations of these basic steps. Common aerobic steps include low kicks, knee-lifts, step touches and jumping jacks to name a few. Instructors can increase their movement repertoire by borrowing steps from other dance forms, such as jazz, folk, modern or ballet, or by using movements from various sports and games. All locomotor movements can be complemented with a variety of arm movements, such as clapping, punching, swinging, circling, flexing

and extending. To aid verbal cueing, instructors should name all of their steps and arm patterns.

Two basic choreographic methods, known as freestyle and structured, are used to combine movement patterns and music. The **structured method** uses choreographed movements that are formally arranged and repeated in a predetermined order, usually performed to the same piece of music each time the routine is used. Examples of structured aerobics programs are those of Judi Sheppard Missett's "Jazzercise" and Jackie Sorenson's "Aerobic Dance."

The **freestyle method** uses movements that are built and sequenced by the instructor during the aerobics class. The pacing is often dependent on the success participants demonstrate with the sequences as well as the complexity of the movement patterns or combinations. Freestyle movements can be sequenced either by using a linear progression or by placing movements into patterns or combinations. A **linear progression** consists of one movement that transitions into another without cycling sequences. By changing only one variable at a time, such as arm or leg movement, direction of movement or rhythm, students can practice movement patterns without the pressure of remembering sequences. Linear progressions are particularly useful for introducing new moves and for adding variations. The following is an example of a linear progression in which only one element of variation is changed at any one time:

Base Movement: Knee-lift in place for 8 counts (four knee-lifts)

Add arms: Arm curls for 8 counts

Add direction: Travel forward for 8 counts; travel backward for 8 counts

Change the arms: Overhead press for 16 counts (still traveling)

Change the legs: Kick (same arms) for

16 counts (still traveling)

Change the arms: Clap for 16 counts (still kicking and traveling)

Combinations are defined as two or more movement patterns combined and repeated in sequence several times in a row. The following is an example of a combination:

Four step-touches in place with upright rows—8 counts

Four knee lifts traveling forward with overhead presses—8 counts

Four heel jacks in place with clapping—8 counts

Four step kicks traveling backward with chest presses—8 counts

According to Copeland (1991), "There are many advantages to using patterns in your choreography. The human mind instinctively arranges events into patterns, so they allow the mind to relax and easily anticipate what will happen next. This repetition allows…students to commit to the movement more fully and to maintain a steady-state workout." However, instructors must select movement patterns carefully. Complex routines can slow down the class and confuse participants, particularly in a beginning or multilevel class.

When using a freestyle approach, it is important to use effective building strategies so that class participants can successfully follow the choreography to maintain appropriate levels of exercise intensity. Copeland recommends that instructors start with a base move, such as marches or step-touches, and change only one element of variation at a time. Examples of elements of variation recommended by Copeland include planes, levers, direction and rhythm. Variations in planes include the horizontal or transverse plane, which divides the body into lower and upper parts and includes rotation around the long axis of the body; the frontal plane, which divides the body into anterior and posterior parts and includes abduction and adduction; and the sagittal plane, which divides the body into right and left sides of the body and includes flexion and extension. An instructor can change the arms from lateral raises (frontal or lateral plane) to arm curls (sagittal plane).

Lever variations refers to the length of a lever or limb (short, long). Changing from an arm-curl (short arm lever) to frontal raises (long arm lever) is an example of a lever variation. Directional variations add the element of travel allowing participants to move forward, backward, left, right, diagonally or in a circle. Variations in rhythm involve changing the rhythm of a movement. For example, varying a step-touch (2 counts in 2 beats) to a step-ball-change (3 counts in 2 beats) changes the rhythm of a similar movement.

Other helpful techniques when teaching freestyle choreography are the repetition- reduction method and the use of rhythmic variations. **Repetition reduction** involves reducing the number of repetitions that make up a movement sequence. For example, if an instructor wanted to use a combination of two kicks and two knee-lifts, he or she might begin the sequence with eight kicks and eight knee-lifts, reducing to four kicks and four knee-lifts, finishing with two kicks and two knee-lifts. This technique allows participants to master each individual movement within a sequence.

The use of **rhythmic variation** allows participants to learn complex movement at a slower pace. This technique emphasizes proper placement or configuration of a movement pattern. For example, if an instructor were teaching a box step (left foot forward, right foot across left foot, left foot backward, right foot to the right), instead of performing individual steps on each beat of the music, 2 counts would be taken for each foot placement, thus taking 8 counts to complete the movement pattern. Once participants have learned the step pattern, it can be performed on the beat.

To keep track of combinations or choreographed routines, it is helpful for instructors to maintain a card file or notebook to record specific movement patterns. Before teaching a new routine or series of combinations to a class, instructors should practice (preferably in front of a mirror) until the movement patterns are memorized, and transitions and cues have been worked out. Practicing routines or combinations in advance helps instructors determine whether the sequence of movement patterns flow smoothly.

A slow progression is important to help participants learn a skill effectively and to avoid musculoskeletal injuries. Instructors must encourage beginners to start slowly and progress gradually. In addition, movements must be selected so that most participants are successful. Some participants will learn new steps more quickly than others. Instructors should be patient and supportive of slower learners, reminding them that they will improve with practice. Instructors should always try to be available before and after class for individual help. It is important that all movement patterns are effectively and safely sequenced to ensure smooth and comfortable transitions. The way instructors sequence movements together should be based on physiological, biomechanical and psychological balance (Copeland, 1991). Intensity and duration are two physiological considerations when sequencing movements. To help class participants maintain heart rates within their training zones, the relative intensity level of each movement must be balanced. For example, if an instructor chooses a high-intensity movement, such as jumping jacks or high-impact lunges, the next movement should be less intense, such as marches. If

an exercise class is of long duration, too many high-intensity movements may fatigue participants before the end of the session.

Biomechanical balance is achieved by balancing the musculoskeletal stress of various movements. For example, if an instructor selects a movement that is performed on one leg at a time, care must be taken to change the support leg before it is overly stressed. Similarly, if a movement is highly stressful to a joint, such as jumping jacks, the next movement should not stress that same joint. Finally, instructors must be cautious of using too many complex movements if they are striving to achieve psychological balance. According to Copeland (1991), "Movement that is too complex is not only frustrating for the student but has a direct effect on the physiological and biomechanical balance. Form, technique and safety can be compromised."

Cueing

Cueing is a crucial part of teaching aerobics classes. It serves as a warning system that allows class participants to follow movement pattern with ease and confidence. The success with which students perform movement sequences in a smooth and continuous manner is dependent on the instructor's ability to effectively cue changes in movement patterns.

When leading aerobics routines, instructors should face the class as often as possible, using mirroring techniques, such as moving to participants' left when directing them to the right. Instructors can only monitor class safety by watching all participants at all times. All cues should be precise and timely. Each cue should be called on the preceding measure to provide the participant with enough time to move smoothly from one step to the next. When beginning a routine, instructors should use rhythmic starting signals, such as "Ready and" to ensure that everyone starts together.

Cues can be given verbally or visually. There are five types of verbal cues: footwork, directional, rhythmic, numerical and step (Griffith, 1982). **Footwork cueing** indicates which foot to move, the left or the right. **Directional cueing** tells participants which direction to move, such as forward or backward. **Rhythmic cueing** indicates the correct rhythm of the routine, such as slow (2 counts) or quick (1 count). **Numerical cueing** refers to counting the rhythm, such as one and two, three, four. Finally, **step cueing** refers to the name of the step, such as step-touch. When leading aerobic exercises, it is best to combine types of cueing. For example, the instructor might cue a sequence consisting of two grapevines and four knee-lifts in place as follows:

First Grapevine
Step cues: "Side, behind, side, touch"
Second Grapevine
Rhythmic cues: "Quick, quick, quick, quick"
First Knee-lift
Step cues: "Step, knee-lift"
Second Knee-lift
Directional cues: "In place"
Third Knee-lift
Footwork cues: "Step right"
Fourth Knee-lift
Numerical cues: "one, two"

As students become proficient at executing movement patterns, they will need fewer verbal cues from exercise instructors. Instead of cueing every movement, instructors can limit verbal cues to transitions between movements. Visual cues are also helpful to communicate movement expectations. The use of visual cues has several advantages, including lowering the risk of instructor voice injury, allowing instructors to communicate in facilities with poor acoustics or with a large number of class

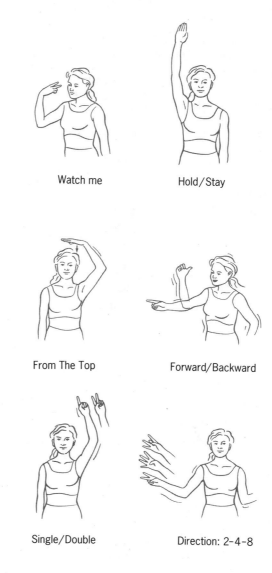

Watch me

Hold/Stay

From The Top

Forward/Backward

Single/Double

Direction: 2-4-8

Figure 8.4
Aerobic Q-Signs
Source: Webb International (1993)

participants, and providing opportunities for the hearing-impaired to join in an aerobics program. There are currently two formalized sets of visual cues in use among exercise instructors (Figs. 8.4 and 8.5).

According to Webb (1989), who promotes a series of hand/arm visual cues called the Aerobic Q-Signs (Fig. 8.4), verbal cues can be used to call out the name of the step while visual cues are used to indicate the direction or number of repetitions. Webb recommends that instructors practice visual cue signs in front of a mirror, making sure that visual cues are given 4 counts before the movement change is to occur. She also suggests that instructors introduce a few signs at a time into their classes so that participants can gradually adapt to their use.

Oliva (1988) promotes visual cues based on the principles of Visual-Gestural Communication and American Sign Language to include persons who are deaf or hard of hearing (Fig 8.5). Oliva maintains that visual cues must be "visually logical" and clearly visible to viewers. For example, instructors should indicate lower body moves by patting the lead leg and a strong distinction needs to be made between moves that travel and moves that simply change direction (within one step

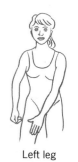

Left leg

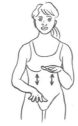

Stay in Place

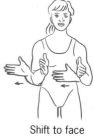

Shift to face
this direction

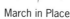

March in Place

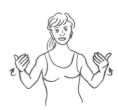

Move it Forward

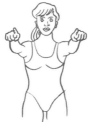

Move it Back

Figure 8.5

Visual Cues for
Exercise Classes
Source: Oliva (1988)

of original position). Specific visual cues that match specific low impact footmoves are available (Oliva 1988). Oliva recommends that visual cues for turns should be indicated directly above the floor space which the turn will cover. Finally, the timing and command sequence for visual cues should be the same as for verbal cues.

The use of verbal and visual previews are particularly useful when introducing a complex movement pattern. Each of these previews is given by the instructor while the class continues to perform the movement that they are currently performing. When using a verbal preview, the instructor explains in detail the next step or arm pattern. When using a visual preview, the instructor demonstrates the next movement sequence, while the class continues to perform the current movement.

When using verbal cues, it is imperative that instructors learn to use their voice properly to avoid vocal injuries. According to MacLellan, Grapes and Elster (1987), voice injuries among aerobics instructors occur from "the improper use of the voice, interference of muscular tension with vocalization, attempts at projection over loud music, and a poor work environment." They recommend the following techniques to prevent voice injury:

1. Keep cues short and avoid unnecessary vocalization.

2. Keep music at a decibel level that does not require instructors to shout over the music.

3. Frequently take small sips of water to keep the vocal mechanism lubricated.

4. Avoid cueing in positions that inhibit abdominal breathing (such as during curl-ups) or constrict the vocal tract (such as when performing push-ups). It is preferable to give the cues before the exercise is executed.

5. When using a microphone speak in a normal voice.

6. Do not lower the pitch of the voice to sound louder as this leads to vocal fatigue (producing a hoarse, weak and strained voice).

7. Avoid frequent clearing of the throat.

SUMMARY

Effectively teaching an exercise class is a challenge to every exercise instructor. Competent teachers carefully design their programs and employ sound teaching principles; they evaluate participant progress through initial testing and periodic retesting; they develop sound strategies to motivate their participants to continue exercising: and they remain abreast of current health, nutrition and fitness information and trends. The extra work that is required to become an effective teacher will be repaid many times over as instructors earn their students' respect by providing safe, fun and well-structured aerobics classes. Demonstrating expertise in the fitness industry will provide instructors with many professional opportunities and with the personal satisfaction of contributing to the well-being of so many aerobic exercisers.

REFERENCES

Bricker, K. (1991). Music 101. IDEA Today 3: 55-57.

Copeland, C. (1991). Smooth Moves. IDEA Today 6: 34-38.

Dishman, R. K. (1986). Exercise Compliance: A New View for Public Health. The Physician and Sportsmedicine 14: 127-43.

Fallon, D. J. and S. A. Kuchenmeister (1977). The Art of Ballroom Dance. Minneapolis, Minn.: Burgess Publishing Company.

Fitts, P. M., and M. I. Posner (1967). Human Performance. Belmont, Calif.: Brooks/Cole.

Franklin, B. A. (1986). Clinical Components of a Successful Adult Fitness Program. American Journal of Health Promotion 1: 6-13.

Griffith,. B. R. (1992). Dance for Fitness, Minneapolis, Minn.: Burgess Publishing Company.

Harris, J. A., A. M. Pittman, and M. S. Waller (1978). Dance A While. Minneapolis, Minn.: Burgess Publishing Company.

Institute for Aerobic Research (1988). Creative Choreography with Candice Copeland. Reebok Instructor News 6: 7.

MacLellan, M. A., D. Grapes, and D. Elster (1980). Voice Injury. Aerobic Dance-Exercise Instructor Manual, San Diego, Calif.: American Council on Exercise, (1987). Magill, R. A. Motor Learning. Dubuque, Iowa: Wm. C. Brown Company.

Mosston, M. (1981). Teaching Physical Education. Columbus, Ohio: Charles E. Merrill Publishing Company.

Nieman, D. C. (1986). The Sports Medicine Fitness Course. Palo Alto, Calif.: Bull Publishing Company.

Oliva, G.A. (1988) . Visual Cues for Exercise Classes. Gallaudet University, Washington, D.C.

Price, J. Hear (1990). Today, Gone Tomorrow? IDEA Today 5: 54-57.

Rasch, P. J. (1989). Kinesiology and Applied Anatomy, Philadelphia, Penn.: Lea & Febiger.

Shyba, L. (1990). Finding the Elusive Downbeat. IDEA Today 6: 27-29.

Siedentop, D. (1983). Developing Teaching Skills in Physical Education. Palo Alto, Calif.: Mayfield Publishing Company.

Webb, T. (1989). Aerobic Q-Signs. IDEA Today 10: 30-31.

Chapter 9

Variations: From Step to Strength Training

ecause exercisers need variety and the fitness industry needs to attract and retain participants, classes of today are much more diverse than in the past. This chapter explores several options to the traditional class, including step training, resistance training, circuit and interval training, funk aerobics, and flexibility training. These "variations" are among the more popular alternative classes accepted by the industry today. Each is described by a different author with specific information regarding class background, fundamentals and design considerations.

Step Training
by Karen Kelly Duncanson
Resistance Training
by Melane Barney
Circuit and Interval Training
by Len Kravitz
Funk Aerobics
by Kathryn Bricker
Water Fitness
by Mary E. Sanders & Nicki E. Rippee
Flexibility Training
by Patricia Kirk

Chapter 9

Variations: From Step to Strength Training

Karen Kelly Duncanson, content specialist and coordinator for this chapter, holds a bachelor's of science degree in physical education from the University of Oklahoma. Active in the fitness industry since 1984, Karen Duncanson promotes fitness through teaching, education, and fundraising events. She currently serves as certification manager for ACE and teaches for the University of California San Diego extension program.

The creation and evolution of step training in the exercise classroom has evolved primarily from the need to provide participants with another type of low-impact activity that is both challenging and interesting. Step training has offered a new dimension to exercise because it is versatile enough to be included in a variety of classes such as aerobic step, combination (low/high plus step), circuit training, interval training and muscular conditioning.

It appears that people who may not ordinarily enter an aerobics class because of the "dancey" or highly choreographed movements are participating in step classes. Some additional reasons may be:

1. Step is conducted in a predictable environment (i.e., no traveling movements across the room, each participant works in his or her own space).

2. The basic movements are designed to be nonintimidating and have generally accepted terminology.

3. The choreography can vary according to the levels of the class from simple arm and leg movements to more complex arm and leg combinations. Although there are various ways to incorporate step into the classroom, this section will focus primarily on the basics of safe and effective movements and combinations.

Research shows that when done properly, step training is an effective means of improving aerobic capacity. Platform height and stepping patterns can significantly increase or decrease the intensity (energy cost/caloric expenditure) of a class (Stanforth, 1991). Some studies indicate an increase in maximal oxygen consumption with no changes in body composition, while others indicate a decrease in body fat, decrease in fat weight and an in-

crease in lean body mass (Velasquez, 1992; & Kravitz, 1991).

Prior to commencing a step training session, it is important that the instructor educate the students about proper body mechanics when assembling and disassembling the platform (see Chapter 3, "Biomechanics and Applied Kinesiology"). Proper body mechanics require that the platform remain close to the participant's body when lowering and lifting the platform. Also while lowering and lifting the platform, the participant must bend at the knees instead of at the waist with straight legs. Instructors must educate students that their platform height is dependent on their individual level of skill, fitness, experience, muscular strength and predisposition to knee-related orthopedic problems when the knee joint is fully loaded (Francis, 1992; Kravitz & Deivert, 1991).

Platform heights can range from 6 to

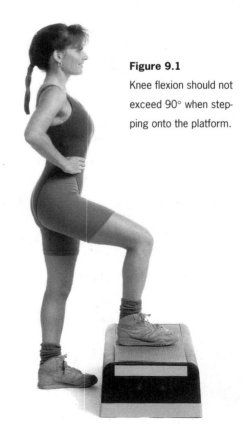

Figure 9.1

Knee flexion should not exceed 90° when stepping onto the platform.

Table 9.1

CORRECT AND INCORRECT STEPPING TECHNIQUES

Do	Don't
When stepping up, do place the entire foot on top of the platform.	When stepping up, do not allow any part of the foot to hang over the edge.
When stepping down, do step down close to the platform to allow the heels to contact the floor (the heel should never be forced down during any movement in which the body is a considerable distance from the platform such as during a repeater or lunge step).	When stepping down, do not bounce or remain on the balls of the feet.
Do step gently and quietly up and down.	Do not pound the feet on and off the platform.
When demonstrating new or difficult movements, especially for beginners or the inexperienced, do encourage them to periodically look at their platform.	Do not constantly focus on the platform or drop the head too far forward while stepping.
Participants should always be able to see their platform in front or in their periphery.	Do not step down with the back toward the platform (participants should never step off the platform with their backs toward the platform).

Source: Francis, 1992; Kravitz & Deivert, 1991.

12 inches, with typical adjustments in 2-inch increments. A good recommendation for the platform height for "healthy knees" is to avoid flexion at the knee beyond 90 degrees (Fig. 9.1) during the first upward step onto the platform (Francis, 1992). It is important that the instructor remember that the platform may be an unfamiliar piece of exercise equipment to participants. Demonstrating proper stepping without the music may be a good way to orient the novice stepper. In addition, basic step movements done at the beginning of class should help participants feel more comfortable. Beginner students may need to look at their platform more often to familiarize themselves with it, but in time these participants should be more confident in their ability and be able to concentrate on proper stepping posture.

Stepping Posture and Technique

To minimize the risk of injury, instructors must constantly remind students about proper stepping posture. Proper body alignment is achieved by: (1) focusing the eyes forward with the neck in neutral position, (2) pulling the shoulders back, (3) moving the pelvis to achieve a neutral position, and (4) relaxing the knees so that they are neither flexed nor hyperextended. Participants should be advised to step by employing a full body lean from the ankle joints, not bending from the waist.

In addition to proper posture, students must be aware of their stepping technique. The teacher is challenged with instructing and reminding students about the "do's and don'ts" of stepping. Table 9.1 presents some guidelines for correct and incorrect stepping techniques.

Class Format

In Chapter 7, "Components of an Aerobics Class," the proper time allotment for each phase of the aerobics class was presented. Be sure to refer to this chapter for the same guidelines when designing a step class.

Warm-up. The bench class should begin with a proper warm-up that prepares the muscles and body for the activity. It is recommended that instructors employ an ac-

Chapter 9
Variations: From
Step to Strength
Training

tive warm-up off the platform that involves the large muscle groups of the lower body, as well as range of motion exercises in the upper body. Since orientation to the vertical movement on the step is a consideration, instructors may progress into some platform stepping drills or other movements that are similar to those that will be incorporated into the class. However, since appropriate music tempo for the warm-up ranges between 130 to 140 beats per minute (bpm), instructors should exercise caution when incorporating these movements on the platform in the warm-up.

An example of a good vertical orientation drill involves marching on the floor for 4 counts, then up on the platform for 4 counts, and back on the floor for 4 counts, repeat if necessary. Flexibility exercises should focus on the low back, hip flexors, hamstrings, gluteals, Achilles/gastrocnemius and soleus muscle groups. As always,

avoid overstretching.

Aerobic Phase—Six Basic Movements. The phase that follows the warm-up is the aerobic stepping segment. Several safe and effective movements can be included in this phase to achieve the aerobic benefit. While there are many movement variations available to the instructor, this segment will focus on six basic movements that can be choreographed to suit the needs of the class.

1. Basic step—This movement is initiated by one leg, the lead leg (Fig. 9.2a). The basic step can begin with the right foot leading up and down on the platform (up to 1 minute) and then transitioning to the left foot for the same amount of time. A variation could be alternating the right and left foot going up on the platform (this requires a "tap step" between the right (R) and left (L) foot). The movement then becomes an alternating tap down (R foot up,

Figure 9.2a-b

The basic step and "V" step variation.

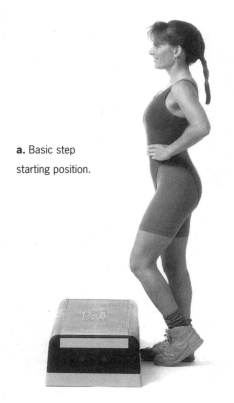

a. Basic step starting position.

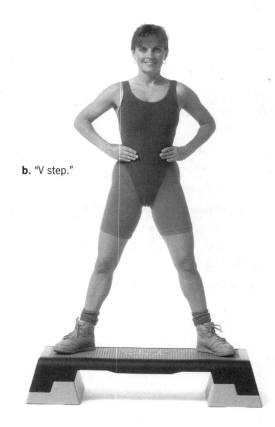

b. "V step."

L foot up, R foot down, L foot tap, L foot up, R foot up, L foot down, R foot tap). Another variation is the "V step" in which the legs appear to make a "V" by widening the movement on the platform and then coming together on the floor (Fig. 9.2b).

2. Travel step with alternating lead—This involves moving in a diagonal direction from one side of the platform to the other. The leg closest to the platform is the first leg up on it. Variations to this movement include a tap up, tap down, knee up, kick, "V step", etc.

3. Over the top—This involves moving from one side of the platform to the other (Fig. 9.3). In this movement, the participant starts from one side of the platform places the inside foot on the bench to walk over the top and get to the other side, then taps down with the foot closest to the platform. The execution is right foot up, left foot up, right foot down, left foot down.

A variation to the "walk-over" would be a propulsion in which the body becomes airborne.

4. Lift step—This movement involves lifting the lower limb in relation to the lower body (Fig. 9.4a-d). Variations of limb movement may include a knee up, hamstring curl, leg side or tap up. Choreography can be designed to alternate between the limbs. Variations of direction include: facing the front with alternating knees, traveling from the right side of the platform (e.g., left knee up) to the left side of the platform (e.g., right knee up), straddling the platform with alternating knees, etc.

5. Lunge—Considered to be a more advanced movement, the lunge starts on top of the platform, the left leg extends to contact the left side, then the entire body rotates to allow the right leg to extend and contact the right side (Fig. 9.5). A variation is to face the front of the platform and alter-

Figure 9.3a-c
Over the top.

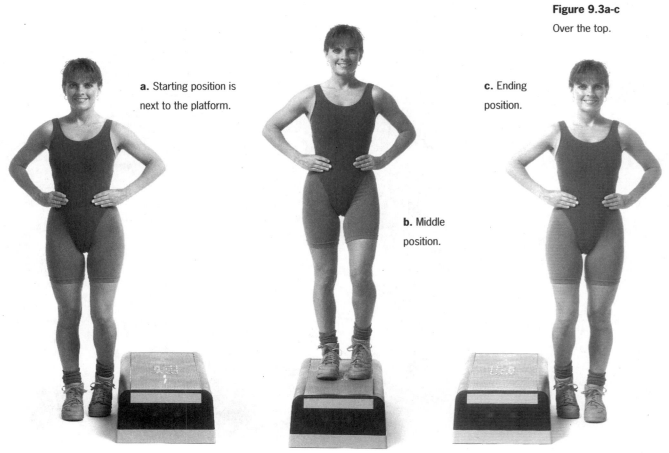

a. Starting position is next to the platform.

b. Middle position.

c. Ending position.

Chapter 9

*Variations: From
Step to Strength
Training*

nate the lunge behind the platform. The lunge is considered a propulsion move that should not exceed 1 minute and should be used with caution.

6. Repeater—This movement involves any alternating step in which the non-weight-bearing phase is repeated for no more than five consecutive times on one leg (Fig. 9.6). Variations can be three to five repeaters and then change to the other leg. To avoid or reduce stress to the supporting leg, avoid doing more than five consecutive repeater movements on the same leg.

Muscle Conditioning and Cool-down. As stated in the introduction, instructors may utilize the platform during muscle conditioning exercises. In this phase, the class focuses on isolation exercises for specific muscle groups (see "Resistance Training" section). Appropriate music tempo should

range between 120 to 130 bpm.

The last phase of the class is dedicated to important stretching and relaxation. Following the guidelines stated in the flexibility section of this chapter, focus should be on stretching the muscle groups that were involved in the aerobic stepping phase. The muscles important in this segment include the same muscle groups involved in the warm-up phase. Music tempos appropriate for stretch and relaxation should be below 100 bpm.

Choreography Considerations

Instructors must choreograph moves in such a way that the progression is smooth and the class is well-organized. Transitions from one move to the next will be more effective if cues are clear, concise, deliberate and timely. Just as in any class, preparation and organization will be apparent in

Figure 9.4a-d
Lift step showing
knee lift variation.

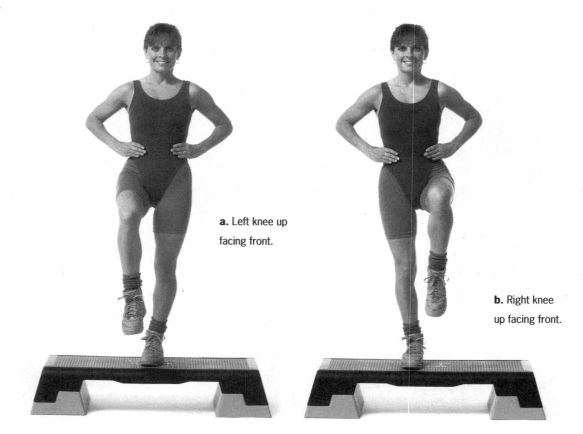

a. Left knee up
facing front.

b. Right knee
up facing front.

the teacher's delivery and instruction of the class. Instructors should practice the moves before teaching the class to ensure a successful delivery. Music speeds for this segment should range between 118 and 122 bpm for optimal cardiovascular benefits. Some reports indicate that movements may be safe up to 126 bpm although musculoskeletal risks may outweigh the cardiovascular benefits. It is always important that the instructor monitor the class to determine the appropriate tempo.

The following choreography guidelines are intended to enhance the safety and effectiveness of a step/training class:

1. To reduce unnecessary stress on the joints, instructors should vary patterns so that turning, pivoting, lunging or repeating movements are not excessive.

2. Movements leading with one leg should not exceed 1 minute in order to reduce stress to that lead leg.

3. When introducing arm movements to the step patterns, instructors should be certain that the participants appear to be comfortable with the foot movements. Arm variations include, but are not limited to:

• low range (biceps curl [Fig. 9.7a], hammer curls, triceps extension [Fig. 9.7b]).

• midrange (lateral raises [Fig. 9.8a], chest presses, upright rows [Fig. 9.8b]).

• high range (shoulder presses [Fig. 9.9a-b], lat pull-downs, single arm forward flexion [Fig. 9.9c]).

4. During the aerobic stepping phase, discourage the use of hand-held weights since the risk of injury to the shoulder girdle outweighs the potential aerobic benefits. Participants should concentrate on proper stepping posture and reserve resistance training for the muscle conditioning phase of the class.

c. Straddle variation.

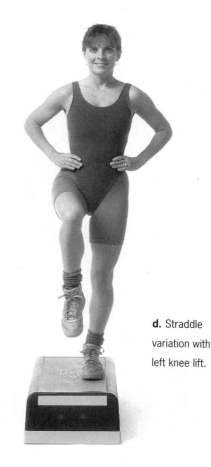

d. Straddle variation with left knee lift.

Chapter 9
Variations: From
Step to Strength
Training

Figure 9.5a-c
Lunge.

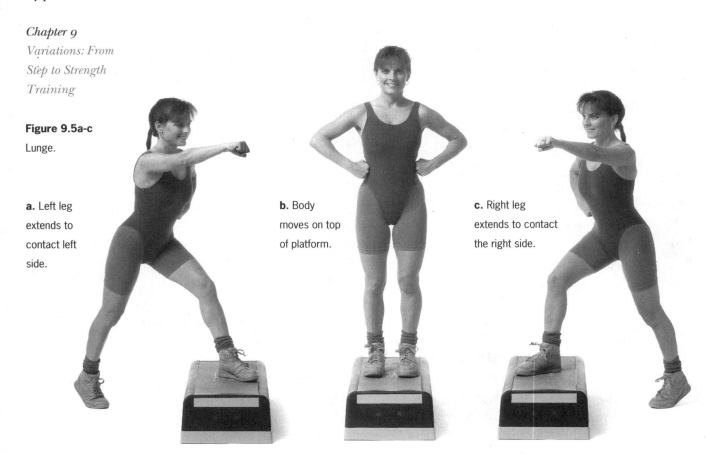

a. Left leg
extends to
contact left
side.

b. Body
moves on top
of platform.

c. Right leg
extends to contact
the right side.

Figure 9.6a-b
Repeater.

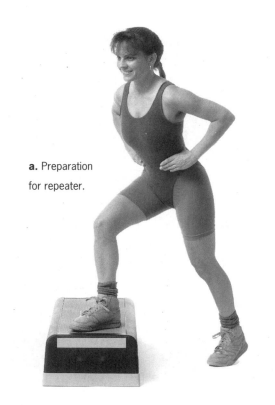

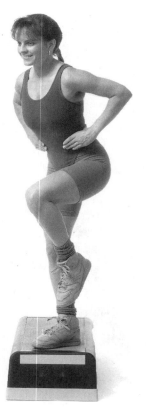

a. Preparation
for repeater.

b. Knee lift
is repeated.

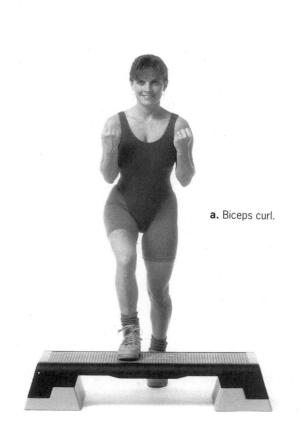

a. Biceps curl.

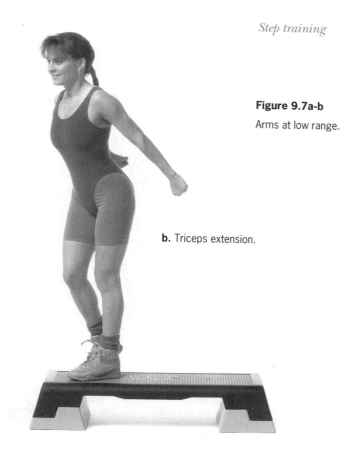

Figure 9.7a-b
Arms at low range.

b. Triceps extension.

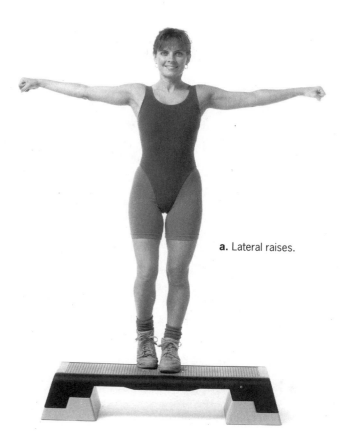

a. Lateral raises.

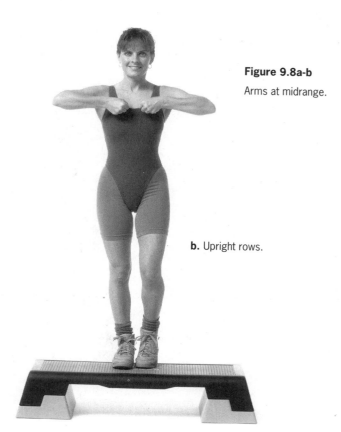

Figure 9.8a-b
Arms at midrange.

b. Upright rows.

Chapter 9
Variations: From
Step to Strength
Training

Figure 9.9a-c
Arms at high range.

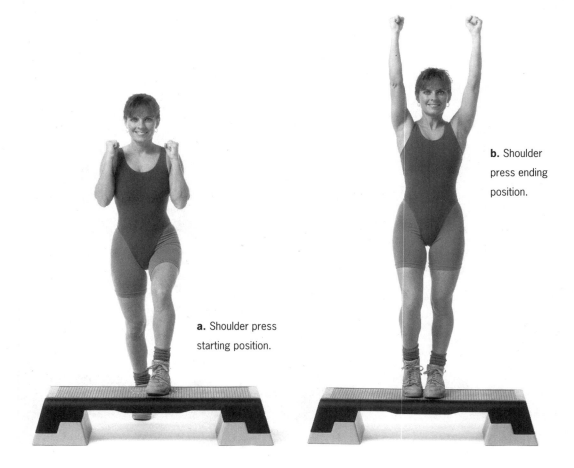

a. Shoulder press starting position.

b. Shoulder press ending position.

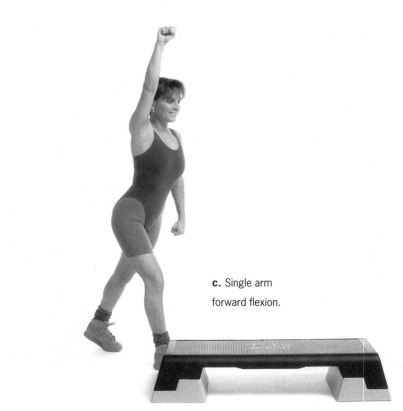

c. Single arm forward flexion.

Table 9.2

STEP REEBOK GUIDELINES

Subject	Guidelines
Platform height	Platform height is dependent on the exerciser's level of aerobic fitness, current skill with step training, and degree of knee flexion when the knee is fully loaded while stepping up. Deconditioned individuals should begin on 4 inches while highly skilled and experienced steppers can use 10 inches. The most common height is 8 inches. Regardless of fitness level or skill, participants should not exercise on a platform height that causes the knee joint to flex deeper than 90 degrees when the knee is fully loaded (when all the body weight is on the leg of the first upward step). Individuals with chronic knee problems should seek their physician's approval to perform step training.
Posture	The head should be up, shoulders down and back, chest up, abdominals lightly contracted and buttocks gently tucked under the hips. Do not hyperextend the knees or back at any time. When stepping up, lean from the ankles and not the waist to avoid excessive stress on the lumbar spine.
Stepping Up	Contact the platform with the entire sole of the foot. To avoid Achilles tendon injury, do not allow the heel to land over the edge of the platform. Step softly and quietly to avoid unnecessary high impacts. Watch the platform periodically to ensure proper foot placement.
Stepping Down	Step close to the platform (no more than one shoe length away) and allow the heels to contact the floor to help absorb shock. Stepping too far back while pressing the heel into the floor could result in Achilles tendon injury. If a step platform requires stepping a significant distance from the platform such as a lunge step or a repeater, do not push the heel into the floor. Keep the weight on the forefoot.
Leading Foot	Change the leading foot (the foot that begins the step pattern) after no more than 1 minute. The leading leg experiences greater musculoskeletal stress than the non-leading leg.
Propulsion Steps	Do not perform propulsion steps (in which both feet are off the floor or platform at the same time) for more than 1 minute at a time. Propulsion steps result in higher vertical impact forces and are considered an advanced technique. All propulsion steps should be performed up onto the platform and not down from the platform. It is therefore appropriate to run or jump up onto the platform, but not down.
Repeaters	To avoid stress to the support leg, do not perform more than five consecutive repeaters (in which the non-weight-bearing leg repeats the movement such as a kneelift) on the same leg.
Arms	Master the footwork before adding the arm movements. Avoid using the arms at or above shoulder level for an extended period of time because this places significant stress on the shoulder girdle. Be sure to frequently vary low-, mid- and high-range arm movements.
Music	Music tempos above 122 bpm are not recommended. Researchers have found that participants are well within their target training zones when using 122 bpm. Technique and safety are seriously compromised when music speeds are too fast.
Weights	The use of weights during the aerobic portion of step training produces little if any increases in energy expenditure or muscle hypertrophy. However, the risk of injuring the shoulder joint is significantly increased when weights are rapidly moved through a large range of motion, especially if the arms are fully extended. Until further biomechanical testing is conducted on the use of hand weights while stepping, it is recommended that weights be reserved for the strength segment of a step training class.

Source: Reebok International (1993).

5. Instructors should practice prudent progression to avoid advancing the students too quickly.

SUMMARY

The basics of safe and effective step training have been presented in this section. Table 9.2 presents a summary of the guidelines presented. There are still countless opportunities for other types of classes that include the platform and it is up to the instructor to design a class according to his or her own creativity. Instructors should remember the basics, practice prudently and use the platform to the best of their ability in order to achieve the type of class that works best for their clientele.

REFERENCES

Caralco, L., et al. (1991). The Metabolic Cost of Six Common Movement Patterns of Bench Step Aerobic Dance. *Medicine and Science in Sports and Exercise,* Abstract 140, Supplement 23:4.

Francis, et al. (1992). Effects of Choreography, Step Height, Fatigue, and Gender on Metabolic Cost of Step Training. *Medicine and Science in Sports and Exercise,* Abstract 69, Supplement 24:5.

Francis, L. (1992). Step Aerobics. *American College of Sports Medicine Certified News,* 2:1.

Franks, D., & Howley, E. (1992). *Health Fitness Instructor's Handbook,* 2nd Edition, Champaign, IL: Human Kinetics.

Kravitz, L., & Deivert, R. (1991). The Safe Way to Step. *IDEA Today,* April, 47-50.

Kravitz, et al. (1991). The Physiological Benefits of Step Training. Peer reviewed and accepted for publication by the *American College of Sports Medicine,* abstract, 1991.

LaForge, R. (1991). What the Latest Research Has to Say About Step Exercise. *IDEA Today,* September, 30-35.

Stanforth, D., et al. (1991). The Effect of Bench Height and Rate of Stepping on the Metabolic Cost of Bench Stepping. *Medicine and Science in Sports and Exercise,* Abstract 855, Supplement 23, 4.

Velasquez, et al. (1992). Changes in Cardiorespiratory Fitness and Body Composition After a Twelve-Week Bench Step Training Program. *Medicine and Science in Sports and Exercise,* Abstract 464, April, 1992.

RESISTANCE TRAINING

Resistance training first made its way into aerobics classes in the early 1980s. Instructors were looking for a safe and effective way to condition various muscle groups in a limited amount of time. Rubber bands and weights were added to existing moves in the floorwork section of classes in order to achieve momentary muscle fatigue in less time and with fewer repetitions. In 1990, the American College of Sports Medicine (ACSM) revised its position stand on the quality and quantity of exercise to include resistance training sessions of "moderate intensity." In addition to aerobic exercise three or more times a week, the ACSM suggests a minimum twice-weekly routine of eight to ten different exercises that condition the major muscle groups of the body. As a result of this recommendation, resistance training in the classroom gained new popularity.

Advantages of Resistance Training

Instructors can be a valuable resource to students by educating them about the benefits of resistance training. These benefits include maintaining or increasing strength and endurance and achieving a more lean and defined body. Although resistance exercise will not necessarily cause a direct improvement of aerobic performance, increase in muscle size and strength have been noted to be concurrent with fat loss.

Recent studies have shown a significant loss of body fat and increase of lean muscle tissue when aerobic and resistance exercises are integrated. Resistance training increases muscle mass, which increases the caloric needs of the additional lean tissue. This, in turn, increases the basal metabolism (the rate at which the body uses calories to perform vital functions, such as breathing, heart rate and digestion). The increased caloric requirement by the body means that while the body is at rest, it will metabolize excess calories while performing all daily activities, enabling an increased utilization of fat for calories and decrease in overall body fat.

Training Considerations

To achieve the benefits of strength and endurance training, muscles must be overloaded in order to produce momentary muscle fatigue. This momentary muscle fatigue must occur within 60 to 90 seconds to be considered effective. Since the classroom situation is different than the weight room, not all training principles can apply. However, instructors should consider the following training guidelines:

1. Exercise speed—Movements should be slow and controlled so that the muscle depends more on even application of its force than on momentum. Ballistic move-

Melane Barney is the owner of Performance Fitness, a provider of Continuing Education through ACE and AFAA, and conducts instructor workshops around the world. She has developed fitness programs for three clubs in Orange County, California, and is a national trainer for Reebok Body Walk. Melane has presented at several fitness conventions and stars in two exercise videos.

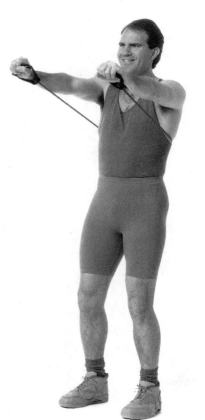

Figures 9.10-9.15 show upper-body resistance exercises.

Figure 9.10
Chest press.

ments are not advised because of the increased potential of injury to the joints and connective tissue.

2. Exercise resistance — It is advisable to select resistance at which participants achieve 70 to 80 percent of the maximum resistance. Since this may be difficult to calculate for everyone, and especially since various types of resistance equipment are available, the focus should be on momentary muscle fatigue. Applying the 60- to 90-second time frame for momentary muscle fatigue, the exercise can be considered effective if the participants experience fatigue after 8 to 12 repetitions. As the muscles become stronger, more resistance will be necessary to still achieve the strength benefits.

3. Range of motion—Each exercise should be performed through the full range of motion around the joint, and emphasis should be placed on the completely contracted position. By working through the full range of motion, the primary movers are strengthened while the antagonistic muscles are stretched, improving both muscular strength and joint flexibility.

Safety Considerations

Special attention must be placed on proper body alignment and technique when using any form of resistance. Knees and elbows should extend, but not to the point of hyperextension or locking. Wrists should remain neutral, neither flexed nor hyperextended. Movements should be controlled on both the concentric and eccentric contractions. Instructors must emphasize proper form and execution of exercises to facilitate good technique.

Instructors should refer to Chapter 3, "Biomechanics and Applied Kinesiology," in this manual for proper body alignment considerations, but the following verbal

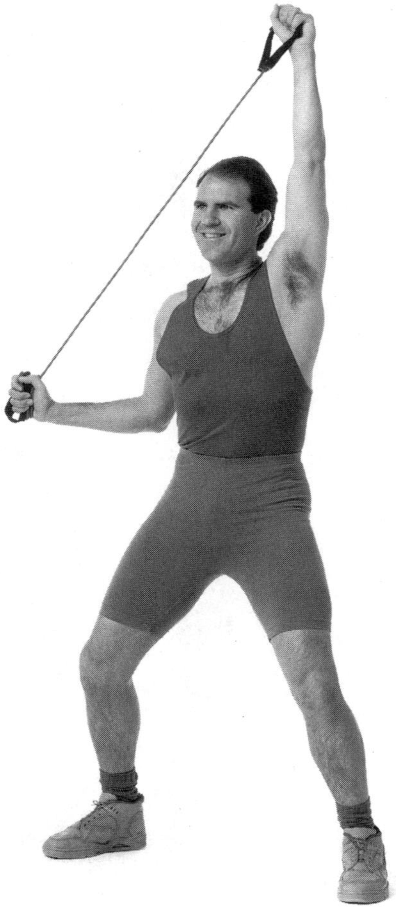

Figure 9.11
Single arm
lat pull-down.

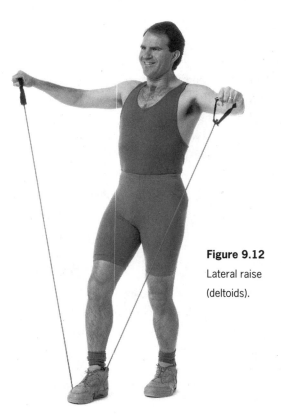

Figure 9.12
Lateral raise
(deltoids).

cues may assist students to achieve a neutral posture:

1. Head neutral, neck relaxed.
2. Shoulders down and back.
3. Chest lifted.
4. Abdominals contracted.
5. Pelvis tilted.
6. Knees relaxed or soft.

Instructors must be aware of the special needs and modifications for students with low-back problems as discussed in the "Musculoskeletal Injuries" and "Special Populations and Health Concerns" chapters of this manual.

Breathing correctly during resistance exercises oxygenates the blood throughout the movement and can help participants focus on the muscle group being worked. Students should be encouraged to exhale on the exertion phase of the movement. Instructors must discourage breath holding during exertion since this could induce the **Valsalva maneuver.**

When using exercise tubing or bands, it is important to check for any signs of wear and tear that could lead to breakage. While performing an exercise, participants must never look directly at the band or tube. Serious injuries can result from a sudden tear or breakage in the band or tube.

Class Design

The class should begin with a warm-up to prepare the body for the upcoming work load. Rhythmic movements should be followed by static stretches to increase and/or maintain flexibility. The warm-up should include movements similar to the exercises that will be performed in class.

After the appropriate warm-up, the participants can begin performing the resistance exercises. The types of equipment available in a typical resistance class include rubberized tubing and bands and free weights. When using the tubing to

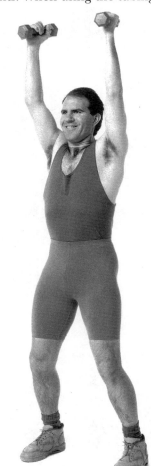

Figure 9.13a-b
Shoulder press with weights.

a. Starting position.

b. Ending position.

Chapter 9
Variations: From
Step to Strength
Training

perform the exercise, it is important to shorten the tube by wrapping it around the hands so that the thumbs can pinch it off and hold it in place. This should help prevent the tightness experienced around the hands when tubes are not held in place. The platform can also be utilized as a prop for sitting or lying to change the angle of the movement.

When designing the resistance training class, it is advisable to proceed from larger to smaller muscle groups. In the upper body, it would be appropriate to start with the larger muscles in the chest and back and then proceed with the shoulders and arms. In the lower body, it would be appropriate to start with the larger muscles of the thighs and then proceed to the muscles in the lower leg. By working the larger muscles first, the most demanding exercises are accomplished while fatigue levels are lowest.

When selecting exercises, it is important to choose at least one exercise for

each major muscle group. This will help to ensure balance and reduce the risk of injury. For time efficiency and smooth transitions, classes should be designed so that all exercises that require a standing position are done at once while all exercises that require sitting or lying are done at once.

Upper-body resistance exercises can be performed by utilizing both weights and tubes while standing (Figs. 9.10–9.15). The platform can be incorporated into the upper-body resistance section to assist participants by sitting or by lying in a supine or prone position (Figs. 9.16–9.18). The hamstring muscle group can be worked by lying prone on the bench, placing the rubber band around the lower leg, and flexing at the knee joint (Fig. 9.19). The inner- and outer-thigh muscle groups can be strengthened by adding ankle weights and rubber bands while in a side-lying position (Figs. 9.20 & 9.21). Additional muscle strengthening exercises can be found in

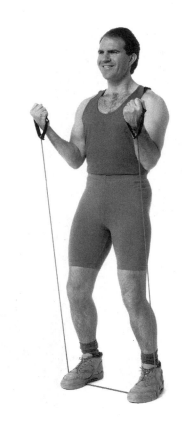

Figure 9.14
Biceps curls utilizing rubberized tube while standing.

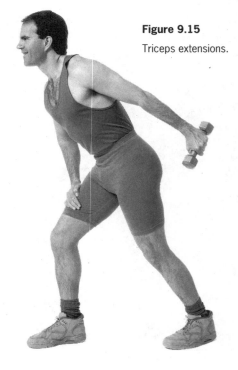

Figure 9.15
Triceps extensions.

Chapter 3, "Biomechanics and Applied Kinesiology," and Chapter 7, "Components of an Aerobics Class."

Additional Considerations

The instructor's communication of correct technique to the participants is essential to the safety and effectiveness of the resistance training class. The following cueing and correctional techniques may assist instructors in the class:

1. Take time before each exercise to assist students in their technique. Verbally explain and physically show proper posture.

2. Start each exercise segment with simple movements and progressively add one element at a time.

3. Remind participants about proper breathing throughout the class.

4. Use words to help participants visualize muscle groups that are being worked.

5. Motivate students with positive feedback.

6. Monitor participants at all times.

7. In the case of a student who is having difficulty moving into correct position, the instructor may try holding his or her hand in the direction where the body part should go. The instructor should then have the student try to touch his or her hand with that body part.

Music Selection

Music selection for resistance training should include songs that have a strong bass. The tempo of the music should be slow enough for the participants to achieve a full range of motion (about 120 to 130 bpm). In designing the choreography, instructors should use the 8 count of the music to their advantage. For example, counting up 2 and down 2 for 2 repetitions works well. Also, changing counts to emphasize either the eccentric or concentric contraction is effective and provides variety.

Resistance training

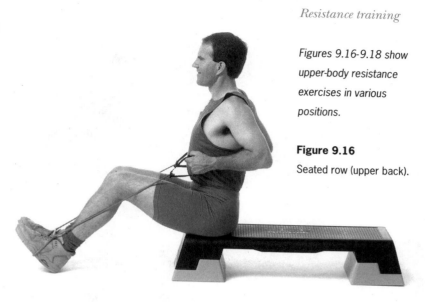

Figures 9.16-9.18 show upper-body resistance exercises in various positions.

Figure 9.16
Seated row (upper back).

Figure 9.17
Dumbbell chest fly.

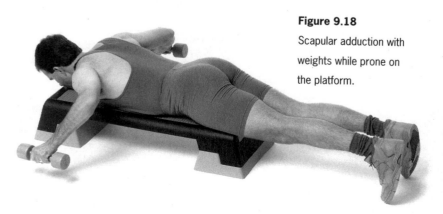

Figure 9.18
Scapular adduction with weights while prone on the platform.

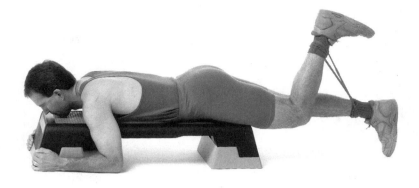

Figure 9.19

Hamstring curl using a rubberized band while prone on the platform.

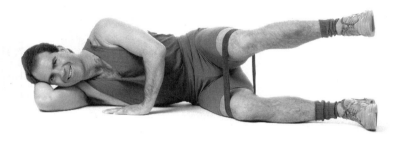

Figure 9.20

Side-lying leg abduction using the rubberized band.

Figure 9.21

Side-lying leg adduction utilizing an ankle weight.

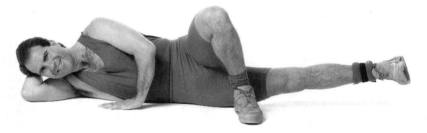

For example, when emphasizing the eccentric contraction, instructors can count up 1, then down 2-3-4 for 2 repetitions.

SUMMARY

Resistance training is an important part of a balanced exercise program. Instructors should understand the principles of strength and endurance training, adhere to safety guidelines, emphasize proper posture, cue appropriately, sequence exercises in a logical manner, and design the class so that it is safe, effective and challenging. When participants enjoy themselves and experience the satisfaction of good results, instructors can be confident that their students will continue to come to class.

SUGGESTED READING

American College of Sports Medicine. (1990). The Recommended Quality and Quantity of Exercise for Developing and Maintaining Fitness in Healthy Adults. ACSM position statement. *Medicine and Science in Sports and Exercise, 22,* 265-274.

Berger, R. (1992). *Introduction to Weight Training.* Human Kinetics: Champaign, IL.

Fleck, S.J., & Kraemer, W.J. (1987). *Designing Resistance Training Programs.* Human Kinetics: Champaign, IL.

Franks, D., & Howley, E. (1992). *Health Fitness Instructor's Handbook,* 2nd Edition, Champaign, IL: Human Kinetics: Champaign, IL.

Westcott, W. (1991). Testing and Evaluation. In M. Sudy (Ed), *Personal Trainer Manual: The Resource for Fitness Instructors,* San Diego: American Council on Exercise.

CIRCUIT AND INTERVAL TRAINING

Circuit training was developed by R.E. Morgan and G.T. Anderson in 1953 at the University of Leeds in England. It is a method of fitness training that attempts to increase muscular strength and endurance while decreasing the percentage of body fat. The term circuit refers to a number of carefully selected exercises arranged sequentially.

In the original format, the circuit comprised nine to twelve stations. This number may vary according to the design of the program. Each participant moves from one station to the next with little or no rest, performing 30 to 45 seconds of 10 to 30 repetitions at each station (Table 9.3). The stations may include exercise machines, hand-held weights, elastic resistance, calisthenics or any combination thereof. By adding aerobic training stations between each circuit, cardiorespiratory endurance may be enhanced as well.

Circuit training can be a complete exercise session by itself or can be integrated into the muscle conditioning segment of the class. Circuit training classes can add variety to the class schedule.

Music

One important element of this program is the music. It would be quite arduous for instructors to continuously watch the clock while changing exercises every 45 seconds, leading the class, and correcting the mistakes of students. The key to keeping the intervals correctly timed is simple—music cueing. Here are some ways to make it work:

1. Make a tape with "fade-ins" and "fade-outs." To do this, record a 45-minute tape of high-energy music with a dubbing deck or two decks. While recording the music, fade the level of the recording very low every 45 seconds and then back to the regular recording level. There should be about a 3-second gap—an opportunity to verbally introduce the next exercise.

2. A second option is to use a voice-over if the stereo system has the capability. After each 45-second interval, announce "stop" or "time to change," followed by "ready, begin" a few seconds later (the voice-over technique tends to be more useful in circuit training that uses exercise machines). In traditional aerobics class formats, the repeated commands tend to become monotonous. An alternative to the voice-over is the use of colorful lights to indicate changes. The use of red and green lights, easily seen by the whole class, works very well in indicating station changes.

3. Use different songs for each station. This may be the most creative music format. Simply record a song for 45 to 55 seconds and then fade it out. Then fade in a new song. This takes a lot more recording time and songs. However, if muscular conditioning stations are alternated with aerobic stations, this approach will give instructors the freedom to alternate preferred upbeat tempo aerobics numbers with slightly slower music for the specific exercise stations.

Administrative Considerations of Circuit Training

Adding a circuit training format or class to a program will require the instructor to consider the following:

1. Room size—Big enough to set-up the different stations as well as to allow for traffic flow of the class.

2. Equipment—The type of equipment available will dictate the type of exercises performed.

3. Class size—Planning for a circuit

Len Kravitz, has a doctorate in health promotion and exercise science at the University of New Mexico and is a regular contributing editor for IDEA Today. He is the author of three books and the producer of four exercise videos.

Figure 9.22

Figure 9.23

Figure 9.24

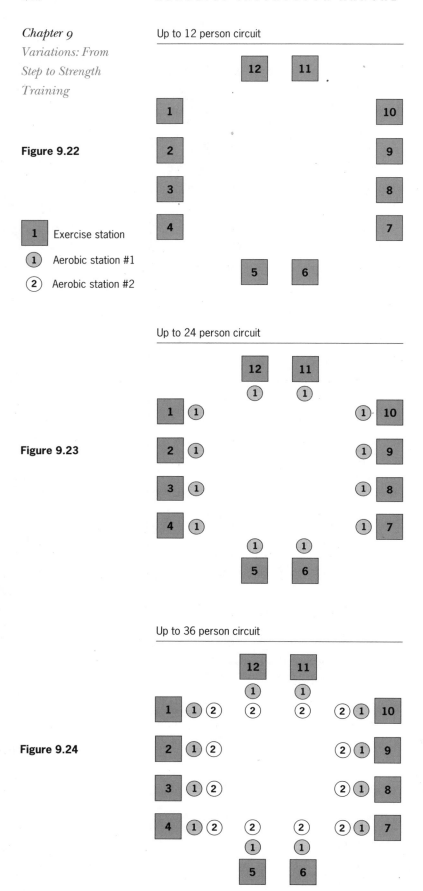

training class may be difficult depending on whether the number of students from class to class is unpredictable.

4. Mainstreaming newcomers—Often new participants to the program are unfamiliar with the exercises and format.

Circuit Training Design

Instructors can be very creative with the circuit design. For instance, assume that there are 12 exercise stations for a particular circuit class. This can accommodate a class consisting of up to 12, 24 or 36 students, and possibly more if needed. A class consisting of at least 12 students would simply alternate from station to station, with or without alternating aerobic stations (Fig. 9.22).

In a class consisting of up to 24 participants (and more than 12 students), instructors might want to place half of the students on each exercise station, with the other half on an aerobic station. With this design, two students actually work together as a team, traveling from one exercise station to the next (Fig. 9.23).

In a class with up to 36 participants (and at least 24 students), instructors might utilize the exercise station and two aerobic stations. This three-person team would alternate between an exercise station, aerobic station #1 and aerobic station #2. The three participants then travel to the next station to repeat this cycle (Fig. 9.24).

Sequencing the Exercise Stations. There are a number of ways to sequence the exercise stations of the circuit. Instructors may wish to sequence opposing muscle groups together. Another popular sequence is to alternate from an upper-body to a lower-body exercise. Depending on the fitness level of the participants and the goals of the class, instructors may have the participants repeat the circuit two or three times.

Table 9.3

BASIC CIRCUIT TRAINING FORMAT

# of Exercise Stations	Length of Each Station	# of Repetitions	% of 1-RM*	# of Circuits Performed
9-16	30-60 seconds	10-30	40-60%	1-3

*When using exercise machines, participants should train with resistance that is 40 to 60 percent of their one repetition maximum (1-RM). One repetition maximum is the maximum weight a person can lift with one repetition. A person may find his/her 1-RM through trials and attempting heavier loads until a specific load can be lifted only once. For example, if the maximum weight a client can do the bench press is 100 pounds, 40 percent would be 40 pounds. Some exercises, such as squats and lunges, are quite effective with little or no weights because of the resistance applied by the weight of the body.

Table 9.4

GENERAL INTERVAL TRAINING GUIDELINES

Energy System	Work Time	Cycles	Sets	Work/Recovery Ratio	Recovery Time	Type of Recovery
ATP-PC	0-30 seconds	8-10	4-5	1/3	0-90 seconds	Passive
Lactic Acid	30-120 seconds	5-6	1-3	1/2	60-240 seconds	Active
Oxidative	2-5 minutes	3-4	1-2	1/1	2-5 minutes	Active

The following is an example of a 12-station exercise circuit with an aerobic station between each station:

1. Chest press/Aerobics
2. Row pulls/Aerobics
3. Quadriceps extensions/Aerobics
4. Hamstring curls/Aerobics
5. Biceps curls/Aerobics
6. Triceps extensions/Aerobics
7. Heel raises/Aerobics
8. Upright rows/Aerobics
9. Squats/Aerobics
10. Lunges/Aerobics
11. Lat pulls/Aerobics
12. Shoulder presses/Aerobics

PRINCIPLES OF INTERVAL TRAINING

Interval training provides a method of completing a greater volume of high-intensity work by performing high-intensity work bouts in shorter segments mixed with recovery periods of less intense aerobic work. The specific duration of the work and rest intervals, number of cycles and sets of intervals, and type of recovery (active versus passive) depends on the energy systems in which training adaptations are primarily desired. Although a certain combination of training variables may stress primarily a particular energy system, training adaptations to some extent are likely to be seen in all three energy systems (see Chapter 1, "Exercise Physiology"). General interval training guidelines for developing the various energy systems are summarized in Table 9.4.

Interval Training in an Aerobics Class

Interval training is a form of conditioning that combines segments of high-intensity work with segments of moderate-to-light intensity work. Interval training has been an integral part of training programs for many years because a variety of sport and recreational activities require short bursts of movement at high intensities. Anaerobic fitness developed through interval training is becoming an increasingly recognized component of physical fitness (along with the more traditional components of aerobic fitness, body composition, muscle strength, and endurance and flexibility). The incorporation of interval train-

Table 9.5

INTERVAL TRAINING DESIGN CYCLE FOR AN AEROBICS CLASS

Type of Work	Length of Time	Heart Rate Intensity	Music (bpm)
Anaerobic	90 seconds	85% and above	162 bpm
Aerobic	3 minutes	70% to 75%	152 bpm

Number of Cycles: 5 to 6; fade in different music selections to mark the changes.

Recommended 1-hour class format:		
	Warm-up	7 minutes
	Interval Training	24 minutes
	Aerobic Cool-down	3 minutes
	Muscle Conditioning	20 minutes
	Cool-down	6 minutes

ing into a general conditioning program can optimize the development of cardiorespiratory fitness as well as body composition management.

The variety and the ease of design for multiple levels of ability that this training method provides are remarkable. The use of music cueing for intensity changes in the interval program has provided an additional motivational element for classes. This section will provide a scope and sequence to clearly understand interval training, the energy systems involved, and how to design a successful interval workout for an aerobics class and a combined step and aerobics class.

Interval Training Design for Aerobics Classes. The following represents a systematic design of interval training to enhance the aerobic capacity of the participants in an aerobics class. A 1 to 2 **work/recovery ratio** has been incorporated, combining a 90-second, high-intensity **work interval** with a 3-minute moderate-intensity recovery interval. The aerobic portion begins with a 3-minute cardiorespiratory warm-up of low-impact movement that gradually increases the heart rate intensity to approximately 70 to 75 percent.

After this 3-minute warm-up phase is complete, the music fades out while music at approximately 162 bpm fades in for the first 90-second work interval. During this high-intensity 90-second work bout, students are encouraged to challenge themselves to achieve at least 85 percent heart rate intensity. High-intensity combo-impact choreography is used during this 90-second work bout. After the 90 seconds is complete, the music fades out while music around 152 bpm fades in and a more moderate style of combo-impact or low-impact aerobics is performed (recovery cycle). The session is repeated five or six times, for up to 24 minutes, followed by a standard aerobic cool-down. The program described consists of a single set of five to six cycles (Table 9.5).

Inherent to an interval training class is the ability to modify for special populations and individuals with health concerns or other limitations (obese, older adult, injury recovery, entry-level student). During the 90-second work interval, the instructor should encourage these students to decrease heart rate intensity to 60 percent by showing them movement modifications. In large facilities, the participants with health

Table 9.6

INTERVAL TRAINING PROGRAM COMBINING STEP/TRAINING AND AEROBICS

Type of Work	Length of Time	Heart Rate Intensity	Music (bpm)
Aerobic-Step	3 minutes	75% and above*	120 bpm
Aerobic-Traditional	3 minutes	75% and above*	150 bpm
Number of cycles: 4 to 6			
Recommended 1-hour class format:	Warm-up	7 minutes	
	Interval Training	24 minutes	
	Aerobic Cool-down	3 minutes	
	Muscle Conditioning	20 minutes	
	Cool-down	6 minutes	

* Decide in advance which type of work will be the moderate and which will be the high intensity for each workout.

concerns or other limitations do brisk walking while the rest of the class does speed walking, jogging or running during the 90-second work period. This period actually becomes a rest-recovery for them, allowing many participants to continue longer than if they remained at 70-percent intensity for the entire session. (In smaller facilities, use more low-intensity, low-impact movement variations of what the class is performing during the 90-second work period.)

The class program just described has been experimentally designed by applying the principles of the energy system. This is only one example of a class, but instructors should follow the guidelines and design other viable programs.

Interval Training Combining Step and Aerobics

The following is another interval training program option that combines step training and aerobics. This program has been demonstrated to increase cardiorespiratory endurance, increase lean body tissue and decrease body fat. With this interval training program, alternate 3 minutes of step training (music at 120 bpm) at a moderate intensity with 3 minutes of combo-impact aerobics (music at 150 bpm) at a high intensity. It is also quite effective to alternate 3 minutes of step training at a high intensity with 3 minutes of combo-impact aerobics at a moderate intensity. Four to six cycles of this program provides a sufficient interval training class (Table 9.6).

Interval/Circuit Training

Interval/circuit training is a variation of circuit training that appears to be successful at overcoming the administrative challenges of traditional circuit training. This program uses a modified approach. The instructor leads each circuit exercise and the entire class follows without moving around the room. With this design, a fluctuating class size is not an issue, and new participants can easily be integrated because all they have to do is follow.

The equipment needed is minimal—a platform, hand-held weights and/or elastic resistance. Although the class participants do not move to various stations, they still go through a form of circuit training because the instructor changes the muscle group or exercise every 45 seconds (or longer).

This program is termed interval/circuit training because it is often advantageous to "vary" the interval length of the stations. For example, one format using a platform has the participants step for 3 minutes followed by 1 minute of a muscular conditioning exercise. The length of time for the intervals depends on the instructor's design. Up to this point in time, no studies have determined any optimal interval lengths, therefore, instructors are encouraged to use their creativity to discover the best format for their students.

SUMMARY

Circuit training and interval training are excellent methods of improving physical fitness. Both provide exciting and positive ways to alter exercise sessions, thereby helping to prevent "psychological burnout" and to increase long-term exercise adherence.

REFERENCES

Fleck, S. (1983). Interval training. *National Strength & Conditioning Association Journal.* 5(5), 40, 58-62.

Fox, E.L. (1975). Frequency and duration of interval training programs and changes in aerobic power. *Journal of Applied Physiology.* 38(93) 481-484.

Gettman, L.R., Ayres, J.J., Pollock, M.L., & Jackson, A. (1978). The effect of circuit weight training on strength, cardiorespiratory function and body composition of adult men. *Medicine and Science in Sports.* 10(3), 171-176.

Gettman, L. R., & Pollock, M.L. (1981). Circuit weight training: A critical review of its physiological benefits. *The Physician and Sportsmedicine.* 9(1), 44-60.

Gettman, L.R., Ward, P., & Hagan, R.D. (1982). A comparison of combined running and weight training with circuit weight training. *Medicine and Science in Sports and Exercise.* 14(3), 229-234.

Haennel, R. (1989). Effects of hydraulic circuit training on cardiovascular function. *Medicine and Science in Sports and Exercise.* 21(5), 605-612.

Hempel, L.S., & Wells, C.L. (1985). Cardiorespiratory cost of the nautilus express circuit. *The Physician and Sportsmedicine.* 13(4), 82-97.

Kravitz, L. (1986). Interval-Circuit Training. *Dance-Exercise Today,* 4(4), 60-62.

Kravitz, L. (1992). The physiological benefits of a combined step and aerobics training program. J. Rippe (Ed.), *IDEA World Research Forum,* Las Vegas, NV: IDEA.

O'Shea, P. (1987). Interval weight training - A scientific approach to cross-training for athletic strength fitness. *National Strength and Conditioning Journal.* 9(2), 53-57.

Peterson, S.R. (1988). The influence of high velocity resistance circuit training on aerobic power. *Journal of Orthopedic and Sports Physical Therapy.* 9, 339-344.

Skinner, J.S., & McLellan, T.H. (1980). The transition from aerobic to anaerobic metabolism. *Research Quarterly for Exercise and Sport.* 51, 234-248.

FUNK AEROBICS

In one shape-shifting decade, MTV has colonized the consciousness of an international youth culture by disseminating African-American music and hip-hop street culture to a global market. Music and dance styles created in neighborhoods and dance clubs are currently broadcast via satellite to 73 countries.

When a star picks up a "street move," everyone starts doing it, including aerobics instructors. As African-American dance styles became readily accessible to the mainstream, the "funk factor" burst onto the international aerobics scene. By 1990 IDEA, the international association for fitness professionals, was featuring entire sections of funk choreography at its conventions.

Early classes, however, often failed to meet the safety and effectiveness parameters of group exercise and were thus discouraged. As the vitality and appeal of the dance form grew, "funky" dance segments started to be included in the aerobic cooldown. Innovative instructors layered the elements of funk style over traditional class components and a blend evolved, creating a viable alternative to traditional aerobics classes.

The style of movement executed in funk aerobics and seen in music videos has a long tradition in American vernacular dance. Its roots can be traced to traditional African dance and rhythms.

Rhythmic Structure

The distinguishing factor in funk movement is its syncopated rhythm. **Syncopation** occurs when the stresses on the normally accented beats are temporarily shifted to unstressed beats or parts of beats. It's "dancing against the grain," as James Brown, the "godfather of soul," describes it.

Normally, rhythms are organized in units of two, with an alternation between stressed and unstressed beats. The stronger beat, the **downbeat**, is followed by a weaker beat, the **upbeat** (♪♩). This is known as duple meter.

Duple meter is derived from kinesthetic sense of internal rhythms. When people walk, they experience a "1-2-1-2" alternation between dominant/nondominant sides of the body. In breathing (inhale/exhale), as well as the heartbeat (contract/relax), they experience a twofold cycle alternating stronger and weaker events. Consequently in the rhythms of music and dance—and language (tick-tock, splish-splash, klick-klack)—an organizational impulse is expressed toward binary division of alternating stresses. When someone alters the pattern of stresses, as in syncopation, the effect is one of spontaneity and surprise, accounting for much of the vitality and appeal of funky rhythms. The following discussion is intended as an introduction to and demonstration of this complex rhythmic concept.

Common time (4/4 meter) is a compound meter based on duple meter (2 beats plus 2 beats equals 4 beats). Its pattern of stresses is normal.

$$\overset{<}{\text{♩}} \quad \text{♩} \quad \overset{<}{\text{♩}} \quad \text{♩}$$
$$1 \quad 2 \quad 3 \quad 4$$

Count 1 is a down beat. As the first beat in a measure, it receives primary emphasis. Count 2 is a weak beat or upbeat. Count 3 is a downbeat receiving secondary emphasis. Count 4 is an upbeat. To experience syncopation, first walk and count in common time:

$$\underset{1}{\overset{<}{\rule{0pt}{0pt}}} \quad \underset{2}{\rule{0pt}{0pt}} \quad \underset{3}{\overset{<}{\rule{0pt}{0pt}}} \quad \underset{4}{\rule{0pt}{0pt}}$$

Now change the emphasis as follows by moving with greater force, dynamics or

Kathryn Bricker has been presenting choreography seminars since 1979. In 1992 she served on the American Council on Exercise role-delineation and item-writing panels and the Reebok Corps. She has written for several exercise magazines and has presented at numerous fitness conventions. Ms. Bricker is an ACE gold-certified aerobics instructor and is an ACE continuing education provider.

amplitude, such as by stamping, clapping or stepping out farther:

<   <
<u>1</u>   <u>2</u>   <u>3</u>   <u>4</u>

<   <   <   <
<u>1</u> and <u>2</u> and <u>3</u> and <u>4</u> and

For lesson number two, syncopate a step pattern, a "jazz square," consisting of four walks performed in a square.

1. Perform first in common time:

<   <
(<u>1</u>   <u>2</u>   <u>3</u>   <u>4</u>)

Count 1 - L foot steps across in front of R

Count 2 - R foot steps back

Count 3 - L foot steps side L

Count 4 - R foot steps front

2. Syncopate the rhythm to "A-1-2-3-4" by adding a hop (R) on "A."

(hops take off on one foot and lands on the same foot)

3. Syncopate again by skipping the pattern.

<   <   <   <
"A - 1 - A - 2 - A - 3 - A - 4."

Table 9.7

NUMERICAL CUEING: EQUAL PARTS:

Counts:	1 and	2 and	3 and	4 and
Steady Beat:	——	——	——	——
Footwork:	out out R L	in in R L	out out R L	in in R L

Table 9.8

NUMERICAL CUEING: UNEQUAL PARTS:

Counts:	A	1-A	2-A	3-A	4
Steady Beat:	——	——	——	——	——
Footwork:	hop R	step-hop L L	step-hop R R	step-hop L L	step R

(hop on "A" then step on the count)

4. Repeat the entire series several times and perform each component two times. That's syncopation!

Numerical Cueing

The rhythmic complexity of funk steps makes numerical cueing an important instructional skill to acquire. When cueing rhythm, each beat in the steady pulse should be counted. Common time (4/4 meter) is counted using one of two methods, in fours ("1-2-3-4") or in eights ("1-2-3-4-5-6-7-8"). If a step is performed half-time to the steady pulse (walk R counts 1-2, L counts 3-4), if there is a hold (no movement) for a beat or beats, each beat is still counted to give a sense of the relative duration of each movement. When a beat is subdivided into two equal parts, such as when stepping double-time to the steady beat, the subdivision is expressed "and" (Table 9.7).

When a beat is subdivided into unequal parts, such as when performing steps of locomotion based on uneven rhythms (skips, slides, gallops), the subdivision is expressed "A." For example, a skip typically begins with a hop on the **anacrusis**, or up-beat, of the preceding measure. The component parts of the skip, the hop and the step are of unequal duration (Table 9.8).

Slides and gallops are similar, but usually begin on the downbeat with a "step-chase-step-chase-step" rhythm, which is counted "1-A-2-A-3-A-4-A." To get a sense of the value of numerical cueing for developing a feeling for syncopation, compare performing and counting a funky march (A-1-A-2-A-3-A-4), and a military-style march (1-2-3-4). In the funky march, as the torso flexes forward at the hip, the knee bends, and the arms swing up on the accented "A" before stepping down on the count; the rhythmic sense is markedly different from the feeling of emphasis on the downbeats in the military-style march.

Movement Vocabulary

The basic steps of locomotion are universal. Walks, runs, leaps, hops and jumps are based on even rhythms. Skips, slides and gallops are based on uneven rhythms. All movement patterns, including those in funk classes, are combinations of one or more of these steps, with spatial, rhythmic or dynamic variations.

Funk's characteristic style is derived from its origins in African dance rhythms. These characteristics include:

1. Propulsive rhythms that "swing."

2. An "into the earth" feeling—flat-footed, crouched forward, with knees and hips flexed.

3. Emphasis on improvisation, pantomime and individual expression.

4. Emphasis on pelvic movements.

5. Highly developed and rhythmic arm patterns.

6. Call-and-response pattern to encourage interaction.

Safety and Effectiveness Issues

Because funk aerobics evolved from a dance form, it has been necessary to adapt it to maintain both the safety and effectiveness of group exercise. The kinesiological principles discussed in Chapter 3, "Biomechanics and Applied Kinesiology" for establishing safe exercise moves should be applied to funk choreography. Also, instructors wishing to emphasize dance skills in conjunction with general conditioning should demonstrate a breakdown of step patterns before the aerobic component. The aerobic segment can then be performed continuously at appropriate intensities.

If step patterns are too complicated to be readily followed, target heart rates cannot be sustained. Care should be given to select movements that meet the desired objectives of group exercise. The angular, disjointed look and ballistic nature of many funk movements make them unsuitable for inclusion in aerobics classes. "Street moves" should be scrupulously screened for safety to determine whether the body is correctly aligned and if the movement is executed with control.

Pattern-building: Breakdown and Sequencing of Components Parts

When building movement patterns, the "parts to whole" approach discussed in Chapter 7, "Teaching an Aerobics Class," applies. Begin with the simplest component, and add or change one element at a time until the pattern is complete. To do this requires effective skills analysis. Funk aerobics offers some unique challenges in this area.

Many of the steps require isolation of body parts to create the angular, disjointed look of funk style. "Roger Rabbit," for example, includes isolation of the rib cage and shoulders while simultaneously performing rhythmically complex steps. Students will attempt to imitate the technical prowess of the instructor, so skill rehearsal in these movements should be included to ensure they are executed smoothly and carefully, without strain or tension. Isolations are also beneficial in teaching the feel of correct posture and placement and should be sequenced in the warm-up.

The rhythmic complexity of syncopation poses particular problems in coordination and timing. Many students have difficulty developing a feeling for syncopation due to exaggerated neuromuscular tension. The best strategy for relaxing them is to progress slowly through the building blocks of rhythmic training.

As discussed earlier, giving numerical cues for a funky march during the warm-up can impart a sense of the preparatory upbeat. Adding syncopated arm patterns to simple step patterns can further develop this rhythmic sense.

During the aerobic warm-up, footwork drills to develop a sense of "preparation in time" are critical. Timing a preparatory knee bend to execute a hop on the upbeat, for example, is a skill required of many funk steps. Instructors should provide simple drills, mixing steps of locomotion based on even rhythms with those based on uneven rhythms.

Sample Drill: Walks and Skips

Because a skip begins on the anacrusis, of the preceding measure, mixing walks (which have even rhythms) with skips (which have uneven rhythms) can develop the sense of timing needed to perform syncopated step patterns.

Walk and count 8 steps forward ("1-2-3-4-5-6-7-8"), then 8 skips back, ("A-1-A-2-A-3-A-4-A-5-A-6-A-7-A-8").

Repeat in fours, then in twos.

Sample Drill #2: Gallops, Walks and Hops

Gallop forward, R foot leading ("1-A-2-A-3-A-4-A-5-A-6-A-7-A-8").

Walk back, L foot leading ("1-2-3-4-5-6-7-8").

Reverse gallops and walks.

Repeat the gallop, switching the lead foot after count "4" by hopping on count "A."

Walk back, 8 times.

Gallop switching the lead foot every 2 counts by hopping on "A."

To assemble blocks of movement for the aerobic component, sequential forms work well. Start with the simplest movement, such as the "base move," and add or change one element of variation at a time so that the progression is easily followed. Elements of variation can be spatial, such as traveling front and back; rhythmic, such

as performing an established movement double-time; or dynamic, such as contrasting the stronger and weaker execution of movements. Continue choreographing movements using the "parts to whole" approach until a simple pattern, block "A," is developed. The following is an example of how a block of 32 counts can be assembled into a funk pattern:

1. Begin with a grapevine movement to the right for counts 1-4.

2. March forward (with both arms punching to the left and right) for counts 5-8.

3. Grapevine to the left for counts 1-4.

4. March backward (with both arms punching to the right and left) for counts 5-8. (the pattern above resembles a "square")

5. March forward (with both arms punching to the right and left) for counts 1-4.

6. Kick, ball-change counts 5 and 6, run right/left for counts 7 and 8.

7. Skip back counts A-1-A-2-A-3-A-4.

8. Jumping jacks (open 2 counts, close 2 counts) for counts 5-8.

9. Reverse all movements by starting on the left side.

Now using the same "parts to whole" approach, another block (block "B") can be developed. Block "B" should be developed considering balance, proportion, contrast and transition between the blocks to make sense. The pattern in which blocks can be joined creating sequential forms, such as a two-part form (A-B-A-B), or a three-part form (A-B-C), is as varied as is the creativity of individual instructors.

The complexity of funk patterns causes many instructors to bias toward their dominant side. Attention should be given to balance between use of the right and left sides of the body. As bipedal animals, an even number of weight transfers will always put people on the same lead foot. To reverse, build patterns with an uneven number of weight transfers, or that end in a neutral (weight over both feet) position.

To do this, perform a "stairstep" to common time as follows:

Step forward R count "1"

Step forward L count "2"

Step back R count "3"

Step back L count "4"

Now replace count "4" with a non-weight-transferring step. Try a touch, a hop and a hold. Perform count "4" double-time, "and-4" by inserting a ball-change. Slide R an uneven number of weight-transfers to the counts "1-A-2-A-3-A-4-A-5-A-6-A-7-A-8." Perform a stairstep ending with a jump on count "4" (remember jumps can take off on one or both feet, but what makes it a jump is the landing in a neutral position).

Music Type and Selection

Purchasing a premixed audiotape produced especially for funk classes by an aerobics music service is the most cost- and time-effective method for acquiring music. The songs are formatted in appropriate beats-per-minute ranges for traditional class components, as well as mixed to provide the consistent phrasing needed for "add-on" choreography.

To produce original tapes, one must have the necessary time, skills and audio equipment. Additionally, all songs should be used only with the proper licenses. To keep up-to-date on music selection, an instructor can read periodicals such as "Billboard Magazine" and "Street Sound," noting which songs are receiving the most "club play" and "radio play."

Terminology can vary, but generally the musical styles most suitable for funk classes are categorized as follows:

1. Rhythm and Blues/Club: 101 to 120 bpm—Broad range of music characterized by a funky bass line. It has a heavy, bottom sound with melody, song structure and lyrics.

2. House: 118 to 124 bpm—Distinctive because of its deep, rich, heavy bass line with jazzy, high-end cymbals or drums. These tracks are often programmed into a synthesizer.

3. Rap: 60 to 110 bpm—Rap artists often sample popular bass lines or riffs from soul classics and rap (talk in rhyme) over them.

4. Hip-hop: 100 to 109 bpm—Lies somewhere between rap and rhythm and blues/club.

SUMMARY

Funk can be a very fun and effective class provided that instructors follow established safety guidelines for movement. Instructors should exercise caution and scrutinize videos and professional workshops to be sure that they adhere to the principles of safety and effectiveness. The spark and spontaneity of a funky rhythm is within everyone, and instructors can learn to effectively facilitate this rhythm in class.

REFERENCES

Lockhart, A. (1977). *Modern Dance: Building and Teaching Lessons,* 5th Ed., Brown Co. Publishers.

Norris, D., & Shiner, R. (1969). *Keynotes to Modern Dance,* 3rd Ed., Burgess Publishing Co.

Polskin, H. (1991). *MTV at 10: The Beat Goes On.*

Public Television. (1990). *Everybody Dance Now, Dance in America.*

Sherbon, E. (1975). *On the Count of One: Modern Dance Methods,* 2nd Ed.. Mayfield Publishing Co.

Stearns, M., & Stearns, J. (1979), *Jazz Dance: The Story of American Vernacular Dance.* Macmillan Publishing Co., Inc.

Chapter 9
Variations: From
Step to Strength
Training

Mary E. Sanders,
M.S., director of
Wave Aerobics in
Reno, Nevada, is
author of "The Art
& Science of Wave
Aerobics." She con-
sults in development
and education for the
water fitness industry.
Nicki E. Rippee,
Ph.D., an associate
professor of physical
education at the
University of Nevada,
Reno, she developed
the exercises for the
"Indian Heartbeat
With Native Ameri-
cans" video. She is the
co-author of the book,
"Is Your Aerobics
Class Killing You?"

Traditionally, exercising in water has been viewed as a "gentle" fitness medium reserved primarily for the casual exerciser, elderly or injured. However, when exercise science and knowledge of water properties are considered, aquatic exercise is a fitness modality that could be ranked second to none.

A wide range of participants, including high-performance athletes, are discovering the effectiveness of water for fitness training. Water exercise can provide a training effect in all the components of fitness: cardiovascular fitness, muscular strength and endurance, flexibility and body composition. Also, because the body is submerged and primarily in a vertical orientation, water provides a unique opportunity for individuals to feel comfortable working at different intensity levels.

Simply taking land movement to the water will not achieve these training benefits. Work on land is created by regulating movement of different muscle groups with minimal need to consider the effects of the environment (air) acting on the body. In water, every movement must be made with regard to the effect of the environment (water) acting on the body. Both instructor and participant must be able to manipulate the properties of water in order to create a workout that parallels work intensities of land.

This section highlights a few of the skills and some of the knowledge aerobics instructors need to understand the water medium, and discusses the differences between land- and water-exercise environments.

The Water Environment

The following section summarizes scientific principles that affect exercise design in the water. The application of these principles is a method for regulating the intensity of exercise. Examples will be used to illustrate these principles by comparing exercise on the land with the exercise in the water.

Resistance/Drag. Viscosity is the friction that occurs between the individual molecules of water, therefore providing a resistance to its flow. Thus, viscosity acts as a resistance to movement. The effects of resistance on the body are directly related to the other properties of water.

Example:

On land—Viscosity has no application in changing exercise intensity because resistance of air molecules is minimal.

In water—Movement requires force to overcome the resistance of water and will create a greater working intensity when other properties of water are applied.

Buoyancy. Buoyancy is the force experienced by the body when submerged in water, creating an upward lift (Fig. 9.25).

Example:

On land—Buoyancy does not apply.

In water—The student must work at a depth that facilitates the application of force without creating the upward lift. In order to maintain complete control of the movement a participant's body composition is the key factor when choosing a working depth.

Action/Reaction. To every action there is an equal and opposite reaction.

Example:

On land—Arm moves can be added to traveling moves as a technique to increase exercise intensity. This is a function of the increased energy cost rather than assistance or resistance of air to the arm movement.

In water—The addition of arm moves also helps regulate intensity in water, not only through increased energy cost of additional muscular recruitment, but also because of the assistance/resistance of water to the movement. For example, pulling the arms backward in the water pushes the body forward (action/reaction).

Speed/Force. Speed is the rate of distance traveled per unit time. Force must be continually applied for an object to accelerate or decelerate.

Example:

On land—In a typical class, locomotion is performed by using the lower body. The speed depends on how fast the legs move and is not affected by the resistance of air.

In water—Assuming a vertical body position and the use of the legs, as force and the resulting speed increases, resistance increases, exponentially resulting in a significant increase of work intensity.

Inertia. Inertia is the tendency of an object to remain at rest or in motion until acted upon by an outside force.

Example:

On land—The body overcomes inertia by causing the muscles to act on the bones to initiate movement or stop movement in order to regulate intensity.

In water—The inertia of the water can be used to regulate intensity creating work or rest by moving either against a water current or with a water current.

Surface Area/Leverage. This includes the body surface size and the length of the arms and legs that are doing the work.

Example:

On land—The use of larger arm and leg movements creates intensity. Changing the surface area of those moving levers in the air has minimal effect on intensity.

In water—The viscosity of water coupled with larger movements and/or changes in the surface area of body parts moving through water can result in dramatic increases in exercise intensity. For example,

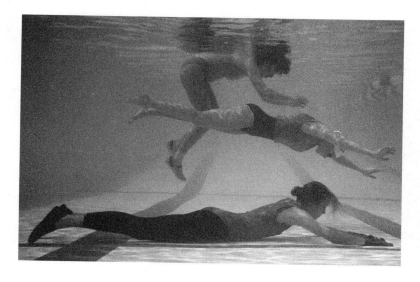

Figure 9.25

Three different reactions to the water environment due to buoyancy.

by changing the hand position from a narrow palm surface slicing through the water to the broad palm surface of the hand pressing in the water increases both resistance and intensity (Fig. 9.26).

Additional Considerations

Water temperature, depth and the equipment used are other important considerations when designing and instructing water-exercise programs.

Temperature. For a water fitness class, the most comfortable temperature for most participants is from 82 to 84 degrees Fahrenheit. The extremely efficient conductive and convective properties of water create a unique challenge to the aerobics instructor to help participants maintain appropriate body temperature for exercising in water. In cooler environments participants can wear clothing specifically designed to reduce heat loss. Instructors should optimize both safety and comfort by closely monitoring water temperature and exercise intensity.

Depth. Shallow water is defined as navel to nipple depth. When the lungs are submerged, it may be difficult to overcome the effects of buoyancy and move with force. Therefore, depths above the nipple

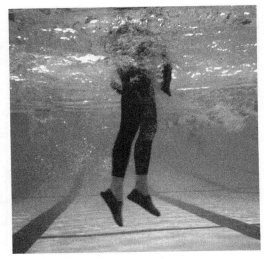

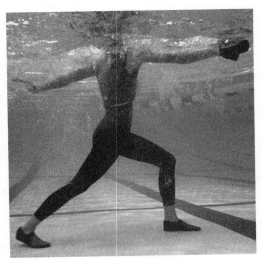

Figure 9.26
Rebound.

a. Up position.

b. Down position.

must be treated as deep water. In shallow water, depths can be artificially manipulated to change the movement dynamics and intensity. Three working positions are used in shallow water:

1. Rebound—pressing forcefully off the ground to move upward (Fig. 9.26).

2. Neutral—lowering the body to armpit depth and working through the water while tapping and sliding the feet softly along the bottom for support (adding some buoyancy) (Fig. 9.27).

3. Suspended—completely buoyant, working the arms and legs without touching the bottom, mimicking deep water (total buoyancy). This position requires skill and practice (Fig. 9.28).

Equipment. Equipment may be added to create overload or provide buoyancy for deep-water exercise programs. Equipment is either held by the participant or attached to the body. Adding equipment enhances the properties of water by increasing buoyancy, resistance or a combination of both. Participants should be taught proper applications and specific safety skills related to equipment.

Measuring Intensity in Water Exercise

There is general agreement that water exercise should follow the same criteria as land exercise for programming in terms of frequency, intensity and time. However, determining intensity in water presents some problems. Earlier information suggests that a working heart rate in water will be an average of 17 bpm slower when compared to a working heart rate on land (Katch et al., 1981). More recent research, however, has demonstrated that this may not be the case in all water exercise. When considering the heart rate issue, a number of variables affect heart rate to the degree that the lower heart rate theory may not be absolutely correct.

While there is general agreement that resting heart rate is reduced by as much as 20 to 30 bpm when standing in waist-deep water, traveling moves have been shown to elevate heart rates within the target range. Water temperature has also demonstrated dramatic effects on heart rate. Exercising in waist- to chest-deep water at cool temperatures between 70 to 80 degrees Fahrenheit produces heart rates of 10 to 15 bpm lower than comparable land exercise. However, the same exercise performed in the water at temperatures between 86 and 88 degrees Fahrenheit elicits a heart rate response similar to land exercise (Beasly,

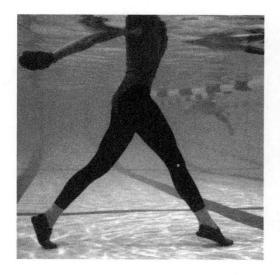 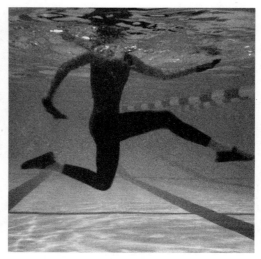

Figure 9.27 (left)
Lowering the body so that the lungs are in the water increases buoyancy.

Figure 9.28 (right)
Complete suspension in the water. Powerful arm and leg action keeps the body balanced.

1989). Additionally, heart rate may be affected by participants anxiety resulting from their lower skill levels, individual participant body composition, the type of clothing worn, the air temperature and the hydrostatic pressure imposed on the lungs at a certain depth of water.

The conflicting research and the wide variety of factors affecting heart rate in water make it difficult to give a definitive conclusion concerning measurement of exercise intensity. It is suggested that the instructor use a variety of methods, including target heart rate, ratings of perceived exertion and the talk test to monitor the participant's intensity levels. Instructors are encouraged to determine the most effective intensity monitoring method suitable for their class. Research has shown that with appropriate class design, water exercise intensity has been sufficient to produce significant improvement in cardiovascular fitness.

Class Design

The exercise class and design relate specifically to the pool design and size, and water depth and temperature. The same scientific exercise principles apply to class design on both land and in water, howev-

er, there are some unique considerations for water.

Warm-up Phase. The warm-up phase is usually 3 to 8 minutes long. The physiological objectives are the same as on land, but there are special considerations for movements that the water environment creates. The participant must have time to adjust to buoyancy, water temperature and balance in this dynamic environment. Suggestions for warm-up include: (1) beginning in a stationary position; (2) a slow speed; (3) working in a soft, flexuous mode; and (4) changing from light to moderate intensity by using short to long levers.

The warm-up must be paced in response to the temperature of the water. A more vigorous warm-up would be used in colder water to enhance muscle warmth and slightly elevate the heart rate. Instructors and participants should work the arms and legs (levers) in various planes around the body in order to rehearse the exercise movements and achieve balance.

The cardiovascular warm-up (2 to 3 minutes) specifically addresses the changes and safety concerns occurring with traveling moves. The objective is to increase intensity to enhance deep muscle temperature and elevate heart rate into the lower end of the training zone. Buoyancy, balance and stabilization of postural alignment are affected to a greater degree in water than on land. In water, participants experience increased resistance during travel moves, which need to be practiced at a lower intensity before the work phase begins.

Work Phase. This phase of the exercise program usually is allotted from 20 to as much as 60 minutes. The conditioning part of the class, the work phase, should be designed to accomplish specific objectives (i.e., aerobic or anaerobic work, caloric expenditure, high resistance muscle work and/or stretching).

The most common aquatic class objective is to perform aerobic exercises for the long-range goal of cardiorespiratory conditioning and fat weight reduction. In this case the physiological overload would consist of multijoint, large-muscle activity while sustaining an exercise heart rate of 60 to 90 percent of maximum heart rate for 20 to 60 minutes. Either an interval or continuous format is appropriate. Since buoyancy decreases or eliminates impact, participants can increase the duration of their work phase without the risk of injury that gravity creates on land.

Intensity Progression. In water, intensity can be changed by manipulating a single, basic move through several variations that change the properties of water acting on the body. These changes create an intensity progression. The following example describes how to apply the concept of intensity progression to the rocking horse movement.

1. The basic movement is performed by rocking forward on the right foot and backward on the left foot. The knees should be slightly flexed when rocking.

2. Short lever arm movements are

added to oppose the forward and backward rocking motion and to slightly increase intensity.

3. The short lever arm and leg movements then extend to become long lever arm and leg movements. This increased action increases drag resistance.

4. To achieve maximum intensity, continue with the speed of the movement, maintain lever extension, and add the element of travel.

To decrease intensity, simply work backward through the same progression, reducing the properties being applied. Use synergistic arm and leg movements to help maintain balance and intensity. Other basic moves that may be manipulated through the intensity progression include jogging, kicking, jumping and scissors. A complete exercise session can be created by adding simple variations to the basic moves. Movement variations create dramatic changes in the effect of water acting on the body, balance and intensity of work.

Cool-down. The aerobic cool-down phase usually lasts 2 to 3 minutes and is water-specific. A gradual reduction in cardiorespiratory function must be balanced with the maintenance of body warmth. As intensity subsides, the cooling effect of water is enhanced, causing a rapid loss of body heat.

Reversing the movements in the warm-up sequence provides an effective format. If the water is cold (<80° F), prevent chilling by transitioning immediately to muscle conditioning, active stretching or by exiting the pool.

Muscular Strength and Endurance Phase. This phase usually lasts 3 to 10 minutes. The purpose of muscle conditioning is to train specific muscle groups. Since the surface areas of various body parts are usually too small to adequately provide an overload for strength and endurance training, it may be necessary to add equipment. Adjustable hand-held paddles and water chutes increase the resistance surface sufficiently to create an overload.

Stretching and Flexibility Phase. This phase lasts from 3 to 6 minutes. Post-exercise stretching is done to improve range of motion of a specific joint. Due to buoyancy, many stretching positions are more readily accomplished in water than on land. For example, buoyancy can assist in a hamstring stretch by causing the leg to be lifted upward. If the water is cold, chilling can be prevented by moving other muscles while stretching. For example, when stretching the upper body, continue to jog lightly.

A brief cool-down of slow, light, buoyant moves such as rocking may end the session. This provision facilitates the transition from water to land by ensuring that participants exit the pool comfortably warm.

Music

Music choices should facilitate movement quality, be entertaining and motivate participants to a desired intensity. However, due to the high resistance and buoyancy of water, it is not always possible to move to the beat as on land. Since water amplifies individual differences, such as body composition, skill, movement speed and timing, counting off steps in choreography is not recommended.

Safety

Safety training for water exercise is very specific and should include basic water assistance, individual safety skills for students and instructors, and instructor safety during deck teaching. Ideally, instruc-

tors should have the safety- and health-related certifications of standard first aid and CPR. Instructors must also understand joint and muscle balance to prevent overuse injuries.

Teaching Water Exercise

On land, the instructor can participate fully in the class while using mirrors and a microphone to assist with demonstration and explanation of the moves. It may be necessary for water instructors to demonstrate movements on the deck without participating directly in the class. Because the water hides the portion of the body submerged, it is more difficult to see movements, and pool acoustics may make audio cues impossible to hear. Teaching and motivation needs outweigh the personal exercise participation of the instructor.

Special care must be taken when teaching from the deck to demonstrate safely while still cueing water-specific moves at appropriate water speeds. Equipment such as a "teaching stool," a waist-high bar or chair for standing support, well-cushioned, nonslip shoes and a water-resistant microphone will help make teaching water moves from the land safer. Microphones are now available that go into the water with the instructor.

Instructors can provide corrective feedback with the view from the deck; however, the best view is achieved by wearing a mask or goggles under water. This allows instructors to check periodically for evaluation of alignment and technique. Ideally, teaching from both deck and water can be combined to protect the instructor and to allow participation in the fun. The more the participants know, the easier it is to teach from the water.

SUMMARY

This has been a cursory look at water fitness. To become adept in aquatic exercise instruction, specialized training and experience are necessary.

The gentle buoyancy of water provides a new freedom of movement that expands beyond the daily effects of gravity. Participants can experience a sense of "play" at their own pace without the fear of injury from falls. Participants may also benefit from the privacy of submersion. Various fitness levels can exercise together by changing the environmental response so that water acts differently on each participant. Water can provide a new setting for cross-training or can be the preferred choice of exercise.

RESOURCES

American College of Sports Medicine (1990). Position Stand: The Recommended Quantity and Quality of Exercise for Developing and Maintaining Cardiorespiratory and Muscular Fitness in Healthy Adults. Medicine and Science in Sports and Exercise. 22:2, pp. 265-274.

American Council on Exercise (1991). Personal Trainer Manual, The Resource for Fitness Instructors, CA: American Council on Exercise.

American Red Cross (1992). Swimming & Diving. Mosby Year Book. pp. 240-243.

Beasley, B.L. (1989). Prescription Pointers, Aquatic Exercise. Sports Medicine Digest. 11(1).

Fawcett, C.W. (1992). Principles of Aquatic Rehab: A New Look at Hydrotherapy. Sports Medicine Update. 7(2), Summer 1992, 6-9.

McArdle, W., Katch, F., Katch, V. (1991). Exercise Physiology, Energy, Nutrition and Performance. Third Edition, Lea & Febiger: Philadelphia, PA.

Miles, D., & Buchanan, P. (1991). The Aquamotion Water Fitness Manual. J. MacDonald, 1048 "C" Palmetto Way, Carpinteria, CA.

Moschetti, M. (1990). Aquaphysics Made Simple. CA. AquaTechnics.

Rippee, N.E., & Sanders, M.E. (1992). Splash into Shape, The newest wave in water workouts. SHAPE Magazine. August, 1992, 68-75.

Sanders, M.E. (1990). The Big Chill is No Thrill. The AKWA Letter. September. 4(3), 1-13.

Sanders, M.E. (1991). Aqua Music. IDEA Today. 9(4), 24-25.

Sanders, M.E. (1992). The Art & Science of Wave Aerobics. Educational video and correspondence course. Producer: In & Under Water 1-800-537-5512.

Sanders, M.E. (1993). Selected Physiological Training Adaptions During Participation in the Wave Aerobics Program. Unpublished Thesis. University of Nevada, Reno; Reno, Nevada 89557-0036.

FLEXIBILITY TRAINING

Over the years, cardiorespiratory and muscular conditioning have been a primary focus of the fitness profession. Although these two components are essential to overall health and fitness, the importance of flexibility in the total fitness program must not be overlooked. As the benefits of flexibility exercise become more apparent, it is necessary to emphasize education and training in flexibility as a significant part of a healthy and fit lifestyle. This is especially important since a large segment of the population is growing older and more susceptible to injury.

Physiology of Flexibility

Enhanced flexibility reduces the risk of injury, helps release muscle tension and soreness, allows more freedom of movement and correction of postural dispositions and promotes physical and mental relaxation. The degree of flexibility a person has may be related to his or her genetics, gender, age and level of physical activity. Some people are naturally more flexible than others, and females are typically more flexible than males. As people grow older they tend to lose flexibility, and they realize that the less active they are the more inflexible they become. With training, however, the degree of flexibility can be increased toward a person's inherent potential.

Flexibility is joint-specific and refers to the degree of range of movement around a joint. Movement may be limited primarily by: the bone structure of the joint, the ligaments encapsulating the joint, the musculotendinous tissues spanning the joint, and neuromuscular coordination. Of these factors, the only one that should be manipulated to increase flexibility is the musculotendinous tissue. The bone structure is obviously self-limiting, and to stretch the ligaments around the joint is extremely

Patricia Kirk, M.S., is the general manager of the Rolling Hills Club in Novato, California. She serves as the chair of the Aerobics Instructor Certification Committee for ACE. Ms. Kirk is also a member of the advisory board of the health and fitness certification program of the University of California, Berkeley.

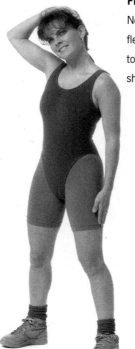

Figure 9.29
Neck stretch. Laterally flex the cervical spine to bring the ear to the shoulder.

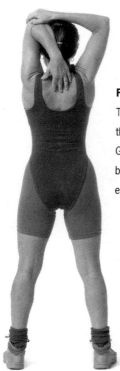

Figure 9.30
Triceps stretch. Point the elbow to the ceiling. Gently press on the elbow so the hand reaches toward the spine.

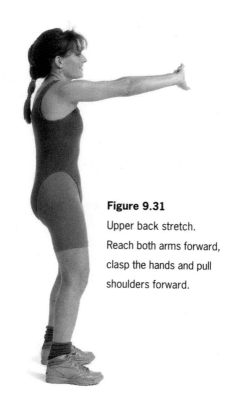

Figure 9.31
Upper back stretch. Reach both arms forward, clasp the hands and pull shoulders forward.

undesirable because ligaments are responsible for the joint's stability. If ligaments are weakened, they predispose the joint to injury.

Inflexibility is believed to be related to acute injury, muscle soreness and postural deviations because of tight musculotendinous tissues surrounding the muscle fibers and spanning the joint. Acute injury and muscle soreness may occur as a result of a quick movement that is greater than the range of motion allowed by these tissues. Postural deviations may also occur as a result of the combination of taut musculotendinous tissues and muscular imbalance, which limit the range of movement. As a result of flexibility conditioning, these connective tissues adapt by lengthening, and thus, increase the range of motion around the joint.

Stretching Techniques

Two types of stretching techniques are most commonly referred to by fitness professionals with respect to increasing flexibility: static and ballistic (or dynamic) stretching. **Static stretching** is the technique most recommended because it is considered the most effective in increasing flexibility and is not generally associated with the risk of injury. A static stretch involves holding a joint in a position that stretches the muscle and connective tissues to their greatest length. It is important to stretch to the point of tension and not to pain. The stretch is typically held for approximately 10 to 30 seconds.

Static stretching is considered the safest and most effective because it does not elicit the neuromuscular response called the **stretch reflex**. Within the muscle and lying parallel to the muscle fibers is a sensory motor receptor called the **muscle spindle**. It is responsible for regulating the changes in the length and tension of the muscle's fibers. The main function of the spindle is to respond to a stretch on the muscle by sending a sensory (or afferent) signal to the spinal cord, then receiving a motor (or efferent) response back to generate a

Figure 9.32
Torso stretch. Support one hand on the hip and reach the opposite hand over the head.

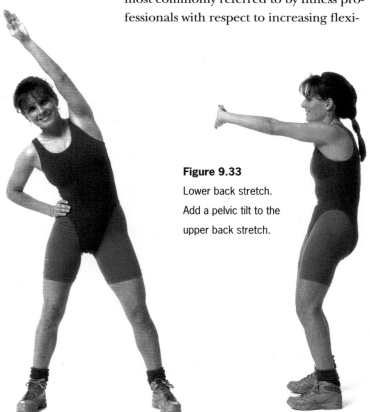

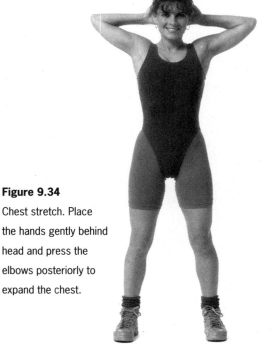

Figure 9.33
Lower back stretch. Add a pelvic tilt to the upper back stretch.

Figure 9.34
Chest stretch. Place the hands gently behind head and press the elbows posteriorly to expand the chest.

reflex action causing the muscle to contract against the stretch; this is called the stretch reflex.

The force and rate of contraction is directly related to the force that was generated by the stretching movement. Thus, if a stretch is performed slowly and gently, the stretch reflex is minimal, if invoked at all.

Static stretching stimulates another type of sensory receptor called the Golgi tendon organ. Unlike the muscle spindle, which lies parallel to the muscle fiber, these lie across several muscle fibers and are located in the tendons connecting the muscle to the bone of the joint. Their main function is to detect the differences in muscle tension particularly on the ligaments. When stimulated by excessive tension, such as caused by a firm stretch or a strong contraction, the **Golgi tendon organ** receptors respond by invoking an inhibitory reflex on the muscle, causing it to relax. The degree to which this stimulates inhibition of contraction is directly related to the force of the stretch. Therefore, a slow,

firm, long stretch will elicit a significant response from the Golgi tendon organ that causes the muscle to relax and, consequently, stretch easily without injury.

Ballistic stretching is characterized by continuous jerking or bouncing movements, and is not recommended as an effective or safe way to stretch. These types of movements result in high-force, fast stretches on the muscle and its connective tissue. These stretches significantly stimulate the stretch reflex. Therefore, the muscle is stimulated to contract with relatively the same degree and rate of force as generated in the stretch. The possibility of injury and soreness is increased because of the near-simultaneous stretch and contraction stimulation of the muscle fiber, which generates a tremendous degree of tension on the fiber.

A third type of stretching technique, called **proprioceptive neuromuscular facilitation** (PNF), seems to be primarily used for rehabilitation in physical therapy or in conditioning for significantly increasing flexibil-

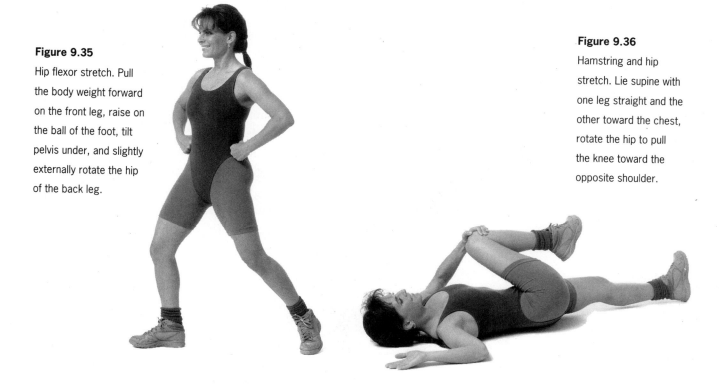

Figure 9.35

Hip flexor stretch. Pull the body weight forward on the front leg, raise on the ball of the foot, tilt pelvis under, and slightly externally rotate the hip of the back leg.

Figure 9.36

Hamstring and hip stretch. Lie supine with one leg straight and the other toward the chest, rotate the hip to pull the knee toward the opposite shoulder.

ity. It is not commonly recommended for group exercise or for the general, unsupervised exercising population. The technique involves statically stretching a muscle immediately after holding a maximal contraction of the same muscle. It is believed that the significant contraction invokes strong responses from the Golgi tendon organ, therefore, causing the muscle to relax that much more for the stretch. Currently, some people believe this technique is extremely effective while others believe that there is no significant proof to support this conclusion. Since PNF exercises were designed to be done with a knowledgeable and experienced professional, classroom PNF is not recommended.

Stretching Methods

Stretches can be performed either passively or actively. A passive stretch is one in which an external force is applied to a muscle group to cause the stretch. An example is using the hands to pull the leg toward the chest while lying supine in order to stretch the hamstring. An active stretch is one by which the body's own movement is causing the stretch—as when reaching an arm up toward the ceiling to stretch the

shoulder and torso.

Passive stretches can be performed between two people by having one person stretch the muscle group of the other person (passive). This can be a very effective means of increasing flexibility. However, it is imperative that the person applying the force be extremely sensitive to the resistance of the muscle group and the responses of the person being stretched so as not to cause injury.

Exercise Recommendations

Flexibility is joint-specific. It is important, therefore, to select a variety of exercises that will provide effective and safe flexibility conditioning for every major muscle group in the body. When recommending exercises, the following should be considered:

1. The individual's current level of flexibility,

2. How much the individual understands about the physiology of flexibility as well as the purpose of the exercise itself, and

3. What the participant is specifically trying to accomplish. All stretches are not appropriate for all people. Certain exercises need to be modified or adjusted to correctly accommodate the individual's particular needs.

A flexibility program should begin with a simple, general, low-intensity warm-up, such as easy walking combined with rhythmic ROM movements for the whole body. Each stretch should begin gently and progress gradually to the more advanced static stretch. The sequence of exercises should work progressively through the

Figure 9.37
Back stretch. Gently pull both knees to the chest, while lifting the head and neck.

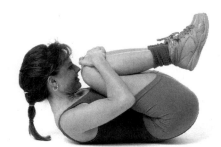

Figure 9.38
Whole body stretch. Lie supine and reach the arms overhead and the legs away from the body.

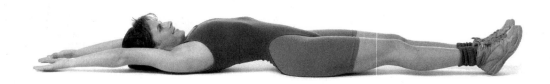

entire body and be specific to each joint and/or muscle group.

Selection of an exercise should depend significantly upon its degree of effectiveness versus its possible risk of injury to the body. The stretch should be performed in the most effective and safest way possible. Accordingly, many stretches are performed more safely while in the supine position versus standing. For example, a supine hamstring stretch is much more effective and is safer than the one performed while standing with the torso flexed at the hip over the legs. Even if supported, this position may compromise the back if students lack body awareness.

Breathing is very important to the process of stretching. Full, deep breaths help to slow certain physiological responses, such as heart rate and blood pressure, while releasing physical and mental tension. This promotes relaxation and may allow for a greater range of motion.

Class Programming

Stretch and flexibility classes are fast becoming a very popular and viable option to the more "traditional" aerobic or group exercise sessions. Due to the heightened awareness of the importance of flexibility to performance, injury prevention and proper posture, much more attention is being given to flexibility programming. It should be an integral part of a facility's mainstream exercise program because it is a necessary complement to the aerobics and muscular conditioning classes. A stretch and flexibility class is an excellent place for the inactive individual to begin an exercise program. Starting with gentle exercise and gradually progressing to more strenuous exercise may help keep a person motivated to continue.

There still seems to be some controversy regarding whether flexibility exercises

are more effective before or after exercise. However, most professionals recommend stretching before and after activity with very specific purposes. The warm-up should include a general, low-intensity activity such as walking combined with rhythmic, easy, full range-of-movement exercises for the entire body. These exercises are primarily responsible for increasing blood flow and enhancing range of movement—or "loosening up." During the cool-down, the stretches should be designed to achieve maximum gains in range-of-motion and include static stretches in order to increase flexibility.

In the stretch and flexibility class, the warm-up is followed by a series of exercises designed to enhance body alignment (placement techniques) and increase flexibility for each major muscle group of the

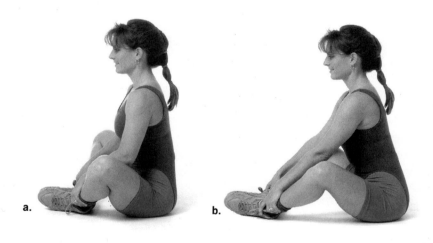

Figure 9.39a-b
Inner thigh stretch.

a. With soles together, pull the heels close to the groin and gently press the elbows on the thighs.

b. Modified stretch. Heels move away from the groin area while stretching.

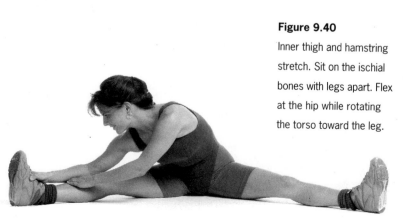

Figure 9.40
Inner thigh and hamstring stretch. Sit on the ischial bones with legs apart. Flex at the hip while rotating the torso toward the leg.

Chapter 9
Variations: From
Step to Strength
Training

body. Each exercise should begin with a gentle range-of-motion stretch and progress gradually to a more dramatic, full range-of-motion static stretch. Throughout each exercise, the instructor needs to encourage proper breathing and body alignment techniques. Sequencing the exercises from head to toe is a very com-

mon approach because it allows the work to begin standing, gradually progress to sitting and finish in the supine position.

From here, the class can progress smoothly into the final cool-down or relaxation phase. A relaxation phase is becoming more common to the cool-down format of all classes because it provides an excellent opportunity to promote stress reduction. Instructors may wish to select any or all of the stretching exercises shown (Figs. 9.29 through 9.42). Instructors should remind students to maintain a neutral spine and lifted torso for stretches performed in a standing or seated position. Additional flexibility exercises are presented elsewhere in this manual (Chapter 3, "Biomechanics and Applied Kinesiology", and Chapter 7, "Components of an Aerobics Class").

Equipment and environment can significantly influence the success of a stretch and flexibility class. Certainly, mats are required for appropriate cushioning against hard surfaces. Towels are a very helpful tool to help relatively inflexible people perform a stretch. For example, if a woman is unable to reach very far toward her feet for a stretch on the hamstring, holding onto a towel around her feet will help provide leverage to the stretch.

Music, as with all aerobic or group exercise classes, plays a very important part in setting the mood and pace for a stretch and flexibility program. Upbeat, percussive music is not conducive to the relaxed physiological state required during stretching. New age, classical, easy rock and jazz are more appropriate selections for this type of program.

The most important aspect to a successful program is that it be enjoyable. Everyone, regardless of his or her fitness level, needs to feel he or she can accomplish the stretches. There should be significant in-

Figure 9.41a-b

Calf, instep and ankle joint muscle stretches. Place both legs straight in front of the body while sitting on ischial bones.

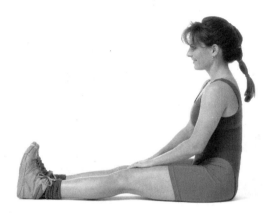

a. Dorsiflex at the ankle joint.

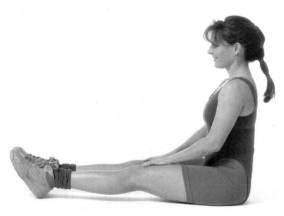

b. Plantarflex at the ankle joint.

Figure 9.42

Relaxation. Lay supine with the eyes closed and the body relaxed. Concentrate on breathing for 1 to 3 minutes.

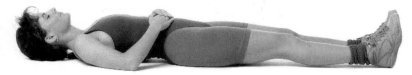

teraction between the instructor and the client, as well as an opportunity for the participants to be social with each other. This will generate a feeling of support and fun, which are very important influences on exercise adherence.

Some fitness professionals say that while cardiorespiratory and muscular conditioning keep us healthy and fit, stretching and flexibility training keep us young and agile. P. Kirk

REFERENCES

American College of Sports Medicine. (1991). *Guidelines for Exercise Testing and Prescription.* Fourth Edition, Lea & Febiger: Philadelphia, PA.

Anderson, B. (1980). *Stretching.* Shelter Publications, Bolines, CA.

deVries, H. (1986). *Physiology of Exercise: For Physical Education and Athletics.* Fourth Edition, Wm. C. Brown: Dubuque, Iowa.

Luby, S.; Faber & Faber. (1986). *Bodysense. The Hazard-Free Fitness Program for Men and Women.* Winchester, MA.

McArdle, W.; Katch, F., Katch, V. (1991). *Exercise Physiology, Energy, Nutrition and Performance.* Third Edition, Lea & Febiger: Philadelphia, PA.

Part III
Individual
Needs

Chapter 10

Adherence and Motivation

By Deborah Rohm Young and Abby C. King

Fundamentals of exercise adherence

- Major factors influencing exercise adherence
- Personal
- Program
- Environmental

Traits of an ideal aerobics instructor

- Punctuality and dependability
- Professionalism
- Dedication
- Sensitivity to the participant
- Willingness to plan ahead
- Recognizing signs of burnout
- Taking responsibility

Strategies that encourage adherence

- Formulate reasonable participant expectations and exercise goals
- Give regular, positive feedback
- Make exercise sessions easy, interesting and fun
- Develop exercise reminders, cues and and prompts
- Encourage an extensive social support system
- Help participants develop intrinsic rewards
- Prepare participants for inevitable missed classes

Exercise and body image

- Maintaining a healthy body image
- Exercise dependence

Given that it is difficult to pick up a newspaper or magazine without finding an article discussing the benefits of exercise, it is little wonder that most Americans know that regular exercise is desirable. Adults are indeed aware of the health and psychological benefits associated with exercise, yet this knowledge is rarely transferred into action—only 10 percent to 20 percent of the adult population regularly exercise. Often adults do not know how to start their own exercise program, where to get sound advice on beginning a program, or are fearful of failing

Deborah Rohm Young, Ph.D., a post-doctoral research fellow at the Stanford Center for Research in Disease Prevention, Stanford University School of Medicine, has written several articles on adherence and has researched the health benefits of physical activity.

Abby King, Ph.D., assistant professor of health research & policy and medicine at Stanford Medical School and senior scientist at the Center for Research in Disease Prevention, has written extensively on the behavioral determinants of exercise.

because of previous experiences with exercise. Aerobics instructors are in a fortunate situation—they do not have to convince people to attend their workout; participants have taken the first step by finding an exercise class and committing themselves to attending at least once. The instructor's challenge is to encourage continued participation.

The most common reasons given for not continuing an exercise program are lack of time and boredom. The time constraint reason is intriguing; those who exercise regularly also cite lack of time as an ongoing problem for them. But these individuals fit regular exercise into their daily schedules. How do they avoid letting their time pressures short-circuit their exercise program? What "tricks" do they use to motivate themselves? Regular exercisers also report facing boredom yet they continue with their program. How are they different from those who let boredom drive them out of aerobics classes?

Researchers who have studied exercise **adherence** issues have begun to formulate answers to these and other questions regarding the motivational aspects of regular exercise. The aerobics instructor who incorporates motivational techniques into each exercise class has a unique opportunity to help participants develop positive attitudes toward regular exercise and to stay involved in exercise throughout their lives.

This chapter will discuss characteristics often found in exercise program participants and dropouts. Knowing about the factors that influence exercise adherence, and specifically who are the least likely to attend regularly and who may drop out, can be crucial in the development and implementation of strategies to maximize adherence.

Numerous studies have confirmed the effectiveness of using such motivational

strategies, but often these strategies are not implemented in the "real world." This chapter will identify characteristics of instructors that help maintain adherence and will detail the strategies necessary to enhance adherence to regular class participation. Additionally, skills needed to help participants maintain exercise programs during "high-risk" times, such as vacations, holidays and when under pressure at work or home will be presented.

MAJOR FACTORS INFLUENCING EXERCISE ADHERENCE

What is exercise adherence? Although exercise adherence has been defined in a number of ways, for the purpose of this chapter it will be defined as the amount of exercise performed during a specified period of time compared to the amount of exercise recommended. The amount of exercise can refer to the frequency, intensity, duration or some combination of these three dimensions.

A surge of research performed in the last 15 years has identified a number of factors associated with exercise adherence. They often have been categorized as personal, program and environmental factors.

Personal Factors. To effectively motivate participants, it is helpful to be aware of characteristics that appear to be associated with exercise adherence as well as dropout. Although not every person exhibiting a particular characteristic may adhere to or drop out from the program, understanding these characteristics may help the exercise instructor to "flag" those potentially at risk and provide them with extra assistance early in the program.

As shown in Table 10.1, some unique characteristics exist in those who tend to adhere to exercise programs. One is that such individuals are more likely to have previously participated in exercise pro-

Table 10.1

CHARACTERISTICS OF EXERCISE ADHERERS AND DROPOUTS

Adherers	Dropouts
Past participation in exercise	Blue-collar occupation
Involvement with youth sports	Smoker
Enjoy physical activity	Overweight
At higher risk for heart disease	Psychological mood disturbances
Perceived good health	Perceived poor health
High self-motivation	Low self-motivation
High exercise knowledge	Low exercise knowledge
Positive attitudes toward exercise	Negative attitudes toward exercise
Perceive exercise benefits outweigh costs	Perceived disruptions in routine from exercise
Sufficient behavioral skills	Activity too intense, too much exertion
Receive social reinforcement for exercise	
Perceived available time	

Adapted from Dishman, R. K., Sallis, J. F., & Orenstein, D. R. (1985). Determinants of physical activity and exercise. *Public Health Reports, 100,* 158-171.

grams. Additionally, physical and psychological/behavioral skills necessary to exercise appropriately and regularly (e.g., physical coordination, good time-management skills); a participant's self-motivation (the ability to persevere without external rewards); an ability to perceive exercise as enjoyable; and the participant's ability to overcome typical barriers to exercise such as travel, injury, illness, competing demands on time and high-stress periods have all been associated with increased adherence to exercise programs.

Although some of these factors may be lacking in some participants and may be difficult to develop, others, such as perceptions of the enjoyability of exercise, are more amenable to change. By asking participants, possibly through a brief questionnaire completed early in the program, what they did and did not like about previous programs in which they may have participated, the exercise instructor can adjust the current program to optimize its enjoyability for the participants. Later in this chapter, additional ways to develop skills that participants need to maintain good

exercise habits are presented in detail.

Individuals identified in the scientific literature to be at increased risk for dropout include smokers, blue-collar workers and the overweight (Table 10.1). By developing a quick checklist, the exercise instructor can ask a new participant about items that may put him or her at increased risk for dropout (Fig. 10.1).

When a participant at increased risk for dropout is identified, extra monitoring is desirable, particularly for signs of overexertion. A high-risk participant trying to exercise at an overly vigorous pace is twice as likely to drop out. Given the strong desire to conform to the larger group, simply telling participants not to overexert themselves may not be enough if the majority of the class is exercising at a high intensity level. If the class consists of participants with varying abilities, it is useful to present both a more difficult and an easier version of each routine. If possible, having a co-leader or experienced class member actually demonstrate a lower-intensity version of the routine at the same time that the higher-intensity version is being demonstrated

Figure 10.1

EXAMPLE OF NEW PARTICIPANT CHECKLIST

Date _____

Name _____ Age _____

Occupation _____ Smoker ____ Yes ____ No

Current health conditions _____

_____

Reason for joining class _____

Previous experiences with exercise ____ Yes ____ No

may decrease the chance that participants will overexert in trying to keep up with the more vigorous routine. Including regular breaks during the workout also may help to maintain exercise involvement for the participant at increased risk for dropout.

It is imperative that the instructor maintain a noncondescending attitude toward all participants, including those with suboptimal health behaviors. Although it may be difficult for some aerobics instructors to understand why individuals do not lose those extra pounds or quit smoking in light of overwhelming health risks associated with these behaviors, it must be remembered that every individual has unique priorities and behavior patterns in life. Rather than chastise for a perceived bad habit, the instructor should praise positive behaviors and provide a good example.

Program Factors. Factors specific to the exercise program can also affect participant adherence. Convenience of the exercise class is often cited as a determinant of adherence. Classes should be scheduled, if possible, during times of the day when most participants potentially have free time. It also is beneficial if classes are scheduled at a variety of times so that there is an alternate class the participant can attend if

unforeseen circumstances require that a participant miss a class.

To maximize adherence, classes should be no longer than 60 minutes. Programs any longer than that are perceived to be too time-consuming by many participants, while programs much shorter are often considered not worth the effort.

If the exercise class is costly or requires special prior preparation, adherence often drops.

The exercise routine itself also impacts adherence. If the routine is either too easy or too hard for the participant, or not varied enough to prevent boredom, chances for dropout are increased. The perceived friendliness of class members can be an additional boost to adherence. When new participants feel welcome, it is easier for them to return to subsequent classes.

Environmental Factors. Environmental factors—the ambiance of the exercise site, cues and reminders for exercise, weather conditions, time limitations and the amount of support and feedback related to exercise —can all influence whether a participant maintains the exercise program.

A well-lit exercise room decorated in a pleasant motif and sufficient size to accommodate the class members, along with an adequate cooling/heating system, is preferable to a hot, dark, smelly, gym-like environment.

It is important to start and finish classes on time; most people are busy these days and a lack of promptness disrupts everyone's daily schedule. This is especially critical during periods of inclement weather when participants may have to rearrange other daily activities to make it to class. Similarly, if exercise must be canceled because of bad weather, give participants plenty of advance notice whenever possible. Setting up a "telephone tree" (where one participant has the responsibility of contacting another in an emergency-type situation) to contact class members quickly may be a worthwhile endeavor for some class situations.

Ongoing support by the aerobics instructor and others through face-to-face, telephone or mail contact is particularly beneficial for adherence. The instructor can encourage attendance by praising participants for daily attendance and for reaching predetermined goals. Telephone and mail contacts can prompt the wayward participant as well as remind all about upcoming exercise "special events," such as fitness challenges or seasonally inspired, adherence-based promotions.

In general, a telephone call to a participant who has missed two consecutive classes is warranted to determine reasons for nonattendance and to provide nonjudgmental support and encouragement. Newsletters that provide exercise tips and promotions for upcoming events are useful in building enthusiasm. With the advent of desktop publishing software, professional-looking newsletters can be achieved at minimal cost.

Support from family and friends is essential for adherence and can be developed by the aerobics instructor with the help of the participant. This can be accomplished by encouraging the participants to talk with others about goals they have set, what has been accomplished during exercise class and rates of progression. Make sure the participants share their newsletters; perhaps even include some interesting facts about participants' families or friends that would pique their interest. Involving others in the exercise program or providing them with knowledge of what is going on in class, as well as goals the participant has set, can encourage outside support and minimize any sabotage that might occur on the part of family members as a consequence of feeling "left out."

TRAITS OF AN IDEAL EXERCISE INSTRUCTOR

An aerobics instructor's attitudes, personality and professional conduct are among the strongest motivating factors often cited for maintaining exercise adherence. Although exercise instructors are responsible for developing and administering a good class, those factors alone will not guarantee optimal adherence. Personal attributes of the exercise instructor can strongly augment his or her ability to effectively motivate the participants. It is often thought that leadership is an innate trait, but leadership skills can be developed even by those not considered "born leaders." Some of the qualities of an effective, adherence-creating exercise instructor are discussed below.

Punctuality and Dependability

Instructors must assure exercise participants that each exercise class will start and end on time. A class that starts late or does not end on schedule is disruptive. Participants also want to know that their regular exercise instructor, not a parade of substitutes, will be there to greet them. Absences should be planned and substitutes scheduled in advance whenever possible.

Professionalism

All participants should be treated with respect. Gossiping about other class members or staff is not only inappropriate, but, if overheard from others, should not be tolerated. Professionalism extends to choice of exercise wear; although it is fine to be decked out in the latest style, be careful to avoid styles that can be perceived as being overly provocative or that may serve as a distraction.

Dedication

Part of being a professional is being dedicated to one's work. Efforts should be made on a continual basis to keep the exercise classes fun and enjoyable for the participants. This means going to workshops to keep up on the latest developments regarding exercise delivery and finding out answers to questions that participants may have on health-related topics. It is imperative to stay abreast of the latest health news and be informed of the scientific basis for health claims.

Sensitivity to the Participants

The ideal exercise instructor recognizes that all participants are unique and come to exercise class for their own reasons. The purpose of class is not to treat all participants similarly; but, rather, to work with the strengths of each individual participant to maximize his or her exercise session. Interacting with participants as individuals, treating them with an open, non-judgmental manner and expressing a willingness to listen are much appreciated.

Willingness to Plan Ahead

Participants appreciate when the exercise instructor provides them with advance notice of events that interfere with regular exercise class, such as holiday closures, intersession breaks or a planned vacation. They also are grateful when the exercise instructor informs them of upcoming events or fitness challenges that are offered in the community. If given enough advance notice, participants may want to specifically train for an event.

Recognizing Signs of Burnout

Talking with other exercise instructors about how to prevent burnout or work through it is invaluable. All exercise leaders will experience this phenomenon at some time or another, and getting another professional's advice will be useful. It is important to schedule regular vacations; it is amazing what a week or two away from work can do to improve one's attitude!

Taking Responsibility

Invariably things will go wrong either with the exercise class itself or with the surroundings (e.g., broken air conditioning system). Taking responsibility for these and making sure that all efforts are made to correct the situation are appreciated by all. In addition, having back-up plans available when such situations arise can prove to be very useful.

STRATEGIES THAT ENCOURAGE ADHERENCE

Motivation depends on a participant's personal resources, abilities and strengths, as well as external factors and circumstances. By assuming otherwise —that only innate personal factors influence adherence—an exercise instructor may "write off" a participant rather than try to teach skills that are lacking.

Rather than placing the blame for non-adherence on the participant, the exercise instructor must view motivation as a joint responsibility shared with the participant. It is also helpful to view the process as a dynamic one; alternative strategies may be needed for different clients at different stages in the exercise program.

Several strategies have been proven successful in motivating participants to regularly attend exercise class. The following strategies can easily be integrated into any exercise class and will help to motivate participants to become regular exercisers. (Some strategies, however, may not be applicable to an exercise instructor's specific program, so the exercise instructor should determine which strategies are appropriate for a given situation and subsequently apply them in an individualized manner.) After the leader has developed a particular strategic plan for adherence, the plan should be reassessed often to determine its continued feasibility and effectiveness.

Formulate Reasonable Participant Expectations

Early on, find out each participant's expectations from the exercise class and help formulate reasonable ones. Expectations must be realistic to avoid disappointment. Although regular exercise provides many benefits, it is not a panacea, and the participant must be informed of what benefits can be expected from the type of exercise being performed in the class. For instance, if a participant expects dramatic weight loss as a result of attending exercise class, he or she will be disappointed if this does not occur. It is preferable to advise the participant that, without a concomitant decrease in caloric intake, actual loss of body fat from physical training is likely to be negligible—only on the average, of about 1.7 percent, (Wilmore, 1983).

More realistic expectations would be weight loss on the order of one-half pound per week, trimmer legs or thighs over time,

or an increased sense of well-being after completing an exercise session.

Set Exercise Goals

When an individual joins an exercise class or program, take the time to develop realistic, flexible, individualized, short-term goals with that person. This can be accomplished by setting up a short interview with a new participant shortly after he or she joins the class. If it is not possible to arrange a specific time for this, have an experienced participant lead the cool-down phase of class and talk to the new participant during that time. Goals that are realistic are important in order to avoid injury and maintain interest.

Although the exercise instructor should help the participant formulate goals, the goals should be set, as much as possible, by the participant rather than the exercise instructor. Short-term goals determined for each exercise session in conjunction with longer-term monthly goals allow for flexibility on a daily basis without jeopardizing the longer-term goals.

Goals can be specific to the exercise process, such as attending a certain number of classes in the coming weeks, or reaching a predetermined target heart rate during class by a certain date. They also can be related to some benefits associated with exercise, such as making new friends or developing a new social network. It is useful to encourage goals related to enjoyment and pleasure from exercise rather than only tangible goals such as weight loss.

Remind participants about their goals periodically during workouts and publicly praise those who have accomplished theirs. If goals are listed and displayed on a chart or are in participant files, they can easily be reviewed and evaluated regularly (e.g., twice a month). When goals are met, assist the participant in making new ones.

If it appears that the participant is unlikely to reach a specific goal, encourage a revised, more realistic goal. This will reduce the likelihood of disappointment or loss of interest associated with not meeting the goal, or potential physical injury that may occur when trying to "catch up" to reach a goal (such as performing too much exercise in too short a time). If a goal cannot be met, brainstorm with the participant reasons why the goal was not met in order to plan more realistic goals in the future. To avoid any potential embarrassment, this should not be done publicly, but rather by talking with the participant during the warm-up or cool-down phase of the program. The exercise instructor can regularly use this format to talk individually with participants and provide personalized instructions.

Consider formalizing the commitment to exercise with participants through written or oral contracts. A contract is often a written agreement signed by the participant and the exercise instructor (and others, if appropriate) that clearly itemizes the exercise goals and the rewards associated with achieving those goals. Contracts can increase the participant's commitment to the exercise program by defining the specific relationship between exercise goals and positive outcomes contingent on meeting those goals. They also involve the participant with the planning of the exercise program, thereby providing a sense of ownership of the program (Fig. 10.2).

Exercise contracts should contain input from both the participant and exercise instructor. They should prepare the contract together during a brief meeting before or after class or have a discussion during a warm-up or cool-down period, as previously described. Responsibilities each has in meeting the terms of the contract can be itemized at this time. Requirements for

class attendance or additional home-exercise workouts and completion of exercise logs are often specified in contracts. The exercise instructor should make certain that the participant has the skills necessary to meet the terms of the contract; beginning with modest goals is one way to ensure this. Precautions should be written into the contract to ensure that the participant does not engage in unhealthy practices to meet contract requirements (e.g., extended exercising over several days to meet a time-based goal, starvation tactics to meet a weight goal).

Exercise goals should be written in a manner so they can be objectively measured, thereby eliminating any questions regarding goal attainment. For example, a goal that specifies attendance requirements over one month (e.g., attend 10 out of 12 possible monthly classes) is preferable to one that states "every attempt will be made to attend as many classes as possible during the month." Make certain that the reward contracted for is delivered after the goal has been met. If the reward is an incentive, such as a T-shirt, ensure that enough are in stock so they can promptly be distributed.

Give Regular, Positive Feedback

As much as possible provide participants with ample, ongoing, positive reinforcement and individual praise. Feedback that is specific and relevant to the participant is known to be a powerful reinforcer. Studies have shown that personalized feedback about progress throughout the exercise session is more successful than feedback delivered in a more general manner (Martin et al., 1984). Feedback can be physiologically oriented in terms of resting heart rate, exertional heart rate or rating of perceived exertion (RPE) (Borg, 1970).

Feedback also can be oriented toward

Figure 10.2

SAMPLE EXERCISE CONTRACT

My Responsibilities:

1. To attend 10 out of 12 exercise classes during the next four weeks.

2. To record my resting heart rate, exertional heart rate and rate of perceived exertion after each exercise class.

3. To exercise out of class for at least 20 minutes one time per week.

4. For any exercise class I have to miss due to illness or other unavoidable reasons, I will:

a. Call my instructor to explain why I missed it. (Instructor's telephone number): _____

b. Plan to make up the missed session by (specify): _____

5. To reward myself at the end of each week that I attend all of my scheduled exercise classes by (example: visiting a museum on an afternoon).

_____

My Aerobics Instructor's Responsibilities:

1. To lead all classes, except when ill, unless advance notice is given.

2. To monitor my progress by evaluating my log sheets.

3. To give me individual feedback regarding my progress.

This contract will be evaluated on: _____
                                       Date

_____
Participant

_____
Exercise Instructor

the exercise behavior itself, such as routine logging of exercise activity. A log sheet can be developed and kept at the exercise facility in which participants can keep a record of resting heart rate, exertional heart rate and RPE each time they attend class. (Fig. 10.3) Recording information only takes a few minutes and can be accomplished immediately after class. Reviewing log sheets at regular intervals (perhaps monthly) provides the participant with important feedback (e.g., how resting heart rate has decreased over time, or how many sessions were attended during the previous month). Log sheets also provide the participants with information about the intensity of their exercise sessions, letting them know if they are working too hard or need to pick up the intensity in order to obtain a good workout.

Incentives, such as T-shirts and visors, can be provided to the participant when certain goals are met. Extrinsic rewards can be particularly important in the early stages of exercise adoption. Incentive-based goals should be set that can be realistically achieved by the majority of participants. Prizes based on attendance rather than large increases in performance are often preferred by participants and can

Figure 10.3

SAMPLE EXERCISE LOG

RPE Scale

6	7	8	9	10	11	12	13	14	15	16	17	18	19	20
	VERY, VERY LIGHT		VERY LIGHT		FAIRLY LIGHT		SOMEWHAT HARD		HARD		VERY HARD		VERY, VERY HARD	

RHR = Resting Heart Rate   EHR = Exertional Heart Rate   RPE = Rate of Perceived Exertion

Target EHR Zone _____

Date	RHR	EHR	RPE	Comments	Out-of-class exercise?
_____	___	___	___	_____	___ Yes ___ No
_____	___	___	___	_____	___ Yes ___ No
_____	___	___	___	_____	___ Yes ___ No
_____	___	___	___	_____	___ Yes ___ No

motivate those experiencing less-than-optimal-success in reaching physiological goals. Fitness "challenges" can provide rewards for different levels of participation by offering alternative prizes for a variety of achievements. Another successful incentive strategy is having participants deposit a sum of money at the beginning of the program, a certain amount of which is forfeited if weekly contract goals are not met. Robinson et al. (1992) found that the group using a deposit strategy had 97-percent adherence to the exercise program over six months compared to 19-percent adherence in a comparable group that did not use this motivational strategy.

Public monitoring of attendance as a means of providing feedback and receiving achievement awards is useful for motivating participants. Posting attendance charts in the exercise room rewards the high attender with a public display of adherence and may motivate the less-than-optimal adherer to attend class on a more regular basis. A chart with a theme, such as "Exercise Around the World," can be devised where daily attendance is worth a certain number of miles, with bonus miles given for not missing class for a specified number of times. When participants "reach" predetermined countries, awards can be given that are representative of that country.

Make Exercise Sessions Easy, Interesting and Fun

As previously mentioned, aspects of the exercise session itself are related to adherence and motivational issues. The exercise routine should be easy to follow; one means of accomplishing this is to break it up into achievable parts so the participant can successfully perform the routine.

One way to guarantee dropouts is to have an exercise routine that the participants cannot follow. It is also helpful to provide ample, positive reinforcement or support while the participants are learning the routine. Varying the routine regularly and providing different types of music that suit the tastes of the class can be useful.

Ask the participants what type of music they prefer and prepare routines to it.

Assess the enjoyment factor of the exercise program on a regular basis, perhaps through the use of the RPE scale or a simple enjoyment assessment scale. Participants should generally be exercising in an RPE range between 12 and 16. If the participants are working in too high an RPE range, they may not be enjoying the exercise; rather, they may be working hard just to keep up with the exercise instructor.

Exercise enjoyment also can be assessed orally during the exercise session with a six-point rating scale, with 1 equaling "extremely unenjoyable" and 6 equaling "extremely enjoyable." The exercise instructor can determine which parts of the exercise class are most favorable to the participants by asking about their enjoyment level throughout different points during class. Look at the faces of the participants —if they're struggling and not having a good time during class, it will be obvious.

If it is evident that some participants are working excessively, lower the intensity of the routine for awhile until the over-workers can "catch their breath" and get back into their exercise comfort zone. As previously mentioned, if the class is of varying abilities, visually provide both a lower-intensity and higher-intensity version of the routine.

The importance of a cheerful, friendly exercise instructor cannot be overemphasized. The participants may enjoy coming to class just to see a friendly face and receive praise for what they accomplish in class. So, instructors should leave their personal problems in the locker room and greet their class with a smile!

Acknowledge Exercise Discomforts

Teach the participants how to tell the difference between the transient discom-forts associated with exercise and what discomforts are potentially a sign of injury or more serious problems. Newcomers to exercise may not be used to the feeling of increased breathing, heart rate and sweating associated with exercise. They must be reassured that these are normal responses and should be expected.

Participants must be informed of potential injuries that may arise and be able to recognize a symptom that warrants attention. Any sudden, sharp pain that does not dissipate or a muscle soreness that does not lessen after a few days may be a sign of injury and should be examined by a health professional. Similarly, the participants must know the signs and symptoms of a heart attack, particularly when the exercisers are of middle and older ages. A dull, aching discomfort in the chest, neck, jaw or arms associated with excessive or clammy skin that is not relieved with rest may be signs of a heart attack; proper medical authorities should be contacted immediately.

It is helpful to ask participants individually how they are feeling and if they are experiencing any unusual discomforts; often these are not offered voluntarily and potential injuries may not be discovered without prompting from the exercise instructor. Personal advice to take it easy for a class or two until a minor ache or pain lessens and follow-up during successive classes lets the participant know the exercise instructor cares and is looking out for the participant's best interests.

Use Exercise Reminders, Cues and Prompts

Encourage the participants to develop prompts or cues in their home or work environments that will promote regular class attendance, such as scheduling exercise in a daily appointment book and laying out exercise gear the night before exercise class.

Posters placed at participants' homes or work environments that depict individuals enjoying exercise may be beneficial in encouraging attendance. A variety of prompts at work, home and the exercise location can help to keep the participants thinking about exercise.

Encourage an Extensive Social Support System

Develop a buddy system among participants so they can call each other to make sure they attend class and have an additional support person to discuss progress and goals. Additional social support for exercise can be encouraged by having participants ask friends or relatives to pitch in by reminding them to attend their exercise classes. Support does not have to be face-to-face; telephone and mail contacts are additional avenues of support that can be utilized. As previously described, newsletters are a useful means for keeping participants informed of class activities, and they add to a sense of belonging. Telephone contacts initiated after one or two missed classes that let the lapsing participant know he or she was missed may encourage a return to class.

Develop Group Camaraderie

It is particularly important for the exercise class members to feel a sense of cohesiveness. This tends to occur spontaneously; however, it also can be facilitated by the exercise instructor if the group does not appear to "gel" on its own. Simple introductions of a new class member, along with a unique "tidbit" about each member, helps everyone become familiar with each other. During exercise warm-up and cool-down, each participant can share an interesting aspect of his or her past, or provide details of a fun weekend activity. Letting the participants talk about themselves when class

time permits encourages the personality of each to shine. Providing interesting, little-known facts about each participant in a newsletter also is beneficial. The social support and reinforcement for exercise developed through group membership is powerful and should be not be overlooked.

By the same token, the exercise instructor must be aware of individual behaviors that threaten to undermine positive group dynamics. Most groups have chronic complainers or generally disruptive individuals. These individuals must be dealt with early to avoid the tendency for them to take charge of the group or monopolize the exercise instructor's time. For a chronic complainer, the exercise instructor should listen attentively and acknowledge that he or she understands the participant's complaint, then agree on a solution with the participant and follow through to make any needed changes. The participant should be informed when the issue has been solved, and the exercise instructor should acknowledge with the participant that there is no more reason to discuss it further.

The disruptive individual should not be given too much attention (since that is probably what he or she wants). If lack of attention does not change the individual's behavior, then the exercise instructor must speak to the individual privately to discuss the interruptions and possible reasons for the disruptive behavior.

Emphasize Positive Aspects of Exercise

Help the participants to generally disregard minor exercise discomforts, recognize their own self-defeating thoughts and counteract them with positive thoughts. Encourage participants to think "good thoughts," such as how refreshing it feels to move about freely, how encouraging other class members are and so on, while performing the exercise routine. Comment on positive aspects of the routine throughout; "here comes the fun part," "looking great" and similar comments keep the participants focused on the positive. Martin et al. (1985) found that those who were told to attend to environmental surroundings and enjoy the outdoors during a class-based running program had greater attendance and were more likely to continue exercising after the formal program ended compared to those who concentrated on increasing their performance during the exercise sessions. Pleasant thoughts that focus on enjoyment of movement and how accomplished the participants will feel when exercise class is over will help the exercise class time move by quickly and enjoyably.

Help Participants Develop Intrinsic Rewards

After the exercise behavior is part of the participant's routine, it is often useful to supplement class rewards and support with a natural reward system that is provided outside of exercise class. Positive feedback on exercise habits provided from family, friends and co-workers transfers some of the positive feedback received during exercise class to other environments as well as provides additional avenues of social support. Encourage the participant to develop a natural reward system that focuses on increased feelings of self-esteem, a sense of accomplishment and increased energy levels instead of merely external rewards. Natural reinforcers add to a sense of personal identification of being an exerciser and will help participants continue to exercise even when they cannot make it to class.

Prepare Participants for Inevitable Missed Classes

It is important to realize that the participant will not be able to attend classes

at some point in a program. Although the participant may be unable to make it to class during vacations, holidays or times of increased work or family pressures, they may still be able to continue a home-based exercise program and should be encouraged to do so. Confidence for exercising in different settings can be built by encouraging participants to add at least one day of exercise outside of class time, preferably using a different mode of exercise (such as brisk walking, swimming or any other type of exercise the participant enjoys). This will give participants experience with an exercise alternative if they must miss a scheduled class. Ask the participants about exercise performed outside of class and praise them when it has been accomplished. When the participant successfully exercises on his or her own, confidence for continuing exercise in general is being built.

Exercising with family or co-workers is ideal for out-of-class exercise sessions. If the participant cannot find someone to exercise with, encourage other class members to meet him or her in an alternative exercise setting. Not only does this add an additional mode of social support for exercise, it also provides participants with an opportunity to problem-solve with their exercise buddies any difficulties encountered with exercise. Additional days of exercise can be included in the exercise contract, and exercise logs of these sessions can be kept to document these sessions. During times when participants are extremely busy, remind them that a shorter workout than normal is still beneficial and will keep them regularly exercising. Although an exercise instructor's primary responsibility is to encourage class attendance, supporting the concept of at least one out-of-class exercise session will ultimately help the participant's overall exercise achievement.

Classes may not be offered in some instances. If classes are provided as part of a university environment, there may be a break in classes due to semester breaks or holidays. By advising the participants in advance, participants can prepare for these breaks. Using the skills mentioned in the previous paragraph will be beneficial during these times. The exercise instructor also can try to arrange exercise alternatives with other exercise classes at different locations in the community so the participants can continue exercising in a similar format.

Prepare Participants for Changes in Instructors

A change in instructors is usually quite disruptive for participants. Unfortunately, little is typically done to prepare participants for this change. Planned change in leadership because of pregnancy leave, travel or a permanent relocation can be smoothed if participants are prepared for the change well ahead of time. If possible, advance introductions of the new exercise instructor are beneficial. Having the regular and new instructor team teach several exercise classes can help prevent fears of a change in format after the regular exercise instructor departs. There will undoubtedly be times of illness for the exercise instructor, so substitutes should be planned for and arranged in advance. It would be a bonus if the exercise instructor could introduce the substitutes to the participants so when they need to be used, the participants are already familiar with them.

Train to Prevent Exercise Defeatism

Prepare participants for the eventual missed class. How slips are handled determine if they will be temporary or permanent. Let the participants know that missing a class is a realistic probability. If participants can predict and prepare for lapses in their exercise program, their occur-

rences will not likely be as disruptive. Certain times make exercise class attendance unlikely (family crises, holidays, illness, extra pressure or deadlines at work). When these can be anticipated and seen as being temporary rather than a breakdown in the success of the exercise program, adherence is more likely to be maintained. Lapses should be viewed as a challenge to overcome rather than as a failure.

Participants can be made aware of the defeatist attitude that accompanies the belief that once an exercise program is disrupted, total relapse or dropout is inevitable. Although breaking the adherence rule does place the participant at a higher risk for dropping out, dropout is not inevitable. If exercise is viewed by the participants as a process in which there will undoubtedly be times that they will be less active than others, when a class is missed they will not consider themselves nonexercisers. Rather, they will catch the next available class or exercise on their own when time permits. Participants also can be encouraged to avoid "high-risk" situations (such as going to a "happy hour" before exercise class) that test their resolve to exercise. Encourage participants to surround themselves with cues that support the exercise behavior. A simple telephone call after one or two missed sessions may bring the participant back to class if he or she understands that missing class is not a sign of failure.

Emphasize an Overall Healthy Lifestyle

Exercise is only one of a number of lifestyle-related activities that participants engage in throughout the week. It is often assumed that those who regularly exercise also practice other healthy behaviors; sadly this is often not the case. Diets of exercisers are generally not any different from the American diet and several studies have been unable to find a decreased smoking prevalence among exercisers (Blair et al., 1990). The exercise instructor has an excellent opportunity to provide accurate information and to encourage the development of additional healthy lifestyle behaviors. Questions regarding diet, weight control and other behaviors will undoubtedly be asked; the exercise instructor, by being well-versed in these topics, can offer sound information with scientific basis.

Finally, the exercise instructor is viewed as a model for a healthy lifestyle and should try to live up to the participants' expectations. Encourage the participants by example; don't smoke or abuse alcohol, maintain a prudent, healthy diet and normal body weight.

EXERCISE AND BODY IMAGE

Cultural norms for attractiveness are often centered on "ideal body types." In the United States, this "ideal body type" has, in recent times, been associated with extreme thinness, particularly in women. While this body type may photograph well for fashion magazines, it is not ideal for most women and is most likely an unattainable and potentially unhealthy goal for many. When women perceive that their bodies are being compared to this unrealistic "ideal," many become dissatisfied with their body shape and fret over any extra pounds in undesirable places.

High levels of physical activity have been associated with a preoccupation with weight and body shape. These unhealthy attitudes may put some individuals, particularly teenaged and young adult women, at risk for developing eating disorders, such as **anorexia nervosa** and **bulimia**, as well as addictions to exercise or overexercise.

The exercise instructor, by being aware of this phenomenon, can encourage participants to accept their own body shape. Remind participants that everyone has their own unique body shape and no amount of exercise is going to change that basic shape. As an instructor, stay away from pointing out specific exercises to "fix" certain body parts since it may lead to a preoccupation or dissatisfaction with that body part. It is better for the participants to focus on the enjoyment of moving and the overall good feelings associated with exercise.

While the exercise instructor will want to encourage regular exercise participation, a small number of individuals may take the exercise habit to the extreme and exhibit signs of exercise **dependence** or **addiction**. Exercise dependence has been defined in a variety of ways; a good definition is when the commitment to exercise assumes a higher priority than commitments to family, work and interpersonal relations (Morgan, 1979).

Excessive exercise may be associated with body image distortions or even more serious disorders, such as anorexia nervosa and bulimia, where excessive exercise is used as an additional method to lose weight or to "purge" calories that have recently been consumed (Brownell and Foreyt, 1986).

Exercise instructors can look for signs of exercise dependence/addiction in their participants, including continuing to exercise in spite of injuries or illness, extreme levels of thinness, a decay in interpersonal relationships, and feelings of extreme guilt, irritability or depression when unable to exercise. If the exercise instructor suspects a participant is exercising to excess or may have an eating disorder, the matter should be dealt with using forethought and sensitivity. The exercise instructor should express concern over what has been observed and ask the participant directly about his or her exercise and eating habits. Chances are that if a disorder exists, the participant has already been confronted about the situation. The exercise instructor should be sensitive and understanding, offering support as well as suggesting that professional guidance be sought. It is helpful if several names and telephone numbers of qualified professionals are available to provide to the participant in need.

SUMMARY

Dropout rates for those beginning an aerobics program can reach 50 percent or more after only six months. Instead of placing the blame for nonadherence on the participant, the exercise instructor must view motivation as a shared responsibility and work with the participant to develop a successful motivational strategy. Extra assistance should be provided to the participant who has been identified to be at high risk for dropout.

Motivation is a dynamic process, and by applying a variety of strategies and reviewing and refining these strategies regularly, achievement of regular exercise can be attained for most participants. Motivational techniques range from structuring appropriate expectations and goals, to identifying short-term benefits and providing specific feedback, to teaching problem-solving skills, to serving as a positive role model and training participants to manage their own reward systems.

Additionally, the convenience and attractiveness of the exercise setting, enjoyability of the exercise class, supportiveness of the exercise environment, as well as personal factors specific to both the exercise instructor and the participant, are also factored into the exercise adherence equation. Understanding and applying the principles of adherence and motivation described in this chapter will help the exercise instructor develop into a more effective teacher and health professional.

ACKNOWLEDGEMENTS

We would like to thank Mary E. Sheehan, M.S., and Catherine M. Norbutas, B. A., for their comments on a previous draft of this manuscript. This work was supported in part by Public Health Service Grant # 5 T32 HL07034 awarded to Stephen P. Fortmann, M.D., and Public Health Service Grant # AG-00440 from the National Institute on Aging awarded to Abby C. King, Ph.D.

REFERENCES

Borg, G. V. (1970). Perceived exertion as an indicator of somatic stress. *Scandinavian Journal of Rehabilitation Medicine, 2*, 92-98.

Blair, S. N., Kohl., H. W. III., & Brill, P. A. (1990). Behavioral adaptations to physical activity. *In C. Bouchard, R. J. Shephard, T. Stephens, J. R. Stephens, B. D. McPherson (ed.), Exercise, Fitness, and Health. A Consensus of Current Knowledge* (pp. 385-398). Champaign: Human Kinetics.

Brownell, K. D., & Foreyt, J. P. (eds.) (1986). *Handbook of Eating Disorders.* New York: Basic Books, Inc.

Cooper, P. J., & Fairburn, C. G. (1983). Binge-eating and self-induced vomiting in the community: A preliminary study. *British Journal of Psychiatry, 142*, 139-144.

Martin, J. E., Dubbert, P. M., Katell, A. D., Thompson, J. K., Raczynski, J. R., Lake, M., Smith, P. O., Webster, J. S., Sikora, T., & Cohen, R. E. (1984). Behavioral control of exercise in sedentary adults: Studies 1 through 6. *Journal of Consulting and Clinical Psychology, 52*, 795-811.

Morgan, W. P. (1979). Negative addiction in runners. *Physician and Sportsmedicine, 7*, 57-70.

Robinson, J. I., Rogers, M. A., Carlson, J. J., Mavis, B. E., Stachnik, T., Stoffelmayr, B., Sprague, H. A., McGrew, C. R., & VanHuss, W. D. (1992). Effects of a 6-month incentive-based exercise program on adherence and work capacity. *Medicine and Science in Sports and Exercise, 24*, 85-93.

Wilmore, J. H. (1983). Body composition in sports and exercise. Directions for future research. *Medicine and Science in Sports and Exercise, 15*, 21-31.

ADDITIONAL RESOURCES

American College of Sports Medicine. (1993). ACSM's. *Resource manual for guidelines for exercise testing and prescription, (2nd edition).* Philadelphia: Lea & Febiger.

Dishman, R. K. (ed.). (1988). *Exercise Adherence. Its Impact on Public Health.* Champaign: Human Kinetics.

King, A. C., Blair, S. N., Bild, D. F., Dishman, R. K., Dubbert, P. M., Marcus, B. H., Oldridge, N. B., Paffenbarger, R. S., Jr., Powell, K. E., & Yeager, K. K. Determination of physical activity and interventions in adults. *Medicine and Science in Sports and Exercise,* 24, S221-S236.

Chapter 11

Special Populations

and Health Concerns

By Scott O. Roberts

The benefits of regular physical activity and exercise are becoming increasingly clear. Individuals who choose to be more physically active, in both their leisure and work activities, lower their risk for developing certain degenerative diseases, such as osteoporosis, diabetes, obesity and cardiovascular disease. The term "health-related fitness" now appears frequently in exercise literature to describe the health benefits of exercise. Instead of defining physical fitness in terms of one's athletic abilities (speed, power and balance), health-related physical fitness is defined

Scott Roberts, M.S., is a clinical exercise physiologist in the Department of Cardiology, Lovelace Medical Center, Albuquerque, New Mexico. An ACSM-certified exercise program director, he is the author of dozens of scientific papers and several books on exercise testing and prescription, children's fitness, fitness and wellness, and the co-author of an exercise physiology textbook. Roberts also has served as a member of ACE's Aerobics Instructor Examination Committee.

by an individual's cardiorespiratory fitness, muscular strength, flexibility and body composition. The shift in emphasis from performance-related fitness to health-related physical fitness has far-reaching implications for aerobics instructors and other fitness professionals.

Exercise is also becoming increasingly recognized as an important therapeutic modality in the rehabilitation of certain acute and chronic health conditions. For example, aerobic exercise is widely recommended and supported as an adjunct treatment for individuals recovering from coronary heart disease. Several recent studies have shown that exercise, combined with risk factor modification, can significantly decrease morbidity and mortality in individuals with known coronary heart disease. Even a modest amount of physical activity, such as daily brisk walking, can reduce the risk of developing heart disease (Table 11.1).

DEFINITION OF "SPECIAL POPULATIONS"

The term "special population" refers to individuals with characteristics that distinguish them from the typical adult exerciser (e.g., older adults, children, pregnant women). These populations have special needs and/or requirements, but do not necessarily have a "health" challenge (see Chapter 12, "Exercise and Pregnancy").

This chapter also addresses needs and requirements for exercise in individuals with selected health concerns. Today, individuals with a wide range of health or medical problems can, in most cases, participate in a variety of fitness activities and enjoy many of the same benefits available to healthy individuals (see Chapter 4, "Nutrition and Weight Control").

Most of the guidelines discussed throughout this book have come from extensive research. However, a great deal

remains to be learned regarding how individuals respond and adapt to exercise. Therefore, fitness instructors should always use conservative approaches when developing exercise programs and leading group exercise for special populations and for those with health concerns.

GENERAL PROGRAM DESIGN CONSIDERATIONS

There are several considerations when designing an exercise program for populations with special needs or health concerns. The major ones follow.

Medical History

The information obtained in a medical history or health-risk appraisal can provide valuable information that can be used in the design of a health promotion or exercise program. More specific medical information regarding a client's past and present medical status can be obtained by reviewing the medical history. A complete and up-to-date health appraisal and medical history is required before designing or leading an exercise program for clients with a known or suspected medical or health problem (see Chapter 5, "Health Screening").

Instructor's Responsibilities

In most situations, fitness instructors do not "prescribe" exercise to clients with special needs. Ideally, the exercise program comes from a physician, nurse or other allied health professional, such as an American College of Sports Medicine (ACSM) certified exercise specialist or exercise program director. However, fitness instructors can, and should, monitor the client's response to exercise, and be able to provide sound advice that will make exercise safer and more effective.

For example, fitness instructors can assist clients with their exercise program by: (1) helping them monitor their progress or lack of progress, (2) providing encouragement and support, (3) offering suggestions for safer exercises and/or exercise moves, and (4) making sure clients follow their exercise prescription for maximum safety and benefit.

Instructors are ultimately responsible for the safety of their clients immediately before, during and immediately following an exercise class. Furthermore, fitness instructors are responsible for leading safe and appropriate exercise classes for the population of clients attending their class. For example, a severely obese client should not be allowed to participate in a high impact aerobics class, nor should someone with a blood pressure problem, who comes to class feeling dizzy and nauseated, be allowed to exercise at all.

Instructors who fail to monitor their clients in a safe and effective manner should be held liable for such actions. Today's public demands a high degree of competency in fitness instructors, and justifiably so. Fitness instructors cannot assume their clients will choose the most appropriate exercise regime based on their current health status and previous exercise experience. Ideally, comprehensive policies for new clients should be established at facilities where fitness instructors are employed. Such policies should ensure that new clients are not allowed to participate in a class until an instructor has had an opportunity to meet the new clients, review a medical history or health-risk appraisal, an exercise prescription (if available), and discuss any problems or concerns the client may have.

Safety and Emergency Considerations

The recent emergence of the field of exercise science, both rehabilitative and health/fitness, has resulted in highly variable, nonstandardized programs. The number of individuals at risk for cardiovascular, pulmonary and metabolic disorders who regularly participate in some form of fitness program continues to rise. Because the fitness industry is relatively unregulated and nonstandardized, directors of programs, as well as fitness leaders, must look to the health-care and health-and-fitness professional associations for guidelines and standards that are reasonable and take into account that which is being done in similar settings. In the absence of specific regulations, litigation will be based on that which is reasonable, prudent and consistent with policies and procedures in similar facilities, such as hospitals, clinics and health-club settings. (see Chapter 14, "Emergency Procedures," and Chapter 15, "Professional Responsibilities").

Client-Physician-Instructor Relationship

To adequately monitor and lead safe and effective exercise programs for individuals with special needs, an instructor will often find it necessary to discuss a client's program with the client's physician. In many cases, clients will come to the instructor with an exercise prescription written by a physician, or from another exercise program or facility. If the instructor has any questions regarding an exercise prescription, he or she should discuss it with the individual who developed the exercise program. To make exercise safe and effective for the individual, the client, physician and fitness instructor all need to communicate with each other on a regular basis.

CARDIOVASCULAR DISORDERS

Heart and circulatory diseases create the largest population of exercisers with a specific health challenge that an aerobics instructor will likely encounter. Fitness instructors must always be aware of the **scope of practice** as it relates to their in-

Table 11.1

SUMMARY OF SELECTED HEALTH BENEFITS ASSOCIATED WITH REGULAR EXERCISE

Reduces the risk of cardiovascular disease	Increases HDL cholesterol
	Decreases LDL cholesterol
	Favorably changes the ratios between total cholesterol and HDL-C, and between LDL and HDL cholesterol
	Decreases triglyceride levels
	Promotes relaxation; relieves stress and tension
	Decreases body fat and favorably changes body composition
	Reduces blood pressure, especially if it is high
	Makes blood platelets less sticky
	Reduces cardiac arrhythmias
	Increases myocardial efficiency by lowering resting heart rate and increasing stroke volume
	Increases oxygen-carrying capacity of the blood
Helps control diabetes	Makes cells less resistant to insulin
	Reduces body fat
Develops stronger bones that are less susceptible to injury	
Promotes joint stability	Increases muscular strength
	Increasing strength in the ligaments, tendons, cartilage and connective tissue
Contributes to fewer low-back problems	
Acts as a stimulus for other lifestyle changes	
Improves self-concept	

From: Anspaugh, D. J. (1991)

dividual education, certification and experience. A discussion related to the basics of programming for this relatively low risk population follows.

Hypertension

Hypertension is one of the most prevalent chronic diseases in the United States, affecting more than 30 percent of all Americans. **Hypertension** is a condition in which the blood pressure is chronically elevated above levels desirable for an individual's age and health. Hypertension is defined as 140/90 mm Hg for individuals younger than 60 or greater than 160/95 mm Hg for those older than 60.

Half of all individuals with high blood pressure don't even know they have it, which is why hypertension is commonly referred to as the "silent killer." It is a serious health problem because people affected by high blood pressure have three to four times the risk of developing coronary heart disease and up to seven times the risk of having a stroke.

The Role of Exercise in Hypertension Control.

Exercise training is now recognized as an important part of therapy for controlling hypertension. Several exercise training studies have confirmed that regular physical activity results in lower blood pressure readings compared to those of sedentary individuals. The causes of the reduction in blood pressure following endurance exercise appears to be related to the vasodilating effect of exercise, which results in a reduction in vascular resistance, as well as the reduction of heart rate at rest. Since most hypertensive clients are obese, non-drug therapy is usually the first line of treatment. A combination of weight reduction, salt restriction and increased physical activity have all been recommended as treatments for reducing and controlling high blood pressure.

Program Design Considerations. Guidelines specific to the hypertensive exerciser include the following. Specific program design considerations appear in Table 11.2.

1. All clients, especially hypertensive clients, should be instructed not to hold their breath and/or strain during exercise (Valsalva maneuver).

2. If weights are used, the resistance should be kept low and the repetitions high.

3. Exercise intensity may need to be monitored by the rating of perceived exertion (RPE) scale, since medications can affect the heart rate during exercise.

4. Have the client report to the instructor any changes in medications, and/or any abnormal signs or symptoms before, during or immediately following exercise.

5. Encourage the client to monitor and track his or her blood pressure before and after exercise.

6. Instruct the client to move slowly when transitioning from the floor to standing, since hypertensive individuals are more susceptible to orthostatic hypotension if on antihypertensive medication.

Fitness instructors who work with hypertensive individuals should know how to "accurately" take blood pressure readings. The American Heart Association has a course and certification program for taking blood pressures. Other sources of instruction might include a community college or university. Some hypertensive clients may be taking hypertensive medication, which can affect the client's response to exercise (see Chapter 5, "Health Screening").

Special Precautions. Both hypertensive and hypotensive responses are possible during and after exercise for individuals with high blood pressure. Factors to consider when working with hypertensive clients include: (1) the clinical status of the client, (2) what medications the client is currently taking, (3) the frequency, duration, intensity and mode of exercise he or she is participating in, and (4) how well the individual manages the hypertension.

Fitness instructors need to discuss all of these factors with their clients and possibly the clients' physician to make sure the exercise program prescribed is safe and effective.

Coronary Artery Disease

Coronary artery disease (CAD) continues to be the leading cause of death in the United States. The majority of heart attacks are caused by the buildup of **plaque** in the arteries supplying blood to the heart muscle (coronary arteries). This process is referred to as **atherosclerosis.** The plaque consists of fatty substances, cholesterol, and other blood and chemical substances. The plaque enlarges over time, progressively narrowing the arterial channel through which blood travels. Eventually, a clot forms and completely closes the vessel, resulting in a heart attack.

Exercise plays an important role in preventing heart disease, as well as in the

Cardiovascular disorders

Table 11.2

SAMPLE EXERCISE PROGRAM FOR HYPERTENSIVE INDIVIDUAL

	Exercise Program
Mode	Dynamic exercise, such as low-impact aerobics, walking, etc. Isometric exercises should be avoided. Weight training should be prescribed, using low resistance and high repetitions.
Intensity	Low-intensity, dynamic exercise is recommended. The exercise intensity level should be near the lower end of the heart rate range (40 to 65%).
Frequency	Clients should be encouraged to exercise at least four times per week. Daily exercise may be appropriate for certain clients.
Duration	Encourage a longer and more gradual warm-up and cool-down (greater than 10 minutes). Total exercise duration should be gradually increased to 30 to 60 minutes.

rehabilitation of individuals with heart disease. The major risk factors for CAD—hypertension, smoking and high cholesterol—are all positively affected by exercise. Furthermore, physical inactivity is now recognized as an additional major risk factor for CAD. CAD can be delayed or prevented by controlling risk factors.

The Role of Exercise in Preventing and Treating CAD. The benefits of habitual physical activity in preventing and treating heart disease are becoming increasingly clear. Physical inactivity is now recognized as a major contributor to the heart disease process. Numerous studies have confirmed that even moderate exercise can produce favorable improvements in cardiorespiratory endurance, and reduced CAD risk factors (Table 11.1).

Program Design Considerations—Working With Low-risk CAD Clients. Low-risk cardiac patients should have established stable cardiovascular and physiological responses to exercise. All clients identified with cardiac risk factors need to have a physician release and referral to exercise. Ideally, low-risk cardiac clients should have a treadmill test to determine their functional capacity and cardiovascular status. The treadmill results can then be used to establish a safe exercise level (Table 11.3).

Additional guidelines specific to the low-risk CAD client include the following:

1. All clients should be screened for heart disease risk factors.

2. Clients who fall into the medium- or high-risk categories should consult with their physician before being allowed to exercise.

3. If a client has heart disease or has recently had a heart attack or heart surgery, the instructor will need to obtain additional information (i.e., medical clearance and guidelines from a physician).

4. Carefully follow the guidelines from the physician.

5. Monitor exercise intensity closely. Make sure the client is keeping within his or her individual heart rate or RPE range.

6. The client must inform the fitness instructor if he or she has any abnormal signs or symptoms before, during or after exercise.

7. The exercise intensity level should be kept low to start, and gradually increased over time.

8. If a client has recently completed a cardiac rehabilitation program, call to get an exit exercise prescription.

Weight Training Guidelines for Healthy Adults and Low-risk Cardiac Patients. The following guidelines were developed by the American Association of Cardiovascular

Table 11.3

SAMPLE EXERCISE PROGRAM FOR LOW-RISK CAD CLIENTS

	Exercise Program
Mode	Dynamic exercise, such as low-impact aerobics, walking, etc. Isometric exercises should be avoided. Weight training should be prescribed using low resistance and high repetitions (see weight training guidelines).
Intensity	Low-intensity dynamic exercise versus high-intensity, high-impact exercise is recommended. The exercise intensity should be gradually increased to 60 to 85% of the heart-rate reserve.
Frequency	Clients should be encouraged to exercise at least three to four times per week. Clients with low functional capacities may benefit from daily exercise.
Duration	Encourage a longer and more gradual warm-up and cool-down (greater than 10 minutes). Total exercise duration should be gradually increased to 30 to 60 minutes.

and Pulmonary Rehabilitation (1991). All clients with CAD should have specific clearance for weight training before beginning such a program.

1. To prevent soreness and injury, initially choose a weight that will allow the performance of 10 to 12 repetitions comfortably, corresponding to approximately 40 to 60 percent of the maximum weight load that can be lifted in 1 repetition. High-risk adults and low-risk cardiac patients should select an initial weight load that can be lifted for 12 to 15 repetitions.

2. Generally, two to three sets of each exercise is recommended.

3. Don't strain! Ratings of perceived exertion (6 to 20 scale) should not exceed "fairly light" to "somewhat hard" during lifting.

4. Avoid breath-holding. Exhale (blow out) on the most strenuous part of an exercise. For example, exhale when lifting a weight stack overhead and inhale when lowering it.

5. Increase weight loads by 5 to 10 pounds when 10 to 12 repetitions can be comfortably accomplished; for high-risk adults and cardiacs, weight can be added when 12 to 15 repetitions can be managed easily.

6. Raise the weight to a count of two

and lower the weight gradually to a count of four; emphasize complete extension of the limbs when lifting.

7. Exercise large muscle groups before small muscle groups. Include devices (exercises) for both the upper and lower body.

8. Weight train three times per week.

9. Avoid sustained handgripping when possible, since this may evoke an excessive blood pressure response to lifting.

10. Stop exercise in the event of warning signs or symptoms, especially dizziness, abnormal heart rhythm, unusual shortness of breath and/or chest pain.

11. Stay moving from one device to another; in other words, don't rest for extended periods between sets.

12. The recommended guidelines for prescribing exercise are those outlined by the ACSM. These guidelines are further discussed in the *Resource Manual for Guidelines for Exercise Testing and Prescription*. Additional information is available through the American Heart Association as well as from other clinical treatises on the practice of prescribing exercise. Although the ACSM guidelines are recommended with these additional references, this list need not be considered complete.

The modes of exercise most frequently prescribed are the use of free weights,

isokinetic, variable resistance or accommodating resistance training devices.

Special Precautions. If a client has had
angina in the past, he or she should always
carry a bottle of nitroglycerine with them.
If clients develop chest pain, they should
stop exercise immediately, and take their
nitroglycerine as prescribed by their physician. If the pain persists, proceed as directed by established emergency policies and
procedures (see "Special Precautions" for
hypertension, and Chapter 14, "Emergency
Procedures").

All instructors who work with low-risk
cardiac clients must be CPR-certified.

METABOLIC DISORDERS

A variety of metabolic disorders can
have an effect on an individual's
ability to exercise. Only individuals who
are clinically stable and have been cleared
to exercise by their physician should be
allowed to exercise in a non-medically supervised setting. Exercise can help control
and/or reverse certain medical disorders,
such as diabetes mellitus, one of the most
common metabolic disorders a fitness instructor will encounter.

Diabetes Mellitus

Diminished secretion of insulin by the
pancreas or an inability to utilize insulin
results in a disease known as **diabetes melli-**

tus. Diabetes is a serious disease if left untreated. Diabetics are at greater risk for numerous health problems, including kidney
failure, nerve disorders, eye problems and
heart disease. Prolonged and frequent elevation of blood sugar can lead to microan-
giopathy (damaged capillaries), which
leads to poor circulation. In addition, diabetics are at greater risk for developing
neuropathy (damaged nerves), which can
lead to permanent nerve damage.

There are two forms of diabetes, insulin
dependent (Type I) and non-insulin dependent (Type II). **Type I diabetes** is caused
by destruction of the insulin-producing
beta cells in the pancreas. Type I diabetics
produce little or no insulin. Type I diabetes
generally occurs in childhood, and regular
insulin injections are required to regulate
blood glucose levels (Table 11.4).

Type II diabetes is the most common
form of diabetes, affecting 90 percent of
all diabetic patients. Type II diabetes typically occurs in adults who are overweight.
Type II diabetics are unable to use the
insulin they produce because of reduced
sensitivity of insulin target cells. Treatment
of Type II diabetes varies, and may include
a change in diet, medication and exercise
therapy.

Effective Diabetic Control. Effective diabetic control is based on long-term regulation of blood glucose levels. Glucose
regulation in Type I diabetics is achieved
through regular glucose assessment, proper diet, exercise and appropriate insulin
medication. For the Type II diabetic, glucose regulation is achieved through a
change in lifestyle centered around proper diet, weight loss/control, exercise and
insulin or oral medications, if needed. A
combined diet and exercise regime results
in weight loss and weight control, improvement in cardiorespiratory fitness, reduced
need for insulin, improved self-image and

Table 11.4

COMPARISON OF TYPE I AND TYPE II DIABETES

	Type I	Type II
Term	Insulin-dependent (childhood onset)	Non-insulin dependent (adult onset)
Onset	Under 20 years old	Over 40 years old
Overweight	Very uncommon	Frequent
Family History	Infrequent	Frequent
Use of Insulin	Always	Not always

Table 11.5

SAMPLE EXERCISE PROGRAM FOR TYPE I AND TYPE II DIABETICS

Exercise Program	Type I	Type II
Mode	Aerobic	Aerobic
Intensity	Low to High	Low
Frequency	5 to 7 days/week	4 to 5 days/week
Duration	20 to 40 minutes	40 to 60 minutes

The golden rules of glucose regulation during exercise are to check blood glucose levels frequently when starting an exercise program, and to be aware of any unusual symptoms prior to, during or after exercise.

a better ability to deal with stress.

The Role of Exercise in Diabetic Control. Exercise plays an important role in diabetic control. One of the major benefits of exercise for diabetics is that it makes the muscle cells more permeable to glucose. Aerobic exercise seems to allow the body to make better use of available insulin. Another important benefit of aerobic exercise is the effect it has on reducing cholesterol levels and weight. With excessive blood glucose elevation, blood fats rise to become the primary energy source for the body. Since diabetics are prone to having higher than normal blood fat levels, they are also at higher risk for heart disease.

Exercise Program Design Considerations. Before beginning an exercise program, diabetics need to speak with their physician or diabetes educator so that a program of diet, exercise and medications can be developed. The primary goal of exercise for the Type I diabetic should be better glucose regulation and reduced heart disease risk. For the insulin-dependent diabetic the timing of exercise, the amount of insulin injected and the injection site are important considerations before exercising. Exercise should be performed daily so that a regular pattern of diet and insulin dosage can be maintained. Since the duration of exercise is lower for the Type I diabetic, the intensity can be slightly higher than the Type II diabetic.

The primary goal of exercise for the Type II diabetic is weight loss and weight control. Eighty percent of Type II diabetics are overweight. By losing weight through the combined effect of diet and exercise, Type II diabetics will reduce the amount of oral insulin medication required. The primary objective during exercise for the Type II diabetic is caloric expenditure. Maximizing caloric expenditure is best achieved by low-intensity, long-duration exercise. Since the frequency and duration of exercise are high for Type II diabetics, the intensity of exercise should be kept low (Table 11.5).

Additional guidelines for both Type I and Type II diabetics include the following:

1. Diabetic clients requiring insulin injections should not be injected in primary muscle groups that will be used during exercise. This regime can cause the insulin to be absorbed too quickly, resulting in **hypoglycemia.**

2. Diabetic clients need to check their blood glucose levels frequently. Clients should work with their physician to determine the right insulin dosage, based in part on the blood glucose levels before and after exercise.

3. Diabetics should be encouraged to always carry a rapid-acting carbohydrate (such as juice or candy) to correct hypoglycemia.

4. Diabetics should be encouraged to

Table 11.6

SAMPLE EXERCISE PROGRAM FOR CLIENTS WITH ASTHMA

	Exercise Program
Mode	Dynamic exercise, walking, cycling and swimming. Upper-body exercises, such as arm cranking, rowing and cross-country skiing, may not be appropriate because of the higher ventilation demands.
Intensity	Low-intensity dynamic exercise versus high-intensity, high-impact exercise is recommended. The exercise intensity should be prescribed based on the client's fitness status and limitations.
Frequency	Clients should be encouraged to exercise at least three to four times per week. Clients with low functional capacities or who experience shortness of breath during prolonged exercise, may benefit from intermittent exercise (two 10-minute sessions).
Duration	Encourage a longer and more gradual warm-up and cool-down (greater than 10 minutes). Total exercise duration should be gradually increased to 20 to 45 minutes.

exercise at the same time each day for better control.

5. Exercise should be avoided during peak insulin activity.

6. A carbohydrate snack should be consumed before and during prolonged exercise.

7. Diabetic clients need to take very good care of their feet. Clients need to regularly check for any cuts, blisters or signs of infection. Good-quality exercise shoes are also very important.

Special Precautions. For the Type I diabetic, potential problems can occur during or following exercise. In addition to hypoglycemia, a lack of insulin may cause **hyperglycemia**. Hyperglycemia occurs when there is insufficient insulin to mobilize glucose, and glucose levels become elevated to dangerous levels. A second potential problem that can occur is when insulin is mobilized too quickly, thus leading to lowering of the blood glucose to a dangerous level. A low blood glucose level is referred to as hypoglycemia.

One of the first rules for the insulin-dependent diabetic is to either reduce insulin intake or increase carbohydrate intake before exercise. For both types of diabetics, exercise should begin one to two hours after a meal, and before peak insulin activity. Usually insulin dosages need to be decreased prior to exercise, since exercise has an insulin-like effect.

RESPIRATORY AND PULMONARY DISORDERS

Considering that proper breathing is a major element of both healthful living and exercise, those with respiratory and lung disorders form a population with special fitness needs.

Asthma

Asthma is a reactive airway disease characterized by shortness of breath, coughing and wheezing. It is due to constriction of the smooth muscle around the airways, a swelling of the mucosal cells and increased secretion of mucous. Asthma can be caused by an allergic reaction, exercise, infections, emotion or other environmental irritants. Approximately 80 percent of asthmatics experience asthma attacks during exercise, a term referred to as **exercise-induced asthma** (EIA). Asthma is not a contraindication to exercise, but before starting an exercise program asthmatics should develop a plan for exercise with their physician.

The Role of Exercise and Asthma. Clients

with controlled asthma should benefit from regular exercise. Although asthmatics are more likely to experience breathlessness during exercise, this should not stop them from exercising. During exercise, some asthmatics will become short of breath due to the cooling effect in the airways caused by the large volumes of inspired air and also because of the evaporation of water in the respiratory tract. This is EIA.

Exercise Program Design Considerations. In addition to the sample exercise program (Table 11.6), the following guidelines are valuable for use with the asthmatic exerciser:

1. Before starting an exercise class, the client must have a medication plan to prevent EIA attacks.

2. The client should have a bronchodilating inhaler nearby at all times and be instructed to use it at the first sign of wheezing.

3. The exercise intensity should be kept low in the beginning, and gradually increased over time.

4. The exercise intensity should be reduced if asthma symptoms occur.

5. Using an inhaler several minutes before exercise may reduce the possibility of EIA attacks.

6. The results of pulmonary exercise testing should be used to design the appropriate exercise prescription.

7. Encourage clients to drink plenty of fluids before and during exercise.

8. An extended warm-up and cool-down period should be encouraged with asthmatics.

9. Clients with respiratory disorders will often experience more symptoms of respiratory distress when exercising in extreme environmental conditions (high or low temperature, high pollen count and heavy air pollution).

Special Precautions. Clients with respiratory disorders need to be carefully followed by their physician. Only clients with stable asthma should exercise. If an asthma attack is not relieved by medication, have the client transported to a medical facility immediately or call an ambulance.

Bronchitis and Emphysema

Bronchitis is a form of obstructive pulmonary disease. **Chronic bronchitis** is an inflammation of the bronchial tubes. The major cause is cigarette smoking; air pollution and occupational exposures play a lesser role.

Acute bronchitis is an inflammation of the mucous membranes of the bronchial tubes. An acute bout of bronchitis can develop following a cold or exposure to certain dust particles or fumes, and resolve in several days or weeks. Chronic bronchitis, however, persists, for a lifetime in most cases. **Emphysema** is another form of chronic pulmonary disease caused by overinflation of the **alveoli.** The overinflation results from a breakdown of the walls of the alveoli, which causes a significant decrease in respiratory function. The classic signs of emphysema are chronic breathlessness and coughing. Bronchitis and emphysema are collectively referred to as **chronic obstructive pulmonary diseases** (COPD).

The Role of Exercise and COPD. Clients with chronic bronchitis and emphysema may benefit from mild exercise training. However, clients with severe COPD may not receive any benefits from aerobic exercise. Clients with COPD need to be carefully screened and followed by a physician. Most clients with COPD do not improve their pulmonary function. However, other benefits, such as reduced anxiety, body weight and stress, and an improved ability to perform normal daily activities can be achieved through exercise in patients suffering from COPD.

Program Design Considerations for COPD Clients. It is unlikely that the majority of fit-

Table 11.7

SAMPLE EXERCISE PROGRAM FOR CLIENTS WITH COPD

	Exercise Program
Mode	Dynamic exercise, walking, cycling and swimming. Upper-body exercises, such as arm cranking, rowing and cross-country skiing, may not be appropriate because of the higher ventilation demands.
Intensity	Low-intensity dynamic exercise versus high-intensity, high-impact exercise is recommended. The exercise intensity should be carefully prescribed based on the client's breathing responses to exercise. The exercise intensity should be kept below the point where any difficulty in breathing is experienced.
Frequency	Clients should be encouraged to exercise at least four to five times per week. COPD clients usually benefit from intermittent exercise.
Duration	Encourage a longer and more gradual warm-up and cool-down (greater than 10 minutes). Total exercise duration should be gradually increased to 20 to 45 minutes.

ness instructors will ever work with COPD clients. However, COPD clients who are stable, and have obtained all the potential benefits from a medically supervised exercise program, should benefit from participating in a non-medically supervised exercise. COPD clients should be encouraged to "do the best they can," because every little bit of exercise they do can result in potential health benefits.

In addition to the sample exercise program (Table 11.7), the following guidelines are valuable in exercise programming for clients with COPD:

1. Before starting an exercise program, COPD clients must have extensive pulmonary tests completed.

2. Only stable COPD clients should be allowed to participate in a nonmedical setting.

3. The exercise intensity and type of exercise should be chosen carefully to avoid developing shortness of breath.

4. The guidelines for working with asthmatic patients should also be considered.

5. Only clients with bronchitis who are fully recovered from an acute bout of bronchitis should exercise.

6. COPD clients should have a bronchodilating inhaler with them at all times and be instructed to use it at the first sign of wheezing.

7. COPD clients should also perform their breathing exercises to help strengthen their respiratory muscles.

8. Upper-body exercises, such as arm cranking or rowing, should be avoided because of the increased strain on the pulmonary system.

9. Some COPD clients may require supplemental oxygen during exercise.

Special Precautions. COPD clients must not smoke. The type and dose of medications should be reviewed with the client's physician, based on the client's response to exercise. If a COPD client's performance in a non-medically supervised program worsens, they should be encouraged to participate in a pulmonary rehabilitation program until such time as their signs and symptoms have improved.

ORTHOPEDIC DISORDERS

The following section looks at the characteristics of and requirements for those with low-back pain or arthritis.

Low-back Pain

Back injuries, including sprains and strains, are the number one disability for people under age 45. It has been estimated that 80 percent of the population will experience an episode of low-back pain some time in their lives. Of that 80 percent, 5 percent will go on to develop chronic low-back pain. **Low-back pain** (LBP) accounts for 10 percent of all chronic health conditions in the United States and 25 percent of days lost from work. LBP has been referred to by medical experts as the most expensive benign health condition in America.

Back injuries translate into millions of lost work days every year and cost billions in medical care, disability payments and legal payments. Reducing back injury rates is a top priority for all employers. In fact, the most common type of workers' compensation claim is a back strain/sprain, which accounts for up to 25 percent of all claims, representing annual payments of $2.5 to $7 billion, including one half of all disability compensation payments annually! In addition, nearly 2 percent of the U.S. work force files back compensation claims.

The Role of Exercise in Preventing and Treating LBP. It appears that physical fitness combined with a healthy lifestyle may help prevent low-back pain. In fact, many physicians feel that the major cause of chronic low-back pain is simply physical deconditioning. More specifically, low endurance of large muscle groups, particularly the back extensors, seems to put one at a greater risk of developing LBP (Table 11.8). Exercises for the low back should be performed on a regular basis to gain maximal benefits.

Program Design Considerations. Exercise participants should be screened for low-back risk factors. Prevention is the key to avoiding LBP. For more comprehensive information on preventing LBP, several informative books are referenced at the end of this chapter.

Some common-sense tips that are helpful in the prevention of low-back pain include the following:

1. Always be aware of proper form and alignment.

2. Always maintain pelvic neutral alignment and an erect torso during any exercise movements.

3. Avoid head-forward positions in which the chin is tilted up.

4. When leaning forward, lifting or lowering an object, always bend at the knees.

5. Avoid hyperextending the spine in an unsupported position.

6. Allow for an adequate warm-up and cool-down period during all exercise classes.

7. Most LBP is caused by muscle weaknesses and imbalances, including tight hamstring and low-back muscle groups, tight hip flexor muscles, and weak abdominal and low-back muscles. Exercises should be routinely performed to improve muscle strength and flexibility.

8. Individuals who experience LBP or have a history of chronic LBP should be advised to consult with a physician and get specific recommendations for exercises.

9. If someone complains of LBP following an exercise class have him or her sit or lie down in a comfortable position and apply ice to the affected area. Following a mild back strain, individuals should be encouraged to take several days off from exercise.

Special Precautions. Chronic low-back pain is one of the most common and costly health ailments for Americans. The high incidence of low-back pain may be primarily due to factors such as obesity, poor posture, anatomical disorders, muscle and ligament strains and poor physical fitness. Exercise is frequently prescribed for the prevention and treatment of LBP. Individuals who complain of low back-pain should first be evaluated by a physician be-

Table 11.8

RISK FACTORS FOR LBP

General	The incidence of LBP increases with age. Poor exercise tolerance, strength, balance of the abdominal and extensor muscles, being overweight or extremely tall all correlate with a greater risk for developing LBP.
Postural/Structural	Postural or structural abnormalities can be identified by physical examination and spinal radiology.
Occupational	One of the most powerful potential risk factors for LBP is lifting. Other occupational risk factors for LBP include twisting, bending, stooping and floor surface conditions. Prolonged sitting, particularly without proper arm and spinal support, is associated with LBP.
Environmental	Cigarette smoking is a risk factor for LBP. Chronic coughing may also be associated with intradiscal pressure.
Psychosocial	A range of psychological factors (including depression and anxiety) and social problems (especially stressful job environments) are associated with an increased incidence of disabling LBP.
Recreational	Golfing and tennis have been slightly associated with an increased risk of disk herniation, possibly because of the twisting activities involved with these sports. Only a minimally significant statistical association has been found between LBP and jogging or cross-country skiing.
Other	Multiple pregnancies have been associated with an increase in LBP, probably due to loss of abdominal tone following pregnancy, the strain of lifting children, and various hormonal effects.

fore starting an exercise program. Other precautions to take when working with LBP clients include: (1) an organized program of physical exercise which emphasizes general fitness, aerobic capacity and specific reconditioning of the muscles that support the spine should be encouraged, (2) the warm-up and cool-down periods may need to be extended, (3) proper lifting techniques should be taught and demonstrated during exercise classes (keep the load close to the body, and always face the weight being lifted), (4) clients should report to the fitness instructor any changes in pain and/or medications, and (5) clients should be instructed to avoid activities that are clearly associated with previous episodes of low-back pain.

Arthritis

Although there are different forms of arthritis, the most common forms are rheumatoid and osteoarthritis. **Osteoarthritis** is a degenerative process caused by the wearing away of cartilage, leaving two surfaces of bone in contact with each other. **Rheumatoid arthritis** is caused by an inflammation of the membrane surrounding joints. It is often associated with pain and swelling in one or more joints. The benefits of exercise include stronger muscles and bones, improved cardiorespiratory fitness and improved psychosocial well-being. Exercise is contraindicated during inflammatory periods because exercise may worsen the process in such cases.

The Role of Exercise for Arthritic Clients. Exercise is recommended for clients with arthritis to help preserve muscle strength and joint mobility, to improve functional capabilities, to relieve pain and stiffness, to prevent further deformities, to improve overall physical conditioning, to re-establish neuromuscular coordination, and to mobilize stiff or contracted joints. Improvement of function and pain relief are

Table 11.9

SAMPLE EXERCISE PROGRAM FOR CLIENTS WITH ARTHRITIS

	Exercise Program
Mode	Non-weight-bearing activities, such as cycling and swimming, are preferred because they reduce joint stress.
Intensity	Low-intensity dynamic exercise versus high-intensity, high-impact exercise is recommended. The exercise intensity should be carefully prescribed based on the client's pain tolerance before, during and after exercise.
Frequency	Clients should be encouraged to exercise at least four to five times per week. Arthritic clients usually benefit from frequent (daily) exercise sessions.
Duration	Encourage a longer and more gradual warm-up and cool-down (greater than 10 minutes). Total exercise duration should start out short—10 to 15 minutes.

the ultimate goals.

Program Design Considerations. A physician or physical therapists should carefully design the fitness program. Exercise should be avoided during an acute arthritic flare. Fatigue is a common complaint in arthritic clients. Exercise programs need to balance rest, immobilization of affected joints and exercise to reduce the severity of the inflammatory joint disease.

In addition to Table 11.9, the following guidelines are valuable in exercise programming for clients with arthritis:

1. Clients with arthritis should be encouraged to participate in classes in which quick or excessive movement can be avoided, such as low-impact or water exercise classes.

2. Exercise sessions should begin at a low-intensity with frequent rests.

3. Exercise intensity and duration should be reduced during periods of inflammation or pain.

4. Arthritic clients may need an extended warm-up and cool-down period.

5. The exercise session should be modified in terms of intensity and duration according to how well the client responds, changes in medication, and the disease and pain levels.

6. Try to tailor the stretching portion of the exercise class to focus on the arthritic joints.

7. Have the client take a day or two of rest if he or she continues to complain about pain during or following an exercise session.

8. If arthritic clients cannot tolerate an aerobics class, suggest other forms of aerobic exercise, such as swimming or cycling.

9. Always stress proper body alignment during exercise.

10. Poor posture can predispose clients to muscle aches and pains that will limit the amount of exercise they can perform.

11. Pain is quite normal in people with arthritis. Try to get clients to work just up to the point of pain, but not past it. Simple movements for healthy people can be quite painful for individuals with arthritis.

12. If certain movements are too difficult, try isometric exercises with arthritic clients. Tubing can also be used to add resistance.

13. It is essential to put all joints through a range of motion at least once a day to maintain mobility.

Special Precautions. Individuals suffering from arthritis generally have very low exercise capacities. Exercise is commonly used for therapeutic purposes to help alleviate joint problems. Rapid or intense exercise movements should be avoided. Other precautions to take when working with arthritic clients include: (1) any changes in their medications, medical plan or response to exercise need to be reported to the instructor, (2) clients with rheumatoid arthritis should not exercise during periods of inflammations, (3) proper body mechanics should always be reinforced, (4) regular rest periods should be encouraged, and (5) the arthritic client should consult with his or her physician if severe pain persists following exercise.

SPECIAL POPULATIONS

As defined earlier, the term special population refers to groups of exercisers with special needs and/or requirements, but who are not necessarily challenged with a high-risk medical disorder. For example, an instructor needs to understand that an older adult is at increased risk for cardiovascular disorders and requires additional attention before even beginning an exercise program, while those that are hearing-impaired definitely have special needs, but otherwise are every bit as healthy as a non-hearing-impaired exerciser.

Hearing Impairment

Nearly 21 million people in the United States are hearing-impaired, making this the largest disability group. Fitness professionals should be aware that hearing impairment is a generic term used to refer to virtually any degree of hearing loss. Of the 21 million impaired, approximately 500,000 individuals are unable to hear any normal conversation, while more than 7 million report significant difficulty hearing normal conversation, even with a hearing aid.

Given the ongoing labeling issue of whether to call a person with a hearing problem either deaf, hard of hearing or hearing-impaired, it is best for the exercise instructor to ask the individual which he or she considers him/herself to be and to respect the client's preference.

Hearing loss is clinically defined by several factors. An individual's hearing profile, or configuration, is reflected by an audiogram that is created by a battery of hearing tests. The audiogram will indicate the degree of hearing loss based on the individual's response at various decibel levels and frequencies.

For the aerobics instructor, the most important information needed to best serve the hearing-impaired relates to how the individual or group has adapted to the disability. Some individuals use sign language as a primary mode of communication, while others use speech and lipreading while some function both ways. Familiarity with and sensitivity to these cultural phenomena enable the instructor to understand and effectively implement the program design considerations below.

Program Design Considerations. An instructor designing an aerobic program for hearing-impaired persons should initially select which of the two groups described above needs to be targeted. Adaptations requested or expected by a signer are likely to be different than those requested or expected by a lipreader. To ensure a successful experience for all, it is necessary to focus initially on one set of needs.

Answering one or more of the following questions will enable the instructor to target the group correctly:

1. If a hearing-impaired client has already requested or enrolled in a program, with which group does he or she identify?

2. Does he or she know other hearing-impaired persons who would like to participate?

3. Is there a chapter of the Self Help for the Hard of Hearing (SHHH), the National Association of the Deaf (NAD) or the Association of Late Deafened Adults (ALDA) in the community?

4. Is there a state school for the deaf or a college program for the deaf in the community?

(If it is a major metropolitan area, chances are good that a large number of people in both groups reside there.)

Once the target group has been determined, the following program considerations can be addressed:

1. An introductory session should be offered to introduce the signers or lipreaders to the facility. If they are signers, a certified sign language interpreter or a hearing-impaired fitness professional should be hired to assist with communication.

2. Music with a strong, distinct beat should be selected. Most hearing-impaired people have some hearing in the lower frequencies. Signers will most likely want the music loud. Lipreaders will probably want it softer at first because they will be concerned about hearing the instructor's verbal cues. As they become more familiar with the class, however, they may want the music louder (see Chapter 8, "Teaching an Aerobics Class").

3. Lipreaders may request an assistive listening device, an electronic aide that allows sound to bypass the airspace between the speaker (instructor) and the receiver (client). Groups such as SHHH or ALDA or a local audiologist can assist the instructor in obtaining such a device.

4. If it is an aerobics class, the instructor must be an excellent visual cuer and thoroughly trained, preferably by someone familiar with hearing-impaired needs.

One final note: it is important to remember that a hearing-impaired person will perceive information overwhelmingly through the eyes. Since one's eyes cannot focus on an exercise movement while concentrating on lipreading or signing, it is crucial to demonstrate then explain, or vice versa, but not to do both simultaneously when demonstrating on exercise equipment.

Older Adults

The U.S. population is getting older. By the year 2030, more than 20 percent of the population will be over the age of 65. This age group represents the fastest growing segment of the population.

Aging is a normal biological process. Although certain physiological changes are inevitable with aging, it appears that the rate of decline of the effects of aging can be reduced or even postponed through exercise. No one can promise that exercise will prolong life, but research certainly suggests that one's quality of life can be improved through regular exercise.

Normal Physiological Changes With Aging. Maximal heart rate is age-related. With age, maximal heart rate declines. The accuracy of estimating training intensity based on heart rate diminishes with age. Other methods of monitoring exercise intensity, such as the RPE scale, should be considered when working with the elderly. Although exercise heart rate declines with age, in healthy older subjects who exercise, stroke volume (or the amount of blood pumped out of the heart per beat) has been shown to increase, and thus overcome the effect of a lowered heart rate.

With normal aging, maximal oxygen uptake declines approximately 8 to 10 percent per decade after age 30. This decline is primarily due to the decrease in maximal heart rate. It is clear, however, that aerobic capacity can be improved at any age. In one study, a group of 49- to 65-year-old sedentary subjects walked and jogged three times a week for 20 weeks. Following the training, the men improved their aerobic capacity by an average of 18 percent. In another study, a 22-percent increase in aerobic capacity was found in a group of 70- to 79-year-old participants. Reduction in aerobic capacity can be altered by exercise training.

With age, bones become more fragile. Serious and often debilitating fractures are common in the elderly. By age 90, as many as 32 percent of women and 17 percent of men will have sustained a hip fracture, and between 12 and 20 percent of this group will die of complications of hip fractures. **Osteoporosis**, or a gradual loss or thinning of bone with aging, is a major concern to the elderly. Weight-bearing and resistance-training exercises are known to help maintain bone mass. The positive effect of exercise in preventing osteoporosis is based on extensive literature documenting the rapid onset and severe bone loss in immobilized individuals and the significant difference in bone density (bone strength) of physically active versus sedentary individuals. Regular physical activity appears to have beneficial effects on the rate of age-related bone loss.

Skeletal muscle mass declines with age, resulting in decreased muscular strength and endurance. For each decade after age 25, 3 to 5 percent of muscle mass is lost.

Significant strength gains are possible in the elderly. The results from a 1988 Tufts University study found that in a group of 60- to 72-year-old untrained men, participating in 12 weeks of strength training (8 repetitions/set, three sets/day, three days/week), knee extensor strength increased 107 percent and knee flexor strength increased 227 percent following 12 weeks of training. This study demonstrated that strength gains do occur in older men, and these gains are associated with significant muscle hypertrophy and muscle protein turnover.

With normal aging, connective tissue becomes stiffer, and joints become less mobile. Loss of flexibility with age may also be the result of underlying degenerative disease processes such as arthritis. Flexibility does decrease with age, however, there is no evidence that the biological processes associated with aging are responsible for this loss. Loss of flexibility is more likely the result of diminishing physical activity. Flexibility can be improved at any age through exercises that promote the elasticity of the soft tissues.

Lean body weight declines and body fat increases with normal aging. The changes in body composition resulting from age are primarily due to a decrease in the basal metabolic rate and physical activity habits of the elderly. Basal metabolic rate declines at a rate of 3 percent per decade. Numerous studies have demonstrated the beneficial effects of exercise on body composition in the elderly.

Program Design Considerations. Before starting an exercise program, elderly individuals should first see their physician. Although many of the principles of prescribing exercise to the elderly are the same for any group, special care should be given when setting up a fitness program for older participants.

The following are considerations for use in the development of a group exercise program for older adults:

1. All movement should be slow to moderately paced. For choreographed routines, steps should be simple and repeated often. Fast transitions from one type of movement to another should be avoided to prevent postural hypotension and subsequent dizziness, falling or fainting.

2. Several modes and positions of exercise should be used. Some positions include standing, sitting, standing with a chair for balance, and floor exercise using a mat. Prior to initiating floor exercise, feedback should be solicited from the group on whether the exercise is desirable. Some

adults feel awkward or embarrassed if they have difficulty getting up from the floor in front of their peers. Instruction in how to get up from the floor may be necessary.

3. A variety of equipment should be used to achieve program objectives and sustain motivation. Examples include wands or dowels, surgical tubing, towels or rubber strips for flexibility and range of motion, Frisbees and low walking beams for balance and coordination, and 1-pound weights for strength.

4. The pressor reflex should be avoided by keeping the overhead position of the arms to a minimum.

5. Special precaution should be taken for all participants who take medications. These include cardiovascular drugs, such as beta blockers, calcium channel blockers, and diuretics, which affect exercise tolerance. Hypotension may develop if a participant exercises soon after taking nitroglycerin. The dose, type and time of administration of insulin may need to be changed to prevent hypoglycemia. Medical approval and ongoing medical consultation for those on prescription drugs is recommended.

6. The exertion level of all participants should be continually monitored. Heart rate monitoring should be taught using the radial or carotid pulse. Permission to rest and to get a drink of water should be given throughout the exercise class. Participants should be told frequently to progress at their own rate.

7. In addition to the instructor, one additional staff member should always be present to observe participants' physical reactions and to assist with any major or minor emergency.

8. The use of layered clothing should be suggested to prevent overheating or cooling. Older adults are less tolerant of the heat and cold.

9. A microphone should be used when conducting a program in a large area if the acoustics are poor. Lower tones can be more readily heard by the older adult.

10. For visual charts viewed from a distance, colors such as yellow, orange and red are seen more clearly.

11. The instructor should be certified in CPR, and a well-defined emergency plan should exist.

Special Precautions. Particular care should be given when prescribing weight-lifting exercises to those with high blood pressure, heart disease or arthritis. Encourage an extended cool-down period, approximately 10 to 15 minutes. Elderly people often have a more difficult time exercising in extreme environmental conditions. Avoid exercising in these conditions if possible. Some elderly individuals with arthritis or poor joint mobility may have to participate in non-weight-bearing activities, such as cycling, swimming, and chair and floor exercises.

Children

An abundance of literature cites the poor physical fitness and health status of American children. One of the most alarming statistics comes from the National Children and Youth Fitness Study, which reported that approximately 20 percent of this nation's children and adolescents between the ages of 5 and 17 are considered obese. This figure is 50 percent higher than 20 years ago. Unfortunately, obese children have a much higher probability of becoming obese adults.

Another alarming health statistic reports that as many as 40 percent of children between the ages of 5 and 8 already exhibit at least one of the following heart disease risk factors: obesity, hypertension and high cholesterol levels.

It is important to get children interested and involved in exercise sport activities

Table 11.10

PHYSIOLOGIC CHARACTERISTICS OF THE EXERCISING CHILD

Function	Comparison to Adults	Implications for Exercise
Metabolic *Aerobic power* *(VO$_2$ max[ml/kg/min])*	Similar	Children are able to perform endurance activities similar to adults.
Anaerobic power	Lower	The ability of children to perform intense activities is lower than adults.
Cardiovascular *Maximal cardiac output*	Lower	Children are limited in their ability to bring internal heat to the surface.
Maximal heart rate	Higher	Maximum HR is between 195 and 215 bpm.
Pulmonary *Maximal minute ventilation*	Smaller	Activities that require large respiratory minute volumes may cause early fatigue.
Thermoregulatory *Sweating rate*	Lower	Greater risk of heat-related illness on hot, humid days.
Acclimatization	Slower	Children require a longer and more gradual acclimatization period.
Body core heating During dehydration	Greater	Children need to hydrate well; must be encouraged to drink fluids.

From: Zwiren, L.A. (1991).

at an early age. Exercise and fitness activities should be enjoyable and appropriate for the age of the child.

The more parents get involved, the more likely children are to become active. The National Youth Fitness Study found that while schools are important to a child's exercise and health habits, home and community environments significantly contribute as well. Children who watch more television, have less active parents, and participate less in community activities tend to score lower on health-related fitness measures.

Exercise training should be considered an important part of health promotion efforts for children. Physical activity needs to become a lifetime pursuit. Educators, parents and fitness professionals can help achieve this goal by teaching children positive attitudes—that fitness is fun—and by making young children aware of the benefits of exercise.

A number of the benefits of regular physical activity for children are listed below:

1. Prevention of cardiovascular disease.
2. Reduction and control of high blood pressure and childhood obesity.
3. Improvement in the ability to perform basic motor skills.
4. Possible prevention of injuries.
5. Improved self-confidence and self-image.
6. Early development of good posture.
7. Greater ease and efficiency in performing motor tasks and sport skills.
8. Better performance on nationwide fitness tests.
9. Early development of coordination and balance.
10. The establishment of fitness as a lifetime interest.
11. Improved flexibility.
12. Favorable improvements in body composition.

Within the last decade, a great deal of

Table 11.11

SAMPLE ENDURANCE TRAINING PROGRAM FOR CHILDREN

	Exercise Program
Mode	Children should be encouraged to participate in sustained activities that use large muscle groups (i.e., swimming, jogging, aerobic dance). Other activities, such as recreational, sport and fun activities that develop other components of fitness (speed, power, flexibility, muscular endurance, agility and coordination) should be incorporated into a fitness program.
Intensity	Exercise intensity should start out low and progress gradually. There are currently no universal recommendations available for the use of training heart rate during exercise for children. Using the Borg Scale of perceived exertion is a more practical method of monitoring exercise intensity with children. Children should report a rating of 2 to 4 on the Modified Borg Scale (Table 11.12).
Frequency	Two to three days of endurance training will allow adequate time to participate in other activities, and yet be sufficient to cause a training effect.
Duration	Since children will be involved in a variety of activities during and after school, a specific amount of time should be dedicated to endurance training. Endurance exercise activities should be gradually increased to 30 to 40 minutes per session. With younger children, it will be necessary to start out with less time.

research has focused on the effects of exercise training in children. From these studies, it appears that children respond to training much the same way adults do (Table 11.10). Studies have demonstrated that important health and performance characteristics can be improved through exercise.

Effects of Endurance Training on Aerobic Capacity in Children. Numerous training studies have demonstrated that young children are physiologically adaptive to chronic endurance exercise. The average improvement in oxygen uptake following training in prepubescent children averages 8 to 10 percent, depending on the mode of training, the intensity of the exercise and the length of training program. Exercise capacity and maximal oxygen uptake increase throughout childhood, regardless of training, thanks to the normal growth and development of physiological systems. The increase in endurance capacity in children is the result of numerous physiological changes.

Endurance Training Guidelines. Sufficient evidence exists that children physiological-ly adapt to endurance training. Lacking, however, is a general consensus on the quality and quantity of exercise required to improve and maintain a minimum level of fitness in children. In 1988, the ACSM published an opinion statement on physical fitness in children and youth, which stated that, "until more definitive evidence is available, current recommendations are that children and youth obtain 20 to 30 minutes of vigorous exercise each day."

Several investigators have recommended that adult standards be used when establishing the intensity of exercise, as well as the frequency and duration of children's fitness programs. These recommendations are supported by Rowland (1988), who found that of the eight studies he reviewed, six had adult standards of aerobic training, showing significant improvements in aerobic power, while no significant improvements were noted in the other two studies.

In addition to the sample endurance training program for children (Table 11.11) the following guidelines are helpful in program development:

1. Although children are generally quite active, children usually choose to participate in activities that consist of short-burst, high-energy exercise. Children should be encouraged to participate in sustained activities that use large muscle groups.

2. The type, intensity and duration of exercise activities need to be based on the maturity of the child, medical status and previous experiences with exercise.

3. Regardless of age, the exercise intensity should start out low and progress gradually.

4. Because of the difficulty in monitoring heart rates with children, the use of a modified perceived exertion scale is a more practical method of monitoring exercise intensity in children (Table 11.12).

5. Children are involved in a variety of activities throughout the day. Because of this, a specific time should be dedicated to sustained aerobic activities.

6. Because it is often quite difficult to get children to respond to sustained periods of exercise, the sessions need to be creatively designed.

Programming Considerations for Group Exercise With Children. While the standard intensity, frequency and duration guidelines for adults may be applied to children there are many factors that are either unique to children or need to be emphasized differently when compared to adult exercise groups. In addition to the age classifications delineated in Table 11.13, the following considerations are valuable in group exercise programming for children:

1. Be sure to match the height of a step exercise platform to the size of the child.

2. Keep class sizes small.

3. Encourage fluid intake before, during and after exercise.

4. All exercise movements should be performed in a slow and controlled manner.

5. Choose music that is both appropriate for the speed of movements and is motivating.

6. Include a brief warm-up and cool-down period.

7. Do not teach a children's aerobic class as one would an adult class. Children are not miniature adults.

8. Children should be properly supervised at all times.

9. Match exercise training programs to the age and maturity level of the child.

10. The intensity of the exercise training should be carefully selected and monitored.

11. Children should never perform sudden, explosive movements.

12. Children should be taught to breathe properly during exercise.

Effects of Resistance Training on Strength Development in Children. Adequate strength is an important part of health-related fitness and optimal physiological function for both adults and children. It is also recognized as an important contribution to

Table 11.12

RATE OF PERCEIVED EXERTION SCALE FOR CHILDREN

	Explanations	Visual Example
0 - Rest	How you feel when you are sitting and resting.	Child sitting in a chair or watching TV.
1 - Easy	How you feel when you are walking to school or doing chores around the house.	Children walking to school, no sweat.
2 - Pretty Hard	How you feel when you are playing on the playground or running around.	Children playing and just starting to sweat.
3 - Harder	How you feel when you're playing sports, playing hard on the playground or working hard.	Children playing sports and starting to sweat.
4 - Hard	How you feel when you are running hard.	Child running hard and sweating profusely.
5 - Very Hard, Maximal	The hardest you have ever worked or exercised in your life.	Child running and ready to collapse at the finish line of a race.

Table 11.13

AGE CLASSIFICATIONS FOR YOUTH EXERCISE

Age Group	Suggested Program
Preschool and Kindergarten (Early Childhood)	Early childhood is a period of rapid growth and development. Games and exercises should focus on the development of basic movements, such as running, balancing, jumping, kicking, throwing and catching.
6 to 9 years	Participation in sports becomes very important to children in this age group, so encourage them to try fun exercises that refine a variety of skills.
9 to 13 years	This age group can handle more adult exercises. Motivating these older kids and keeping them interested is the challenge with this group.

improved motor performance, self-image and athletic performance. Unfortunately, by examining the literature, it is apparent that strength, specifically upper-body strength, is poor among children.

It was once thought that young children were not capable of increased strength through resistance training because they lacked adequate concentrations of testosterone. Although certain hormones are an important contribution to the development of strength, especially maximal strength, it is not the most important means through which children develop strength. The primary mechanisms responsible for strength development in children is through increased motor unit recruitment and coordination, with perhaps some change in muscle hypertrophy. There is now substantial evidence demonstrating significant increases in strength following structured resistance training in children; these increases are similar to those observed in older age groups. Furthermore, the safety and efficacy of resistance training programs for prepubescent children has also been well-documented.

In addition to improvements in muscular strength, other fitness- and performance-related effects of resistance training include: (1) increased flexibility, (2) improved physical performance, (3) improvements in body composition, (4) improvements

in cardiorespiratory fitness, (5) reductions in serum lipids, and (6) reductions in blood pressure. With further research, additional benefits may be discovered.

Recommendations for Resistance Training. A wealth of data demonstrates that strength gains do occur in children following structured resistance training programs. Although the exact mechanisms responsible for the increases in strength, as well as the lack of information on the long-term effects of prepubescent strength training are not completely known, some form of resistance training should be a regular component of children's fitness programs.

The following guidelines are helpful in designing resistance training programs for children:

1. Children should be encouraged to participate in a variety of activities that involve repetitive movements against an opposing force.

2. Before children are allowed to lift free weights, proper lifting technique needs to be demonstrated. Start with small, one-half- to 1-pound dumbbells. Perform a variety of upper- and lower-body exercises.

3. Most exercise equipment is designed for adults. If children cannot be properly fitted for the machines, they should not be used.

4. Other forms of resistance training,

such as manual resistance training, can be used with children. With manual resistance training, the resistance is provided by a partner. Children take turns applying resistance during different movements.

Example—Hip Abduction: one child lies on the ground while the other child applies resistance to the leg being raised (abducted).

5. Isometric training can also be utilized with children.

Example—Bent-over Lateral Raises: one child bends at the waist and tries to raise his or her arms up, while the other child applies the resistant force. These exercises can also be done individually.

6. Exercise tubing can be purchased in different resistances, or made from scratch. All resistance exercises should be performed in a slow, steady, sustained manner. Use a specific count during the initial movement, the hold phase and then return to the resting phase.

7. Additional programs include:

Pulling Activities: tie a rope to a wall and have children pull themselves toward the wall while sitting on a piece of carpet; or pull a weighted sandbag toward him or herself.

Pushing Activities: push-ups, throwing a medicine ball.

Hanging: child hangs from a bar, hang and swing, child slowly releases from an assisted pull-up (eccentric work).

8. Resistance training should be but one component of a comprehensive fitness program.

Special Precautions. It is important to remember that children are not small adults, and thus they should not be treated as such. Other special precautions to take when working with children include: (1) avoid having children exercise in extreme environmental conditions, (2) children should have a medical examination before starting any form of structured exercise program, (3) children should be properly supervised at all times, (4) exercise training programs need to be matched to the age and maturity level of the child, (5) the intensity of the exercise training must be carefully selected and monitored, (6) children should never perform single maximal lifts or sudden explosive movements, and (7) children should be taught to breathe properly during exercise.

SUMMARY

This chapter has presented important information on how to modify exercise sessions for individuals with selected medical and/or health conditions. Overwhelming and convincing evidence exists that exercise plays an important role in the prevention and treatment of certain degenerative diseases, such as osteoporosis, diabetes, obesity and cardiovascular disease. Today's fitness instructors need to become educated and trained to work with a variety of individuals, including those with known or suspected medical and/or health conditions. The special populations segment of the fitness industry will continue to grow, offering fitness instructors an excellent opportunity to become specialists in this area.

ACKNOWLEDGEMENT

The author wishes to acknowledge Gina Oliva of Gallaudet University for contributing the "Hearing Impairment" section of this chapter. Gina is available as a resource to the fitness industry on issues related to exercise in the hearing-impaired.

REFERENCES / SUGGESTED READING

American Association of Cardiovascular and Pulmonary Rehabilitation (1991). *Guidelines for Cardiac Rehabilitation Programs.* Champaign, IL: Human Kinetics Books.

American College of Sports Medicine, (1993). *Resource Manual for Guidelines for Exercise Testing and Prescription.* Philadelphia, PA: Lea & Febiger.

Anspaugh, D. J., Hamrick, M. H., & Rosato, F. D. (1991). *Wellness: Concepts and Applications.* St. Louis, MO: Mosby-Year Book Publishers.

American College of Sports Medicine (1991). *Guidelines for Exercise Testing and Prescription,* Fourth Edition. Philadelphia, PA: Lea & Febiger.

Bar-Or, O. (1989). Trainability of the Prepubescent Child. *The Physician and Sportsmedicine,* 5, 64-82.

Deobil, S. J. (1989). Physical Fitness for Retirees. *American Journal of Health Promotion,* p. 85-90.

Frontera, W. R., Meredith, C.N., O'Reilly, K.P., et al. (1988). Strength conditioning in older men: skeletal muscle hypertrophy and improved function. *Journal of Applied Physiology,* 64(3), 1038-1044.

Frymoyer JW, Pope MH, Clements JH, et al. (1983). Risk factors in low back pain: an epidemiological survey. *Journal of Bone Joint Surgery,* 65A, 213-218.

Hagberg, J. M., et al. (1989). Cardiovascular responses of 70-79 year old men and women to exercise training. *Journal of Applied Physiology,* 66, 2589-2594.

Marcus, R. (1989). Understanding and Preventing Osteoporosis. *Hospital Practice,* p. 189-218.

Pope MH and B Fleming. Biomechanics of Low Back Pain. (1990). *Surgical Rounds for Orthopaedics,* p. 35-42.

Roberts, S. O., & Staver, P. (September, 1992). Fit Kids. *American Health Magazine,* p. 70-75.

Roberts, S.O., Roberts, R.A., & Hanson, P. (Editors) (1994). *Clinical Exercise Testing and Prescription.* Boca Raton, FL: CRC Press.

Roberts, S.O. (1994). Developing Strength in Children: A comprehensive approach. Reston, VA: National Association of Sport and Physical Education.

Roberts, S.O. (with) Weider, B. (1994). *Resistance and Weight Training for Young Athletes.* Chicago, IL: Contemporary Books.

Roberts, S. O. (1993). Trainability of Children: current theories and training considerations. In (M. Leppo, Ed.). *Childhood Fitness: A Multidisciplinary Approach.* Reston, VA: American Alliance of Health, Physical Education, Recreation and Dance.

Rowland, T. W. (1985). Aerobic responses to endurance training in prepubescent children: critical analysis. *Medicine Science in Sports and Exercise,* 17, 493-497.

Seals, D. R. & Hagberg, J. M. (1984). The effect of exercise training on human hypertension: a review. *Medicine and Science in Sports and Exercise,* 16(3), 207-215.

Strong, W. B. (1990). Physical Activity and Children. *Circulation,* (81)5, 1697-1701.

U.S. Department of Health and Human Services. *Healthy People 2000 - National Health Promotion and Disease Prevention Objectives.* DHHS Publication No (PHS) 91-50212. U.S. Government Printing Office. Washington, D.C. 20402.

Zwiren, L.A. (1993). Exercise Prescription for Children. *Resource Manual for Guidelines For Exercise Testing and Prescription.* Philadelphia, PA: Lea & Febiger.

Chapter 12

Exercise and Pregnancy

By Camilla B. Callaway

regnancy is a time for joy, a time for planning and a time for health consciousness. It is also a time when a pregnant student needs good information and guidance regarding exercise. An instructor should be aware of the unique physical and physiological conditions that exist during pregnancy. The adaptations the pregnant body makes for the growth and birth of a baby require continual exercise modifications and adaptations to ensure exercise effectiveness and safety. The objective of the American Council on Exercise is for instructors to be knowledgeable of the special needs of

Camilla Callaway, M. Ed., received her master's degree in Exercise Science from Colorado State University in 1980. She holds certifications from both the American Council on Exercise and the American College of Sports Medicine. Presently, she lectures to expectant mothers and prenatal educators on pregnancy and exercise through the Swedish Employee Wellness Center's Educational Department. She has also been an active volunteer with various committees with the American Council on Exercise.

pregnant women and to provide classes that are well-designed, effective, challenging and, above all, safe. Accordingly, the main purpose of this chapter is to enable instructors to develop such exercise programs for pregnant students and to educate instructors on important issues regarding exercise and prenatal conditions.

BENEFITS

Many benefits are associated with exercise during pregnancy. A realistic, comprehensive, well-designed exercise program may help relieve some of the common problems associated with pregnancy, such as musculoskeletal irritants, constipation, swollen extremities, leg cramps, varicose veins, insomnia, fatigue and excessive weight gain. Exercise during pregnancy may improve posture, reduce backaches, facilitate circulation, reduce pelvic and rectal pressure and increase energy levels. Exercise may assist in controlling gestational diabetes (Clapp, 1992; & Artal, 1992). With a modified exercise program, pregnant women may maintain aerobic fitness, along with muscular strength and flexibility. The sense of well-being often associated with regular exercise programs can be very comforting during the stressful moments of pregnancy. Exercise may increase body confidence and help to ease negative feelings that often accompany pregnancy, weight gain and preconceptions of labor and delivery.

CONTRAINDICATIONS

The safety of the mother and **fetus** is the primary concern in any exercise program during pregnancy. Medical supervision of an exercise program throughout pregnancy is imperative. Each pregnant participant should be evaluated by her primary care physician and advised regarding her personal prenatal exercise

program before returning to class. The student's physician is the most appropriate person to evaluate her fitness status in relation to her pregnancy. Many programs require a signed physician consent-to-exercise form before the student can begin an exercise program. It is inappropriate for an instructor to assume the responsibility of prescribing a prenatal exercise program without physician approval. The first trimester is most crucial in the formation of the fetus, therefore prenatal health care and education should start immediately. Early education on pregnancy and exercise could be handled with a prenatal information packet available for newly pregnant students. Suggested contents for this packet is the American College of Obstetricians and Gynecologist (ACOG) guidelines for pregnant and **postpartum** exercisers. ACOG **contraindications**, both relative and absolute, warrant the participant's concern and physician consultation.

ACOG's relative contraindications include the following: chronic hypertension or active thyroid, cardiac, vascular or pulmonary disease, should be evaluated carefully in order to determine whether an exercise program is appropriate (ACOG, 1994).

ACOG's absolute contraindications include the following: pregnancy-induced hypertension, preterm rupture of membranes, preterm labor during the prior or current pregnancy or both, incompetent cervix/cerclage, persistent second- or third-trimester bleeding and intrauterine growth retardation. A student should also be made aware of the warning symptoms that indicate the need to cease exercise and consult her physician immediately. The list includes pain of any kind, uterine contractions occurring every 15 minutes or sooner, vaginal bleeding or amniotic fluid leakage, dizziness or faintness, shortness of breath, palpitations or tachycardia, persistent nausea or vomiting, back pain, pubic or hip pain, walking difficulty, general edema (swelling), numbness in any body part, visual disturbances or decreased fetal activity (Artal, 1991).

PHYSIOLOGICAL ADAPTATIONS

Research in the pregnancy and exercise area is still in its infancy and is very controversial. There is limited research related to the effects of exercise during pregnancy and the postpartum period, and ethical considerations make certain research impossible. At present, it is best to use moderation when defining the safety limits of exercise.

When instructors prepare beginner students for aerobics classes, they often inform them of the short-term effects of exercise. They discuss how the body will heat up and feel hotter, that since they are using more oxygen their breathing rate will increase, and that their heart rate will rise to help move the much-needed oxygen and nutrients to the working muscles via the blood or circulatory system. What this simplistic statement briefly describes is the adaptations of exercise and the adaptations of pregnancy.

Pregnancy and exercise adaptations instigate many of the same or similar bodily functions. Indeed, all of the increases in functions that exercise promotes—respiratory rate, cardiac output, stroke volume, heart rate, oxygen consumption, blood volume, body temperature, metabolic rate and glucose consumption—are also increased by pregnancy alone. Thus, when exercise and pregnancy are combined, the interaction can produce physiological results that are quite complex and often difficult to predict (Clapp, 1992).

The main goal of exercise is to provide the working muscles with the amount of oxygen and nutrients needed to sustain the new energy level and to find a new, steady equilibrium able to sustain a higher level of functional capacity. Pregnancy takes the body into a new state of activity geared toward the growth and development of the baby. Energy is spent enabling the cardiovascular system, the respiratory system and the reproductive system to each adapt to the necessary level of function required to grow a new life in 40 weeks. Resting oxygen consumption increases gradually and reaches a level near term approximately 20 to 30 percent above prepregnancy levels (Wolfe, 1989; & Artal, 1992). Resting heart rate increases approximately 7 beats per minute (bpm) in the first trimester, peaking at approximately 15 bpm above the prepregnancy rate near the third trimester (Artal, 1992).

A pregnant woman's body is in a constant state of work. The short-term effects of exercise are already present. Now pregnant, she must elevate the components of the oxygen transport system and the metabolic rate to a new, higher level to perform her regular exercise program. Prenatal students usually reduce exercise performance to complement the increased work load under which their body is now functioning. Most studies agree that exercise programs should be moderate in intensity and duration and low in impact.

ADDITIONAL CONCERNS

Blood returning to the heart from the body is known as venous return. Due to increase in blood volume and sensitivities to postural positions, venous return may be impaired or disturbed during pregnancy. **Supine hypotension** is an example of such a disturbance. In the supine position (lying on the back), the weight of the uterus presses against blood vessels, especially the inferior vena cava. This pressure occludes the vessels causing a restriction in the blood flow, which may, in turn, cause a reduction in blood pressure, cardiac output and blood flow to the fetus. Students should be advised to avoid the supine position after the first trimester (ACOG, 1994).

Instructors often have to remind pregnant women that they are supposed to gain weight during pregnancy. Average pregnancy weight gains are between about 27 and 34 pounds; body fat increases an average of 4 to 5 percent (Artal, 1992; & Clark, 1992).

Weight gain increases the work load on the cardiovascular system, the respiratory system and musculoskeletal system; but prevention of normal weight gain may be detrimental since weight gains are predictive of fetal birthweight. Nutritional diets should be designed to provide for the baby's development and appropriate weight gains. Lactating caloric and nutritional needs are still great during the postpartum period. New mothers should not restrict calories for the purpose of quick weight loss. Current research shows that lactation is well-maintained during postpartum physical activity if exercise is gradually introduced and mothers consume a sufficient amount of nutrients (Schelkun, 1991).

FETAL RISKS ASSOCIATED WITH EXERCISE

During exercise, the oxygen transport system analyzes the actions taking place and reacts to provide for the higher level of activity. As a result of this hormonal influence, the blood flow is reallocated to the working muscles. This reallocation of the blood flow causes a reduction in the blood flow to the fetus. During the exercise bout, maternal temperature and metabolic rate will most likely be elevated.

As a result, potential risks to the fetus include **hypoxia** (low oxygen), **hyperthermia** (high temperature), **hypoglycemia** (low blood sugar) and **dehydration** (low water). At this time, most researchers feel that exercise at moderate intensity, duration and frequency poses no problem, but increasing to higher levels could put the fetus at risk in several ways (Uzendoski, 1989; & Huch, 1990).

Blood flow to the uterus is a function of intensity and duration. The higher the intensity or the longer the duration the greater the oxygen need at the muscle site, thus the greater the reduction of blood flow to the fetus. Research has shown the fetus can adjust safely to reductions of blood flow resulting from moderate exercise bouts (Uzendski, 1989). With the reduction of blood flow comes a reduction in what is being transported to the fetus (i.e., oxygen and nutrients), as well as what is being transported away from the fetus (i.e., carbon dioxide, heat and waste products). The following protective adaptations are responses to the decreased blood flow experienced during moderate intensity and duration exercise: an increased hemoglobin level, exercise-induced **hemoconcentration** that provides a higher percentage of oxygen to a lower level of blood volume, an improved ability for oxygen to be released from the hemoglobin present and a postexercise increase in blood flow to the fetus to compensate for the reduced flow during exercise (Schick-Boscheotto, 1991). The risk of greatest concern is temperature regulation. The fetus rids its heat through its blood flow to the placenta. Fetal temperature is contingent upon maternal temperature, fetal metabolic rate and uterine blood flow, with the greater effect stemming from maternal temperature. The higher the intensity of an exercise bout, the higher the maternal temperature and the higher the fetal temperature. Hyperthermia is known to be **teratogenic** (capable of causing birth defects) (McMurray, 1990).

A major concern is for the central nervous system, but other concerns are spontaneous abortion, lower birth weights, increased uterine contractions and **uteroplacental insufficiency**.

Temperatures above 38.9 degrees centigrade (102 degrees fahrenheit) early in pregnancy may cause birth defects, especially to the central nervous system. The type and severity of fetal damage depends on the timing, dosage and duration of the heat exposure (Jones, 1985). Maternal core temperatures are slightly higher than prepregnancy levels and resting fetal temperatures are slightly higher than the mirrored maternal temperature. Retrospective studies searching for a common factor in neural development defects found that heat (hyperthermia) was a major cause. Neural tube defects have been cited due to sensitivity to temperature rises of 2.5 degrees centigrade (4.5 degrees fahrenheit) during the first trimester (Jones, 1985; & Mc Murray, 1990).

It is not uncommon for temperatures to be well above 38.9 degrees centigrade (102 degrees fahrenheit) during high-intensity, long-duration exercise, and this is further increased if the environment includes high temperature or high humidity. For obvious safety reasons, maternal exercise temperatures should be kept below 38.9 degrees centigrade (102 degrees fahrenheit). Maintaining adequate hydration and wearing appropriate clothing will help to dissipate heat and keep temperature down during exercise (ACOG, 1994).

It is important to remember that early pregnancy (during the first trimester), when the mother-to-be feels very little change to her body, is the most critical phase of her pregnancy regarding heat

sensitivity and fetal development. To help prevent overheating during exercise, pregnant students should be advised: (1) to exercise in a cool, well-ventilated, low-humidity environment, (2) to drink plenty of cool water to avoid dehydration, which will contribute to temperature increase, and to (3) maintain a moderate intensity and duration. Less common risks to the fetus during exercise include premature labor and fetal growth retardation. Overstimulation of the uterus, caused by an increase in the hormone norepinephrine, as well as dehydration or hyperthermia, could contribute to the risk of premature labor (Huch, 1990; & Artal, 1991). Impaired fetal growth is possibly caused by decreased glucose stores induced by maternal hypoglycemia. Nutritional goals should reflect the needs of fetal development as well as the maternal exercise program (Clark, 1992).

MUSCULOSKELETAL SYSTEM ADAPTATIONS AND DYSFUNCTIONS

It takes a thoughtful and purposeful plan to teach an effective fitness class. Each exercise instructor intellectually determines the movements in a class. These everyday decisions become more complicated when working with pregnant students. The challenge for instructors is to design and choose exercises that will allow success, comfort and safety for the pregnant student.

Many studies conducted on pregnancy and exercise express concern for increased risk of injury vulnerability. Factors such as added-weight-gain-induced postural realignments, increased joint laxity and muscular imbalances could predispose students to certain irritations and injuries. An understanding of these factors and other alterations to the musculoskeletal system will enable instructors to wisely choose and modify various exercises for the benefit of their pregnant students.

Joint Laxity

To make room for the growth of the fetus and eventually its birth, space is essential. To facilitate the expansion of the uterine cavity the hormone **relaxin** begins to be released during the first trimester. It relaxes the musculoskeletal system by softening ligaments, loosening joints and stretching muscles and tendons. A gentle but effective expansion occurs, providing more space.

Elevated estrogen levels contribute to the relaxin effect and continue this effect through the postpartum lactating period, when relaxin levels have been reduced. The by-product of this hormonal activity is a vulnerable musculoskeletal system.

The ligamentous laxity reduces joint stability, which could increase the chance of sprains, an injury resulting from the overstretching or tearing of a ligament or joint capsule. The loosened joint may eventually become hypermobile.

Postural Realignment

As weight is gained and hormonal influences deepen, postural alignment is altered. The abdominal wall is expanded forward, causing the woman's skeletal structure to lean slightly forward. If not counterbalanced by an anterior pelvic tilt, she could, in theory, topple forward. The pelvis does tilt anteriorly, changing the center of gravity and increasing the lordotic curve of the lumbar spine. The upper back is also realigned due to the increased weight of the breast tissue. The chest and shoulders are pulled forward and inward, increasing the kyphotic curve of the thoracic spine. A forward neck often accompanies these postural deviations and an extreme exaggeration of the vertebral column's normal "S" curve results. This is

known as a kyphotic lordotic postural alignment and is further explained in Chapter 3 "Biomechanics and Applied Kinesiology" (Artal, 1990; & Jacobson, 1991).

Muscle Imbalances

When posture is not in the ideal alignment muscle imbalances are likely to arise. The common muscle imbalances identified in pregnancy are either "tight" (scapula protractors, levator scapula, thoracolumbar area, hip flexors, tensor fascia lata, piriformis, hamstrings, adductors and calves) or "weak" (scapula retractors, low lumbar paravertebral, gluteus maximus and medius, abdominals and quadriceps) (Wilder, 1988).

Muscle imbalances play a dominant role in choosing floor-work exercises for class. Prenatal classes should be designed to reduce these muscle imbalances, which will, in turn, help reduce the postural deviations. When dealing with muscle imbalances, it is more effective to first relax the tightened muscles through stretches and mobility exercises and then follow with strengthening exercises for the weaker muscle groups.

When students are unable to perform certain exercises because of discomfort or irritation, an instructor should react to the short-term situation by modifying exercises to reduce such difficulties. When discomfort or irritations persist, the student must realize that she may need to cease the activity in order to rest the area and to prevent further aggravation. In all cases, the student should communicate concerns to her physician. In severe cases in which discomfort becomes chronic, consulting a physical therapist specializing in prenatal care should be considered.

Dysfunctions and Irritations

The following section provides a summary of common dysfunctions and irritations, including backaches, pelvic-floor weakness, **diastasis recti**, ligament strain, pubic pain, **sciatica**, muscle cramps, nerve compression and overuse syndromes. While suggestions of exercise modifications are touched upon, detailed exercises are found later in this chapter.

Backaches. The most frequent complaint during pregnancy is backaches. About one half of pregnant women develop pain in the low-back area. For a long time, this lumbosacral pain has been considered a side effect of pregnancy that one has to endure. Now it is believed that better body mechanics, exercise, massage, relaxation and physical therapy can help reduce and possibly prevent backaches.

As noted previously, postural realignments during pregnancy contribute heavily to the incidence of backaches. The typical posture of a pregnant woman is characterized by an exaggerated curved lower back, rounded upper back and a forward head.

Exercises appropriate for this situation should focus on reducing the improper alignment. Mobility and stretching exercises should emphasize relaxing and lengthening the back extensors, hip flexors, shoulder protractors, shoulder internal rotators and neck flexors. Strengthening exercises focused on the abdominals, gluteals and scapula retractors will reinforce their ability to support proper alignment.

Gentle reminders to students are helpful to maintain proper alignment throughout each section of class whether it be low-impact, aqua or floor work. To practice maintaining a neutral pelvis, instruct students to strengthen the muscles that tilt the pelvis posteriorly (i.e., the abdominal and gluteal muscle groups). The gluteal muscles should be pulled downward and together with an upward pull of the abdominals. This motion should reduce the anterior pelvic tilt position.

Various cues, such as heads up, shoulders back, buttocks tight, belly buttons up or abdominals hugging baby may communicate alignment to students. Even a simple question, "How does that low back feel?" may stimulate better posture. Breaks during class for pelvic tilts and other back-relaxer exercises can be pleasant aides.

Aside from postural alterations that bring on back pain, other factors that may contribute to the condition are increases in relaxin, hypermobility of the sacroiliac joint, improper body mechanics, **vascular disturbances** (a particular cause of nighttime back pain), **transient osteoporosis** from dietary calcium deficiency and psychosocial stress (Hummel-Berry, 1990).

Pelvic-Floor Weakness. The five layers of muscle and fascia attached to the bony ring of the pelvis are commonly referred to as the **pelvic floor**. From superficial to deep layers, they are as follows: the superficial outlet muscles, urogenital triangle, pelvic diaphragm or levator ani muscles, smooth muscle diaphragm and endopelvic diaphragm. They support the pelvic organs like a sling to withstand all the increases in pressure that occur in the abdominal and pelvic cavity and provide **sphincter** control for the three **perineal** openings (Noble, 1988).

There are fascial connections between the levator ani muscles, the sacroiliac ligaments, the hip rotator muscles and the hamstrings. This connection allows weaknesses of the pelvic floor muscles to refer stress to these areas. Pelvic-floor weaknesses can cause the pelvic alignment to falter and thus irritate the sacroiliac joint and the hip joint (Wilder, 1988). It is crucial that these muscles function competently. In addition, prolapse of the bladder, uterus or rectum may develop if muscles become too weak to support the pelvic organs. Finally, urinary **incontinence** can often be initiated during pregnancy because of pelvic-floor weakness.

Kegel exercises are designed to strengthen the pelvic floor and assure its proficient function. (see exercise prescription section). The benefits of strengthening the pelvic floor are: providing support for the heavy pelvic organs; preventing prolapse of the bladder, uterus and rectum; supporting pelvic alignment; reinforcing sphincter control; enhancing circulation through a congested area of the vascular system; and providing a healthy environment for the healing process after labor and delivery (Dunbar, 1992).

Diastasis Recti. The partial or complete separation of the rectus abdominis muscle as a result of the linea alba widening and finally giving way to the mechanical stress of an advancing pregnancy (or during delivery) is known as **diastasis recti** (Wilder, 1988). The linea alba, a tendinous fiber that merges the abdominal muscles with the fascia, extends from the xiphoid process to the symphysis pubis (see Chapter 2, "Fundamentals of Anatomy").

Diastasis recti is most common during the third trimester and immediately postpartum and is attributed to the following influences:

1. Maternal hormones. **Relaxin, estrogen** and **progesterone** encourage the connective tissue to become less supportive. There is a loosening effect upon the abdominal fascia and a reduction of the cohesion between the collagen fibers.

2. Mechanical stress within the abdominal cavity. This varies according to fetus size and number, placenta size, the amount of amniotic fluid, the number of previous pregnancies and the amount of weight gain. The abdominal musculature is designed to function in a vertical direction of shortening and lengthening, but pregnancy needs are for the abdominal wall to expand horizontally, and it is not normally elastic in the transverse direction. This incompatible situation introduces unbearable mechanical stress that can end in functional failure for the abdominal wall. After a slow deformation of the soft tissue, the final separation is often caused by a sudden forceful action, such as jackknifing out of the bed without proper body mechanics.

3. Weak abdominal muscles. A correlation may exist between diastasis recti and weak abdominal muscles. Women with strong abdominal musculature are considered more prepared to resist this condition (Boissonnault, 1988). Other predisposing factors include heredity, obesity, multiple-birth pregnancy, a large baby, excess uterine fluid and a lax abdominal wall from former pregnancies.

Proficient prenatal instructors may test for diastasis recti. The most common test is performed by placing two fingers horizontally upon the suspected location while the student lies supine with knees bent. Have her perform a curl-up. If the fingers are able to penetrate the location there is probably a split. The abdominal muscles can be felt to the side of the split. The degree of separation is measured according to the number of finger widths of the split. Finger width is equated to centimeters. A separation of more than 2 centimeters above the umbilicus or 1 centimeters below the umbilicus is considered a diastasis. Any separation or widening is cause for modifications to the exercise program (Bursch, 1987; & Wilder, 1988).

Ironically, certain types of abdominal exercises may actually introduce susceptibility. Exercises to avoid are those that put direct pressure on the linea alba from within, due to uterine resistance, and from without, due to the gravitational resistance. Because of this pressure, it is suggested that abdominal curl-ups be performed in a semirecumbent position rather than supine.

When a separation occurs it is frequently detected by the student noticing an unusual bulge along the center line of her abdominal wall. Instructors should advise students to watch for such occurrences. Consulting a physician is necessary to confirm the occurrence and to be advised as to how to continue the exercise program.

Round, Inguinal and Broad Ligament Irritations. The round, inguinal and broad ligaments are the most common ligaments to be irritated or strained during pregnancy. The **inguinal ligament** is formed as the fascia of the internal oblique, the external oblique and transversus abdominis blend together at their lower margin. It runs between the pubic tubercle and the anterior superior iliac spine. As the abdominal wall expands, the inguinal ligament is also stretched. It continues to be stretched throughout the pregnancy, slowly adapting with the abdominal-wall expansion. This constant state of tension can easily turn into a spasm with an increase in abdominal pressure resulting from a cough, sneeze or laugh.

Workouts must be flexible to the present state of ligamentous tension. On days that the student feels vulnerable, intensity of the workout and stretch put on the ligament should be reduced. Sensitivity is common with abdominal exercises and inner- and outer-thigh exercises. When performing abdominal exercises try to relieve the tension by keeping the knee and hip joints bent, the knees rolled to the side and the curling height low. With hip abduction and adduction the knee and hip joints should again be slightly bent. This places the inguinal ligament in a more relaxed position and also reduces the leverage of the leg. Avoid quick shifts of body position, especially changing from right to left side-lying positions. Prepare the body to change positions by warming joints with pelvic tilts, maintaining proper alignment

and using arms to help lift the body from the floor. The round and broad ligaments directly support the uterus within the pelvic cavity. The **round ligament** connects to both sides of the uterine fundus and extends forward through the inguinal canal and terminates in the labia majora (Fig. 12.1). The round ligament may be irritated with extreme stretches above the head, rapid twisting movements, or jackknifing off the floor or bed. Before initiating such activities, the area should be properly warmed. The use of proper mechanics for lying down and rising up will also prevent strain on the round ligament (Fig. 12.2). Lifting heavy loads from the floor to high shelves may cause strain. In the exercise arena, women may experience discomfort when the round ligament is jostled from jogging or jumping. If irritation is felt at the onset of exercise, the warm-up period may need to be lengthened. An effective warm-up for

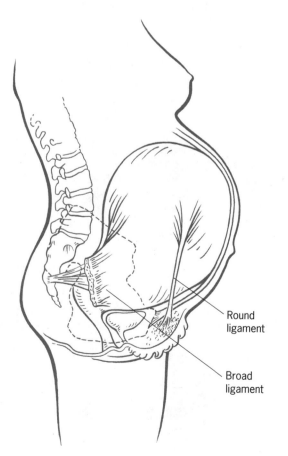

Figure 12.1

Round and broad ligaments.

Round ligament

Broad ligament

Chapter 12
Exercise and
Pregnancy

the inguinal ligament, the round ligament and the abdominal wall may contain torso range-of-motion activities, pelvic tilts and an effleurage massage. (An effleurage massage is a very light, stroking movement, done here by placing the fingertips upon the pubis and sliding them upward along the linea alba, then sliding them down both sides of the abdominal wall near the round ligament location, gently rubbing along the inguinal ligament and meeting at the pubis to begin the circular motion again). The largest ligament supporting the ovaries, as well as the uterine tubes, uterus and vagina, is the **broad ligament**. It connects the lateral margins of the uterus to the posterior pelvic walls. The pull it receives from the enlarged uterus can cause a severely arched and aching low back.

Focus in class on this ligament should be relaxation. Pelvic tilts, the cat stretch, trunk flexion exercises, self-massage of the low back plus torso range-of-motion movements can all help to relieve tension in the broad ligament as well as in the back extensor muscles. Help encourage students to avoid exaggerating the arch of the low

back, to maintain good postural alignment and to use good body mechanics.

Pubic Pain. As the growth of the fetus demands more space, the pelvis accommodates by expanding. Unfortunately, this expansion does not happen without consequence. The loosened ligaments that allow this necessary expansion also allow increased motion. The irritation of the pubic **symphysis** caused by the increased motion at the joint is called symphysitis (Wilder, 1988). This irritation may be worsened by exercise. Ice (RICE technique) may be used to relieve immediate irritation (see Chapter 13, "Musculoskeletal Injuries" for RICE guidelines). A physician consultation is advised and physical therapy may be ordered. Pelvic belts, which compress the pelvis and minimize motion in the symphysis pubis and sacroiliac joint, may be prescribed in severe cases. Partial symphyseal separations and complete dislocations are possible during pregnancy, as well as pubic stress fractures. They usually result from delivery and therefore, are of more concern for postnatal students.

When pubic pain occurs with students, efforts to alleviate irritation will determine the choice of activity and exercise. Exercises using hip adduction and abduction,

Figure 12.2a-c
Proper body mechanics for rising up from the side-lying position to the sitting position.

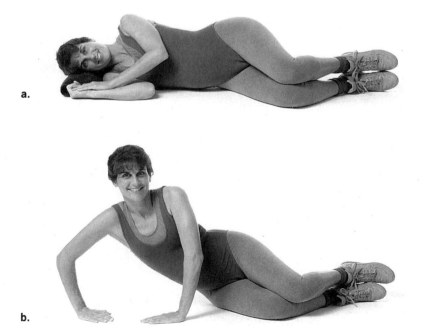

a.

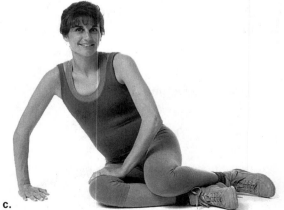

b.

c.

and, to a lesser extent, hip extension, can cause further irritation of the pubis. The relationship of the tendons to the hip joints during hip abduction, adduction and extension, may cause excessive movement of the pubis, which intensifies the pain. Appropriate modifications are to reduce hip joint exercises to a level of tolerance or to avoid pain completely. Perform standing hip abduction and extension exercises to reduce symphysis pubis irritations. Reduce impact and weight-bearing factors of aerobic activities and suggest aqua aerobics, swimming or stationary biking.

Shoe quality is important to mention to these students; walking, jogging or dancing in worn-out shoes can worsen joint irritations. If relief is not successful, students should be advised to cease all pain-producing activity.

Sacroiliac Joint. Fifty percent of all back pain is related to lumbosacral pain (Hummel-Berry, 1990). The sacroiliac joint functions to resist the anterior pelvic tilt accentuated by the increase in lumbar lordosis due to the uterine growth and pregnancy weight gain. To facilitate the passage of the fetus through the pelvis relaxin is released to soften the normally rigid ligaments of the sacroiliac joint and symphysis pubis. The postural adjustments, pulling the pelvis anteriorly, in conjunction with the hormonal relaxation effect, ultimately combine to force the sacroiliac ligaments to give, to stretch and to possibly become hypermobile (Daly, 1991).

Symptoms of sacroiliac dysfunction include pain during the following activities: prolonged sitting, standing or walking; climbing stairs; standing with weight on one leg; or twisting activities (Lile, 1991). The pain is usually unilateral (on one side) and in some cases radiates to the buttocks, lower abdomen, anterior medial thigh, groin or posterior thigh (Daly, 1991). Students may complain of having pain in the sacroiliac area when they stand up out of a chair or when they get out of bed. The pain is felt at the sacroiliac joint, then radiates into the buttocks, but it does not radiate down the leg as characteristic with sciatica.

Exercises should be chosen to add strength and support to the sacroiliac area, and to facilitate pelvic stability. If the lumbosacral angle (the angle between the

Figure 12.2d-f
Proper body mechanics for getting up from the floor.

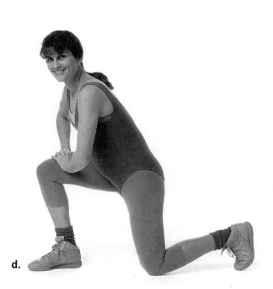

d.

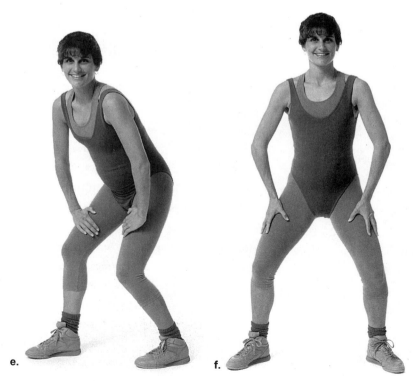

e.

f.

lumbar vertebrae and the sacrum) is reduced, pain will usually be reduced. The gluteal muscles add the most direct support, but endurance exercises for the abdominals are also helpful. Abdominal endurance assists in preventing the anterior pelvic tilt that is straining the sacroiliac joint and ligament. Suggestions for class include accentuating proper postural alignment, using abdominal compression exercises throughout class, and using standing hip extension and abduction exercises. All of the preceding actions should incorporate pelvic stability (refer to hip exercises in floor-work section of this chapter). Participants with severe cases should be advised to see their physician who may order a consultation with a physical therapist specializing in backs or obstetrics for additional treatments and orthotic devices.

Sciatica. Pressure placed upon the sciatic nerve from fetal position or postural structures can produce nerve irritation that is extremely painful. A woman experiencing pain that radiates from her buttocks down to her legs is probably experiencing sciatic nerve irritation. Exercise can do little to relieve this situation. Students may be advised to note previous activities that preceded the irritation and in the future avoid that activity or review the body mechanics used during an aggravating activity. Pelvic tilts may offer some immediate relief by shifting the irritating pressure away from the nerve. After experiencing a sciatic nerve irritation, the gluteal and hamstrings muscles will respond by tightening. Gently stretching these muscles can help to relax them out of this protective response.

Nerve Compression Syndromes. More than 80 percent of pregnant women have some degree of swelling during their pregnancy. Soft-tissue swelling may decrease the available space in relatively constrained anatomical areas. The result of this constricted space and fluid retention is nerve compression syndromes or, less commonly, compartment syndromes. Nerve compression syndrome is possible in many areas that have a compressed nerve compartment. The most prevalent nerve problem during pregnancy is carpal tunnel syndrome. It results from compression of the median nerve within the wrist. Complaints of numbness and tingling sensations of the thumb, index and middle fingers are characteristic. Avoiding hyperextension and maintaining the wrist joint in its neutral position is suggested. A related nerve compression syndrome is tarsal tunnel syndrome or posterior tibial nerve syndrome, which involves cramping and compression of the calf. Complaints may stem from numbness of the inside of the ankle to the medial plantar aspect of the foot. Thoracic outlet syndrome results from compression and aggravation of the brachial plexus. Tingling and numbing sensations may be felt down the arms and hands. Postural deviations with internally rotated shoulders can aggravate the situation. Exercises to encourage shoulder external rotation and stretches to reduce shoulder internal rotation should be added to the workout regime to balance the muscles. Weight of the breast tissue needs to be supported with a strong bra to reduce any forward pull of the shoulders.

During class always facilitate circulation with moving, pumping muscles. Joint range-of-motion exercises, especially at the wrist and ankle joints, help reduce fluid retention and should be included in class.

Another suggestion is to avoid long periods of standing and sitting; take breaks at work to walk around if sitting, or sit and elevate the feet, if standing. This helps to reduce stagnate circulation from lack of movement. While working at a desk for long periods of time use a box to periodically elevate the feet.

The same suggestion is useful for long periods of standing. Advise students to lie on their left side with feet slightly elevated, such as side-lying on a sofa with feet elevated on the sofa arm, whenever possible. This position is the most efficient at facilitating the venous return and reducing fluid retention (swelling). Drinking plenty of water and reducing salt intake may prevent excessive fluid retention. Severe swelling and fluid retention can indicate other medical conditions related to pregnancy besides contributing to nerve compression. Therefore, such a condition should be reported immediately to the primary physician.

Overuse Syndromes. Weight gain, postural changes and hormonal influences create a perfect environment for producing overuse syndromes. Many common overuse syndromes associated with exercise are intensified by these adaptations of pregnancy. Chondromalacia, a gradual degeneration of the articular cartilage that lines the back surface of the patella, can become irritated and inflamed because of the poor alignment stress placed upon the knee joint. Pain can become incapacitating. Classes should include strengthening exercises for the quadriceps muscles to add support to the knee joints, and extra attention should be given to maintaining proper knee alignment during these exercises. Hyperflexing the knee when bearing weight can accentuate the aggravation. Alignment is an especially important issue in stepping activities in which the repetitive motion could easily result in improper alignment as the student becomes fatigued.

The feet may become flatter and more pronated due to weight gain. When the feet are not striking properly, it can cause further alignment deviations in the hips and knees. Plantar fasciitis, an inflammation of the plantar fascia, the broad band of connective tissue running along the sole of the foot, may result from the improper foot placement. Advise students to avoid wearing worn or unsupportive shoes.

Muscle Cramps. Awaking abruptly to a muscle cramp can be very painful and frustrating. This is not an uncommon experience for pregnant women and many pregnant women do not know how to relieve them. Advise students to avoid extreme pointing of the toes (plantarflexion), high heels and tight shoes. All of these may stimulate muscle cramping. To relieve a muscle cramp, put the muscle in a stretched position and hold it there until the sensation subsides. For example, with a hamstring cramp straighten the knee, for a calf cramp straighten the knee and dorsiflex the foot, and for a foot cramp dorsiflex the foot and spread the toes.

EXERCISE CLASSES AND PROGRAMS FOR PREGNANT WOMEN

Whether a pregnant exercise student wishes to be integrated into an exercise class of nonpregnant women—perhaps a class she has already been in—or joins a class especially designed for pregnant women, it is the exercise instructor's responsibility to be aware of any pregnant woman's new physical status and to make appropriate individualized adjustments for that student.

If, for instance, an exercise class meets midday in a poorly ventilated area of a club located in a humid locale, and a regular student tells the instructor about her new pregnancy, the instructor will want to talk to the student—whatever her fitness level—about the dangers of hyperthermia and suggest alternative classes.

Similarly, pregnant women in higher altitude locales should be cautioned about hypoxia, while those who have been in high-impact aerobics classes should be

Chapter 12
Exercise and
Pregnancy

steered into less jarring programs.

For many instructors in large-city environments, the greatest challenge may well be just knowing who, if anyone, is pregnant in a class. Many women well into their second trimester may not "show." So unless an instructor actually mentions to her class from time to time her need to know about pregnancies, she may not find out about any for quite awhile.

Specialized classes for pregnant women obviously have several benefits over integrated classes. Participants can be individually monitored better for such things as strain, discomfort and fatigue. In addition, the prenatal exercise class is a natural support group with discussions of many pregnancy-related issues and help in maintaining stress control, self-esteem and body confidence.

In both specialized and integrated classes, however, there should be communication between the instructor and pregnant women about a range of subjects, including sufficiency of warm-up time, needed modifications of exercises, intensity of movements, perceived exertion, weight gain and comfort and pain levels.

Instructors should always be mindful of possible conditions such as hyperthermia, hypoxia, hypoglycemia and musculoskeletal injuries. Any exercise activity should be stopped if the student finds it overly diffi-

cult to perform, if it causes discomfort, pain or embarrassment from feeling big and clumsy.

Floor Work

All exercises should be done with a smooth and controlled speed and a range of motion that allows one to maintain proper alignment and comfort. If any exercise stimulates discomfort it should be immediately discontinued. Special attention should be given to teaching proper body mechanics when lying down and rising up from the floor (Fig. 12.2).

Neck. Neck range-of-motion activities help to reduce tension. After muscles are warmed, stretch the sternocleidomastoid, levator scapula and the upper trapezius to further relieve tension and reduce the forward head position associated with poor postural alignment. During this segment it is important to keep some movement in the legs to facilitate circulation. Complete the neck stretches with an examination of proper head and neck alignment (refer to discussions related to spinal alignment in Chapter 3, "Biomechanics and Applied Kinesiology").

Shoulder Girdle. To correct suspected muscle imbalances, begin with a warm-up and stretch of the scapula elevators, scapula protractors and shoulder internal rotators. Balance this with scapula retraction of the rhomboids, middle trapezius and lower trapezius exercises. Body placement during scapula retraction exercises can reduce the chance of low-back extension; a slight lunge such as used when stretching the calf muscles is perfect. The abdominals and gluteals function as pelvic stabilizers and need to be incorporated in this workout to prevent hyperextension of the lower back. Shoulder external rotation exercises improve postural alignment by widening and opening the chest area. These also

Figure 12.3
Back alignment may be facilitated by placing a towel roll just under the tailbone to slightly tilt the pelvis anteriorly.

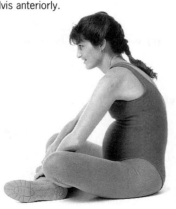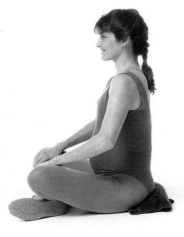

reduce the constriction of the brachial plexus, a negative element associated with thoracic outlet syndrome.

Shoulder and Elbow Joints. The workout of the anterior, middle and posterior deltoids, pectoralis major and the latissimus dorsi may proceed as usual. The biceps and triceps also do not need extensive modification. Maintaining functional ranges of motion during exercises, especially when weights are being used, will help prevent overlengthening muscles, tendons and ligaments of vulnerably loose joints. Body placement and positioning, chosen for various exercise performances, should facilitate circulation and promote proper alignment. Many arm exercises can be performed in combination with other exercises, such as standing leg work or stretches. If performed in a sitting position, back alignment may be facilitated by placing a towel roll just under the tailbone, which will tilt the pelvis slightly anteriorly and adjust for the rounded back (Fig. 12.3). Sitting on the edge of a bench may be another comfortable sitting position while focused on the shoulder and elbow joint muscles.

Wrist Joint. A small amount of time should be allocated to wrist range of motion to promote circulation in a tight compartment area. Finger motion may also be performed to reduce the swelling of this stagnate, peripheral, circulatory area. These movements can be used during arm

exercises or choreographed into the aerobic segment.

Low Back. These muscles are often tight and strained from the weight of the uterus pulling the abdominal wall and pelvis forward, resulting in the exaggerated lumbar lordosis posture. The class goal for this area is to relax these muscles to improve posture and decrease possible back pain. Range-of-motion exercises may be used to warm these muscles, followed by stretches to encourage them to lengthen and relax. Back range of motion consists of flexion, extension, lateral flexion and rotation. The many possible exercises and stretches include side bends, twists, standing back roll, pelvic tilts, pelvic rotation, pelvic side lifts, cat stretch, lateral rolls, tail wags, modified press-up, cross backs, knee to chest stretch and knee rolls (Fig. 12.4).

Abdominal Wall. This area, in particular, seems to be of concern to instructors. The concern is probably derived from attempting to maintain abdominal strength while avoiding supine hypotension and diastasis recti. Concern is definitely warranted since most abdominal workouts are performed in the vulnerable supine position. Exercising in the supine position may induce supine hypotension syndrome and place immense mechanical stress on the abdominal wall, especially along the linea alba. Positioning students in a semirecumbent position removes the constricting uterine pressure from the inferior vena cava and

Figure 12.4
The cat stretch.

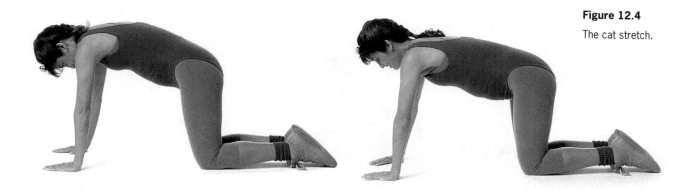

aorta blood vessels and reduces the direct gravitational strain on the linea alba. Many of the conventional abdominal exercises may be easily modified into the semirecumbent position (Fig. 12.5). For additional support to the linea alba, the abdominal wall may be splinted with crossed arms and hands (Noble, 1988). Stress to the inguinal ligament is reduced when the hip and knee joints remain flexed and rolled to the side, as with the semirecumbent position. Besides the usual curl-up abdominal exercises, experiment with various pelvic-tilt and abdominal-compression exercises. This group of exercises is essential for maintaining postural alignment and pelvic stability. They may be performed in a variety of positions, ranging from standing to the all-fours position. Abdominal compression should be combined with other exercises throughout class to help maintain proper pelvic alignment.

Pelvic Floor. Introducing Kegel exercises to students is mandatory. There are numerous routines for performing Kegel exercises. For example, begin with an isometric contraction of the pelvic floor, feel the muscles lift and tighten, hold it for a slow count of 10, then relax the muscles for another count of 10 and repeat again. Another exercise is to imagine an elevator going up and down, as the pelvic floor is lifted. Stopping the elevator on each floor is a variation that requires more muscle control (Nurse Practitioner, 1985; & Noble, 1988).

Kegel exercises can be placed in class along with abdominal and gluteal exercises. It is just a matter of cueing them appropriately. For example, initiate a semirecumbent curl-up, lift for 2 counts, hold for 2 counts, incorporating a Kegel during the hold for 2, then lower for 2 counts and repeat the sequence again. Suggest each student choose a cue to remind themselves to Kegel outside of class; when they brush their teeth, talk on the phone, cough, sneeze or laugh, they can be cued to Kegel. A suggested workout program of initially four daily sets of 10, working up to four daily sets of 25, seems reasonable. Kegel exercises should not be used to prevent natural urination (Wilder, 1988).

Hip Flexors. The hip flexor muscles are often tight as a result of the prenatal posture. The fact that people tend to spend a large part of their day sitting causes them to shorten. Therefore, the emphasis in class is to stretch and relax them.

Hip Extensors. The role of the hip extensors is to oppose the hip flexors' pull of the pelvis anteriorly and to assist the abdominals in their role of tilting the pelvis posteriorly. In assisting with the posterior pelvic tilt, it also helps alleviate the strain being placed on the sacroiliac joint. Standing may be a more comfortable position for gluteus maximus workouts, since it seems to place less stress on vulnerable areas. The common all-fours and side-lying positions often place strain on the symphysis pubis, inguinal ligament, sacroiliac joint and the lumbar spine, and therefore may be replaced with the standing position. To facilitate support for the sacroiliac joint, hip extension exercises are used to strengthen the gluteal muscles. In order to recruit more muscle fibers from the gluteal muscle group, perform hip extensions while the hip joint is abducted, adducted or externally rotated (Fig. 12.6). Abdominal compres-

Figure 12.5

The semirecumbent position easily replaces the supine position for abdominal exercises.

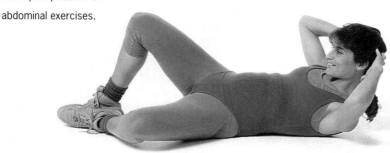

sion should be included in the exercises to assist in maintaining pelvic stability.

Hip Abduction. To promote more fiber recruitment of the gluteal muscles, perform hip abduction while the hip is extended and/or externally rotated in addition to the neutral position. This is another exercise that offers indirect muscle support to the sacroiliac joint. Incorporating abdominal compression will assist in maintaining a stable pelvis. A towel roll may be used to support the neck and the abdominal wall, and thus maintain body alignment when lying sideways (Fig. 12.7). If the inguinal ligament or the symphysis pubis is sensitive, the hip and knee joints should be flexed during hip abduction. This repositioning reduces the leverage weight and puts the inguinal ligament in a more relaxed position. Standing may be a more comfortable position for hip abduction. If irritation still occurs, then that exercise should be deleted from the workout until comfortable performance can be achieved.

Hip Adductors. Because of the anterior tilt position of the pelvis, the tendons of the hip joint muscles are pulled slightly forward. The hip adductors, inner-thigh muscles, may become tensed and strained in this new alignment. During hip adduction exercises, strain may occur in nearby vulnerable areas, such as the symphysis pubis, the groin area or the inguinal ligament. If exercises cause a significant amount of stress on these areas, the student may complain of discomfort during or after class. Modifications for hip adductor work may relieve the stress. Sidelying hip adductor exercises may be conducted with minute variations, such as use of a towel roll to promote body alignment (Fig. 12.8). By bending the hip and knee joints, less stress is placed on the inguinal ligament, symphysis pubis and hip joint because of the more relaxed position and reduced leverage. Preference for whether the top leg goes behind or over the working leg, as well as whether the torso lies touching the floor or is lifted and supported by a towel roll, varies

Figure 12.6

Standing hip exercises. These exercises should all be performed in conjunction with a posterior tilt of the pelvis triggered by abdominal and gluteal contractions.

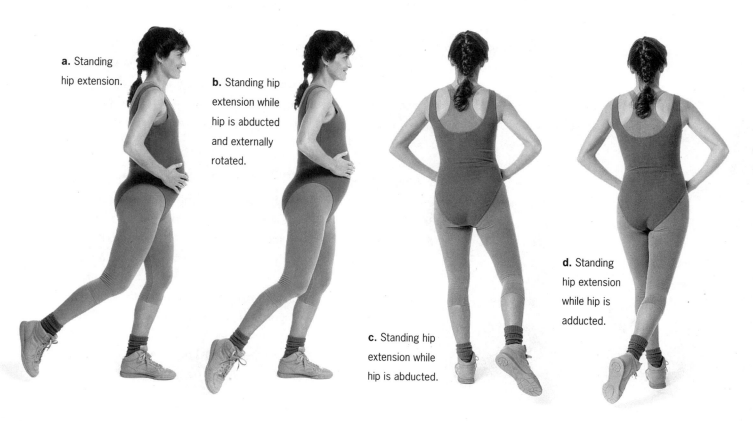

a. Standing hip extension.

b. Standing hip extension while hip is abducted and externally rotated.

c. Standing hip extension while hip is abducted.

d. Standing hip extension while hip is adducted.

Chapter 12
Exercise and
Pregnancy

among students. All positions should be manipulated to maintain alignment. The butterfly sitting position for hip adduction may be used as an alternative position (Fig. 12.9). It is less intense, but possibly less irritating to those sensitive to most hip adduction exercises. The supine position is not recommended for hip adduction workouts because of supine hypotension repercussions. If irritation becomes chronic with every adductor exercise, then adductor exercises should be deleted from the workout until comfortable performance can be achieved.

Quadriceps/Knee Extension. An important muscle group to strengthen is the quadriceps. The daily body mechanics of a pregnant woman are of utmost importance due to the easily strained back and joints. Strength in this muscle group better equips her for the squatting and bending necessary in her daily activities. Things such as getting out of a chair take on new dimensions with the pregnant body. The abdominal wall may limit the ability to lean forward and stand, thus legs and arms must assist more to rise. Exercises that incorporate daily activities are most helpful. They not only train the muscles, but also educate students on proper body mechanics when performing simple activities with a sometimes awkward pregnant body. Pretending to be picking up a 2-year-old, taking groceries out of the car, opening lower drawers, vacuuming or any other daily scenario may be utilized. Safety for the knee joint is the same as with all populations, but remember a greater weight load is be-

ing carried. Deep knee bends or squats past 90 degrees of flexion should be avoided. Students should remain around a comfortable 45 degrees of flexion. Avoid hyperflexion of the knee while bearing weight because of the extreme pressure this places on the knee joint.

Hamstrings/Hip Extensors and Knee Flexors. The hamstrings may be tighter during pregnancy due to postural adaptations, such as the anteriorly tilted pelvis. Range-of-motion activities and stretches may be implemented to reduce tightness. The common supine hamstring stretch may be replaced with a standing or side-lying hamstring stretch to avoid discomfort and supine hypotension.

Ankle Joint. The main goals for this joint are to facilitate circulation and maintain flexibility. Warm-ups should include stimulation of the calf muscles and the anterior lower leg muscles. Ankle range-of-motion activities may help reduce swelling in the ankles by promoting venous return. Avoid extreme plantarflexion or pointing of the toes in all exercises. This can easily initiate a calf muscle cramp, which may be relieved by dorsiflexing the ankle to stretch the calf muscles. A pleasant activity for cool-down or relaxation is self-foot massage. The pregnant woman's feet are overloaded with her natural weight gain, and a massage can be very soothing.

Aerobic Exercise

The prenatal aerobics program must reflect the new state of the woman's cardiovascular system, respiratory system, reproductive system, metabolic rate and the fetal developmental needs. The competing demands on these systems between exercise and pregnancy must be recognized and adjusted for.

In 1985, ACOG devised guidelines for exercising during pregnancy (Table 12.1).

Figure 12.7

A towel roll may be used to support the neck and to facilitate proper alignment.

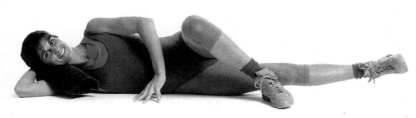

The purpose of these guidelines was to meet the concerns of a new population of pregnant women in the fitness boom. Women wanted to continue their exercise programs but were eager to know what effects, if any, it would have on their babies' safety. Physicians were not always prepared for this question. ACOG devised an exercise prescription for pregnant women that would satisfy the American College of Sports Medicine's (ACSM) recommendations for healthy adult cardiorespiratory fitness, but would not place the fetus at risk for hyperthermia, hypoxia or hypoglycemia. ACOG's guidelines meet the minimal requirements of the ACSM recommendations for cardiorespiratory fitness. In 1994, ACOG revised the guidelines for exercising during pregnancy (Table 12.1) with the understanding that, in the absence of medical complications, women who engage in moderate physical activity can maintain their cardiovascular and muscular fitness during and after their pregnancy. ACOG's prescription has become the standard of care for exercising during pregnancy.

Many studies disagreed with the restrictions of the 1985 guidelines, indicating that they may not be appropriate for the athletic population or the very sedentary population. The following recommendations provide a safe workout program that will maintain cardiorespiratory fitness levels.

The aerobic-exercise warm-up should gradually increase muscle temperature through general body movement and joint range-of-motion activity. Give special emphasis to stimulating those areas under mechanical stress from pregnancy—the abdomen, pelvis, back and hips.

The rate of perceived exertion scale (RPE) may be used to monitor exercise intensity. Fairly light to somewhat hard (12 to 14 on the 6- to 20-point Borg scale) is a recommended range for pregnancy. RPE may prove a more reliable method for measuring workout intensity because of changes in the maternal resting heart rate and maximal heart rate (Pivarnik, 1991; & White, 1992).

The final form of a student's prenatal exercise program should be individualized and physician-approved. This information should be passed on to the instructor and his or her supervisor. When conducting a prenatal exercise class or advising prenatal students, it is recommended that all programming and information be consistent with the ACOG guidelines. Of special note are the importance of a good warm-up period and the use of low-impact aerobic exercises.

Water Exercise

The favorite exercise modality from a research standpoint is most likely water activities. Hyperthermia is a primary factor of concern with pregnancy and exercise, and in the water, body temperatures appear to rise less and dissipate sooner (McMurray, 1990). Because of the hydrostatic effects of water, submaximal exercise in water is associated with a smaller **plasma** volume decrease than that with exercise on land, which may result in better maintenance of uterine and placental blood flow (Watson, 1991).

Temperatures could negate the benefits. Pool water should feel cool when first

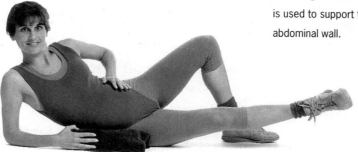

Figure 12.8

Hip adduction is performed with both the knee and hip joints bent to reduce the leverage of the leg. A towel roll is used to support the abdominal wall.

Table 12.1

ACOG GUIDELINES FOR EXERCISE DURING PREGNANCY AND POSTPARTUM

Recommendations for Exercise in Pregnancy and Postpartum

There are no data in humans to indicate that pregnant women should limit exercise intensity and lower target heart rates because of potential adverse effects. For women who do not have any additional risk factors for adverse maternal or perinatal outcome, the following recommendations may be made:

1. During pregnancy, women can continue to exercise and derive health benefits even from mild-to-moderate exercise routines. Regular exercise (at least three times per week) is preferable to intermittent activity.

2. Women should avoid exercise in the supine position after the first trimester. Such a position is associated with decreased cardiac output in most pregnant women; because the remaining cardiac output will be preferentially distributed away from splanchnic beds (including the uterus) during vigorous exercise, such regimens are best avoided during pregnancy. Prolonged periods of motionless standing should also be avoided.

3. Women should be aware of the decreased oxygen available for aerobic exercise during pregnancy. They should be encouraged to modify the intensity of their exercise according to maternal symptoms. Pregnant women should stop exercising when fatigued and not exercise to exhaustion. Weight-bearing exercises may, under some circumstances, be continued at intensities similar to those prior to pregnancy throughout pregnancy. Non-weight-bearing exercises such as cycling or swimming will minimize the risk of injury and facilitate the continuation of exercise during pregnancy.

4. Morphologic changes in pregnancy should serve as a relative contraindication to types of exercise in which loss of balance could be detrimental to maternal or fetal well-being, especially in the third trimester. Further, any type of exercise involving the potential for even mild abdominal trauma should be avoided.

5. Pregnancy requires an additional 300 kcals per day in order to maintain metabolic homeostasis. Thus, women who exercise during pregnancy should be particularly careful to ensure an adequate diet.

6. Pregnant women who exercise in the first trimester should augment heat dissipation by ensuring adequate hydration, appropriate clothing, and optimal environmental surroundings during exercise.

7. Many of the physiologic and morphologic changes of pregnancy persist 4 - 6 weeks postpartum. Thus, prepregnancy exercise routines should be resumed gradually based on a woman's physical capability.

Contraindications to Exercise

The aforementioned recommendations are intended for women who do not have any additional risk factors for adverse maternal or perinatal outcome. A number of medical or obstetric conditions may lead the obstetrician to recommend modifications of these principles. The following conditions should be considered contraindications to exercise during pregnancy:

- Pregnancy-induced hypertension
- Preterm rupture of membranes
- Preterm labor during the prior or current pregnancy or both
- Incompetent cervix/cerclage
- Persistent second- or third-trimester bleeding
- Intrauterine growth retardation

In addition. women with certain other medical or obstetric conditions, including chronic hypertension or active thyroid, cardiac, vascular or pulmonary disease, should be evaluated carefully in order to determine whether an exercise program is appropriate.

Source: ACOG (1994). Reprinted from Exercise During Pregnancy and the Postpartum Period with permission from American of Obstetricians and Gynecologists.

entered. If it feels like bath water, it is probably too warm (Karsenec & Grimes, 1984).

The pressure of water appears to lessen fluid retention and swelling, two common discomforts of pregnancy. The prone position in swimming actually facilitates optimum blood flow to the uterus, by redistributing the weight of the uterus away from the inferior vena cava and the aorta. A positive attribute of water classes is the buoyancy effect of water, which increases comfort by supporting their weight and reducing their clumsiness and trouble with balance. This wonderful weightless feeling can be a major relief to the pregnant woman. Water exercises can be easier on the musculoskeletal system, with minimal strain placed on the joints of the body. Swimming and other water-oriented movements place muscles in a more relaxed, non-weight-bearing position, allowing relief to those muscles bearing extra mechanical stress and pressure from the pregnancy.

Strength and Endurance Training

Strength training can be safe during pregnancy if a student remembers the standard safety rules of weightlifting. Safety suggestions for working with weights are to stay in control of the weights, move through a functional range of motion, breathe during the lifts, use slow, appropriate speeds for the exercise and avoid the Valsalva maneuver and the supine position (Work, 1989; & Sinclar, 1991). Problems could arise if the student tends to jerk, swing, speed or basically be out of control when she is lifting. Form is of the utmost importance during pregnancy because of the effect of relaxin. Functional range of motion should match prepregnancy range to protect the joints from injury or irritation. The supine position is to be avoided to reduce the risk of supine hypotension. Women should train with light weights 2 to 5 kilograms (5 to 10 pounds) and decreased repetitions. Overhead lifting should be avoided to prevent irritation or injury to the low back (Artal, 1992). Endurance training is recommended for pregnant students to help prepare them for carrying, lifting and nurturing their infant. In the weight room, endurance training can be achieved by reducing weights to

a resistance that allows 15 or more repetitions. The safety rules for strength training noted above should be applied to endurance training.

Programming Suggestions and Modifications

The following suggestions and modifications may be implemented as needed to further individualize programming for the prenatal exerciser. Design longer warm-ups to soothe vulnerable areas, such as the inguinal, round and broad ligaments. Always demonstrate and emphasize proper alignment to be used throughout class. Keep legs moving while standing to stimulate sluggish venous return. Choose positions to give a student the best workout within her comfort zone while maintaining proper body alignment. Supine positions may be replaced with semirecumbent positions and prone positions with an all-fours position or an elbows-and-knees position. All of these positions may be easier with the use of towel rolls or pillows to help maintain body alignment. Changing positions often in class may facilitate circulation, but be aware that moving simply from the left side to the right side can be a strain if good body mechanics are not used. There are an infinite number of floor-work exercises for each muscle of the body. Use cre-

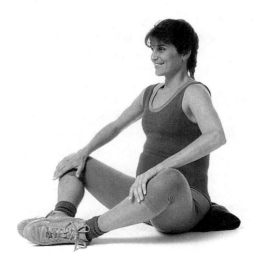

Figure 12.9

The butterfly sitting position for hip adduction.

ativity to discover exercises to train muscles without causing discomfort for the pregnant student. Experiment with methods to challenge students appropriately. Muscle groups may be worked in a weight-bearing or non-weight-bearing position to vary the resistance. When working legs and arms use short levers by flexing knees, hips and elbows to create less stress and strain on vulnerable ligaments and joints. The most demanding instructional area is the abdominal wall. Taking a conservative approach to this muscle group can provide a workout that increases the strength needed for maintaining proper posture, the pushing phase of delivery and deterring diastasis recti. Lastly, introduce pregnant students to Kegel exercises.

The prenatal exerciser presents many interesting challenges to a fitness instructor. From the initial warm-up through the final cool-down numerous factors must be considered to make an exercise program both safe and effective for the pregnant exerciser. Table 12.2 summarizes an entire prenatal class format in the form of substitute instructor guidelines.

POSTNATAL EXERCISE

Returning to exercise after delivery is like going backward through pregnancy. The situation is similar to the relationship between a warm-up and cool-down; they mirror each other, but in reverse. So all the things a woman does to prepare and endure pregnancy continue to be done in the postpartum period to slowly return to prepregnancy status. If the postnatal student is advised before delivery, certain postnatal exercises may begin at home after the delivery. When the new mother feels ready and receives her doctor's approval, she may return to her class. The first priority after delivery is to bond with one's baby. The second priority

is to start Kegeling as soon as possible. The pelvic floor has been traumatized during delivery, by either severely stretching or by an episiotomy. Kegels after delivery may be a little scary, since the incision may be felt. Postoperative nurses should assure patients that Kegeling will help the healing process of the pelvic floor. Before thinking about doing other exercises, such as sit-ups, the pelvic floor should be rehabilitated.

Suggest that students gradually return to exercise activities. Short walks will enable postpartum students to get some fresh air and release tension. If they have been in bed for awhile, it is sometimes hard to rest even though they are exhausted. Short walks may release stored energy and tension and enable them to rest comfortably. General body movement, range-of-motion activities or isometric muscle contractions followed by stretching are other ways to relieve tension or energy buildup. The preceding suggestions could be done in the bed, bath or shower.

Posture and back pain are still a concern in the postpartum period. The weight of the uterus is no longer pressing against the abdominal wall, but the abdominal wall is now loose and nonsupportive to the low back. For low-back health, continue the low-back exercises and range-of-motion activities discussed in the floor-work section of this chapter. Back extension, through the press-up exercise, may be added in the postpartum period. The use of good body mechanics is crucial during this hectic, new period. Poor body mechanics, postural adjustments, in combination with the fatigue experienced by a new mother, can easily predispose her to back pain. Breast weight is increased for lactation, which pulls the shoulders and scapula forward, exaggerating the thoracic kyphotic (cuddling) posture. Prior to delivery, students should be instructed on shoulder external rotation

Table 12.2

PRENATAL CLASS FORMAT (SUBSTITUTE INSTRUCTOR GUIDELINES)

Please! *Watch each individual student* for signs of stress, strain, discomfort fatigue and/or disgust. Always be prepared to show modifications of exercises for each student's personal needs. The instructor must ask her if she needs modifications.

Warm-up	General movements to increase muscle temperature.	
	Normal joint range of motion (ROM): Neck, shoulders, wrist, pelvis, hips, knees and ankles.	
	Emphasis on back, pelvis and hip joints.	
	Stimulate postural alignment.	
	Keep movements slow, controlled, comfortable.	
	Gradually increase ROM.	
Nonimpact Aerobics	Intensity	Heart rate—100 to 140 bpm.
		Breathing rate, conversational.
		Perceived exertion, fairly light to somewhat hard.
		Perspiration level—glowing.
	Duration	Depends on each participant's fitness level.
	Mode	Nonbouncy, nonjerky, rhythmical.
		Contract-relax, smooth, flowing.
		Large, controlled ROM of arms and legs.
		Maximize traveling, minimize standing in place.
		Avoid quick changes of direction.
Cool Down I	Easy pumping leg movement to facilitate circulation (Ankle ROM, anterior lower leg stimulated).	
	Stretches—easy positions, not to maximum resistance.	
Body Work (Muscular strength, endurance and flexibility)	Positions	Varied to promote circulation (standing, sitting or side-lying).
	Upper Body	Deltoids, triceps, pectorals, biceps, middle and lower traps (stimulate scapular retraction and posture here and throughout class).
	Lower body	Quadriceps, hips (extension, abduction and adduction in controlled repetitions, keep knees and hips slightly bent to eliminate strain to commonly irritated areas).
	Abdominals	Avoid supine position.
		Slow repetitions, smaller ROMs, low lift, knees and hips bent, predominately from side.
		Pelvic tilts with emphasis on lower abdominals.
	Additional	Exhale during contraction, inhale as relaxing.
		Remember modifications for those with diastasis recti.
		Pelvic tilts as well as back ROM exercise (e.g., cat stretch) are welcomed throughout class whether standing, sitting or lying.
Cool Down II	Final stretching, low-back stretch.	
	Relaxation, visualizations, deep breathing.	
	Neck ROM and stretches.	
	Normalize circulation for standing.	

and scapula retraction exercises for the postpartum period.

Postpartum students are usually very anxious to begin abdominal workouts. Pelvic tilts and abdominal compression exercises may be initiated soon after delivery. It is advisable to tighten the pelvic floor during abdominal exercises. Abdominal compression may place pressure upon the pelvic floor if it is loose, causing it to stretch and weaken. As the pelvic floor begins to normalize, various curl-up exercises may be gradually added. Diastasis recti is still a concern after delivery. Students should be advised to examine their abdominal wall for this abnormality. Noble's splinting abdominal exercises are a cautious first choice for early abdominal curl-up exercises (Noble, 1988). To balance the abdominal workout, complete it with back extension and scapula retraction exercises. The prone position may be uncomfortable in the postpartum period because of the weighted breast. The all-fours position and the elbow-and-knees position should be avoided until the pelvic floor has healed and normalized. The over-stretched vaginal opening may be vulnerable in these latter two positions. The standing position or side-lying position may be used for hip extension, abduction and adduction exercises.

The suggested time for returning to aerobic activities is after the students postpartum doctor's appointment. This commonly takes place six weeks after delivery. Before this appointment, walking for aerobic fitness benefits is suggested. Factors that may determine postpartum return include complications of labor and delivery, uterine involution, pelvic-floor healing, pre-pregnancy fitness levels and self-motivation. Initially, non-weight-bearing aerobic activities are suggested. As the body heals and strengthens, weight-bearing aerobic activities may be added. When a student returns to her prenatal class, advise her to gradually re-enter, to prevent doing too much too soon, a common cause for muscle soreness and overuse injuries. Remind the student to listen to her body, exercise comfortably hard but not to overdo it. For additional information on postpartum exercise guidelines, refer to ACOG's guidelines.

REFERENCES

American College of Obstetricians and Gynecologists. (1994). *ACOG Technical Bulletin.* Washington, D.C.

American College of Sports Medicine (1990): The Recommended Quantity and Quality of Exercise for Developing and Maintaining Cardiorespiratory and Muscular Fitness in Healthy Adults. *Medicine and Science in Sports and Exercise.* 22 :265-274.

Artal, R. (1992). Exercise and Pregnancy. *Clinics in Sports Medicine.* 11 (2).

Artal, R. et al. (1990). Orthopedic Problems in Pregnancy. *The Physician and Sportsmedicine,* 18(9).

Artal, M.R. et al. (1991). *Exercise in Pregnancy.* Baltimore: Williams and Wilkins.

Boissonnault, J.S. & Blaschak, M.J. (1988). Incidence of Diastasis Recti Abdominis During the Childbearing Year. *Physical Therapy,* 68(7).

Bursch, Gail S. (1987). Interrater Reliability of Diastasis Recti Abdominis Measurement. Polyform Products Inc., 67(7).

Clapp III, J.F. et al. (1992). Exercise in Pregnancy. (S294-S300). *Medicine and Science in Sports and Exercise.* 24(6).

Clark, N. (1992). Shower Your Baby With Good Nutrition. (39,40,45) *The Physician and Sportsmedicine.* 20(5).

Daly, J.M. et al. (1991). Sacroiliac Subluxation: A Common, Treatable Cause of Low-Back Pain in Pregnancy. *Family Practice Research Journal,* 11(2).

Dunbar, A. (1992). Why Jane Stopped Running. (4,5) *The Journal of Obstetric and Gynecologic Physical Therapy.* 16(3).

Huch, R. & Erkkola, R. (1990). Pregnancy and exercise—exercise and pregnancy. A short review. (208-214) *British Journal of Obstetrics and Gynecology.* 97.

Karsenec, J. and Grimes, D. (1984). *Hydrorobics.* Leisure Press.

Hummel-Berry, K. (1990). Obstetric Low Back Pain: Part I and Part II. *The Journal of Obstetric and Gynecologic Physical Therapy*. 14(1) 10-13 and 14(2) 9-11.

Jacobson, H. (1991). Protecting the Back During Pregnancy. *AAOHN Journal*, 39(6).

Jones, R. et al. (1985). Thermoregulation During Aerobic Exercise in Pregnancy. *Obstetrics and Gynecology*. 65(340)

Lile, A. & Hagar, T. (1991). Survey of Current Physical Therapy Treatment for the Pregnant Client With Lumbopelvic Dysfunction. *Journal of Obstetric and Gynecologic Physical Therapy*. 15(4).

McMurray, R.G. et al. (1991). The thermoregulation of pregnant women during aerobic exercise in the water: A longitudinal approach. *European Journal of Applied Physiology*. 61.

McMurray, R.G. and Katz, V.L. (1990). Thermoregulation in Pregnancy, Implications for Exercise. *Sports Medicine*, 10(3).

Noble, Elizabeth. (1988). *Essential Exercises for the Childbearing Year*, Third Edition. Houghton Mifflin Company Boston.

Nurse Practitioner. (1985). Kegel Exercise. (33-34) *Nurse Practitioner*.

Pivarnik, J.M. et al. (1991). Physiological and perceptual responses to cycle and treadmill exercise during pregnancy. (470-475) *Medicine and Science in Sports and Exercise*. 23(4).

Schelkun, P.H. (1991). Exercise and Breast-Feeding Mothers. (109-114) *The Physician and Sportsmedicine*. 19(4).

Schick-Boschetto, B. & Rose, N.C. (1991). Exercise in Pregnancy Review. *Obstetrical and Gynecological Survey*. 47(1).

Sinclair, M. (1992). In training for motherhood? Effects of exercise for pregnant women. *Professional Nurse*. May.

Uzendoski, A.M. et al. (1989). Short Review: Maternal and Fetal Responses to Prenatal Exercise. *Journal of Applied Sport Science Research*. 3(4).

Watson, W.J. et al. (1991). Fetal Responses to Maximal Swimming and Cycling Exercise During Pregnancy. (381-386) *Obstetrics and Gynecology*. 77(3).

Wilder, E. (1988). *Obstetric and Gynecologic Physical Therapy*. Churchill Livingstone. New York, Edinburgh, London, Melbourne.

Wolfe, L.A. et al. (1989). Physiological Interactions Between Pregnancy and Aerobic Exercise. (295-351) *Medicine and Science in Sports and Exercise*. Supplement.

Work, J.A. (1989). Is Weight Training Safe During Pregnancy? *The Physician and Sportsmedicine*. 17(3).

SUGGESTED READING

Artal, M.R., Wiswell, R.A., and Drinkwater, B.L (Ed.) (1991). *Exercise in Pregnancy*. Baltimore: Williams and Wilkins.

Noble. (1988). *Essential Exercises for the Childbearing Year*, Third Edition. Houghton Mifflin Company Boston.

Sol, N. (1991). Modifications of Health Conditions and Special Populations. In M. Sudy (Ed), *Personal Trainer Manual: The Resource for Fitness Instructors*. (pp. 335-356). San Diego: American Council on Exercise.

Wilder, Elaine. (1988). *Obstetric and Gynecologic Physical Therapy*. Churchill Livingstone. New York, Edinburgh, London, Melbourne.

Part IV
Instructor
Responsibilities

Chapter 13

Musculoskeletal Injuries

By Marjorie J. Albohm

The injuries and conditions commonly associated with aerobic exercise can be extremely disabling. If not prevented or treated properly, they can stop a person from participating altogether. To prevent aerobic exercise injuries, the various causes of such injuries and their proper management must be thoroughly understood. The primary cause of aerobic exercise injuries is overuse—placing too much stress on one area of the body for an extended time. When stress is applied the body can either adapt by becoming stronger, or it can fail and break down

Marjorie J. Albohm, M.S., A.T., C., is coordinator of sports medicine and director of orthopaedic research at the Center for Hip and Knee Surgery, Mooresville, IN. She is a faculty member at the Indiana University School of Medicine. The sixth woman in the nation certified by the National Athletic Trainers Association, she has served on the medical staff at the 1980 Winter Olympic Games and the 1987 Pan American Games, and at many other national and international events.

(Fig. 13.1). Excessive, repeated stress causes failure, which usually results in **chronic injury.** Chronic problems have a gradual onset, without history of a specific incident of injury. They last for several weeks, often becoming neither better nor worse. There may be symptoms of discomfort, swelling, or limited motion.

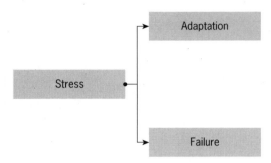

Figure 13.1

Overuse syndrome

If a chronic injury continues to be stressed, it may become an **acute injury,** which occurs when an area already stressed and weakened is pushed beyond its limits and further injured. Acute injury has a more sudden onset, usually characterized by a specific incident at a point in time. The symptoms are specific pain, specific swelling, limited motion, and inability to use the injured area in a normal function. Shin splints, for example, are considered a chronic overuse problem. However, if they are ignored and activity levels are not reduced, the continual stress to the shin area can cause a stress fracture, which may become an acute problem. Acute injuries may also occur without being related to chronic injuries, as in an ankle sprain. This specific injury can be the result of sudden impact, a fall or incorrect movement that immediately disables the person.

It is important to recognize the various causes of stress placed on the body during aerobics so that activities can be modified to avoid straining a particular area to failure. The locations that receive the most stress in aerobic exercise are either the most active or subject to the most stress, they are the shoulders, feet, ankles, lower legs and the knees.

FACTORS ASSOCIATED WITH INJURY

There are many factors associated with injury in an aerobics class. A class with a low rate of injury will have a safe workout environment, proper footwear, proper exercise technique, and good instructional supervision. These factors are discussed below. Other factors, such as a good warmup and proper exercise progression, are discussed in Chapter 7.

Floor Surface

Exercising on nonresilient surfaces is a common cause of injury. Some surfaces absorb two and a half times a person's body weight during dance exercise. An unyielding surface, such as concrete, will not absorb shock effectively, and so the feet, shins, and knees will receive more stress. The ideal floor surface provides both cushion and stability. Injuries are highest on a concrete floor covered with carpet. Wood floors over airspace, which are slightly springy, are the best surfaces. Heavily padded concrete floors covered with carpet also seem to reduce injuries.

If classes must be held on inadequate floor surfaces, instructors should tailor routines accordingly. For example, on a surface such as a thick carpet that may improve shock absorption but sacrifices stability, the routine should reduce or eliminate the twisting or sliding movements that may cause participants to catch their feet in the carpet and fall or twist an ankle. On a nonresilient surface, such as limited carpet over concrete in a church basement or recreation center, the instructor should use low-impact routines during the aerobics segment. (See Chapter 7 for a discussion of low-impact aerobics.) If the program and budget permits, foam mats can be provided to participants for running and jumping activities. Only high-quality mats should be used, however. A slick surface, seams, or low spots resulting from point-pressure breakdown can cause participants to trip.

Platform Surface

Due to the increased popularity in step aerobics it is important to consider the platform surface with respect to safety and injury prevention. Surfaces must be covered with "nonslip" materials. Platforms should be constructed with slightly resilient materials allowing them to "give" with body weight and impact.

Shoes

Shoes are as important as floor surfaces for shock absorption and injury prevention. In addition to dissipating the impact of weight-bearing physical activity, the athletic shoe is designed to provide external support to prevent lateral instability and related foot, ankle, and knee injuries. A single shoe suitable for all fitness-related activity is obsolete. While running shoes and court shoes may be better than none at all, aerobic-exercise shoes are really preferable; they are essential for preventing activity related injuries. A good aerobics shoe will have the following features:

Shock absorption. For aerobic exercise, the most important feature of a shoe is its ability to absorb shock, especially in the forefoot and heel areas where much of the impact occurs. The midsole portion of the shoe is the heart of the cushioning system and should contain a layer of high-density, shock-absorbing material. The surface area of the heel should also contain such material since this location receives considerable impact during step aerobics.

Because shock-absorbing qualities are built into the shoe, this feature is sometimes difficult to assess in the store. The best test is to try on the shoes and jump up and down, both on the toes and flat-footed. The sensation of impact with the floor should be firm, but not jarring. Ask the salesperson about special absorbing materials, which should extend to the toes.

Because the arch absorbs shock, shoes should also provide support to the inside long arch (innerlongitudinal arch) and to the ball of the foot (metatarsal arch) (Fig. 13.2). The insole (sock liner) of the shoe provides a contoured foot bed which is designed to provide proper arch support and shock absorption. The quality and design of insoles vary significantly from shoe to shoe. Too high an arch will be uncomfortable, and too little will not cushion the arch against shock impact. Evaluate and inspect the insole before shoe purchase.

Participants with certain foot types or activity patterns may need additional shock-absorbing material or arch support. Com-

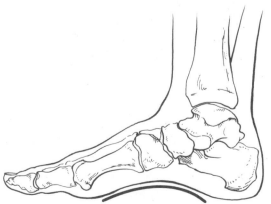

Figure 13.2

Arch support for aerobics shoes.

mercial inserts are available at local athletic footwear stores, or custom orthotics may be prescribed. It is advisable, however, to consult a medical specialist trained in managing foot and ankle problems before adding inserts to aerobic shoes. Unnecessary support or cushioning can create foot instability and cause injuries rather than prevent them.

Lateral support and stability. Many features of a shoe contribute to its stability. The shoe must have an outsole wide enough to provide a solid platform for the foot. A rigid heel counter is necessary to hold the foot in place and provide stability to the ankle. The upper material of the shoe should be supportive and should be reinforced at the forefoot to keep the foot from slipping sideways. The shoe should feel generally stable during all phases of aerobic exercise, including jumping on the toes, jumping from side to side, and twisting with the foot flat on the floor.

Flexibility at the ball of the foot. The ball of the foot is the only area in which an aerobics shoe should be flexible. General flexibility or flexibility in the rear-foot is not desirable. Some manufacturers add rubber toe guards to keep the toe area stable. It is important to check that these guards do not inhibit the flexibility of the shoe. An aerobics shoe should bend in the same place a foot bends—in the ball of the foot, about one third of the way down from the toes.

Fit and comfort. Overall fit and comfort are extremely important, but they are also extremely subjective. The shoe should be long enough that the toes do not touch the end, even when the foot spreads or swells slightly during prolonged exercise. The shoe should be wide enough to accommodate the foot comfortably in both the forefoot and heel, and it should be free of irritations or pressure points.

High Top vs. Low Top. Mid-cut and high-top shoes offer the potential for increased stability, lower incidence of heel slippage, and better accommodation of orthotic devices. However, consumers must not be mislead into thinking that they will provide additional stability. Although hightop aerobics shoes may provide a feeling of additional support to the ankle, it is unlikely that they will significantly prevent ankle sprains. A high-top shoe may not be strong enough to keep the ankle from withstanding force and turning inward or outward.

What may be the right aerobics shoe for one person may be wrong for another. People with high-arched feet tend to require greater shock absorption, while people with flat feet tend to require shoes with greater support and heel control, and heavier participants may require shoes with firmer midsoles. The best approach is for both instructors and participants to try on several shoes from reputable manufacturers and to buy shoes suitable for their own activity patterns, floor surfaces, and foot types.

Frequency and Length of Participation

High-intensity activity, done frequently over a long time, will have a cumulative

Figure 13.3

A squat that produces an angle at the knee joint of less than 90 degrees is considered high-risk.

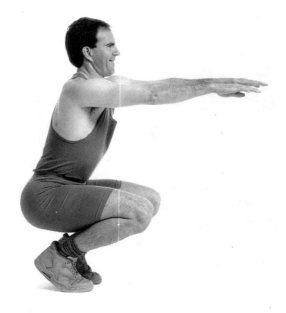

stressful effect on the body. Injury rates increase when people exercise more frequently. Also, the longer someone participates in aerobic exercise, the greater the chance of injury. Instructors are more affected than students because they usually exercise more frequently over a longer period. To prevent injury, it is advisable to participate in classes no longer than one hour and no more than three to four days per week. Beyond that level the risk of injury increases.

Exercise Technique

Improper exercise technique may also contribute to overuse stresses. Unilateral high jumping or kicking in excessive repetition may create greater stress than the lower extremities can accommodate. Instead, the instructor should emphasize lower jumps, hops, or jogging. Alternate left and right sides after each repetition during weight-bearing activities, and limit repetitions to no more than four on each side at one time. Perform every exercise through its full range of motion, unless otherwise indicated. Remember, high-impact activities do not significantly increase aerobic output, but they do increase injury risk. Weight-bearing activities may have to be modified if injury symptoms develop.

Modifications. It is often simple to modify exercise movements to prevent injury. Any exercise that consistently causes discomfort or pain should be eliminated or modified. Assess the mechanics and technique of new exercises before they are introduced to a class. Listen to participants' comments about exercises and watch their techniques at all times. Discuss common injury problems with participants before they occur to emphasize prevention.

Some individual modification of movements may be necessary if a participant has a particular condition or injury. Again, movements that cause pain or discomfort to the injured area should be eliminated and alternative exercises should be provided. For example, if weight-bearing activity is painful, suggest low-impact or nonimpact aerobic exercise activities, as well as swimming and biking.

High-Risk Exercises

Several high-risk exercises and techniques should never be performed in an aerobics class. These exercises are frequently linked with the injuries described later in this chapter. Follow the suggested modifications to ensure safety.

Full squats adversely affect the knee joint by stretching it to a fully opened position that supports the entire body. This position puts extreme stress on the supporting ligaments of the joint, weakening it over time and possibly causing chronic degenerative problems in the knee. Modification: keeping the knees at a 90-degree angle or greater and the hamstrings parallel to the floor is a safe and effective way to condition the thigh muscles. Performing squats with less than a 90-degree angle at the knee joint is a high-risk exercise (Fig. 13.3).

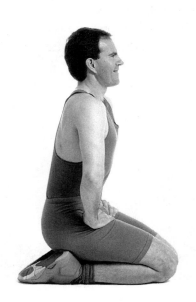

Figure 13.4

Knee sitting—a contraindicated position.

Chapter 13
Musculoskeletal
Injuries

Additionally, make certain that the knee is directly over or slightly behind the toes to avoid patellofemoral problems. Perform this exercise with a slow, controlled descent and a moderate speed ascent.

Knee-sitting (Fig. 13.4) produces effects similar to that of full squats. The knee joint is stretched open under the stress of body weight. This position stretches the ligaments and can produce joint instability. A participant with any history of knee problems should never perform this exercise. Modification: Refer to alternative quadriceps stretching exercises to ensure safety.

Back hyperextension exercises (Fig. 13.5) put abnormal stress on the low back (lumbar spine), causing possible vertebral fractures or dislocations over time. Avoid arching the back to any degree more than that produced by raising the chest while keeping the abdomen in contact with the floor. Modification: Substitute back extension exercises for hyperextension exercises. These may include simple "press-up" exercises (Fig. 13.23).

Hurdler's stretch (Fig. 13.6) is commonly performed in many classes and places a great deal of stress on the medial ligament in the knee of the back leg. When the medial ligament is overstretched, pain and joint instability may occur. Modification: The following exercise can accom-

plish the same effect without risking injury: Sit with one leg in front and the opposite knee bent toward the body; lean the upper body forward to the point of tightness, and hold.

Full neck circles may cause excessive movement of the cervical vertebrae and may contribute to degenerative changes in them. This exercise may also cause dizziness in some participants. Modification: Specific flexion and side-to-side lateral movements of the low neck accomplish the same purpose as full neck circles, without the risk.

Straight-leg sit-ups (Fig. 13.7) should never be performed in an aerobics class. Sit-ups in this position place great stress on the iliopsoas muscles. Strong to begin with, their overdevelopment may cause low-back pain and the development of an abnormal lumbar curve. Modification: To strengthen the abdominals, do curl-ups with the knees bent, abdominal crunches, and reverse curls.

Forward trunk flexion with hyperextended knees (Fig. 13.8) places the body in a potential injury-producing situation. The hamstrings are in an extreme stretch and are pulling the knees into a hyperextended position that places them under extreme stress. The position also compresses the intervertebral discs of the spine. Low-back pain may result as well as posterior knee pain. Rotating the trunk

Figure 13.5

Back hyperextension—a contraindicated exercise.

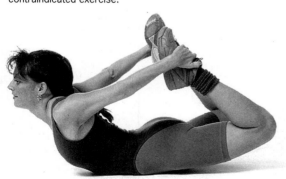

Figure 13.6

Hurdler's stretch—a contraindicated exercise.

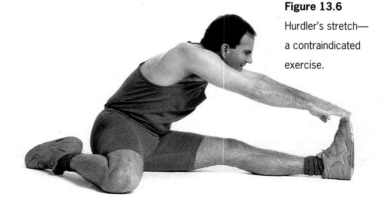

in this position, as in windmill exercises, can be even more dangerous because it creates increased pressure on the discs. Modification: The modified hurdler's stretch or the supine hamstring stretch may be safer alternatives.

A grand plié (Fig. 13.9) may cause excessive stress on the knees and the surrounding musculature if done incorrectly. This stress may be felt on the medial side or on the anterior aspect of the knee if weight is not distributed properly. The ligaments may stretch and, over time, gradual degenerative changes may affect the bony surfaces. This exercise may be appropriate for a ballet class, but it should be avoided in an aerobics class. Modification: Participants can perform partial pliés, not utilizing a full squat, without risk of injury. Remember to keep the knees aligned directly over or slightly behind the toes, not forward of the toes to prevent patellofemoral disorders. Perform these exercises in a controlled manner.

The plough (Fig. 13.10) puts great stress on the cervical and thoracic vertebrae, compressing some of the vertebrae and causing the supporting ligaments of others to stretch. Extending the legs overhead adds the load of the body's weight to these stressed areas. Although some participants may choose to do this yoga exercise on their own, it is not appropri-

ate for a large dance-exercise class. Modification: The low back and trunk may be stretched through simple, controlled trunk rotation exercises. The hamstrings may be stretched through the modified hurdler's stretch.

Contraindicated Techniques

It is important to remember that proper technique is essential to prevent injuries. Proper exercise techniques must always be taught, emphasized, and practiced. Remember, students tend to mimic the instructor's style. Keep all movements controlled. Avoid ballistic movements which often rely on momentum rather than controlled muscular contractions.

When performing step aerobics be sure that the platform height is appropriate for each participant's skill level. Make certain that all exercises are performed through a full range of motion. Step exercises should be performed with complete knee extension with each step. Repetitive movements in a constant flexed-knee position may lead to patellofemoral disorders.

Be cautious when utilizing hand-held weights during step exercise. Be sure that minimum resistance is utilized (1 to 2

Figure 13.8

Forward flexion with
hyperextended knees—
a contraindicated
exercise.

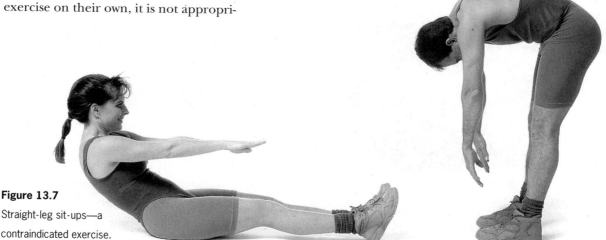

Figure 13.7

Straight-leg sit-ups—a
contraindicated exercise.

pounds) and that all movements are performed with proper technique in a slow, controlled manner.

Quality of Instruction

A good instructor is as important as all the other injury-prevention factors. Proper aerobics instruction and proper direct supervision of participants is of primary importance in reducing the risk of injury. Good instructors must be trained in exercise physiology, anatomy, kinesiology, basic first aid, and injury management. They must have a thorough understanding of all aspects of aerobics. They determine technique, intensity, and effective injury prevention. Mirrors surrounding the dance floor are an excellent device to help participants and instructors monitor exercise technique and form. (See teaching techniques in Chapter 8).

To ensure safety, a thorough medical history should be obtained from each participant. It should document previous significant injuries or illnesses, current medical restrictions, and problems encountered with previous exercise. At-risk participants should obtain a medical release from their physician before they enter the class. (Chapter 5, "Health Screening")

Figure 13.9

Grand plié is contraindicated when the upper leg falls below a line parallel to the floor as shown.

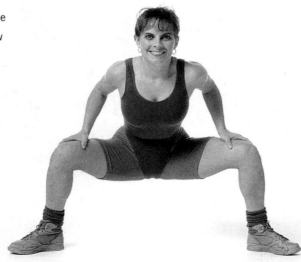

Each aerobics class should begin with a slow warm-up period emphasizing stretching and muscle flexibility. The aerobics phase should begin gradually, slowly raising the heart rate, and usually continuing for 20 to 30 minutes. For most participants, aerobic benefits are minimal after 30 minutes, and injury risk is greatly increased. Heart rate should be frequently monitored throughout the aerobic activity, and participants should often be reminded to breathe properly. Strength exercises should include biceps, triceps, abdominals, quadriceps, hamstrings, abductors, abductors, and gluteal.

A cool-down is necessary to lower the heart rate and help prevent muscle injury and soreness. A gradual decrease in intensity and a gradual change of body position are necessary during this phase to prevent lightheadedness or faintness. If the class has been exercising on the floor, they should stand up slowly. The instructor should emphasize relaxed, deep, even breathing to return heart rates to normal. (See Chapter 7 for a discussion of warm-up and cool-down.)

GENERAL INJURY GUIDELINES

Even with good aerobics shoes, a resilient floor surface, and proper exercise technique, injuries will happen occasionally in a dance-exercise class. Remember that only a physician can diagnose an injury and prescribe specific treatment. There are, however, general guidelines for managing injuries among participants.

RICE. Swelling, caused by bleeding or inflammation in and around the injured area, is the body's response to injury. If swelling is controlled and minimized, the injured area is less painful and normal movement can be resumed sooner.

Swelling is best controlled by the treatment of Rest, Ice, Compression and Elevation (**RICE**). Resting may be accomplished by modifying an activity (for example, switch from weight-bearing to non-weight-bearing activities after an injury to feet or legs) until symptoms subside. Ice, compression and elevation (ICE) should be applied for 20 to 30 minutes at a time, as often as possible, during the first 48 to 72 hours after injury. If the injury is chronic, ICE should be applied after every activity session or whenever swelling occurs.

Acute Injuries. When a participant has an acute (new) injury such as an ankle sprain, the instructor can recommend RICE and advise the person to see a physician immediately. Before returning to class, the participant should provide a written physician's clearance for resuming exercise activity.

Chronic Injuries. A participant who has a chronic problem, with a gradual onset of symptoms, should be advised to use the RICE treatment and to avoid any activity that causes pain in the affected area. If specific symptoms persist for three to five days or suddenly worsen, the participant should see a physician immediately. If a participant asks for the name of a physician specializing in sports injuries, the instructor should always provide two or three names, not just one. Participants should make their own choices.

Warning Signs. If any of the following signs and symptoms persists for more than three to five days, the participant should not be allowed to continue full participation in the class without seeing a physician and obtaining a medical clearance:

1. Specific point-tender pain on or around a bony area. If an area of pain one or two fingers wide is located directly on or close to a bone, suspect a fracture. This principle applies to all areas of the body. The participant should have the area x-rayed as soon as possible.

2. Radiating pain. Any time pain moves (travels or radiates) up or down a body part, a nerve or nerves are probably involved. The pain may feel like tingling or like pins and needles. This sensation may occur any time the affected body part is used, or just during physical activity. The pain usually does not remain constant but comes and goes.

3. Neurological signs. Muscle weakness in a specific muscle or muscle group may indicate neurological impairment. The person will feel that one area is considerably weaker than the corresponding part. Also, any sign of disorientation, dizziness, fainting, blurred vision, or nausea may indicate a neurological problem.

4. Swelling. Swelling in any area, in any amount, indicates that a particular body location is being overstressed. Swelling may occur after an acute injury or with a chronic injury. The amount of swelling may vary among people with the same problem. The fact that swelling is present, not the amount, is most important.

5. Discoloration. Common "black-and-blue" areas may be simply the result of incidental impact. If, however, there is an extremely noticeable area of discoloration associated with an acute or chronic injury, a physician should be consulted. This condition means that a considerable amount of bleeding into surrounding tissues has occurred.

6. Movement impairment. Any time

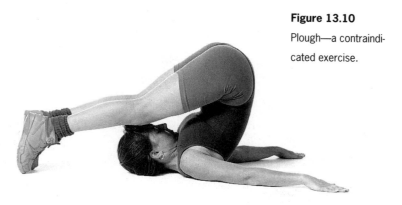

Figure 13.10

Plough—a contraindicated exercise.

Chapter 13
Musculoskeletal
Injuries

normal movement is impaired, limiting the range of motion, the affected body part should be rested. Pain or discomfort that causes limitation of movement indicates that some problem is present. Never let anyone participate whose movement is impaired in any way, such as by limping.

COMMON AEROBICS CLASS INJURIES

Most injuries in a dance-exercise class occur to the foot, ankle, shin, low back, and knee. The following is a description of the problems an instructor will most likely see in class, followed by general guidelines for prevention and treatment.

Neuroma (Interdigital, Morton's)

Interdigital nerves travel between the metatarsal bones in the foot and enable the toes to function normally. A **neuroma** is an entrapment of part of an interdigital nerve that usually occurs between the third and fourth toes (Fig. 13.11), where the branches of the nerve cross in an "X" pattern. The entrapped nerve causes swelling that results in sharp, radiating pain traveling to the ends of the involved toes. The area directly over the affected nerve will be sore during weight-bearing, running, and jumping activities, and when activity is performed on the ball of the foot.

Prevention. To prevent a neuroma, shoes for daily wear and for exercise must be the proper width to prevent compression of the metatarsal arch and interdigital nerves. Wearing narrow dress shoes over time may cause a neuroma. Shoes worn during exercise must be well padded in the metatarsal area. Exercises should not be performed on the ball of the foot or on unyielding surfaces.

Treatment. ICE should be applied for 20 to 30 minutes after any weight-bearing activity. It might be helpful to place a pad on the bottom of the foot, slightly behind the area of tenderness. Even with proper rest, modification of activity, and treatment, this problem often does not improve. In some cases, a podiatrist or orthopedic surgeon may recommend surgery.

Metatarsalgia

Metatarsalgia is a general term describing pain in the ball of the foot. Pain is usually felt under the second and third metatarsal heads (Fig. 13.12), caused by bruising the joints in these areas. Metatarsalgia differs from a neuroma in that the pain is more general in the area of the metatarsal heads and usually no sharp pain radiates to the end of the toes. Metatarsalgia occurs gradually and is aggravated by extreme repeated force or impact on the ball of the foot, such as in running or jumping. At first, specific pain may be felt only during activity. As this problem progresses, pain may be felt during normal weight-bearing and even non-weight-bearing activities.

Prevention. Wear shoes that are supportive and well padded in the metatarsal area. Exercise on resilient surfaces and avoid repetitive impact activities, especially

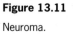

Figure 13.11

Neuroma.

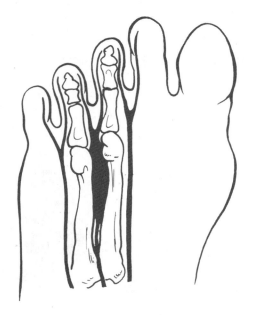

impact to the ball of the foot.

Treatment. A pad placed directly behind the affected metatarsal heads may relieve some pressure to the area. ICE should be applied to the metatarsal area after exercise. If pain continues even when not exercising, stop all running and jumping activities.

Plantar Fascitis

The plantar fascia is a broad band of connective tissue found on the bottom of the foot, running the length of the sole of the foot (Fig. 13.13). **Plantar fascitis** is an inflammation of this band of tissue caused by stretching or tearing, usually near the attachment at the heel.

The plantar fascia is put under a great deal of stress during weight-bearing activity. When weight is shifted to the ball of the foot and a push-off motion is performed, as in running or jumping, that stress greatly increases. Pain is felt in a specific area on the bottom of the foot, back toward the heel. This pain may radiate toward the ball of the foot. There is less pain during non-weight-bearing activity. Typically, the foot feels very tender the first thing in the morning and becomes gradually less painful with movement.

Repeated irritation of the plantar fascia is likely to cause the formation of a sharp, bony growth (**bone spur**). People with a mild high arch are more likely to experience this problem.

Prevention. Shoes must have adequate arch supports to prevent this problem. The shoe and arch support should be flexible to avoid additional stress to this area. High-intensity running or jumping on unyielding surfaces should be limited. Stretching the calf and Achilles tendon daily will also help to prevent this problem.

Treatment. When symptoms begin to occur, add an arch support to both activity

shoes and dress shoes. Apply ICE in the arch area after activity and whenever pain is present. Any shoe that causes pain in the arch should be avoided.

If symptoms do not improve or if they worsen, rest the arch until there is no pain during normal activities. Limit weight-bearing activities, and substitute non-weight-bearing activities such as swimming or cycling. Persistent pain should be examined by a physician or sports podiatrist.

Stress Fractures

Stress fractures occur in major weight-bearing locations of the body, especially the foot (metatarsal bones) and lower leg (tibia). A **stress fracture** is an impending fracture due to excessive stress (overuse) of a bone. This repeated stress causes the bone to begin to break down.

Stress fractures occur gradually. There is usually a specific area of pain directly over the affected bone. Sometimes the pain will be sharp and radiating. The affected area is always tender to the touch. The pain is progressive and will gradually become more intense as weight-bearing activities continue. Pain will be most severe during running and jumping activities.

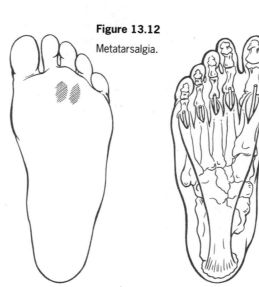

Figure 13.12
Metatarsalgia.

Figure 13.13
Plantar fascia.

Pain may also remain after exercise, during standing or walking.

Stress fractures are often difficult to diagnose accurately because they initially do not appear on an X-ray. It may be necessary to obtain a bone scan to identify a stress fracture. Pain may persist in varying degrees for four to twelve weeks. If this problem is ignored, complete fractures may occur.

Prevention. Avoid repetitive activities on unyielding surfaces, wear proper shoes, and increase exercise intensity gradually. If a previous injury has required rest, return to normal activity slowly and gradually.

Treatment. If a stress fracture is suspected, repetitive jumping and excessive running should be avoided because they will cause increased pain. Shock-absorbing arch supports may be added to relieve stress. A doughnut-type pad placed on the area may relieve pressure on the point of extreme tenderness. ICE should be applied after activity or any time pain is present. Non-weight-bearing activities may be substituted if weight-bearing activities are too painful. This type of fracture will heal gradually, and when all symptoms have

disappeared, full weight-bearing activities can gradually be resumed.

Achilles Tendinitis

The Achilles tendon is a narrow tendinous extension of the calf musculature that attaches to the heel (calcaneus) (Fig. 13.14). Repeated, forceful stretching will create small tears in the fibers of the tendon, causing it to become inflamed and resulting in **Achilles tendinitis.** This chronic overuse problem has a gradual onset and is often caused by jumping and running without proper warm-up stretches. The tendon will be sore to the touch directly over the affected area and there will be pain and stiffness when the foot is dorsiflexed (toes moved toward the shin), which moves the tendon. Symptoms will progressively worsen if the problem is ignored.

Prevention. Changing from regular dress shoes, especially high heels, to flat aerobics shoes places a great deal of stress on the tendon. Therefore, thorough, daily stretching of the calf muscles (gastrocnemius/soleus) and Achilles tendon is necessary and will help prevent this problem. Mild stretching after exercise may also help prevent muscle and tendon soreness.

Treatment. As soon as any symptoms are experienced, begin applying ICE to the affected area. Also, increase the amount of mild stretching to the calf area. If symptoms progress, limit activity. Do not perform any exercises that cause pain in the tendon area. Rest usually will greatly improve this condition.

Shin Splints

Shin splints is a general term applied to any pain or discomfort that occurs on the front or side of the lower leg, in the region of the shin bone (tibia) (Fig. 13.15). Shin splints may have various causes, including faulty posture, poor shoes, fallen arches,

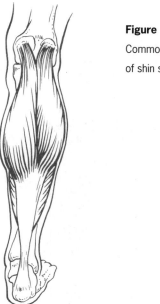

Figure 13.14

Achilles tendon.

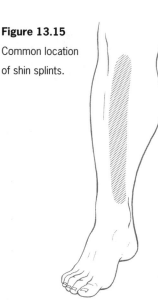

Figure 13.15

Common location of shin splints.

insufficient warm-ups, muscle fatigue, poor running mechanics such as extensive pronation, training too fast or too soon, and exercising on unyielding surfaces. Many people consider shin splints one of the most common and disabling conditions in dance exercise.

Shin splints are characterized by pain in the shin on one or both legs. There may be a specific area of tenderness or swelling directly over the affected bone. This symptom is also common with a stress fracture. Pain and aching will be felt in the front of the leg after activity and sometimes during activity, as the condition worsens. If shin splints are ignored and the participant attempts to "run through" them, a stress fracture will almost always occur that will present additional pain and disability and limit activity for several months.

Prevention. To prevent shin splints, increase activity gradually, wear shoes with good shock-absorbing features, and avoid repetitive weight-bearing activities on unyielding surfaces. When running or jumping, land flat-footed or toe-heel, respectively, to minimize impact.

Stretch the calf muscles and strengthen the anterior tibial (front shin) muscles daily and before each class.

Treatment. Apply ICE to the shin area after activity. If pain persists, activity should be limited. Any time bruising, swelling or specific point tenderness occurs in the affected area, all activity should be stopped. Any non-weight-bearing activities that do not cause pain to the shin area can be continued. Shin splints usually respond well to rest. When symptoms have subsided, activity may be resumed gradually.

Ankle Sprains

A **sprain** is an injury to a ligament, which is a band of fibers connecting one bone to another bone. In the ankle,

sprains usually occur on the outside of the joint, most often involving the lateral ligaments. These injuries are caused by an extreme inward (inversion) movement of the ankle, forcing it beyond its normal range of motion (Fig. 13.16). Sprains are acute injuries classified by degree of severity. A mild sprain (first degree) involves minimal stretching of ligament fibers. A moderate sprain (second degree) involves tearing of some ligament fibers, with the ligament still intact. In severe sprain (third degree), the ligament is torn completely in two or more pieces. Most ankle sprains in aerobics classes are mild or moderate.

When a sprain occurs, pain will be felt directly over the injured ligament. Swelling will occur around the injured ligament and spread throughout the joint. There may be some discoloration in the ankle and foot. Normal motion will be limited by swelling in the joint.

Prevention. Avoid slick dance surfaces or heavily padded surfaces where the foot sinks into the padding, causing the participant to trip. Match the shoe to the floor surface: Use a shoe with good outsole traction for smooth surfaces, and one with less traction for carpeted surfaces. If mats are used for the aerobics segment, make sure they are large enough that participants won't fall off the edge.

Common aerobics class injuries

Figure 13.16

Inversion ankle sprain.

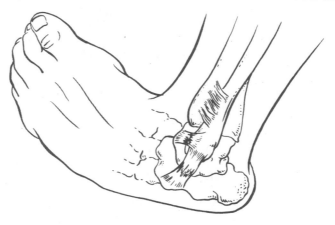

Treatment. Use RICE immediately and continue for 48 to 72 hours after the injury. ICE should be applied three to four times each day. Weight-bearing activity should be limited. See an orthopedic surgeon for x-rays to rule out a fracture and to receive an accurate diagnosis.

Meniscus (Cartilage) Tears

A meniscus is a gristly substance that lines the top surface of the tibia. It cushions the area where the upper leg bone (femur) rests on the tibia. There are two menisci in each knee: medial and lateral (Fig. 13.17). Tears can occur in either, although the medial meniscus seems to be injured more frequently.

Meniscus tears are commonly caused by sharp, twisting movements of the knee, forceful flexion (bending) and extension (straightening) of the knee (as in a forced squat), or a sharp hyperextension of the knee. An unstable foot plant or improper exercise technique may cause this injury.

When a meniscus is torn there is a specific incident of injury. Pain may be felt "inside" the knee. It is difficult to flex and extend the knee, which may lock or catch. It may feel as though it will give way. Movement requiring quick change of direction and squatting (deep knee-bend position)

will be difficult if a meniscus is torn. There may be swelling around and behind the knee. Because the menisci have a very poor blood supply, they usually do not heal.

Prevention. To prevent meniscus tears, emphasize proper body control in exercises that require balance. All change-of-direction movements must be performed in a controlled manner. Avoid squats, hurdler stretches, and other movements that bend and twist the knees. Make certain the muscles of the thigh (quadriceps and hamstrings) are well-conditioned. These muscles help support the knee during various dance-exercise activities.

Treatment. If a meniscus tear is suspected, limit any painful, weight-bearing exercises. Apply ICE after activity and whenever the knee hurts. See an orthopedic surgeon to obtain a specific diagnosis and the proper treatment prescription. In some cases activity may be resumed after injury, and in others, surgery may be necessary.

Chondromalacia

Chondromalacia is a gradual degenerative process in which the articular cartilage that lines the back surface of the patella, or kneecap (Fig. 13.18), becomes softer and rougher. Although the exact cause of this problem is unknown, it may result from poor running or jumping mechanics, an abnormal position of the patella, foot pronation, excessive flexing and extending of the knee with heavy resistance (weight training), or excessive running and jumping on unyielding surfaces.

Chondromalacia may occur more frequently in girls and women because of the wider female pelvis that creates a wider angle as the femur meets the tibia at the knee. This increased angle may place the kneecap in a more outward or lateral position and cause excessive rubbing of the undersurface of the patella.

Figure 13.17

Medial and lateral menisci.

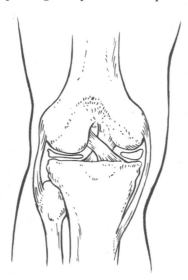

Chondromalacia produces general pain around the patella. A grating, grinding sound or sensation may be heard and felt as the affected knee is flexed and extended. Walking up and down stairs will hurt.

Swelling may or may not be present. This condition begins gradually and progressively worsens when stressful activities are continued.

Prevention. To prevent chondromalacia, avoid high-resistance, lower-extremity weight training and excessive repetitive weight bearing activity on unyielding surfaces. Become conditioned gradually and wear shoes with good shock absorption and arch support during all weight-bearing activities.

Treatment. As symptoms of chondromalacia begin to appear, apply ICE after any activity. Limit weight-bearing activities and extreme flexion and extension movements of the knee. Single straight-leg raises are recommended to maintain strength in the quadriceps (anterior thigh) without further irritating knees. Chondromalacia responds very well to rest, so decrease activity. When symptoms have subsided, resume weight-bearing exercise gradually.

Iliotibial Band Syndrome

The iliotibial band is a thick, wide band of tissue running on the outside of the thigh, from the top of the hip down across the knee and attaching slightly below the knee on a bony prominence (Fig. 13.19). This band may become irritated through overuse, excessive running, or poor running mechanics. At times the band may move and snap back and forth during bending and straightening of the knee. This causes additional irritation where the band crosses the knee joint.

Iliotibial band syndrome is characterized by an area of tenderness on the lateral side of the knee, where the band crosses the knee. Local swelling may be present, but is not always a key symptom with this condition. Pain and swelling increase if excessive bending and straightening of the knee continue.

Prevention. Utilize and emphasize proper movement mechanics. Stretch the lateral muscular structures of the hip and upper thigh daily.

Treatment. Use ICE when symptoms are present. Corrective orthotics may help to improve running mechanics. Perform iliotibial band stretching exercises daily. Gradually modify activity until symptoms subside.

Muscle Strains

A muscle **strain** is a stretching or tearing of muscle tissue either in the main part of the muscle or in the tendon unit. This injury produces varying degrees of pain and disability, depending upon the extent of the tear. A mild, first degree strain involves a minimal stretching of muscle fibers. A moderate, second degree strain involves some tearing of muscle fibers, and a severe, third degree strain involves a total tearing and separation of the muscle allowing no active muscle function.

Muscle injuries are characterized by a specific area of pain, directly over the affected muscle tissue. In mild strains this

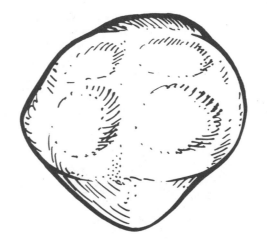

Figure 13.18
Undersurface of patella.

Chapter 13
Musculoskeletal
Injuries

pain might only be felt during exercise when the muscle is contracted or stretched. In moderate and severe strains this pain will be present during normal daily activities and sometimes even at rest. Mild strains usually occur within the belly of the muscle while more serious strains may occur in the tendinous unit. General exercise may be continued if the injured area does not present extreme symptoms or limit normal movement. It is important to remember that muscle injuries may take a long time to heal. It is not unusual to have some symptoms linger six months or more depending on the severity of the injury.

Prevention. Proper stretching of all muscle groups utilized during physical activity is essential to prevent muscle injury. These major muscle groups should be specifically and thoroughly stretched prior to all activity. In addition, it is still believed that a proper warm-up prior to activity also helps to prevent muscle injury.

Treatment. Use ICE for as long as symptoms remain. Perform mild stretching exercises with the affected muscle if the exercises can be accomplished without pain. Modify activity to prevent further irritation to the injured area.

Muscle strains can occur in any muscle group of the body but very often occur in the quadriceps, hamstrings, and adductor muscles of the thigh. In addition, the gastrocnemius/soleus muscles (calf) and Achilles tendon are vulnerable to strain. Remember to stretch these muscles thoroughly prior to physical activity.

Upper Extremity Injuries

Although upper extremity injuries do not commonly occur in aerobics classes, they may occur in other exercise and work-related activities and may affect aerobic-exercise performance.

It is necessary to understand that the shoulder is designed for mobility. Exercises designed to develop the dynamic, and static stabilizers of the shoulder must be performed to prevent significant shoulder injury and promote movement efficiency.

When the shoulder stabilizers are weak overuse symptoms and shoulder dysfunction may occur. Recent research has emphasized the importance of eccentric overload to support and stabilize the shoulder during deceleration phases of movement. Although eccentric strengthening may be difficult to achieve with manufactured equipment and machinery, it can be accomplished through the use of surgical tubing exercise routines.

Rotator Cuff Injuries

A common upper extremity injury involves the rotator cuff muscles. The rotator cuff is a group of four large muscles that surround the shoulder joint. These muscles act not only to stabilize the head of the humerus in the glenoid fossa, but also act eccentrically during deceleration to pro-

Figure 13.19
Iliotibial band syndrome.

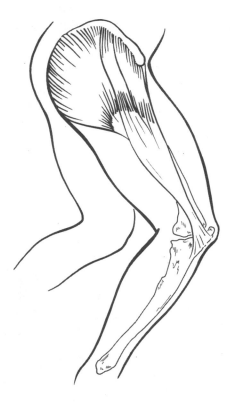

tect the static stabilizers of the shoulder.

The rotator cuff muscles can tear if
there is a violent pull to the arm, forceful
twisting, or a fall on an outstretched arm.
Injury also commonly results from extreme
shoulder external rotation and abduction.
Strains of the rotator cuff may also be
caused by repetitive overuse stress being
applied to the muscles of the shoulder
through throwing, weightlifting, or work-
related activities.

Prevention. Thorough stretching of the
muscles of the shoulder prior to exercise is
essential in preventing strains to this area.
Gradual strengthening of these muscles
through a planned resistance-training program will aid in preventing injury. Remember to include eccentric conditioning to
ensure proper stabilization. Avoid repeated heavy-load resistance repetitions with
isolated muscle groups.

Treatment. Utilize the treatment of ICE
as long as symptoms are present. Modify
activity appropriately to avoid additional
stress to the injured area. Avoid internal
and external shoulder rotation movements if painful. Resume restrengthening
gradually, beginning with range of motion
exercise and progressing to limited resistance exercises.

Bursitis

Bursa are pad-like, fluid-filled sacs located throughout the body where friction

might occur, such as where muscle tendons
cross over bones. Bursa reduce that friction. Overuse of muscles and tendons at
these friction sites, or constant pressure
directly on the bursa, can irritate a bursa
sac, causing **bursitis**. Bursitis can occur anywhere in the body, but it most often occurs where overuse or pressure is greatest.
In aerobics the knees, hip, shoulder, and
elbow are the most commonly affected areas. Pain and stiffness begin gradually in
the area of the affected bursa. There is
usually no visible swelling at first, but
swelling occurs as the condition worsens.

Prevention. To prevent bursitis, gradually add any external resistance (such as
hand or arm weights) when performing
upper-body movements, and use proper
technique with all exercise movements.

Treatment. Apply ICE after any activity.
Try to determine what has caused the additional stress on the particular body part,
and remove or reduce that stress. When
normal movement is reduced and visible
swelling is present, activity involving the
affected area should be stopped. Bursitis
responds very well to rest. Once symptoms
have subsided, activity may be resumed
gradually.

Lateral Epicondylitis (Tennis Elbow)

Epicondylitis is an inflammation of a
bony prominence commonly known as an
epicondyle. The bony prominence on the

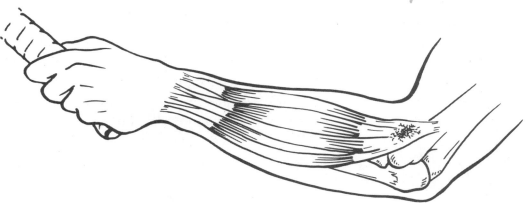

Figure 13.20

"Tennis Elbow."

outside of the elbow serves as an attachment for muscles which go down the forearm into the wrist. Through repeated stress, some fibers of these muscles may become irritated, pull off of their attachments, and cause inflammation of the lateral epicondyle. This condition is commonly called **"tennis elbow"** because it often occurs among tennis players and racquet sports participants (Fig. 13.20). In reality, however, it can occur in any sport, physical exercise, or even work-related repetitive movements. Although tennis elbow is not usually caused by aerobic-exercise activities, participants may come to class with this problem and exercise modifications may need to be made to accommodate their symptoms.

Symptoms include an area of specific point-tenderness directly over the lateral epicondyle of the elbow. An aching sensation will be noticeable in the elbow and may radiate down into the forearm. Pain may be experienced when the arm and elbow are extended and the hand and wrist supinate and pronate.

Prevention. Prevention of lateral epicondylitis includes stretching the muscles of the upper arm, forearm and wrist. It is

also important to gradually strengthen and condition these muscles. Avoid any forceful repetitive movements involving flexion and extension and/or supination and pronation of the hand and wrist.

Treatment. Apply ICE to the elbow area after activity. If symptoms are present avoid any upper arm and forearm movements which may create pain in the area of the lateral epicondyle. Modify biceps and triceps resistance training to avoid pain. Be particularly careful when utilizing hand-held weights in flexion and extension movement.

In addition, the use of a tennis elbow support brace worn on the upper forearm (below the elbow) has been found to be beneficial for relief of symptoms and management of this problem. This device may be utilized during physical activity as well as during rest. It is important to remember that tennis elbow occurs gradually, and once it is in an acute stage, it may take several months, and even up to one year, to resolve.

Carpal Tunnel Syndrome

Carpal tunnel syndrome results from an irritation and swelling in the base of the wrist. It is most frequently characterized by an aching pain in the wrist with sharp, burning pain, tingling, and weakness radiating in the thumb, index finger, middle finger, and even into the ring finger on occasion. Nerves traveling through the wrist to the palm of the hand and fingers pass through very narrow spaces or tunnels. Sometimes this area becomes irritated and the nerves become trapped or compressed in one of these tunnels, causing this pain (Fig. 13.21).

Carpal tunnel syndrome is commonly caused by repetitive and forceful grasping with the hands, constant pressure in the palm and wrist area, and/or repetitive

Figure 13.21

Carpal tunnel syndrome.

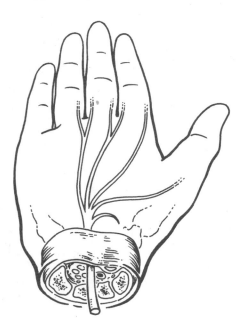

bending of the wrists. In many cases, it is difficult to know exactly what activity has actually caused the problem.

It is unlikely that aerobics will cause carpal tunnel syndrome. However, participants may come to class with this problem and it is necessary to understand the condition and modify activity appropriately.

Prevention. Avoid repetitive and forceful grasping of items. Avoid repetitive overuse stress to the hand and wrist area. If performing repetitive wrist flexion and extension exercises during work-related activities take frequent breaks to relax the hand and wrist area to avoid irritation.

Treatment. Apply ICE to the wrist and hand area after any activity. Rest the area whenever possible. Utilize wrist braces or splints whenever possible to immobilize and rest the affected area.

In addition, avoid any exercise techniques which may cause additional discomfort to this area. Be particularly careful when performing wrist and forearm resistance training such as with hand-held weights. When supporting body weight during push-ups or other floor work be careful to avoid additional stress to the hand and wrist area.

It is important to remember that carpal tunnel syndrome may take a long time to resolve. Additional trauma or irritation to the area must be avoided at all time.

Low-back Pain

The low back is composed of five lumbar vertebrae and their attaching ligaments, which provide the major support to this part of the spinal column. Extensive musculature surrounds this area to provide additional support. The low back is a site of frequent problems caused by congenital abnormalities, poor posture, postural deviations, and poor body mechanics (incorrect lifting and sitting postures). Lack of trunk flexibility and weak abdominal muscles also contribute to **low-back pain**.

The muscles of the trunk act like "guy wires" supporting a telephone pole. The development and maintenance of strength in these muscles, specifically in the lumbar extensor muscles, is of great importance in providing support and stability to the low back. Strengthening exercises should focus on the muscles involved in trunk extension. Instructors must emphasize pelvic stabilization to ensure strength gains when performing these exercises.

Common aerobics class injuries

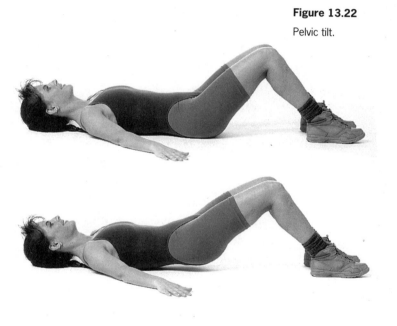

Figure 13.22
Pelvic tilt.

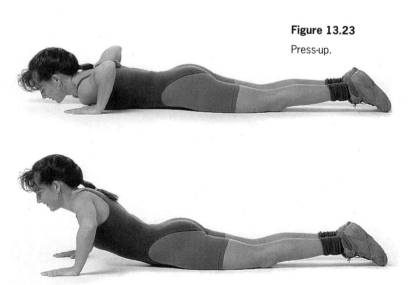

Figure 13.23
Press-up.

Chapter 13
Musculoskeletal
Injuries

Pelvic stabilization is extremely important in both the prevention of low-back disorders and in the execution of mechanically sound movement skills. The effect of pelvic stabilization on lumbar extension strength is well documented. If the pelvis is unrestricted and free to move, the hip extensor muscles, primarily the hamstrings and gluteals, will perform most of the work rather than the lumbar extensor muscles.

Without pelvic stabilization, exercises performed to strengthen the musculature of the low back will not be as effective. Recent research has confirmed the importance of pelvic stabilization during exercise to strengthen the lumbar extensors. When the lumbar extensors are isolated through pelvic stabilization, large improvements in strength may be expected. Additional research has shown the importance of increased levels of lumbar extension strength in relieving low-back pain.

Congenital low-back abnormalities may become apparent when abnormal stresses, such as sudden twisting, are applied to the back. The abnormalities produce mechanical weaknesses that may make the low back vulnerable to injury during physical activity.

Faulty posture or faulty body mechanics put a tremendous strain on the muscles and ligaments of the low back. Lifting heavy objects incorrectly—using the back instead of the legs—is an example of the poor body mechanics that must be corrected to maintain a healthy back.

A sprain or strain to the low back is an acute problem with a specific incident of injury. Sudden violent twisting, extension, or hyperextension movements may injure the ligaments and muscles of the back.

Someone who once experienced an injury to the low back will usually have chronic low-back pain. The vertebrae may be misaligned or they may move in abnormal directions, putting pressure on the nerves and creating muscular weaknesses and radiating pain. These problems occur more often and become more severe with age. The numerous small injuries and postural mechanical deviations create a progressive degeneration over time, and extreme low-back pain may occur, aggravated by any sudden movement. Jumping and running jar and compress the vertebrae of the back, and low-back pain may be experienced after these physical activities.

Regardless of the cause or exact struc-

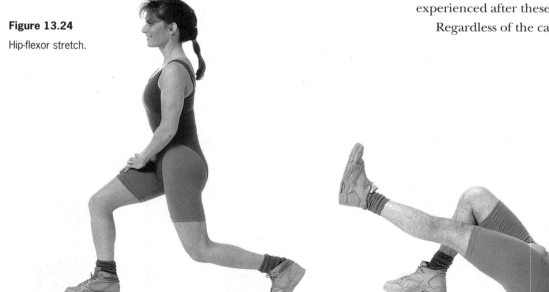

Figure 13.24

Hip-flexor stretch.

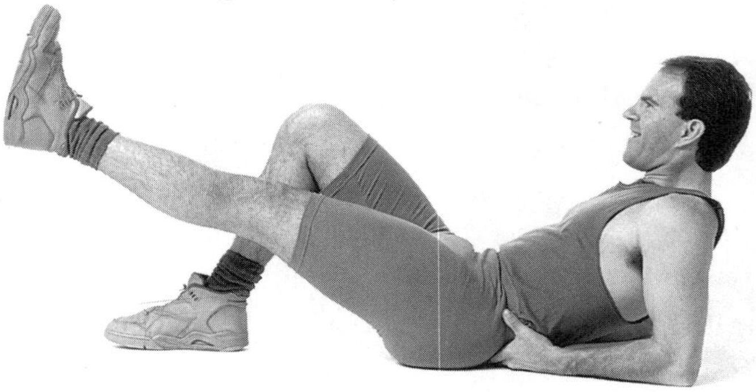

Figure 13.25

Single-leg raise.

ture involved, low-back pain is extremely disabling. The muscles surrounding the affected area go into spasm to protect the back, and the person experiences severe stiffness and immobility. If pain and discomfort persist, it is important to have the back thoroughly evaluated by a physician. Fractures, dislocations, or degenerative disease may be present in the vertebrae, thus requiring that physical activity be restricted or modified.

Prevention. To prevent back problems, keep all of the muscles of the trunk strong. Primary movements of the back are flexion and extension, as well as lateral side-to-side movement and rotation. The musculature surrounding the back supports and protects it. The abdominal muscles and the psoas muscles flex the lumbar spine. Abdominal strength aids in maintaining proper vertebral and postural alignment, and in supporting the low back. Oblique muscle strength is extremely important to low-back support. The oblique muscles contribute greatly to the support of the lumbar area. These muscles should be conditioned as aggressively as the abdominal muscles. The psoas muscles are already extremely strong, and overdevelopment could produce an abnormal lumbar curve. Instead, these muscles should be stretched

to increase their flexibility. Hamstring flexibility is also extremely important to prevent postural deviations and abnormal stresses on the low back. Trunk flexibility should be emphasized to produce maximum range of motion in the back.

Treatment. If low-back pain is extremely severe and disabling, stretching exercises can help relieve muscle spasm. Lying down produces the least strain on the back. To relieve spasm, lie on the back, and slowly and alternately bring the knees to the chest. The pelvic tilt (Fig.13.22) can also be helpful. Lie on the back with knees bent. Press low back to the floor. Raise the hips straight up and hold for 3 to 5 seconds.

When acute symptoms have subsided, flexibility and strengthening exercises may be added. These may include the following:

1. Press-up (Fig. 13.23a-b). Lying face down, place hands under shoulders in the press-up position (Fig. 13.23a). Straighten elbows and push the top half of the body up as far as pain permits (Fig. 13.23b). It is important that the pelvis, hips, and legs remain as relaxed as possible. Maintain this position for 1 to 2 seconds, then lower torso to the starting position.

2. Hip flexor stretch (Fig. 13.24). Stand with one leg extended, knee bent,

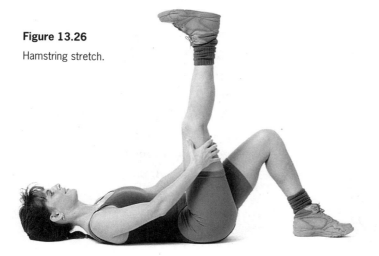

Figure 13.26

Hamstring stretch.

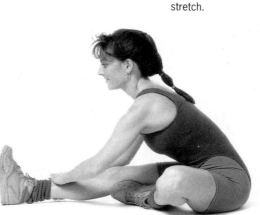

Figure 13.27

Alternate hamstring stretch.

the other leg behind. Shift body weight downward toward extended leg.

3. Single leg raise (Fig. 13.25). To strengthen the quadriceps, lie on the back, one knee straight and one knee bent toward the chest. Raise the straight leg as far as possible. Return slowly. Change legs after 10 repetitions. This exercise can be performed with or without weights.

Never do double leg raises lying on the back. This position puts the psoas muscles in extreme tension and causes abnormal pressure on the lumbar spine area. It may even create an abnormal lumbar curve. The low back must always be kept flat during all exercises performed while lying on the back.

4. Hamstring stretch (Fig. 13.26). On the back, grasp one thigh and pull it gently toward the chest (the opposite leg is bent). Alternate legs.

5. Alternate hamstring stretch (Fig. 13.27). Sit on the floor with one leg bent, knee toward the chest, the other leg straight. Lean forward, trying to touch the legs. All stretching must be gradual (**static**), not bouncy (**ballistic**). The stretch should always be felt in the belly of the muscle and not in the muscle-tendon unit. Make certain that the stretch is felt in the hamstring muscle(s) and not in the low back.

6. Abdominal curls (modified sit-ups) (Fig. 13.28). On the back with knees bent, feet flat on floor, hands across chest, and elbows out straight, raise the shoulders off the floor toward your knees. Repeat. It is

not necessary to raise the chest and upper trunk completely to a sitting position during an abdominal curl. These final degrees of movement are wasted effort because they do not cause further contraction of the abdominal muscles. When the hands are placed behind the head during an abdominal curl, be careful not to pull the neck and create stress on the cervical vertebrae.

Never perform an exercise that creates any pain in the low-back area. Be especially cautious during leg lifts and abdominal curls. Avoid fast, extreme twisting movements that strain the back. Practice good posture, good exercise technique, and proper body mechanics.

SUMMARY

Preventing injury and providing a safe exercise environment are the keys to the future of dance exercise.

Most aerobics class injuries are caused by overuse; Too much stress placed on one part of the body over an extended time. The areas most frequently injured are the shoulder, foot, ankle, lower leg, knee, and low back.

A chronic injury, such as shin splints, occurs gradually with no specific incident of injury. If not treated properly, a chronic injury may become acute. For example, if repeatedly stressed, a shin splint may become a stress fracture. More often an acute injury, such as a sprained ankle, has a more sudden onset and usually is characterized by a specific injury incident.

The best way to prevent injury is to dance on a floor surface that is both stable and resilient, wear good aerobics shoes, follow proper exercise technique (including a warm-up and cool-down), and avoid exercises with a high rate of injury.

When injuries do occur among participants, the instructor must know how to manage them properly. It is not the in-

Figure 13.28

Abdominal curl.

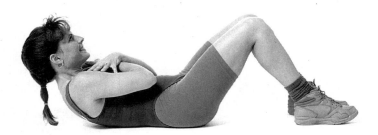

structor's role to diagnose or treat injuries. Instead, the instructor should always refer the participant to a physician. The instructor may suggest that rest, ice, compression, and elevation (RICE) are helpful for many common injuries and explain how to apply the procedures. If certain warning signs (including pain, swelling, weakness in a specific muscle or muscle group, extreme discoloration, or impaired movement) persist for more than three to five days, the instructor should require the participant to obtain medical clearance before returning to class.

REFERENCES

Mosher, C. (1984). "Rhythm and Moves." *Women's Sports and Fitness*, December: 24-27.

Richie, D.H., S.F. Kelso, and P.A. Bellucci. (1985). "Aerobic Dance Injuries: A Retrospective Study of Instructors and Participants." *The Physician and Sportsmedicine*, February: 134-35.

SUGGESTED READING

Albohm, M.J. (1981). *Health Care and the Female Athlete*. North Palm Beach, Fl: Athletic Institute.

Arnheim, D. (1987). *Essentials of Athletic Training*. St. Louis, MO: Times Mirror/Mosby.

Ritter, M.A., and M.J. Albohm. (1987). *Your Injury: A Common Sense Guide to the Management of Sports Injury*. Indianapolis, IN: Benchmark Press.

JOURNALS

The Physician and Sportsmedicine, McGraw-Hill, Inc., Minneapolis, MN.

Chapter 14

Emergency Procedures

By Sandra L. Niehues and Larry P. Brown

Every day the possibility exists that someone in an aerobics exercise class could become the victim of a medical emergency. By carefully screening all participants (see Chapter 5 "Health Screening"), instructors can be reasonably certain that the participants in their classes are free of medical conditions that make vigorous activity unsafe. However, some participants may have an underlying disease that appears for the first time in an exercise setting. Factors related to personality and motivation also can lead to sudden illness or injury. For example, unfit, sedentary participants

Sandra L. Niehues, M.A., A.T.,C. is the director of guest communications for the Golden Door and Rancho La Puerta health resorts. As a certified athletic trainer, she has provided medical care to high school, college, Olympic and professional athletes. Larry P. Brown, M.A., P.T., A.T.,C. is the owner of Camarillo Orthopaedic & Sports Physical Therapy. He is a physical therapist and a certified athletic trainer and contributes significantly to his field as a teacher, and researcher.

commonly try to do too much, too soon, too fast. Even experienced exercisers may try to compete with others in the class and push themselves beyond reasonable and safe limits.

Emergencies may also result from physical hazards such as a wet floor. Problems can even occur if a class is overcrowded or if the environment is too hot or humid. A wise instructor is aware of the possible hazards and is prepared to act purposefully and appropriately when an emergency occurs.

This chapter is intended to familiarize instructors with potential medical emergencies and to provide basic guidelines for dealing with them. It is not intended as a complete resource, nor as a substitute for **cardiopulmonary resuscitation (CPR)** training, which is a requirement for certification by the American Council on Exercise. When faced with a medical emergency, instructors should never exceed their training and capabilities and should not allow anyone in the class to do so. It is not the instructor's role to diagnose an injury or to offer medical advice. If there is any doubt about the seriousness of the participant's condition, it is always wise to err on the side of caution and call for help.

The authors hope that the information provided here will encourage instructors to seek basic first-aid training through the American Red Cross. Instructors who want to develop their skills even further are advised to enroll in a community college emergency medical technician (EMT) course.

EMERGENCY BASICS

Every fitness facility, no matter how large or small, should have an emergency plan for all employees to follow if a crisis occurs. Each employee should receive a copy of this plan and should initial it to signify a complete understanding of its contents. The plan should include contin-

gencies for evacuation in the event of fire or natural disaster, as well as procedures for any life-threatening situations. Telephone numbers for police, fire, emergency medical system and poison control should be included in the written plan as well as posted in plain view near each telephone.

Equipment

Three items every facility should have in case an emergency occurs are a fire extinguisher, a telephone and a well-stocked first-aid kit. The fire extinguisher should be easily accessible and in proper working order. It should be serviced at appropriate intervals and all employees should be trained in its operation. The telephone should have direct dialing capabilities. If the facility only has a pay telephone, the instructor should carry proper change. In areas where 911 emergency service is available, most pay telephones can be accessed without paying first; however, do not assume that all pay telephones can be accessed in this manner.

The first-aid kit should be well-stocked and regularly maintained. Each employee should be familiar with its contents and understand the use of each item. A first-aid kit should contain the following:

1. Assorted bandage materials
2. Sterile gauze pads
3. 4-inch and 6-inch elastic wraps
4. Liquid soap
5. Topical antibiotic cream (Bacitracin is preferred)
6. Tongue blades
7. Triangular bandages
8. Splinting material
9. Ammonia inhalants
10. Sphygmomanometer (blood pressure cuff)
11. Stethoscope
12. Penlight
13. Scissors

14. Paper bag

15. Chemical coldpack

Chemical coldpacks can be used immediately after an injury occurs; however, these packs do not get very cold nor stay cold for very long. Ice is better. If not available at the club, try to make arrangements in advance to get ice from a nearby market or restaurant to help save time when an emergency occurs.

If an item in the first-aid kit has been used, it should be replaced as soon as possible so it will be available the next time it is needed.

Assessment of an Unconscious Victim

A rescuer who comes upon an unconscious victim must immediately be able to institute life-saving treatment. Appropriate action can only result when proper assessment is performed. The following section will describe how to conduct the primary survey of an unconscious victim.

Primary Survey. The primary survey is designed to discover and correct any immediate life-threatening problems. Begin the survey as soon as the victim is reached. During the primary survey talk, feel and observe.

Spend the first 10 seconds of the primary survey assessing the scene and determining what took place and what the victim was doing before the collapse. Was the victim exercising or just finished? Try to be aware of the possible cause of injury. Look for medication bottles lying near the victim.

Spend the next 50 seconds determining the status of the victim. Begin by assessing responsiveness. If the victim doesn't respond to talking or shouting, send someone to call for help right away.

The next step in the primary survey is to establish an airway. Use the head-tilt method or modified jaw-thrust technique (see Appendix D on CPR), if head or spinal injury is suspected. Next, look for signs of respiration. See whether the chest is rising and falling. Listen for sounds of breathing and feel with the cheek for respiration. Because well-conditioned people may breathe only six to eight times per minute, take a full 5 seconds to check for respiration. If there are no signs of breathing, give two full, slow ventilations.

Next, take 5 to 10 seconds to check the carotid artery for evidence of circulation. If there is a pulse and no breathing, begin rescue breathing. If there is no pulse, begin CPR. If the victim is bleeding severely, begin treatment immediately.

If the victim is awake and talking, he or she has a patent airway and adequate circulation. Once the instructor has checked for severe bleeding his or her primary survey is complete.

Also check to see if the participant is wearing a medical alert tag; if so, show it to the emergency rescue team when it arrives.

Accessing the Emergency Medical Services. The **emergency medical services (EMS)** may be activated in many areas by dialing 911. In communities without a centralized dispatch number, calling police, fire or ambulance emergency numbers will activate the system. On the telephone, instructors should be prepared to give their name, and the sex and approximate age of the victim, the nature of the condition (i.e., consciousness, unconsciousness, bleeding, convulsions, abdominal pain), as well as the location and telephone numbers of the facility. Be sure to allow the emergency dispatcher to hang up first.

Secondary Survey and Diagnostic Signs. Instructors trained on the paramedic or EMT level may take a more complete evaluation of the person, called the secondary survey. This involves checking for additional unseen injuries once the victim is out of immediate danger.

Diagnostic **vital signs** may give important clues to a victim's problem. Monitoring these signs at various intervals will give valuable information about the victim's condition and whether it is worsening or improving. The instructor may take vital signs during or after the secondary survey. The specific situation will determine the appropriate time. The following is a brief description of each diagnostic sign.

The pulse is the wave of pressure that occurs each time the heart beats. In adults, the average pulse is 60 to 80 beats per minute (bpm). In children, the rate is higher, around 80 to 100 bpm. Extremely fit persons may have resting heart rates as low as 40 bpm, and someone who has been exercising before collapsing may have a pulse rate as high as 200 bpm. Take the pulse at the carotid artery and count the number of beats in a 60-second period. If the carotid artery is not accessible, use the radial artery at the thumb side of the wrist.

The instructor must assess not only the rate of the pulse, but the quality as well. Quality refers to the sensation of the pulse to the palpating fingers. In a normal person, the pulse should feel full and strong. With certain illnesses, it will feel weak. In others, it may feel bounding, similar to the sensation during exercise. Knowing whether the pulse is rapid or weak, full and bounding, absent or irregular is very important; however, knowing whether any change in the pulse has occurred is even more important. Therefore, assess and record the rate and quality of the pulse initially and again at regular intervals.

The respiratory rate of a normal adult is usually 12 to 20 breaths per minute. Extremely fit persons, however, may only breathe six to eight times per minute. Those engaged in strenuous exercise will have a much higher respiratory rate than normal. As with the pulse, the number of respirations per minute and the quality of the respirations are equally important in establishing a diagnosis. Respirations may be shallow, deep, gasping or labored. They may even be accompanied by coughing or frothy sputum. Observe and record the findings.

Skin color and temperature will be affected by various emergency conditions. A victim's skin color may be a variety of shades, ranging from pale, white, grayish and ashen, to normal, blue, yellow or bright red. To the touch, the skin may feel hot and dry, normal, or cold and clammy. Note whatever conditions are found.

The pupils of a normal person should be equal in size and react equally when exposed to light. Assess the pupils by observing their size and then observing their action when a light is passed across each eye. Look for constriction of the pupils when the light is present and dilation when the light is removed. If a penlight is not available, access pupillary reaction by covering the eyes one at a time and seeing whether the pupils constrict equally once they are again exposed to light.

The level of consciousness of a victim can range from being alert, responsive and oriented, to a state of deep coma. It is the best indicator of the status of the nervous system. Whether the victim lost consciousness immediately, rapidly or gradually is information the rescue team will want. Record this information along with the rest of the vital signs.

Caring for a Conscious Victim

The instructor should first introduce him- or herself and ask the victim's name. Then communicate the following:

1. Training appropriate to the situation: "My name is so-and-so, and I am trained in advanced first aid."

2. What's going to happen next: "I am going to check your injury. Help has been

called and is on the way."

3. What the problem is, even if it is only superficial: "It seems you have a cut over your eye."

4. What the victim should do: "It is important to lie still right now. Please do not move."

The instructor must show the victim that he or she is in control, but never act until he or she has evaluated the entire situation.

CARE OF SUDDEN ILLNESS

If participants are screened properly, and if those who are at risk have received medical clearance from their physician to exercise, serious illness such as a heart attack should be rare in an exercise class. However, because of the potential life-threatening nature of some medical conditions, instructors should be familiar with the signs of illness and be prepared to act quickly.

Myocardial Infarction

Myocardial infarction, or heart attack, occurs when a blood vessel leading to the heart becomes so narrow that the muscle fibers supplied by the vessel receive inadequate oxygen and die.

The most common sign of a myocardial infarction is squeezing or crushing chest pain under the sternum. The victim may also feel pain between the shoulder blades or perceive the pain as radiating to the jaw, down the left arm or down both arms. Often, the victim may assume the cause of the problem is merely indigestion.

Other signs of myocardial infarction include sudden onset of weakness, nausea and sweating without any apparent cause. In the course of the attack, it is common for complications to arise, such as abnormal heart rhythms and faintness. The victim's lungs may fill with fluid, making

breathing difficult, or cardiogenic shock may set in. (Cardiogenic shock occurs when damage to the heart affects its ability to pump blood through the body and adequately oxygenate tissues.)

Many times, cardiac arrest (cessation of the heart's pumping action, necessitating immediate CPR) is the first sign that a heart attack has taken place.

The physical findings for a myocardial infarction vary. The pulse may be elevated as a result of the injury itself, or as a normal response to fear and anxiety. In some cases, the pulse may be abnormally slow. Cardiac rhythm is usually regular but may be irregular. Frequently the victim may be short of breath, but sometimes respiration may be normal. The skin may be either dry or moist and usually will appear pale and gray. The most consistent finding in a victim experiencing a myocardial infarction is fear accompanied by an overwhelming sense of impending doom.

Treatment. Call for help immediately. Place the victim in a semireclined position and loosen all restrictive clothing. Take vital signs, especially pulse, blood pressure and respirations. Record the time they were taken. This information will be valuable to the emergency rescue team. All victims of myocardial infarction will be very frightened; calm reassurance may be the best treatment an instructor can render until help arrives.

Angina Pectoris

When the heart's need for oxygen exceeds the available supply due to a restricted coronary artery, the pain that occurs is called **angina pectoris**. Angina is usually brought on by physical exertion or periods of physical or emotional stress. Unlike the pain from a myocardial infarction, the pain from angina is relieved when the heart's need for oxygen meets the available supply. Rest from the offending activity will relieve the pain because the heart's need for oxygen then decreases. **Nitroglycerin** will also relieve the pain because it diminishes the work of the heart, again reducing the need for oxygen.

The pain may be identical to that of a heart attack, with the following exceptions:

First, pain from an anginal attack lasts only from a few seconds to a few minutes, but pain from a myocardial infarction can last 30 minutes or longer.

Second, an anginal attack does not lead to death because no part of the heart muscle dies. Unfortunately, death is a common occurrence with a myocardial infarction. Because the signs of angina and myocardial infarction can be similar, call for emergency help whenever a participant is experiencing prolonged chest discomfort.

Treatment. If a participant in an exercise class is experiencing an anginal attack, have the person stop exercising immediately. Inquire if there is a history of heart problems and if so, find out if any medications have been prescribed. If the victim has nitroglycerin, make sure he or she takes it. Nitroglycerin should help ease the temporary pain. However, resumption of the activity should not be allowed. A participant who is experiencing angina and is not on medication should visit a physician. It would be wise to require a victim who has experienced an angina attack for the first time to provide a doctor's note giving written approval to continue exercising before allowing him or her to return to class.

Cerebrovascular accident

A **cerebrovascular accident**, or a stroke, occurs when the brain loses function in one of three ways: when a clot forms in an artery in the brain, blocking the normal passage of blood; when a clot formed elsewhere in the body lodges in a blood vessel in the brain, again blocking the normal passage of blood; or when an artery in the brain ruptures, for whatever reason, causing bleeding into the tissues. This bleeding alone can cause brain damage or may trigger spasms of the ruptured artery, further interrupting blood flow.

Strokes caused by blood clots are often the result of atherosclerotic changes and usually occur in older persons. Strokes caused by ruptured blood vessels can affect all age groups, including children.

A stroke caused by a blood clot in an artery of the brain is manifested by a decrease in normal body functions, usually without pain or seizures. A stroke caused by a blood clot formed elsewhere is manifested by sudden loss of consciousness with possible convulsions or paralysis. If the cause of the stroke is a ruptured artery, the manifestations include headache and rapid loss of consciousness. In all cases, the final manifestations will depend on the area of the brain damaged. They may include paralysis of one or both extremities, impaired speech or vision, dizziness, convulsions, or decreased consciousness ranging from coma to simple confusion. Occasionally the only manifestation of a stroke will be a headache.

Treatment. Treatment for a stroke should begin with a call for help. If the victim is unconscious, make sure a proper airway is maintained. Place the victim on his or her side so that secretions can drain, preferably with the paralyzed side down. Take diagnostic vital signs, especially noting blood pressure and the regularity or irregularity of the pulse and respirations, because this information may give the emergency rescue team enough clues to determine the extent of the stroke. Treat the victim gently and avoid excessive handling. Do not give anything by mouth, keeping in mind the throat may be paralyzed. Remember that stroke victims may be able to hear and understand everything going on around them, even though they give the appearance of being unconscious and unable to speak.

Seizure Disorders

Seizures or convulsions may occur as a result of epilepsy, high fever, head injuries, allergic reactions, meningitis, hypoglycemia, eclampsia (a condition affecting pregnant women), withdrawal from alcohol or drugs, or any condition resulting in diminished oxygen to the brain. A seizure may be mild, almost impossible to notice, or it may be violent. The latter type, known as a grand mal seizure, is a dramatic event that comes on suddenly, with an abnormal burst of brain-cell activity and uncontrollable jerky contractions of the skeletal muscles.

There are three phases of a grand mal seizure. During the first, or preictal phases, the victim senses a seizure is about to begin and is usually somewhat disoriented. The ictal phase, which is the actual convulsive phase, occurs next. Along with violent contractions, the victim may lose bowel and bladder control as well. The third phase called the postictal phase, occurs after the violent contractions cease. The victim will be somewhat disoriented, usually very depressed and often embarrassed.

Treatment. Emergency care during a seizure should focus on preventing the victim from becoming injured. Do not try to restrain the victim during the seizure. Instead, protect the victim's head, arms and legs by removing surrounding objects.

Do not place objects in the victim's mouth, such as tongue blades or other bite blocks to prevent "swallowing" of the tongue. Such attempts often cause injury and provide no true medical benefit for the victim.

If help has not arrived by the time the seizure is over, try to reorient the victim. When help arrives, tell the rescue team what the seizure looked like and how long it lasted. If the victim was taking any prescribed medication, give this to the team to take along with them to the hospital.

Diabetes Mellitus

Diabetes mellitus is a disease characterized by a deficiency in the body's ability to use sugar (glucose) as an energy source, particularly following the ingestion of food. This deficiency results in a high level of glucose in the blood, a condition known as hyperglycemia. Diabetes is caused by a lack of the hormone **insulin.**

In people without diabetes, insulin is released from the pancreas when glucose levels increase. This release of insulin promotes the uptake of glucose into the body's cells. In diabetics, however, insulin availability is insufficient, and the glucose level remains elevated.

There are two major classifications of diabetes: insulin-dependent and non-insulin-dependent. Insulin-dependent diabetes, also known as juvenile-onset diabetes, occurs in people under 20 years of age. Non-insulin-dependent diabetes, or adult-onset diabetes, occurs in people over 40 years of age, most of whom (80 percent) are obese. Of the 11 million diabetics in the United States, 90 percent are non-insulin-dependent. Insulin-dependent diabetics need daily insulin injections to control their glucose levels, while non-insulin-dependent diabetics rely on oral medication and diet.

Fortunately, diabetes mellitus can be controlled with diet, medication and exercise. Diabetics must balance the amount of medication they take with the amount of food they ingest because some sugar is present in all foods. Diabetics must also take into consideration the amount of insulin or other oral medications in the body and the amount of exercise to be performed. When the proper balance between the level of insulin and the level of glucose in the blood changes, one of two emergency situations may occur: insulin shock or diabetic coma.

Insulin Shock. **Insulin shock**, or hypoglycemia, occurs when the diabetic has taken too much insulin or oral medication, has not eaten enough food to balance the amount of insulin in the bloodstream, or has exercised excessively. In each case there is an excessive drop in the level of glucose in the blood. An emergency situation develops when the brain receives insufficient glucose. Insulin shock can occur very suddenly and although not common, unconsciousness may occur which could result in brain damage if not corrected immediately (see below).

A person in insulin shock will exhibit the following symptoms: profuse sweating; normal respirations; pale skin; a full, rapid pulse; normal blood pressure; dizziness and/or headache; disorientation or confusion, and fainting, with possible unconsciousness.

Diabetic Coma. Although this is an emergency situation, it is rarely encountered and usually involves the insulin-dependent diabetic. **Diabetic coma**, or hyperglycemia, occurs when there is insufficient insulin available for the cells to use glucose as their energy source. As a result, cells begin to break down fat to satisfy energy needs. The breakdown of fat markedly increases the acidity of the blood and if fluid loss is sufficient, diabetic coma results. A diabetic coma will occur in the uncontrolled diabetic and in the diabetic who has not taken sufficient insulin and who has undergone some physiological stress, such as infection. Unlike insulin shock, a diabetic coma develops very slowly over a period of a few days.

The victim of a diabetic coma will exhibit various levels of unresponsiveness as well as the following signs: dry, cool skin; sunken eyes due to dehydration; rapid, deep, sighing respirations; a weak, rapid pulse; normal or slightly low blood pressure; vomiting and abdominal pain; and a sweet or fruity odor on the breath.

Treatment. If a diabetic participant suddenly becomes confused or changes moods, suspect insulin shock. Although both types of diabetics encounter insulin shock, insulin-dependent diabetics are most likely to experience hypoglycemia. Give the victim a fast-acting sweet beverage or food; orange juice is preferable, followed by a nondiet cola and then candy.

Although unconsciousness is not common in the diabetic, remember never give an unconscious victim fluids. Place granulated sugar under the victim's tongue to produce the desired result.

The victim of a diabetic coma needs insulin and must be transported to an emergency facility as soon as possible.

The following points are important for instructors to remember about diabetes:

1. Know who in the class is diabetic and what type of diabetes is present.

2. Look for a Medic-Alert bracelet or necklace that identifies the diabetes.

3. Insulin shock is the most common problem encountered with diabetics.

4. Always have some form of fast-acting sugar available.

5. Make sure the diabetic exerciser is regularly testing his or her blood glucose level and taking appropriate action if it is too high or too low.

Hyperventilation

Hyperventilation (rapid breathing) occurs most frequently as a response to psychological stress. The victim experiences the sensation of not being able to get enough air, even though a greater than normal volume of air is exchanged. The main problem with hyperventilation is the carbon dioxide is being blown off very rapidly, which increases the pH of the blood and causes the body to experience **alkalosis**, an increase in the bicarbonate concentration of the body fluids.

It is common for the hyperventilation victim to feel dizzy and faint or to experience numbness and tingling in the hands and feet. Stabbing chest pain is frequently a result of increased respirations. Vital signs will show increased pulse and respiratory rates, with the blood pressure remaining normal.

Treatment. During an episode of hyperventilation, most people will be terrified of dying. In this situation, be calm and reassuring. To increase carbon dioxide in the blood, have the victim breathe into a paper bag. If a bag is not available, cupping the hands over the mouth and nose will usually allow the victim to reclaim enough carbon dioxide to return the blood to its normal pH level.

It is important to know that some serious physical problems can bring on hyperventilation because it is one of the best ways the body can decrease the acidity of the blood. Hyperventilation can occur when acid is ingested into the system, or as a result of diabetic coma when the breakdown of fat as an energy source increases the acidity of the blood. It also can occur as a result of cardiac arrest when inadequate tissue perfusion causes the acidity of the blood to rise. Hyperventilation may occur when blood clots migrate and get lodged in the lung. If the instructor suspects that hyperventilation is caused by any of these problems, he or she should call for emergency assistance immediately.

Shock

In a normally functioning person, all parts of the body receive an adequate supply of oxygen and nutrients through the cardiovascular system. For the body to function optimally, this regular perfusion of blood to the tissue must not be interrupted. Each body system has a different level of tolerance to the lack of adequate perfusion. The heart, brain and peripheral nervous system are the most sensitive. If deprived for more than a few minutes, they can become permanently damaged. When all parts of the body receive inadequate flow of blood, **shock** develops. If adequate perfusion is not restored, death will occur.

Shock develops when the cardiovascular system fails when: damage to the heart affects its ability to pump blood through the system; severe blood loss occurs, resulting in inadequate circulation volume; or dilation of the capillaries enlarges the capacity of the cardiovascular system, making the normal volume of circulation blood insufficient to fill the system.

Types of Shock. There are eight different types of shock. Septic shock, which results from a severe bacterial infection and metabolic shock, which occurs in people who have been ill for a long time, will probably never be seen in an aerobics class. The other six types of shock are discussed briefly below.

1. Hemorrhagic shock, or hypovolemic shock, results from severe blood loss. Bleeding may be external from fractures or lacerations, or it may be internal from rupture of organs or major vessels. This type of shock often accompanies severe burns because loss of plasma can also lead to loss of blood volume. Hemorrhagic shock may be seen with crushing injuries from damage to numerous blood vessels.

2. Respiratory shock occurs when the supply of oxygen to the tissues becomes inadequate. A blocked airway or punctured lung can produce respiratory shock, as can any other condition that hinders breathing.

3. Neurogenic shock occurs when blood vessels become paralyzed and then dilate as a result of spinal-cord injury or head

trauma. The blood vessels fill with blood, causing insufficient circulating volume.

4. Psychogenic shock is normally referred to as simple fainting. Fear, anxiety, bad news, severe pain or the sight of blood may trigger fainting. There is a momentary decrease in the blood supply to the brain when a sudden dilation of blood vessels causes the blood to pool in other parts of the body. The body goes limp and falls to the ground. Immediately after collapse, the condition automatically reverses. Blood flows back to the brain and it resumes functioning. The most important concern after fainting is whether injuries were sustained by the victim during the fall.

5. Cardiogenic shock occurs when the efficiency of the heart as a pump significantly diminishes; that is, the pressure of the circulating blood is insufficient for the tissues to receive adequate oxygenation.

6. Anaphylactic shock results from a severe allergic reaction to a toxin from medication, ingestion of a food substance, an insect sting, or inhalation of dust or pollens. Signs of anaphylactic reaction include skin changes, such as flushing, itching, burning and swelling. Respiratory changes, such as coughing, wheezing and difficulty breathing, may also occur. Circulatory changes, such as decreased blood pressure, weakened pulse or dizziness, may be noted. Treatment for anaphylactic shock should be immediate transportation of the victim to an emergency care facility.

In the early stages of shock, victims may exhibit restlessness and anxiety that should be recognized immediately as a sign that shock may be developing. The victim may complain of thirst or feel nauseated and then vomit. Upon examination, the shock victim will exhibit a weak and rapid pulse. The blood pressure will be low and steadily decrease (assume systolic pressure of 100mm Hg or less to be an indication of

developing shock). The skin may be cool and clammy. There may be profuse sweating. Respirations will be weak, shallow, irregular or difficult. The face may turn pale or slightly blue from inadequate oxygenation. A dull, lusterless stare can be seen in a shock victim, with the pupils often dilated. The person may be unconscious.

Prevention of Shock. Shock cannot be properly treated in the field by laypersons. However, instructors can give care to prevent shock by attempting to optimize the efforts of a compromised cardiovascular system. There are four steps to remember:

1. Establish an appropriate airway. Allow the victim to find the position in which he or she can breathe best. This will generally be supine, but in cardiogenic shock, the victim may feel more comfortable in a semireclined position.

2. Control the bleeding. Control external bleeding with compression as described in later sections of this chapter. Control internal bleeding by splinting fractures and avoiding rough and excessive handling.

3. Elevate the lower extremities 12 inches to help reduce pooling of blood and encourage venous return to the heart. A person who feels lightheaded should be allowed to sit down or lie down to avoid fainting. If the person has been exercising rigorously and the heart rate is very high, a gradual cool-down period should be encouraged. The instructor should stay close to the participant in case fainting occurs.

4. Cover the victim with a blanket to help maintain body temperature.

Assess diagnostic vital signs during or after the secondary survey and every 5 minutes thereafter. Keep a record of this information for the emergency rescue team. Never give a shock victim or an unconscious victim anything to eat or drink. If inadequate perfusion continues, irreversible shock will occur and the victim will die.

Recognition of the development of shock, proper care and effective treatment, and prompt transportation to an emergency care facility may save the victim's life.

CARE OF WOUNDS AND BLEEDING

Wounds are breaks in the tissues, either external or internal (open or closed). An open wound is a break in the skin or mucous membrane. A closed wound involves underlying tissues without a break in the skin or a mucous membrane.

Open Wounds

Open wounds range from those that bleed profusely but are relatively free from infection to those that bleed only mildly but have greater potential for infection. Often a victim will have more than one type of wound.

Abrasions are scrapes of the skin's surface. Bleeding from an abrasion is usually limited to blood oozing from ruptured small veins and capillaries. However, contamination and infection are dangers because dirt and bacteria may have been ground into the broken tissues.

Incisions, or cuts in body tissues, are commonly caused by sharp objects or edges. The degree of bleeding depends on the depth and extent of the cut. Deep cuts may involve blood vessels and cause extensive bleeding. Cuts may also damage muscles, tendons and nerves. The destruction of tissue is greater in **lacerations**, which are ragged wounds, than in incisions.

Punctures are produced by pointed objects such as nails, pens or pencils. External bleeding is usually minor, but the puncture object may penetrate deep into the body, damaging organs and soft tissues and causing severe, internal bleeding. Puncture wounds are more likely to become infected than other wounds because they are not usually flushed out by external blood loss. Tetanus organisms and other harmful bacteria, which grow rapidly in the absence of air and in the presence of warmth and moisture, can be carried deep into the body tissues by penetrating objects.

Avulsions involve the forcible separation or tearing of tissue from the body. Heavy bleeding usually follows immediately. A finger, toe, or in rare cases, whole limbs, may sometimes be successfully reattached to the body by a surgeon if the severed part is sent with the victim to the hospital.

First Aid for Open Wounds

If the wound is minor and does not bleed profusely, the instructor may need only hold the wound edges together and bandage it. To prevent transmission of blood-borne diseases, such as hepatitis or AIDS, a person giving first aid should wear protective gloves before attending any open wound.

At times, however, it may be difficult to decide whether a wound needs medical care and suturing. Below is the American Red Cross list of open-wound conditions that usually require medical treatment after emergency care has been provided:

1. Blood spurting from a wound, even if controlled initially with first aid.

2. Persistent bleeding despite all control efforts.

3. Any incised wound deeper than the outer layer of skin.

4. Any lacerations, deep punctures or avulsions.

5. Severed or crushed nerves, tendons or muscles.

6. Lacerations of the face or other body part where scar tissue would be noticeable after healing.

7. Skin broken by a bite (human or animal).

8. Heavy contamination of a wound.

9. A foreign object embedded deep in the tissue.

10. Foreign matter in a wound, not possible to remove by washing.

11. Any other open wound where there is doubt concerning the treatment needed.

Controlling Severe Bleeding

The adult human body contains approximately 6 quarts of blood, which is normally capable of clotting in 6 to 7 minutes. A healthy adult can lose up to 1 pint of blood without harmful effects, but the loss of more than 1 quart can be life-threatening. Hemorrhage from major blood vessels in the arms, neck and thighs may occur so rapidly and extensively that death takes only a few minutes. Hemorrhage must be controlled immediately. In most medical emergencies, only restoration of breathing takes priority over the control of bleeding.

External bleeding may occur after an external injury or an internal injury in which blood escapes into tissue spaces or body cavities. External bleeding can be divided into arterial, venous or capillary; however, such classification is of little value because in a large wound, blood may escape at the same time from all three types of vessels.

In capillary bleeding, such as in an area of scraped skin, blood and serum ooze to the surface. Blood from a vein is dark red with a steady flow. Arterial blood is bright red, flows in spurts, and is not likely to clot unless it is from a very small artery or blood flow is slight. When completely severed, arteries tend to constrict and seal off. In an emergency, the important consideration is the amount of bleeding and how to control it, not the source.

Internal bleeding may result from a direct blow, fractures, strains, sprains or diseases such as bleeding ulcers. When vessels are ruptured, blood leaks into tissue spaces and body cavities. Internal bleeding should be suspected in all cases that involve penetrating or crushing injuries of the chest and abdomen.

The signs and symptoms of excessive blood loss include weakness or actual fainting; dizziness; pale, moist and clammy skin; nausea; thirst; fast, weak and irregular pulse; shortness of breath; dilated pupils; ringing in the ears; restlessness; and apprehension. The victim may lose consciousness and stop breathing. The number of symptoms and their severity is generally proportional to the speed and quantity of blood loss. Control bleeding by direct pressure, elevation and compression of pressure points. Once it has been controlled, place the victim in a reclining position, encourage him or her to lie quietly, and begin treatment for shock. Apply pressure directly to the bleeding site with the palm of the hand. A tourniquet should be applied only when every other method has failed to control excessive bleeding.

Direct pressure. The simplest and preferred method of controlling severe bleeding is to place a dry, sterile dressing over the wound, applying pressure directly to the bleeding site with the palm of the hand. If a sterile dressing is not available in an emergency, use the cleanest cloth available. In the absence of a dressing or cloth, use a bare hand until a dressing is available. If the first dressing becomes blood soaked, apply another one on top of it, using firmer hand pressure. Never remove the initial dressing. To do so would disturb the clotting process, which takes approximately 6 minutes.

A pressure bandage can be applied over the dressing to hold it in place while additional emergency care is given. Place the center of the bandage directly over the dressing on the wound and maintain a steady pull while wrapping the ends of the bandages around the injured area.

Unlike bandages for other wounds, a bandage to control severe bleeding should be tied over the dressing to provide additional pressure to the area. Do not cut off the circulation. The instructor should be able to feel a pulse on the side of the injured area away from the heart. If applied properly, the bandage can remain undisturbed for at least 24 hours.

Elevation. If a head or extremity wound is bleeding profusely, apply direct pressure on a dressing over the wound, and elevate the wounded part. The force of gravity will lower blood pressure in the affected part and reduce blood flow. Do not use elevation on any suspected fractures that are not splinted.

Closed Wounds

Most closed wounds are caused by external forces, such as falls, contusions from blunt objects and automobile accidents. Many closed wounds are small and damage soft tissue only. Fractures of the limbs, spine and skull, as well as damage to vital organs in the chest or abdomen, may occur in more severe wounds.

Pain and tenderness are the most common symptoms of a closed wound. Usual signs include swelling and discoloration of soft tissues and deformity of limbs caused by fractures or dislocations. It is wise to suspect a closed wound with internal bleeding and possible rupture of a body organ whenever a powerful force exerted on the body has produced severe shock or unconsciousness. Even if signs of external injury are obvious, internal injury should be suspected when any of the following general symptoms are present:

1. Cool, pale, clammy skin.

2. Rapid but weak pulse.

3. Rapid breathing and dizziness.

4. Pain and tenderness in a body part where injury is suspected, especially if deep pain seems out of proportion to the outward signs of injury.

5. Restlessness.

6. Excessive thirst.

7. Vomiting, coughing of blood, or passage of blood in the urine or feces.

Emergency Care. Carefully examine the victim for fractures and other injuries to the head, neck, chest, abdomen, limbs, back and spine. If internal injury is suspected, get medical care as soon as possible. If a closed fracture is suspected, immobilize the affected area before moving the victim. Carefully transport the victim in a lying position, giving special attention to the prevention of shock. Watch the victim's breathing and take measures to prevent airway blockage or uncontrolled bleeding. Do not give fluids by mouth to anyone suspected of having internal injury, regardless how much he or she complains of thirst.

Blisters

Blisters are caused by friction that results from skin layers and accumulation of fluid between them. Avoiding friction will prevent blisters. Shoes should fit properly and be broken in gradually. Socks should always be worn to keep the feet clean and to help reduce friction. Dusting the feet with a magnesium carbonate-based powder, or applying a skin lubricant such as petroleum jelly, or applying thin adhesive felt over possible blister sites may also be effective.

Blisters always carry the possibility of severe infection from contamination. A blister that appears to be infected requires medical attention. In general, a blister should be left intact and protected from further injury by either a small doughnut pad or a covering lubricant and dressing. If a large blister is in danger of tearing, it should be punctured with a sterile needle. First scrub the skin area over and around the blister with soap and water, or some other antiseptic. Then introduce a sterilized needle under the skin approximately one-eighth of an inch outside the raised tissue. Next, compress the blister with sterile gauze to drain fluid. The skin provides natural protection for the sensitive skin below, so leave it on for several days. Apply an antibiotic ointment to the area and cover with a sterile dressing. Check the blister frequently for infection.

When a blister has been torn, the following approach may be indicated:

(Remember to wear sterile gloves for any procedure involving body fluids.)

1. Cleanse the blister and surrounding area with soap and water; then rinse with an antiseptic.

2. Using sterile scissors, cut the torn blister halfway around its perimeter.

3. Apply antiseptic or antibiotic ointment to exposed tissue.

4. Lay the flap of skin back over the treated tissue and cover with a sterile dressing.

5. Within two to three days, or when the underlying tissue has hardened sufficiently, remove the dead skin by trimming it as close as possible to the perimeter of the blister.

INJURIES TO THE MUSCULOSKELETAL SYSTEM

Because musculoskeletal injuries are so frequent, it is important to evaluate them properly and master the skills necessary for initial emergency care. Appropriate emergency care of fractures and dislocations not only decreases immediate pain and reduces the possibility of shock, but also improves the chances for rapid recovery and early return to normal activities.

Fractures

A **fracture** is any break in the continuity of a bone, ranging from a simple crack to severe shatter of the bone with multiple fractures fragments. In the initial evaluation of a fracture, the most important factor is the integrity of the overlying skin and soft tissues. Thus, fractures are always classified as open or closed.

In an open fracture, the overlying skin has been lacerated by sharp bone ends protruding through the skin, or by a direct blow breaking the skin at the time of the fracture. The bone may be visible in the wound. The wound may be only a small puncture or it may be a gaping hole exposing much bone and soft tissue. In a closed fracture, the bone ends have not penetrated the skin, and no wound appears near the fracture.

It is extremely important to determine at once whether the fracture is open or closed. Open fractures are often more serious than closed fractures because they may be associated with greater blood loss. There is greater risk of infection because the bone has been contaminated by exposure to the outside environment. For these reasons, describe all fractures to emergency personnel as open or closed so that proper treatment can be undertaken upon arrival at the hospital.

An injured person complaining of musculoskeletal pain must be suspected of having a fracture. While bone ends protruding through the skin or gross deformity of a limb make recognizing fractures easy, many fractures are less obvious. The instructor must know the seven signs of a fracture; the presence of any one should arouse suspicion of a fracture.

These seven signs are deformity, tenderness, inability to use the extremity, swelling and ecchymosis (discoloration), exposed fragments, crepitation (grating noise), and false motion.

All of these signs need not be present for the diagnosis of a fracture. Do not manipulate the limb to elicit them. Inspection of the limb with clothing removed may show deformity, swelling, discoloration or exposed bone fragments if there is a fracture. A victim's unwillingness to use the affected limb indicates guarding and loss of function. Palpation over the injured bone elicits point tenderness. Any of these signs is sufficient to assume limb fracture and initiate emergency care.

Treatment. Emergency management of fractures begins after the vital functions are assessed and stabilized. Completely cover all open wounds with a dry, sterile dressing. Apply local pressure to control bleeding. Once a sterile compression dressing is applied to an open fracture, manage it the same way as a closed fracture. Notify emergency personnel of all open wounds, dressed or splinted.

Emergency personnel will splint all fractures before the victim is moved, unless life is immediately threatened. While waiting for their arrival, place a rolled towel on either side of the extremity so that it is not moved further. Splinting facilitates transportation of the victim and helps prevent the following:

1. Motion of fracture fragments that produces pain.

2. Further damage of muscle, spinal cord, peripheral nerves and blood vessels by broken bone ends.

3. Laceration of skin by broken bone ends that would convert a closed fracture into an open one.

4. Restriction of distal blood flow from pressure of the bone ends on blood vessels.

5. Excessive bleeding into the tissues at the fracture site.

A splint is simply a device to prevent an injured part from moving. For properly trained personnel, the general rules for splinting are:

1. Remove clothing from the area of any suspected fracture or dislocation.

2. To rule out circulatory or neurological injury, check for a pulse distal to the site of injury and for sensation to a light touch or the ability to move the fingers or toes. If there is no pulse or no sensation, act as if there were a medical emergency and inform emergency personnel when they arrive.

3. Immobilize the joints above and below the fracture with a splint.

4. During splint application, move the limb as little as possible.

5. Do not straighten a severely deformed limb. Splint the limb in the position of deformity.

6. In all suspected neck and spine injuries, do not move the injured person.

7. Cover all wounds with a dry, sterile dressing before applying any splint.

8. Pad the splints to prevent local pressure.

9. Do not move or transport victims before splinting extremity injuries.

10. When in doubt, splint.

Soft-Tissue Injuries

Injuries to participants in exercise classes and recreational activities generally involve soft tissue. Fractures occur, but far less often than sprains, strains and overuse syndromes. Since soft tissues do not show on the x-rays, sport and recreational injuries often present diagnostic problems. Also, if ignored, athletic injuries can become increasingly disabling. Unfortunately, a victim's response to such an injury is often denial, but attempting to continue the activity in spite of the symptoms (though only slightly disabling) can result in use of compensatory mechanisms that may alter gait or other body activities. Such changes may cause problems worse than the original injury.

Strains and Sprains. Although the terms "strain" and "sprain" are frequently used interchangeably, they are not the same. A **strain** is an overstretching or tearing of a muscle, tendon or the musculotendinous junction. A **sprain** is an overstretching or tearing of a ligament or joint capsule.

An injury to a musculotendinous unit is usually dynamic (not requiring an outside force), caused by the victims themselves. All musculotendinous units are susceptible to strains, but those frequently strained include hamstrings, quadriceps, calf and shoulder girdle muscles. Strains can result from poor flexibility, improper warm-up and cool-down, or sudden, violent contractions of a muscle.

Strains are classified in order of severity. First-degree strains are mild and involve a minimum of torn fibers. Mild tenderness around the area is usually accompanied by some swelling. Second-degree strains involve moderate tearing of tissue and cause greater pain, swelling and deformity of muscle. Third-degree strains are severe, involving a complete tear of the connective tissue and require a physician's attention.

Sprains, like strains, range from minor tears or stretching to complete disruption of the ligament or joint capsule. Because ligaments attach bone to bone, sprains result when a joint is forced to move in an abnormal direction (one for which it was not intended). On the other hand, strains, which involve a muscle or tendon, usually result from an unaccustomed amount of force. Most sprains occur to hinge joints; that is, joints designed to function in one plane. The knee and ankle are the most frequently sprained joints. Preventive measures include conditioning, stretching and avoiding overextensive muscle use, especially in an exercise class in which the excitement of participating may override one's caution.

Tendinitis. **Tendinitis** is the most common overuse syndrome, and has been described as an inflammatory response to microscopic trauma. After repetitive activity, the tendon or its sheath eventually breaks down, producing inflammation that causes pain and tenderness. Any tendon is a potential site for this injury, but the most common areas are the ankle (Achilles tendon), in and around the knee (iliotibial band and patellar tendon), the elbow and the lower front of the leg (shin splints). Tendinitis can often be prevented through use of proper equipment, such as special footwear, and by preparing the musculoskeletal system for the specific demands to be placed on it. Because overuse syndromes tend to develop when demand exceeds the strength of the musculoskeletal system, proper strength conditioning is necessary.

Bursitis. A bursa is a sac-like structure that aids motion by lubricating sites of potential friction, such as where a tendon or ligament rubs over a bony prominence or other body structure. Bursae are most commonly found in the shoulder, hip, knee and ankle. **Bursitis** (inflammation of a bursa), may be caused at first by a direct blow to, or repetitive action of this fluid-filled sac. Subsequent overuse of the joint, including some activities of daily living, can cause the bursa to remain inflamed. Although this injury is less common in athletes than sprains, strains or tendinitis, once the bursa is aggravated, recurrent irritation is far more likely.

Contusions. A **contusion** (bruise) is an injury that crushes soft tissue but does not break the skin or bone. The usual cause is a direct blow. The intensity of a contusion can range from superficial to deep for soft tissues, and may even include underlying bone. The extent to which a person may be hampered by a contusion depends on the location and the force of the blow.

Treatment of Common Soft-Tissue Injuries. Treatment of soft-tissue injuries can be as simple as applying a bandage or as complicated as requiring several operations and months of rehabilitation. Regardless of the severity of the injury, initial management includes a few simple steps to decrease pain, swelling and inflammation. These steps are important to avoid complicating the injury and to allow better assessment of the situation.

Proper and immediate first aid consists of **RICE** — rest, ice, compression and elevation. After a traumatic event to the body, the area of injury swells. Swelling is a natural reaction to protect the wounded area; however, it slows healing time and can be very painful. The RICE method lessens pain and swelling, thereby speeding the healing process.

Have the victim rest the affected area, either completely (by staying off a sprained ankle, for example) or partly (by shifting from a high-impact to a low-impact exercise activity, or by refraining from exercise), depending on the nature and severity of the injury.

Apply ice for 20 to 30 minutes to the injured area every 2 to 3 hours immediately after a soft-tissue injury occurs, with the exception of fractures. This prolonged icing constricts the capillaries of the lymphatic system at the injured site, slowing the release of fluid, and thereby controlling the swelling. The best procedure is to put crushed ice in a moist towel, place it on the injured area, and secure it with an elastic wrap. Plastic bags filled with ice are more convenient but cooling is less effective because they are not moist.

Compression can be used with or without ice. While icing, secure the moist cold-pack firmly with an elastic wrap or bandage. Between icings, apply a dry elastic wrap over a foam compression pad or by itself. The compression further constricts the release of excessive fluids by the body and provides the injured area with some support. It is important to wrap not only the involved area but also the area above and below it, leaving no skin exposed. Wrapping the entire area will provide even compression and greater protection to the injury. Tell the victim to periodically release the wrap and not to sleep with it in place unless instructed to do so by a physician.

Elevation means placing the injured area higher than the heart, a position that allows gravity to drain fluid and prevent excess accumulation. For example, with a sprained ankle, it is far more beneficial to lie on the back with the entire leg raised and supported, than it is to sit in a chair and rest the foot on a stool. Have the victim sleep with the injured part elevated as long as the swelling persists.

With acute injuries, never apply heat or wrap the area tightly enough to cause skin discoloration, numbness or tingling. Do not allow the victim to walk or run off an injury. After 36 to 48 hours and stabilization of the injury (swelling stops), treatment may vary. That some sports-medicine advisers advocate heat while others suggest cold (after two days) is confusing, but this inconsistency has nothing to do with the initial management, which always consists of cold. If swelling has not lessened in 48 hours, seek medical advice.

HEAT STRESS

The amazingly complex human body is often compared to an engine with a thermostat, a useful analogy with one crucial difference—the human thermostat cannot always "turn off the heat." Humans produce heat in many ways—cellular metabolism, muscular activity, ingestion of food and hormonal actions. People pick up heat from the sun's rays or reflections, particularly off sand and snow.

Heat injury is 100-percent preventable.

Nonetheless, cases of **heat exhaustion** and death from **heat stroke** continue to occur.

Physiological Response to Heat

When it is hot, an exerciser or athlete's work becomes much more difficult. Almost all athletes experience some type of heat stress, either from the external environment or from internal heat generated by their own metabolism. Most heat stress is associated with summer activities, but it is not unusual for winter-sports participants to generate enough heat to produce a heat-stress effect.

Whatever the source, the body acts to protect itself against accumulation of heat. It possesses remarkable thermoregulatory mechanisms that adjust the inner environment to meet the demands of the outer environment, to enable the athlete to perform optimally anywhere.

To maintain thermal equilibrium, the heat gained by the body must be offset exactly by the amount dissipated. This delicate balance is controlled by the thermoregulatory mechanism, which involves circulation, sweating, neuroimpulses and endocrine responses. For example, when a drop in temperature occurs, "cool" signals are transmitted to the brain that cause blood vessels to constrict, thus preserving heat. Conversely, if the temperature rises, an opposite chain of reactions is set in motion, ending with sweating and a cooling effect as the sweat evaporates.

Sweating provides the body with the main line of defense against overheating. Sweating to regulate body heat is a reflex response to a thermal stimulus. Sweat comes from sweat glands in the skin that emit a hypotonic solution (lower concentration of salt than contained in blood) on the skin for the purposes of evaporation. The total quantity of sweat produced is precisely controlled by the body's thermoregulatory requirements. It is estimated that an acceptable rate of sweating is approximately one-half quart per hour, or 3 percent of the person's body weight. When this level is exceeded, the body reduces the amount of sweat it produces, particularly if fluid replacement is ignored.

In cases of heat stress, the natural defenses have been overwhelmed, and thirst, fatigue, visual disturbances, heat cramps and exhaustion may be looked at as physiological cries for help.

When the body cannot withstand the strain of heat stress, the person will show signs of thermoregulatory imbalance—cessation of sweating, feeling extra tired, groggy or thirsty—that, if recognized, are simple to correct. Immediately stop the victim's activity, move him or her to a cool environment and summon a doctor.

The body must also have fluid replacement. Otherwise it will be prone to developing one of the three major heat syndromes: heat cramps, heat exhaustion, and the most serious and sometimes fatal, heat stroke.

Heat Stress Syndromes

Heat injury results when demands of the environment exceed the capabilities of the body's regulatory mechanisms. The temperature regulatory system controls the body's heat to balance heat production and heat loss. If, because of thermal disturbances, the thermostat deviates from a desired condition, the regulatory center directs a response to correct the deviation.

Heat Cramps. Normal muscle contractions require a strict balance of salt and water within the muscles. Excessive perspiration may cause water and salt loss. Some experts believe cramps are due to excessive fluid loss (dehydration), muscle fatigue, or overheating, while others believe electrolyte (salt) imbalance causes the painful muscle spasms. **Heat cramps** occur in people who sweat profusely, and, like most heat disorders, they usually take place at the beginning of a warm-weather season before an acclimatization period. Cramps most often occur in the lower leg muscles, such as the calves, but may also occur in the hamstrings, quadriceps and abdominal muscles.

Once cramps have developed, have the victim rest from the activity, begin stretching and apply cold, moist ice to the muscles involved. Drinking water may help reverse the cramps.

Heat Exhaustion. Heat exhaustion is a more severe heat syndrome, which is caused by a decrease in blood volume and water, or by salt depletion from excessive sweating. Normally fit persons who are involved in extreme physical exertion in a hot environment can develop heat exhaustion. Under these conditions, the muscles and brain require greater blood flow, and at the same time, the skin needs increased blood flow to radiate heat from the skin in the form of sweat. When the cardiovascular system is inadequate to meet demands of the muscles, brain and skin, heat exhaustion results.

Heat exhaustion has a low mortality rate. It is characterized principally by the signs of peripheral vascular collapse or shock. Weakness, faintness, dizziness, headaches, loss of appetite, nausea, pale skin, vomiting and postural syncope (fainting) may occur. Victims are usually sweating profusely, and their body temperatures are normal or mildly elevated. The pulse is usually weak and rapid.

Replenishment of fluids and electrolytes and prolonged rest in a cool, ventilated environment are the best treatment. Rest diminishes the demands of the circulatory system. Rehydration and electrolyte replacement are best achieved over several hours. Intravenous solutions may be necessary if the victim cannot tolerate oral fluid replacement.

Heat Stroke. This is a true medical emergency with a high mortality rate. In heat stroke, all the mechanisms for cooling have failed to the extent that severe elevation of body temperature occurs. It may occur suddenly without being preceded by other clinical syndromes, or it may progress from water-depletion-induced heat exhaustion.

In heat stroke, the hypothalamus loses control, and body temperature rises to levels that damage cells and organs throughout the body. The central nervous system (brain and spinal cord), however, is the most sensitive to heat damage. Central nervous system dysfunction may manifest itself initially by irritability, poor judgement, bizarre behavior, confusion, psychoses, and possibly seizures and coma. The victim may also have an unsteady gait and a glassy stare. The skin will be hot and dry as sweating ceases to avoid further dehydration, and the pulse will be rapid and strong.

Treatment of heat stroke must begin as soon as the disorder is recognized; the victim's prognosis is directly related to how quickly the body's temperature is returned to near normal. Call for help immediately. Remove the victim's clothing to allow skin exposure to air, and cool the body by using ice on the skin surface, immersing in a cool bath, or applying cool, damp towels or sheets. If a fan is available, use it. Once the victim is in the hospital emergency room, physicians will be able to provide more definitive treatment.

Preventing Heat Stress

Heat stress syndromes are obviously related to climate, determined by temperature and humidity. Since the environment cannot be controlled, other factors must be, especially physical conditioning and acclimatization.

Acclimatization. The body's adaptation to heat stress and increased capacity to work in high temperatures and humidity is called **acclimatization**. Since the body can adjust to the stress of repeated exposure to the heat, it is usually best to slowly increase the level of heat or intensity of the work done in a hot environment.

Most people will require four to ten days of exposure to extreme heat for acclimatization. When it is hot, one simple method of heat acclimatization is to reduce the normal workout by 50 percent on the first day. With each successive day, increase the amount of work done in the heat by 5 to 10 percent. In this way, acclimatization should occur in a week or so with no major problems, as long as there is proper intake of nutrients, electrolytes and fluids.

Fluid Replacement. Over the last 15 years, producers of fluid-replacement drinks have made many claims based on minimal facts. According to the advertising claims, each drink has some unique quality that will replace body water and salt lost in sweat. This advertising has led to confusion among persons unable to distinguish between valid claims and unsupported promotional statements.

The most important item in preventing heat injury is water. Small amounts of electrolytes may be added, but it is the consumption of adequate water that radically reduces the incidence of heat-related injuries. The role of fluid during exertion is crucial in maintaining the homeostasis of the body. With a decline in the body's water, neither the circulatory system nor the thermoregulatory system can meet the demands placed on it by the stress of exercise or a warm environment.

Sweat is quite dilute when compared with other body fluids. In other words, more water than electrolytes is removed from the body in the form of sweat. The remaining electrolytes become more concentrated in the cells of the body. As far as the cells are concerned, there is an excess of electrolytes in the body. So, during prolonged, heavy sweating, the need to replace body water is greater than any immediate demand for electrolytes. No empirical or scientific evidence has demonstrated that electrolytes intake during exercise will enhance performance or eliminate occasional muscle cramps. Even after heavy sweating, the need to replace electrolytes is generally satisfied by a balanced diet.

Exercisers and athletes should be encouraged to take in as much fluid as desired during workouts or races, but to avoid large amounts at any one time. The drinks should by hypotonic (dilute) or just cold, plain water, with little or no sugar. Fluids should be consumed in volumes of 3 to 10 ounces every 10 to 20 minutes. Prehydration of 10 to 20 ounces approximately 30 to 60 minutes before a workout is extremely beneficial. After activity, modest salting of food and ingestion of drinks with essential minerals can adequately replace the electrolytes lost in sweat.

SUMMARY

A wise instructor will be prepared to respond appropriately to emergency situations. All instructors should have training in cardiopulmonary resuscitation (CPR), and many will want additional training in first aid through the American Red Cross.

Every fitness business should have the following:

1. Written emergency plan that is read and initialed by all employees.

2. Fire extinguisher.

3. Telephone with clearly posted emergency numbers.

4. Well-stocked first-aid kit.

In a medical emergency, the instructor's first task is to discover and correct any immediate life-threatening problems and to send someone to call for help. If a victim's breathing is obstructed, first establish an airway. If there is no pulse, begin CPR. Next, control any severe bleeding by elevating the wound and applying direct pressure with a sterile dressing.

The most common injuries in an aerobics class involve the musculoskeletal system: strains and sprains, tendinitis, bursitis, contusions and fractures. Immediate treatment for most injuries is rest, ice, compression and elevation (RICE).

The primary treatment for fractures includes immobilizing the injured part and then treating any open wounds for contamination. Following these steps before seeing a physician may help reduce pain and swelling, and shorten the recovery time.

Although sudden, serious illness is not common in aerobics classes where participants have been properly screened, the potential always exists. An instructor familiar with the signs of such emergencies as a heart attack, stroke, seizure, diabetic coma and insulin shock will be able to act quickly and effectively and, perhaps, to save a life.

Exercising in a hot, humid environment can place great stress on the body's thermoregulatory system. All heat stress is 100-percent preventable through adequate fluid replacement, acclimatization and avoiding exercise if heat and humidity become excessive.

However, if body water lost through sweat is not adequately replaced, the participants may develop heat cramps, heat exhaustion or heat stroke. Heat stroke is a medical emergency, and treatment must begin immediately.

Aerobics instructors are not medical experts, and they should never exceed their training and capabilities. It is not the instructor's role to diagnose an injury or to offer medical advice. Instead, the instructor should be prepared to provide immediate emergency aid, call for help when necessary and refer participants with less serious problems to their physician. If there is any doubt about the seriousness of a participant's illness or injury, it is always wise to err on the side of caution and call for help.

SUGGESTED READING

American Academy of Orthopaedic Surgeons. (1987). *Emergency Care and Transportation of the Sick and Injured.* Chicago: American Academy of Orthopaedic Surgeons.

American Red Cross. (1992). *The American Red Cross First Aid and Safety Book, 1st edition.* Little Brown & Co.

Henderson, J. (1978). *Emergency Medical Guide.* 4th ed. New York: McGraw-Hill.

Strauss, R. H., ed. (1991). *Sports Medicine.* Philadelphia, London, Toronto: W. B. Saunders.

Thygerson, A. L. (1991). *The First Aid Book.* Englewood Cliffs, N.J.: Prentice-Hall.

Chapter 15

Legal and Professional Responsibilities

By David K. Stotlar

ost people who teach or administer aerobics programs have been trained as physical educators or exercise specialists. Often their experience with the law, if any, has been limited to cases involving common sports injuries. However, the rapid expansion of the aerobics industry has created new forms of legal liability. The purpose of this chapter is to explain basic legal concepts that concern aerobics instructors and to show how these concepts can be applied to reduce injuries to program participants, thus reducing the likelihood

David K. Stotlar, Ed.D., is director of the School of Kinesiology and Physical Education at the University of Northern Colorado, where he teaches sport law, sport administration and finance. He has served as a consultant to school districts, sports professionals, attorneys, and international sports administrators, and has been published extensively on sports law issues.

that an instructor or studio owner will be involved in a lawsuit.

LIABILITY AND NEGLIGENCE

The term **liability** refers to responsibility. Legal liability concerns the responsibilities recognized by a court of law. Every instructor who stands in front of a class faces the responsibilities of knowing capacities and setting limitations of participants before they begin an exercise program.

Studio owners and managers have the added responsibility of ensuring that the facilities and equipment are appropriate and safe. Aerobics professionals cannot avoid liability any more than they can avoid assuming the responsibilities inherent in their positions. However, those liabilities may be reduced through adherence to the appropriate standard of care and the implementation of certain risk-management principles.

The responsibilities arising from the relationship between the aerobics instructor and the participant produce a legal expectation, commonly referred to as the standard of care. **Standard of care** means that the quality of services provided in a fitness setting is commensurate with current professional standards. In the case of a negligence suit, the court would ask the question, "What would a reasonable, competent and prudent aerobics instructor do in a similar situation?" An instructor or studio owner who failed to meet that standard could be found negligent by a court of law.

Negligence is usually defined as "failure to act as a reasonable and prudent person would act under similar circumstance." For the aerobics instructor, this definition has two important components. The first deals specifically with actions: "Failure to act" refers to acts of omission as well as acts of commission. In other words, an instructor can be sued for doing something that

should not have been done, as well as for not doing something that should have been done. The second part of the definition of negligence pertains to the appropriateness of the action in light of the standard of care, or a "reasonable and prudent" professional standard. If other qualified instructors would have acted similarly under the same circumstances, a court would probably not find an instructor's action negligent.

To legally substantiate a charge of negligence, four elements must be shown to exist. As stated by Arnold, they are: (1) that the **defendant** (person being sued) had duty to protect the **plaintiff** (person filing the suit) from injury, (2) that the defendant failed to exercise that standard of care necessary to perform that duty, (3) that such failure was the proximate cause of the injury, and (4) that the damage or injury to the plaintiff did occur.

Consider this situation: A participant in an aerobics class badly sprains her ankle while following instructions for an aerobic-dance routine. The movement that led to the injury consisted of prolonged and excessive hopping on one foot, something not recommended by reasonable and prudent aerobics instructors. If the participant sues the instructor for negligence, the following questions and answers might surface in court: Was it the instructor's duty to provide proper instruction? Yes. Was that duty satisfactorily performed? Probably not. Did actual damages occur? The plaintiff's doctor concluded that they did. Was the instructor's failure to provide safe instruction the direct cause of the injury? It probably was.

AREAS OF RESPONSIBILITY

The duties assigned to fitness professionals vary from one position to another and from organization to organization. Overall, there are seven major areas of responsibility: health screening, testing and programming, instruction, supervision, facilities, risk management, and equipment. Each area poses unique questions for the professional that are important even to the beginning instructor. The American Council on Exercise (ACE) has developed a statement on ethics that is quite helpful in guiding the actions of fitness professionals (see Appendix D).

Health Screening

A fitness professional's responsibility begins when a new participant walks in the door.

Most prospective participants will be generally healthy people with the goal of improving their personal health and fitness level. Others, however, may come as part of their recovery from heart attacks or other serious health conditions. Therefore, it is imperative that instructors compile a medical history for each participant (see Chapter 5, "Health Screening") to document any existing conditions that might affect performance in an exercise program.

But responsibility does not end with collecting information. The health history and other data must be examined closely for information that affects programming decisions. Instructors have been charged with negligence for not using available information that could have prevented an injury. Every club or studio needs to establish policies and procedures to ensure that each participant's personal history and medical information are taken into account in designing an exercise program.

Fitness Testing and Exercise Programming

Many states require "medical prescriptions" to be developed by licensed medical doctors. Once the medical prescription is developed, a physical therapist is legally allowed to administer and supervise its implementation. The purpose of an exercise "prescription" is to induce a physiological response within a patient that will result in a clinical change in a given condition. As a result, fitness professionals are usually limited to providing exercise programs, not exercise prescriptions which may be construed as medical prescriptions under these circumstances. Although the difference between the terms "program" and "prescription" may seem like a technicality, it may be important in a court of law.

Fitness testing presents similar issues. The health and fitness level of the client, the purpose of the test, and the testing methods should all be calculated before test administration. The use of relatively simple tests, such as a skinfold caliper to measure percentage body fat, would not normally pose significant legal problems. On the other hand, the use of a graded exercise test on a treadmill with a multiple-lead electrocardiogram could expose an unqualified instructor to a charge of practicing medicine without a license. Therefore, it is important that the test be recognized by a professional organization as appropriate for the intended use, be within the qualifications and training of the instructor, and that an accepted protocol (testing procedure) be followed exactly.

Instruction

To conduct a safe and effective exercise program, fitness professionals are expected to provide instruction that is both adequate and proper. Adequate aerobics instruction refers to the amount of direction given to participants before and during their exercise activity. For example, an instructor who asks a class to perform an exercise without first demonstrating how to do it properly could be found negligent if a participant performs the exercise incorrectly and is injured as a result. Proper instruction is factually correct. In other words, an instructor may be liable for a participant's injury resulting from an exercise that was not demonstrated or demonstrated improperly or from an unsafe exercise that should not have been included in an aerobics routine.

In the courtroom, the correctness of instruction is usually assessed by an expert witness who describes the proper procedures for conducting the activity in question. Therefore, the instructional techniques used by an aerobics instructor should be consistent with professionally recognized standards. Proper certification from a nationally recognized professional organization, as well as appropriate documentation of training (degrees, continuing education, etc.) can enhance an instructor's competence in the eyes of a court, should he or she ever be charged with negligence.

In addition to providing adequate and proper instruction, fitness professionals should also be careful not to diagnose or suggest treatment for injuries. This includes not only injuries received in the instructor's exercise class, but also those injuries acquired by other means. When participants ask for advice, it may be best to suggest they call their doctor. In general, only physicians and certain other health-care providers are allowed to diagnose, prescribe treatment and treat injuries. An instructor can provide first aid, but only if he or she is qualified to do so.

Simple advice for a sprained ankle once resulted in a nasty lawsuit. When a participant sprained her ankle during a fitness routine, the instructor told her to go home and ice the ankle to reduce the swelling. Because the ice made the injury feel much better, the participant kept her foot in ice water for two to three hours. As a consequence, several of her toes had to be amputated because of frostbite.

This example may be extreme, but it serves as a valuable warning. There are several ways the instructor could have avoided this tragedy. First, the instructor could have advised the participant to see a physician. While this approach protects the instructor, it would be costly if every participant who suffered a sprained ankle had to see a doctor. Second, the instructor could have provided a more precise description of the first-aid ice treatment. The third and best approach would be a combination of the first two; the instructor would provide specific instructions (both written and verbal) on the first-aid procedures recommended by the American Red Cross and suggest that if the injury did not respond well, then the participant should seek the advice of a physician.

Supervision

The instructor is responsible for supervising all aspects of a class. The standards that apply to supervision are the same as those for instruction: adequate and proper. A prerequisite to determining adequate supervision is the ratio of participants to instructors and supervisors. A prudent instructor should allow a class to be only as large as can be competently monitored. The participant-instructor ratio will, of course, vary with activity, facility and type of participant. An exercise class of 30 may be appropriate in a large gymnasium, but too many for an aqua class. Adequate and proper supervision may be different for a class of fit 20-year-olds than for a class of 55-year-old beginning exercisers.

General or nonindividualized supervision can be used when the activity can be monitored from a position in general proximity to the participants. For example, in an aerobics class a conscientious instructor can give enough attention to all participants through general but systematic observation to keep them relatively safe. On the other hand, a series of fitness tests administered to a participant before an exercise program calls for specific, or individualized, supervision. The person qualified to administer the testing must provide continuous attention in immediate proximity to the participant to ensure safety. Whether general or specific, required supervision should be based on one's own judgment of the nature of the activity and the participants involved, compared with what other prudent professionals would do under the same circumstances.

Facilities

Safety is the basic question for a fitness facility. Is the environment free from unreasonable hazards? Are all areas of the facility appropriate for the specific type of activity to be conducted in that area? For example, aerobic activity requires a floor surface that will cushion the feet, knees and legs from inordinate amounts of stress. Similarly, workout areas or stations of a circuit training class should have adequate free space surrounding them to ensure that observers will not be struck by an exercising participant.

Some facilities provide locker room and shower facilities. These areas must be sanitary, the floors must be textured to reduce accidental slipping, and areas near water must be protected from electrical shock. Although aerobics instructors may not be responsible for designing and maintaining the exercise facility, any potential problem should be detected, reported and corrected as soon as possible. Until then, appropriate warning signs should be clearly posted to warn participants of the unsafe conditions.

In some cases, an instructor may be assigned to teach in an area that is unsafe

or inappropriate for the activity. Under these circumstances, a prudent instructor would refuse to teach and would document that decision in writing to the club or studio management so that constructive action may be taken.

Equipment

For a program that uses exercise equipment, the legal concerns center primarily on selection, installation, maintenance and repair. Equipment should meet all appropriate safety and design standards. If the equipment has been purchased from a competent manufacturer, these standards will probably be met. However, some organizations may try to save money by using homemade or inexpensive equipment. If an injury is caused by a piece of equipment that fails to perform as expected, and the injured party can show that the equipment failed to meet basic safety and design standards, the club or studio would be exposed to increased liability.

It is also important that trained technicians assemble and install all equipment. Having untrained people assemble some types of machinery may void the manufacturer's warranty and expose the program to additional risks. A schedule of regular service and repair should also be established and documented to show that the management has acted responsibly. Defective or worn parts should be replaced immediately, and equipment that is in need of repair should be removed for service.

Instructors and supervisors should instruct each participant on equipment safety. In addition, each instructor and participant should be required to examine the equipment before each use and report any problems to the person in charge.

Another equipment-related situation arises when participants ask their instructor about which shoes to wear or what exercise equipment to purchase for home use. An exercise professional should be extremely cautious when giving such recommendations. Before an instructor is qualified to give advice, he or she should have a thorough knowledge of the product lines available and the particular characteristics of each product. If this condition cannot be met, an instructor should refer the participant to a retail sporting-goods outlet. Otherwise, the instructor could be held liable for a negligent recommendation. An instructor who makes a recommendation based solely on personal experience should clearly state that it is a personal and not a professional recommendation. Instructors who are receiving money for endorsing a particular product must be particularly careful not to portray themselves as experts giving professional advice.

Risk Management

One of the duties of professionals in the fitness industry is to effectively manage risk. The process of **risk management** is more than just avoiding accidents; it encompasses a total examination of risk areas for the fitness professional. Each of the responsibilities identified above presents various levels of risk which should be assessed. The steps involved in a comprehensive risk-management review included the following:

1. Identification of risk areas.
2. Evaluation of specific risks in each area.
3. Selection of appropriate treatment for each risk.
4. Implementation of a risk-management system.
5. Evaluation of success.

Risk management is an important professional duty. Too often, it is considered merely a process by which to avoid lawsuits. Professionals in the fitness industry should approach risk management as a way as to provide better service to their clients. With this philosophy, risk management can become a method of conducting activities, not just a way to avoid legal trouble. The end goal is to have a safe, enjoyable experience for clients.

GUIDELINES

The following guidelines reflect the general areas described in preceding sections of this chapter and are intended to provide aerobics instructors with criteria necessary for reducing injuries to participants and the accompanying legal complications.

Health Screening

Each client beginning a fitness program should receive a thorough evaluation. Specific risk-management criteria may include:

• Evaluation is conducted prior to participating in exercise.

• Screening methods concur with national guidelines (ACE, ACSM, etc.).

Programming

Primary responsibilities of all fitness instructors include program design and exercise selection. Specific risk-management criteria may include:

• Health history is used appropriately in program design.

• Programs and tests selected are recognized by a professional organization as appropriate for the intended use.

• Programs and tests are within the qualifications and training of the aerobics instructor.

• Accepted protocols are followed exactly in all programs and procedures.

Instruction

A fitness professional must provide instruction that is both "adequate and proper." To fulfill this standard the following criteria would apply to instruction:

• Instructions or directions given to clients prior to and during activity which are sufficient and understandable.

• Conformance to "standard of care" (what a reasonable and prudent instructor would provide in the same situation).

Supervision

Aerobics instructors must perform their supervisory duties in accordance with the professionally devised and established guidelines:

• Continuous supervision is provided in immediate proximity to the client to ensure safety.

• Larger participant group is supervised from the perimeter of the exercise area to ensure that all participants are in full view of the instructor.

• Specific supervision is employed when the activity merits close attention to an individual client.

Facilities

The basic issue regarding facilities centers on the safety of the premises. The central issue is whether the environment is free from unreasonable hazards. Examples of risk-management criteria include:

• Floor surface is appropriate for each activity.

• Free area around equipment is sufficient for the exercise.

• Lighting is adequate for performance of the skill and for supervision.

• Entries and exits are well marked.

Equipment

In the equipment area, the legal concerns center primarily on selection, maintenance and repair of the equipment. A risk-management plan should examine the following points:

• Equipment selected meets all safety and design standards within the industry.

• Assembly of equipment follows manufacturer's guidelines.

• A schedule of regular service and repair is established and documented.

• Caution is exercised in relation to recommending equipment.

• Homemade equipment is avoided if at all possible.

ACCIDENT REPORTING

Regardless of the safety measures provided, some injuries are going to occur in the conduct of fitness activities. When someone is injured, it is necessary for the instructor to file an accident report.

The report should include the following information:

• Name, address and phone number of the injured person.

• Time, date and place of the accident.

• A brief description of the part of the body affected and nature of the injury. (e.g., "cut on the right hand.")

• A description and model number of any equipment involved.

• A reference to any instruction given and the type of supervision in force at the time of the injury.

• A brief, factual description of how the injury occurred (no opinions as to cause or fault).

• Names, addresses and phone numbers of any witnesses.

• A brief statement of actions taken at time of injury (e.g., first aid given, physician referral or ambulance called.).

• Signatures of the supervisor and the injured person.

Accident reports should be kept for three to five years, depending on each state's **statute of limitations**. If the person was injured in a formal class setting, it may also be helpful to file a class outline or lesson plan with the accident report. In addition, a yearly review of injuries can be helpful in reducing accidents causing injuries to clients.

SELECTION OF APPROPRIATE RESPONSE FOR RISKS

The most common approaches for the treatment of potential risks are: avoidance, retention, reduction and transfer.

Avoidance—This simply means that the activity is judged to be too hazardous to justify its use. Some examples of this include contraindicated exercises such as full squats and straight-leg sit-ups.

Retention—In some instances, instructors will simply want to budget for the situation. This might include paying for the cost of an emergency room visit for an injured client. It's much cheaper than litigation!

Reduction—Instructors should continue to compare their instruction, facilities, equipment and procedures to national standards. Implementing changes constitutes reduction.

Transfer—This usually is accomplished through insurance. Fitness personnel and clubs should have viable programs of insurance that will cover the cost of legal defense and any claims awarded. Read the coverage carefully because company policies vary considerably. The general types of coverage that should be obtained include:

• **General liability**—covers basic trip and fall type injuries.

• **Professional liability**—covers claims of negligence based on professional duties.

• **Disability insurance**—would provide income protection in the event of an injury to the instructor.

• **Individual medical insurance**—provides hospitalization and major medical coverage.

Aerobics instructors and personal trainers who are independent contractors should pay special attention to their coverage. They should make sure that if they work for clubs all aspects of coverage are understood and included in the written agreements for services.

Duties also include enforcing conduct and ensuring adherence to safety guidelines. Clearly written safety guidelines for each type of activity should be posted in appropriate areas of the facility and rigidly enforced by the supervisor.

Of particular importance are the policies and procedures for emergencies. All employees should be thoroughly familiar with them and should have actual practice in carrying out an emergency plan. For example, every club or studio should conduct a "heart attack drill," requiring all staff to carry out emergency plans and procedures such as those recommended by the American Heart Association. The program manager should maintain records of these simulations.

Many exercise program instructors and supervisors are needlessly exposed to liability because they permit indiscriminate use of the facility. Supervisory personnel should restrict the facility to people who have a legitimate entitlement. Each staff member should have a list of the people scheduled to use the equipment and facilities during specific time periods, and the supervisor should allow access only to those people. This policy should be enforced with the same vigor as the safety procedures.

IMPLEMENTATION OF A RISK— MANAGEMENT SYSTEM

Implementation is a management function. Daily attention must be given to all subject areas identified above. This process is normally called a safety audit and should be conducted regularly. Many professionals in the field develop safety check lists, while clubs often have professional consultants conduct safety audits.

Regardless, a systematic evaluation of the risks in fitness and aerobics is essential for safe program operation.

Waivers and Informed Consent

The staff of many programs attempt to absolve themselves of liability by having all participants sign a liability **waiver** to release the instructor and fitness center from all liability associated with the conduct of an exercise program and any resulting injuries. In some cases, these documents have been of little value because the courts have enforced the specific wording of the waiver and not its intent. In other words, if negligence were found to be the cause of injury, and negligence of the instructor or fitness center was not specifically waived, then the waiver would not be effective. Therefore, waivers must be clearly written and include statements to the effect that the participant waives all claims to damages, even those caused by the negligence of the instructor or fitness center.

Some fitness centers use an informed consent form. While this document may look similar to a waiver, its purpose is different. The **informed consent** form is used to make the dangers of a program or test procedure known to the participant and thereby provide an additional measure of defense against lawsuits.

Obtaining informed consent is very important. It should be an automatic procedure for every person who enters the program, and it should be done before every fitness test. The American Council on Exercise suggests the following procedures:

1. Inform the participant of the exercise program or the testing procedure, with an explanation of the purpose of each. This explanation should be thorough and unbiased.

2. Inform the participant of the risks involved in the testing procedure or program, along with the possible discomforts.

3. Inform the participant of the benefits expected from the testing procedure or program.

4. Inform the participant of any alternative programs or tests that may be more advantageous to him or her.

5. Solicit questions regarding the testing procedures or exercise program, and give unbiased answers to these inquiries.

6. Inform the participant that he or she is free, at any time, to withdraw consent and discontinue participation.

7. Obtain the written consent of each participant.

BASIC DEFENSES AGAINST NEGLIGENCE CLAIMS

It is important for instructors to know and understand that they are not without protection under the law. Several defenses are available for use by fitness professionals as defendants in litigation in fitness-related personal injury cases.

Assumption of Risk

This defense is used to show that the client voluntarily accepted dangers known to exist with participation in the activity. The two most important aspects of this definition are "voluntary" and "known danger." If the client does not voluntarily engage in a program or test, this defense cannot normally be used. Also, if the participant was not informed of the specific risks associated with the program or test, then he or she cannot be held to have assumed them. The best way to prove that a client was knowledgeable of the risks involved is to utilize informed consents and **assumption-of-risk** documents described earlier.

Contributory Negligence

This defense means that the plaintiff played some role in his or her own injury. Although this legal doctrine is viable in only a few states (check applicable state law), it provides a total bar to recovery for any damages. An example might consist of a client exceeding the designated maximum heart rate in a prescribed exercise program. A salient factor would also be whether an instructor was there to monitor the client, or if the client were exercising alone and following program guidelines.

Comparative Negligence

In this defense, the relative fault of both the plaintiff and the defendant are measured to see who was most at fault for the injury. The result is an apportionment of guilt and any subsequent award for damages. The court (or jury) determines the percentage of responsibility of each party and then prorates the award. This can be useful if a client is somewhat to blame for his or her own injury.

Act of God

Although this defense is not often used in fitness and sport law cases, it may be of interest. It involves injury caused by unforeseeable acts of nature. The foreseeability aspect is the most crucial. If, during an exercise session, an earthquake opened the floor and a client were engulfed, it may be applicable.

OTHER LEGAL CONSIDERATIONS

Aerobics instructors are providers of a special service. As a result, professionals in this field must be familiar with the special aspects of the law that are most frequently encountered in the conduct of an aerobics instructor's business.

Contracts

Fitness personnel must have an adequate knowledge of legal **contracts** to perform their tasks, to get paid and to avoid costly legal battles with clients and/or clubs. Some instructors will want to work as individuals, not affiliated with one particular club, while others may want to be employed by a club or fitness center, yet specialize in one-on-one instruction.

Whatever the nature of the work arrangement, an instructor must be aware of the essentials of contract law. Basic contract law indicates that the following elements are necessary to form a binding contract:

• an offer and acceptance—mutual agreement to terms.

• consideration—an exchange of items of value.

• legality—acceptable form and subject under the law.

• capacity—such as majority age and mental competency.

The general considerations which should be addressed in contracts for use with clients, as well as contracts between exercise professionals and clubs for which they intend to work, should include the following:

• identification of the parties (trainer and client/club).

• description of the services to be performed (fitness training and consultation).

• compensation ($X.oo per hour, day, month or class, and payment method).

• confidential relationship (agreement by each party not to divulge personal or business information gained through the relationship).

• business status (confirmation of employment status).

• term and termination (express definition of the length on the contract and the conditions under which termination is allowed by either party).

Employment Status

As noted above, another prominent concern for many fitness professionals deals with employment status: **independent**

contractor versus employee. Both of these terms can apply to the those who work in a fitness center. However, only the independent contractor status applies to self-employed personal trainers working independently from a club. However, most clubs still require independent contractors hired by the club to follow club rules.

Clients who hire a personal trainer do not intend, for the most part, to hire that person as an employee, but prefer to lease their services for a brief period of time. Hence, most self-employed personal trainers are independent contractors and not employees of their clients.

In some instances, owners of fitness centers or clubs have used the term independent contractor for employees. Club owners are often motivated to hire independent contractors in place of regular employees because the company does not have to train, provide medical or other benefits, arrange for social security withholding, or pay into worker's compensation or unemployment funds for independent contractors. Club owners also find an advantage in having independent contractors because it is more complicated, from a legal standpoint, to fire existing employees than it is to simply not renew contracts with independent contractors.

A legal dichotomy exists between regular employees and independent contractors. Most commonly, the courts have considered 10 questions or "tests" to determine if the business relationship in question between a club and a fitness professional is that of a regular employee or an independent contractor. These tests are:

1. The extent of control which, by agreement, the employer can exercise over the details of the work. The existence of a right to control is indicative of an employer-employee relationship.

2. The method of payment, whether by time or by the job. Generally, those persons scheduled to be paid on a regular basis at an hourly or weekly rate have been considered as employees. Conversely, those paid in a single payment for services rendered have more easily qualified as independent contractors.

3. The length of time for which the person is employed. Individuals hired for short periods of time (a few days or weeks) have more often been seen as independent contractors, whereas employment periods that extended upward of a full year have been ruled as establishing an employer-employee relationship.

4. The skill required for the provision of services. When the worker needs no training because of the specialized or technical skills which the employer intends to utilize, the independent contractor status has prevailed. On the other hand, if an employer provides training to a recently hired individual, that person will more than likely be judged to be an employee.

5. Whether the person employed is in a distinct business or occupation. If a worker offers services to other employers or clients, a status of independent contractor would probably be found. If, however, the worker only intended to provide services for one employer, and failed to offer the services to others as an independent business, the employee status could be found.

6. Whether the employer of the worker provides the equipment. If independent contractor status is desired, aerobics instructors will have a better chance getting it if they provide their own equipment.

7. Whether the work is a part of the normal business of the employer. Court rulings have favored classifying individuals as regular employees when services rendered are integral to the business of the employer. Supplemental, special or one-time services are more likely to be provid-

ed by independent contractors.

8. Whether the work is traditionally performed by a specialist in similar businesses. Employers and employees must examine their field of business to gain an understanding of current practices and align themselves with the prevailing trends.

9. Intent of the parties involved in the arrangement. The courts will attempt to enforce intent of the parties at the time the agreement was executed. If a professional thought that he or she were hired as an independent contractor, as did the club, it would influence the court's determination. Therefore, a clear understanding of the arrangement is a must.

10. Whether the employer is engaged in a business. The intent here is to protect clients from being construed as employers when a personal trainer is hired to perform work of a "private" nature. This is most common when one-on-one trainers sell their services to private citizens rather than to clubs or corporations.

The process of determining employment status is marked by careful analysis of the facts and the weighing of interpretations on both sides of the issue. All of the issues addressed above have been used in court cases dealing with this matter, each with varying degrees of authority. It is, therefore, imperative that all fitness professionals and club owners understand and examine these factors when initiating agreements.

Copyright Law

One of an exercise instructor's major legal responsibilities is compliance with **copyright** law. All forms of commercially produced creative expression are protected by copyright law, but music is the area most pertinent to exercise instructors.

Simply stated, almost all musical compositions that one can hear on the radio or television or buy in the music store are owned by artists and studios and are protected by federal copyright law. Whether an instructor makes a tape from various songs on the radio, or from tapes he or she has purchased does not matter; the instructor who uses that tape in a for-profit exercise class—legally speaking, a **public performance**—is in violation of copyright law.

Performance Licenses. To be able to use copyrighted music in an exercise class, one must obtain a performance license from one of the two major **performing rights societies,** the **American Society of Composers, Authors and Publishers (ASCAP)** or **Broadcast Music, Inc. (BMI).** These organizations vigorously enforce copyrighted law for their memberships and will not hesitate to sue a health club, studio or free-lance instructor who plays copyrighted music without a license.

Accordingly, most clubs and studios obtain a **blanket license** for their instructors. The license fees for the clubs are determined either by the number of students who attend classes each week, by the number of speakers used in the club, or by whether the club has a single- or multi-floor layout.

Instructors who teach as individual contractors at several locations may have to obtain their own licenses. They should check with the clubs where they teach to see if each club's blanket license covers their classes. If free-lance instructors teach at several different locations with their own tapes, they will have to obtain their own performance licenses.

Given that the fees for either getting licenses or paying damages for copyright infringement may be prohibitive, independent instructors, in particular, may want to consider other options. One is to create rhythm tapes of their own using a drum machine, an electronic instrument that can range in sophistication from toy to professional recording device. A professional model is not needed, however, to make an appealing rhythm tape. A local musical instrument store owner or salesperson could probably steer the instructor to someone who could help create such a tape.

Other options include buying tapes expressly made for fitness and aerobic exercise classes, which the copyright holder expressly permits to be used in a class, or asking exercise class students to bring their own recordings for the workouts, in effect using them for the clients' own noncommercial use.

Obtaining Copyright Protection. Some exercise instructors may want to obtain copyright protection for certain aspects of their work. The following are several examples of what an instructor may want to copyright:

Pantomimes and choreographic work— If an instructor creates more than a simple dance routine, and publicly distributes (through a dance notation system), performs or displays the choreography, it can be copyrighted.

Books, videos, films—If a choreographed work by an instructor is sold to a **publisher**, video distributor or movie studio, that business entity will own the copyright for the material and the instructor will be compensated with either or both an advance and a certain portion of the proceeds (royalties). Through negotiation with the producing or distributing company, the instructor may be able to retain certain rights to the material.

Compilations of exercise routines—If an instructor makes an original sequence of routines, it may be protected by copyright and licensed to others for a book, video, film or other presentation form.

Graphic materials—If an instructor creates pictures, charts, diagrams, informational handouts or other graphic materials for instructional aids or promotional

material, these too may be copyrighted.

For copyright information or applications, write to:

Register of Copyrights
United States Copyright Office
Library of Congress
Washington, D.C. 20559

Liability Insurance

Every exercise instructor will want to assess his or her liability insurance needs. An instructor employed at a club should inquire about the general liability policy and any other liability insurance the owner might have.

Independent contractors may not be covered by a club's general policy and, if not, should ask the club if they can be added by special endorsement.

Many nonprofit groups, such as churches and recreation centers, may not have coverage that includes their contract instructors. The instructors at these venues should probably have their own general liability coverage.

General liability coverage will cover an accident where a student trips over a loose floorboard or falls and breaks an arm. What about a student hurting herself in a routine that she says was improperly demonstrated? For this kind of claim, exercise instructors would be wise to have professional liability insurance.

Since professional standards in the exercise field are becoming the norm, the expectations of students (and courts, as well) is rising to include all facets of exercise-class management, from screening participants correctly to adequately supervising them.

Professional liability insurance will not cover an instructor for copyright infringement claims or offer protection in suits involving libel, slander, invasion of privacy or defamation of character. These sorts of actions would be covered by a personal injury policy.

Instructors seeking affordable liability policies should check with professional groups, such as IDEA, ACSM, NCSA, and AFAA, or discuss their needs with insurance agents who may suggest liability coverage be added on the instructor's residence insurance as a "business pursuits rider."

Liability insurance is a must for exercise instructors. They should not begin a class anywhere without knowing what the insurance coverage is and what is excluded. The key thing for instructors to do if they are not given adequate insurance information by a club supervisor is to ask specific questions related to a club's liability insurance policy.

Americans with Disabilities Act

Fitness professionals can be affected by legislative mandates beyond insurance regulations. One of the more recent laws that affect the profession is the **American with Disabilities Act,** which became law in 1992. Modeled after the Civil Rights Act, it prohibits discrimination on the basis of disability. The law provides for equal treatment and equal access to programs for disabled Americans. (Previous legislation—Section 504 of the Rehabilitation Act of 1973—required barrier-free access to all publicly funded facilities.)

The new act extends the same provisions to all areas of public accommodation, including businesses. Therefore, it is essential that fitness professionals make sure that their buildings, equipment and programs are available to persons with disabilities. Employers must also provide reasonable accommodations for employees with disabilities, including adjusted work stations and equipment as necessary. Therefore, whether a disabled person is an employee or a client, steps must be taken to ensure that the professional and business environ-

ment is one that respects the dignity, skills and contributions of those individuals.

Scope of Practice in the Profession

Aerobics instructors are generally in the business of providing exercise leadership and exercise-related advice. They are not normally physicians, physical therapists, or dietitians (although some may be certified or licensed in these areas).

The primary area in which the scope of practice comes into question is generally the health history or wellness history form. As described earlier, this form is used as a general screening document prior to the client's entry into a fitness program. Fitness law expert David Herbert says that "wellness-assessment documents should be utilized for…determination of an individual's level of fitness… *never* for the purpose of providing or recommending *treatment* of any condition." Use of such a form in recommending treatment could constitute the practice of medicine without a license.

Another area of interaction between fitness professionals and clients that can cause issues related to the scope of certain professional practices is in dietary and nutritional counseling. According to the American Dietetic Association, a little more than half of the states have statutes that regulate or license nutritionists. In the other states, anyone is able to profess to be a nutritionist. Laws in particular states should be examined to ensure that health-care practice statutes are not violated by fitness professionals who may be surpassing their training and expertise. If a client has complex dietary questions, referral should be made to a registered dietitian (R.D.) or other qualified health-care professional.

Similarly, exercise instructors are not psychologists, marriage counselors or physical therapists and therefore should not provide advice or counseling on issues related to a clients emotional and/or psychological status. Clients should always be referred to licensed practitioners in these and other related areas.

SUMMARY

No program, regardless of how well it is run, can completely avoid all injuries. In an attempt to reduce both injuries to participants and the accompanying legal complications, an aerobics instructor would be wise to adhere to the following guidelines:

1. Obtain professional education, guided practical training under a qualified exercise professional, and current certification from an established professional organization.

2. Design and conduct programs that reflect current professional standards.

3. Formulate and enforce policies and guidelines for the conduct of the program in accordance with professional recommendations.

4. Establish and implement adequate and proper procedures for supervision in all phases of the program.

5. Establish and implement adequate and proper methods of instruction in all phases of the program.

6. Post safety regulations in the facility and ensure that they are rigidly enforced by supervisory personnel.

7. Keep the facility free from hazards and maintain adequate free space for each activity to be performed.

8. Establish and document inspection and repair schedules for all equipment and facilities.

9. Formulate policies and guidelines for emergency situations, rehearse the procedures, and require all instructors to have current first-aid training and CPR certification.

By applying the recommendations presented above, aerobics professionals can help reduce the probability of injury to participants. Should legal action result from an injury, the facts of the case would be examined to determine whether negligence was the cause. A properly trained, competent and certified instructor conducting a program that was in accordance with current professional standards would probably prevail.

REFERENCES

Arnold, D.E. (1983). *Legal Considerations in the Administration of Public School Physical Education and Athletic Program.* Springfield, IL: Charles C. Thomas, Publishers.

Herbert, David L. (1989). *"Appropriate Use of Wellness Appraisals,"* Fitness Management, September, p.23.

Nygaard, G., and T.H. Boone. (1989). *Law for Physical Educators and Coaches,* Columbus, OH: Publishing Horizons.

SUGGESTED READING

Gerson, Richard F. (1989). *Marketing Health and Fitness Services.* Champaign, IL: Human Kinetics Publishers.

Herbert, D. L., and W.G. Herbert. (1989). *Legal Aspects of Preventative and Rehabilitative Exercise Programs,* Second Edition. Canton, Ohio: Professional and Executive Reports and Publications.

Koeberle, B.E. (1990). *Legal Aspects of Personal Training.* Canton, Ohio: Professional and Executive Reports and Publications.

Patton, Robert W. (1989). *Developing and Managing Health/Fitness Programs.* Champaign, IL: Human Kinetics Publishers.

Appendix A
American Council on Exercise
Code of Ethics

The American Council on Exercise (ACE) is a not-for-profit organization committed to the promotion of safe and effective exercise. ACE accomplishes its mission by setting certification and education standards for fitness instructors and through public education and research. Since 1985, ACE has certified more than 68,000 group fitness instructors and personal trainers in 66 countries, making it the largest not-for-profit fitness certifying organization in the world. ACE sets forth this code of ethics to communicate the quality instruction and service the public can expect to receive from ACE-certified fitness instructors.

AMERICAN COUNCIL ON EXERCISE CODE OF ETHICS

ACE-certified Professionals are guided by the following principles of conduct as they interact with clients, the public and other health and fitness professionals.

ACE-certified Professionals will endeavor to:

- Provide safe and effective instruction.

- Provide equal and fair treatment to all clients.

- Maintain an understanding of the latest health and physical activity research and its applications.

- Maintain current CPR certification and knowledge of first-aid services.

- Comply with all applicable business, employment and copyright laws.

- Uphold and enhance public appreciation and trust for the health and fitness industries.

- Maintain the confidentiality of all client information.

- Refer clients to more qualified fitness, medical or health professionals when appropriate.

Appendix B
Group Fitness Instructor Certification Exam Content Outline

The purpose of this exam content outline is to set forth the tasks, knowledge and skills necessary for group fitness instructors to perform their job responsibilities at a minimum professional level. This includes, but is not limited to, teaching the components of fitness to apparently healthy individuals in a group exercise setting. Please note, not all knowledge statements listed here in the exam content outline will be addressed on each exam administered.

It is the position of the American Council on Exercise that the recommendations outlined here are not exhaustive to the qualifications of a group fitness instructor but represent the minimum level of proficiency and theoretical knowledge essential for a group fitness instructor to: screen and evaluate prospective clients; design a safe and effective exercise program; instruct clients in correct exercise technique to avoid injury; and respond to the typical questions and problems that arise in a group exercise setting.

These recommendations apply only to group fitness instructors training healthy individuals who have no apparent physical limitations or special medical needs. It is not ACE's intent to provide recommendations for instructors delivering specialized programs for highly trained athletes, pre and postnatal women, older clients, individuals with physical handicaps, the morbidly obese, or individuals known to have coronary heart disease.

AMERICAN COUNCIL ON EXERCISE EXAM CONTENTS

Exercise Science	Basic physiology; cardiorespiratory, musculoskeletal, neuromuscular, metabolic, and environmental
	Basic anatomy
	Basic kinesiology
	Correct training techniques
	Basic fitness test terminology and procedures
	Physiological and anatomical considerations of special populations
	Basic psychological issues affecting exercise adherence
	Basic nutrition and weight management
Exercise Programming	Components of a class given the class objective
	Incorporation of safe and effective movements
	Design of different types of group exercises classes
	Modifications or adaptations
	Music selection
	Selection, modification, and adaptation for special populations
	Equipment related to class design
	Establishment of a safe exercise environment
	Choreographic techniques

Instructional Techniques	Techniques to monitor exercise intensity
	Teaching strategies to modify incorrect movements
	Modification of group and individual performance
	Correct cueing
	Use of music and sound equipment
	Teaching methodologies
	Injury prevention
	Emergency procedures: first aid, cardiopulmonary resuscitation (CPR), and evacuation plans
	Principles of fitness testing
Professional Responsibility	Current legal principles and issues
	American Council on Exercise Code of Ethics
	Accepted business standards and practices
	Emergency procedures: first aid, cardiopulmonary resuscitation (CPR), and evacuation plans
	Insurance needs related to group exercise instruction
	Professional growth

Exercise Science

TASK 1:

To demonstrate knowledge of basic cardiorespiratory physiology by applying correct cardiorespiratory physiological principles in order to develop and instruct safe and effective exercise.

Knowledge:

1. Knowledge of normal and abnormal static and dynamic exercise, including heart rate, blood pressure, and oxygen consumption.

2. Knowledge of cardiorespiratory physiology terms as they apply to endurance training (e.g. cardiac output, stroke volume, oxygen consumption, ventilation, respiration, and aerobic capacity).

3. Knowledge of the principles of training as they apply to cardiorespiratory endurance (e.g. overload, specificity, reversibility, progression, frequency, training effect, and adaptation).

4. Knowledge of the benefits of endurance training (e.g. improvement in aerobic capacity, weight control, and reduced stress levels, body fat, and risk of heart disease).

5. Knowledge of the risk factors for coronary artery disease and their impact on normal cardiorespiratory function.

6. Knowledge of the relationship amongst heart rate, exercise intensity, and oxygen requirement.

TASK 2:

To demonstrate knowledge of basic musculoskeletal physiology by applying correct musculoskeletal physiological principles in order to develop and instruct safe and effective exercise.

Knowledge:

1. Knowledge of the major components of muscular fitness (e.g. muscular strength,

endurance, and flexibility).

2. Knowledge of training principles for improving muscular strength, endurance, and flexibility.

3. Knowledge of the following terms pertaining to muscular fitness: training effect, resistance, overload, specificity, repetitions, sets, frequency, rest periods, progression, and muscle atrophy and hypertrophy.

4. Knowledge of the potential benefits of muscular strength and endurance training (e.g. injury prevention, optimal leisure and work performance).

5. Knowledge of the various methods of using resistance during muscular fitness training: body weight, gravity, bands, hand weights, and leverage.

6. Knowledge of the risks associated with performing the Valsalva maneuver during resistance training.

7. Knowledge of static and dynamic stretches and the risks and benefits of each method.

8. Knowledge of hypermobility, flexibility, and tightness and their relationship to joint mobility.

9. Knowledge of the relationship of joint mobility and muscular flexibility.

10. Knowledge of the risks associated with muscular strength training: improper body mechanics and lifting techniques that may result in acute and chronic overuse injuries.

11. Knowledge of the different muscle fiber types and their individual characteristics.

12. Knowledge of how osteoporosis and osteoarthritis affect the skeletal system.

TASK 3:

To determine knowledge of basic neuromuscular physiology by applying correct neuromuscular physiological principles in order to develop and instruct safe and effective exercise.

Knowledge:

1. Knowledge of key terms in neuromuscular physiology: motor neurons, motor unit, and neuromuscular junction.

2. Knowledge of the roles of Golgi tendon organs and muscle spindles in the regulation of muscle contraction (e.g. reflex, contraction, and stretch reflex).

3. Knowledge of motor skills with respect to agility, balance, and coordination.

TASK 4:

To demonstrate knowledge of metabolic physiology by applying correct metabolic physiological principles in order to develop safe and effective exercise.

Knowledge:

1. Knowledge of the fundamentals of metabolic physiology, including anaerobic metabolism (ATP-CP system and glycolysis), oxidative metabolism, and fatty acid oxidation.

2. Knowledge of aerobic and anaerobic metabolism and the roles of each during various physical activities.

3. Knowledge of the roles of carbohydrates, fats, and proteins as fuel for aerobic and anaerobic exercise.

4. Knowledge of the following definitions: kilocalorie, caloric expenditure, caloric deficit, caloric intake, and energy balance.

TASK 5:

To demonstrate knowledge of anatomy by identifying correct anatomical structures in order to develop and instruct safe and effective exercise.

Knowledge:

1. Knowledge of the basic components of the cardiorespiratory system (e.g. heart, vessels, lungs).

2. Knowledge of the general anatomy of the heart, cardiovascular system, and the cardiorespiratory system.

3. Knowledge of the chambers of

the heart.

4. Knowledge of the circulatory pathway through the cardiorespiratory system.

5. Knowledge of the major components of the musculoskeletal system (e.g. bone, muscle, ligaments, tendons).

6. Knowledge of the function of the different joints of the body.

7. Knowledge of the major muscle groups and bones.

TASK 6:

To demonstrate competence in the area of basic kinesiology by applying correct kinesiological principles in order to develop and instruct safe and effective exercise.

Knowledge:

1. Knowledge of the following anatomical and directional terms: anterior, posterior, medial, lateral, dorsal, ventral, plantar, superior, inferior, prone, and supine.

2. Knowledge of the anatomical planes: sagittal, frontal, and transverse.

3. Knowledge of the fundamental movements from the anatomical position (e.g. abduction, adduction, elevation, depression, flexion, dorsiflexion, plantar flexion, and rotation).

4. Knowledge of the types of muscular contractions: isokinetic, isometric, isotonic (eccentric and concentric).

5. Knowledge of normal (good) postural alignment and the normal curvature of the back: kyphosis and lordosis.

6. Knowledge of abnormal curvatures of the back: excessive kyphosis, excessive lordosis, and scoliosis.

7. Knowledge to differentiate agonist, antagonist, and synergist and to pair opposing muscles.

8. Knowledge of the principle of muscle balance.

9. Knowledge of healthy back exercises: back range of motion (flexion, extension, and rotation), abdominal strength, pelvic

stability, and scapular retraction.

10. Knowledge of the actions and applications of the major muscle groups (e.g. trapezius, pectoralis major, rotator cuff muscles, biceps, triceps, deltoids, rectus abdominis, internal and external obliques, transversus, erector spinae, latissimus dorsi, gluteus maximus, gluteus medius, quadriceps, hamstrings, gastrocnemius, soleus, anterior tibialis, posterior tibialis, hip adductors, hip abductors, and iliopsoas).

11. Knowledge of the potential risks associated with certain exercises (e.g. double leg raises, full squats, full neck circles, hurdler's stretch, knee hyperflexion while bearing weight, plough exercise, and trunk hyperextension).

12. Knowledge of the factors that affect movement: neurological, proprioceptive, biomechanical, and kinesthetic awareness.

Skills:

1. Skill in identifying joint type, action, and normal degree of range of motion.

2. Skill in identifying common muscle imbalances and their causes which contribute to abnormal postural alignment.

3. Skill in developing exercises to promote pelvic and scapular stability.

4. Skill in educating participants on proper body mechanics.

5. Skill in designing safe exercises for all major muscle groups.

TASK 7:

To demonstrate an understanding of the principles of exercise programming by applying correct training techniques in order to develop and instruct safe and effective exercise.

Knowledge:

1. Knowledge of the various components of a conditioning program (e.g. warm-up, cardiorespiratory conditioning, muscular conditioning, and cool-down).

2. Knowledge of the components of an

exercise program, including frequency, intensity, duration, mode of activity, and progression.

3. Knowledge of the various methods of determining and monitoring exercise intensity, including target heart rate (THR), Borg's rating of perceived exertion (RPE), and the talk test.

4. Knowledge of the major components of physical fitness, including cardiovascular endurance, muscular endurance, muscular strength, flexibility, and body composition.

5. Knowledge of the current American College of Sports Medicine (ACSM) guidelines for improving and maintaining cardiorespiratory endurance and muscular fitness with reference to mode of activity, intensity, duration, and frequency for various levels of fitness.

TASK 8:

To demonstrate an understanding of fitness test terminology and results by identifying correct modifications and recommendations in order to develop and instruct safe and effective exercise based upon fitness results.

Knowledge:

1. Knowledge of the various methods of fitness assessments, including submaximal and maximal aerobic capacity tests, muscular strength and endurance tests, and body composition tests.

2. Knowledge of the rationale for the determination of aerobic capacity, muscular strength and endurance, flexibility, and body composition.

Skill:

1. Skill in applying the results of the fitness assessments to the development or modification of an exercise.

TASK 9:

To demonstrate an understanding of the various physiological and anatomical

considerations of special populations by identifying correct modifications and recommendations in order to develop safe and effective exercise.

Knowledge:

Special Populations: General

1. Knowledge of the benefits of regular exercise for specific conditions such as coronary artery disease, hypertension, diabetes mellitus, musculoskeletal disorders (including rheumatoid arthritis, lower-back problems, and osteoporosis), obesity, and asthma.

2. Knowledge of modifications necessary for a participant with a medical condition who has been cleared by a physician or appropriate medical personnel.

Special Populations: Older Adults

3. Knowledge of physiological processes and exercise implications for older adults, including the musculoskeletal, cardiorespiratory, metabolic, and psychosocial systems.

4. Knowledge of musculoskeletal, cardiovascular, respiratory, and metabolic health concerns common to older adults, including suitable exercise programs.

5. Knowledge of appropriate motivational reinforcement techniques of older adults.

Special Populations: Pregnant and Postpartum Women

6. Knowledge of the American College of Obstetricians and Gynecologists (ACOG) recommendations for exercise during pregnancy and the postpartum period, as well as contraindications and warning signs to cease exercise.

7. Knowledge of the risks associated with exercise and pregnancy due to the following hypoxia, hyperthermia, hypoglycemia, and dehydration.

8. Knowledge of musculoskeletal adaptations due to pregnancy weight gain, hormonal changes, and postural changes.

Special Populations: Children

9. Knowledge of the special concerns

of working with children, including thermoregulation, anaerobic capacity, intensity monitoring, and safety.

10. Knowledge of musculoskeletal, cardiovascular, respiratory, and metabolic concerns of children involved in exercise programs.

11. Knowledge of youth fitness testing methods.

12. Knowledge of the importance of program design, including: (1) gradual increase in exercise intensity, (2) improvement in adequate muscular strength and flexibility, (3) proper body mechanics, and (4) appropriate clothing and equipment.

Skills:

General

1. Skill in identifying health problems or risk factors that interfere with a participant's ability to exercise safely in class and that may warrant physician referral, such as a recent injury, diabetes, obesity, pregnancy, musculoskeletal problems (including arthritis), hypertension, asthma, and previous difficulty with exercise (including exercise-related chest discomfort, dizzy spells, and extreme breathlessness).

Older Adults

2. Skill in modifying the exercise program in terms of intensity, duration, frequency, and mode.

3. Skill in identifying aging characteristics and exercise implications for the older adult.

4. Skill in designing appropriate exercise programs regarding the aging process and health concerns.

5. Skill in designing effective exercise activities and motivational reinforcement for older adults.

Pregnant and Postpartum Women

6. Skill in designing exercises to accommodate postural changes associated with pregnancy (e.g., lordosis, pelvic widening).

7. Skill in adjusting frequency, duration, intensity, and mode of activity for pregnant women.

8. Skill in monitoring exercise levels during pregnancy using HR, RPE, and respiration rate.

9. Skill in modifying muscular training programs with respect to pregnancy-induced musculoskeletal adaptations.

10. Skill in making appropriate modifications necessary to pregnant and postpartum participants accepted in a regular group exercise class.

TASK 10:

To demonstrate a basic understanding of various psychological issues by correctly relating them to group exercise program design in order to optimize exercise adherence and the well-being of participants.

Knowledge:

1. Knowledge of motivational techniques used to optimize exercise adherence and other healthy lifestyle behaviors.

2. Knowledge of the issues related to body image.

3. Knowledge of the issues related to self-efficacy and obsessive/compulsive behavior in a group exercise setting.

4. Knowledge of the principles of the learning theory with respect to effective teaching in a group exercise setting.

TASK 11:

To demonstrate an understanding of basic nutrition by applying correct nutritional recommendations in order to provide appropriate information to apparently healthy individuals.

Knowledge:

1. Knowledge of the six categories of nutrients, their functions, and current dietary guidelines according to the U.S. RDA.

2. Knowledge of special nutritional needs as they apply to osteoporosis and anemia.

3. Knowledge of nutritional misinformation and misconceptions (e.g. salt tablets and protein powders).

4. Knowledge of cholesterol, lipoproteins, and triglycerides.

5. Knowledge of supplements and ergogenic aids (e.g. bee pollen and caffeine).

6. Knowledge of the toxic effects of over-supplementation of vitamins.

7. Knowledge of hydration with water versus "sports drinks."

8. Knowledge of special dietary needs with respect to referral to a registered dietician.

9. Knowledge of the signs and symptoms of atypical eating behaviors (e.g. anorexia, bulimia, and compulsive overeating).

Skill:

1. Skill in identifying special dietary needs for the purpose of referral to a registered dietician.

TASK 12:

To demonstrate knowledge of environmental physiology by applying correct physiological principles in order to develop safe and effective exercise.

Knowledge:

1. Knowledge of concepts from environmental physiology that may affect exercise performance, including heat, humidity, altitude, cold, and pollution.

2. Knowledge of the physiological responses to variations in environmental conditions (e.g. changes in temperature, heart rate, blood pressure).

3. Knowledge of the physiological adaptations that result from acclimatization.

4. Knowledge of recommendations and precautions for exercising in heat, humidity, cold, altitude, and pollution.

TASK 13:

To demonstrate knowledge of weight management by applying sound nutritional and exercise principles in order to provide appropriate information to apparently healthy individuals.

Knowledge:

1. Knowledge of safe and effective weight-loss methods.

2. Knowledge of the number of pounds per week recommended for unsupervised, safe and effective weight loss.

3. Knowledge of the definition of kilocalories as applied to caloric intake and expenditure.

4. Knowledge of the different protocols of fat weight loss and/or body composition change (e.g. diet and exercise combined, diet alone, etc.).

5. Knowledge of the concepts of energy balance, energy imbalance, and set point theory.

6. Knowledge of the different methods of determining ideal body weight (e.g. height/weight, charts, scale, body composition).

7. Knowledge of extreme approaches to weight loss (e.g. fasting, spot reducing, diet pills, drugs).

Exercise Programming

TASK 1:

To determine the content of each class component in order to plan safe and effective group exercise sessions with respect to the objective for the class by adhering to accepted standards of practice.

Knowledge:

1. Knowledge of the components involved in an aerobics class: warm-up, pre/post-cardiorespiratory conditioning, cardiorespiratory conditioning, cool-down, muscle conditioning, and flexibility exercises/final cool-down.

2. Knowledge of the components of a circuit training class: warm-up, pre/post-cardiorespiratory conditioning, cardiores-

piratory/strength training, flexibility exercises, and final cool-down.

3. Knowledge of the components of an aerobic interval training class: warm-up, pre/post-cardiorespiratory conditioning, interval cardiorespiratory/muscular conditioning, cool-down, flexibility exercises, and final cool-down.

4. Knowledge of the major components of a resistance class: warm-up, muscle conditioning, and flexibility/final cool-down.

5. Knowledge of the major components of a stretch class: warm-up and flexibility exercises/final cool-down.

Skill:

1. Skill in determining the content, combination, and sequence of various types of group exercise classes.

TASK 2:

To demonstrate the ability to design a class by incorporating appropriate movements for each component of a class in order to provide a safe and effective exercise session.

Knowledge:

1. Knowledge of basic anatomy.

2. Knowledge of basic exercise physiology.

3. Knowledge of basic applied kinesiology.

4. Knowledge of safe and effective movements for each component of an exercise class.

Skills:

1. Skill in selecting safe and effective movements for each component of the exercise class.

2. Skill in designing a safe and effective exercise class by applying knowledge of anatomy, physiology, and kinesiology.

TASK 3:

To demonstrate competence in designing exercise sessions of various modes used in group exercise by adhering to accepted

standards of practice in order to plan safe and effective exercise.

Knowledge:

1. Knowledge of interval, circuit, and resistance training and low-impact, high-impact, flexibility, aqua, and step/bench exercise.

Skill:

1. Skill in applying different modes of activity and associated exercises to the design of an exercise class.

TASK 4:

To demonstrate competence in the design of an exercise class by planning appropriate modifications or adaptations to activities in order to provide safe and effective exercise.

Knowledge:

1. Knowledge of the physiological effects and appropriate precautions to take with respect to the following substances: beta blockers, diuretics, antihypertensives, antihistamines, tranquilizers, alcohol, diet pills, cold medications, caffeine, and nicotine.

2. Knowledge of modifications and adaptations for participants with medical conditions who have been cleared for exercise by a physician or appropriate medical personnel.

3. Knowledge of modifications and adaptations for special populations: pregnant and postpartum women, children, and senior citizens.

4. Knowledge of modifications and adaptations for participants desiring increased exercise intensity.

Skills:

1. Skill in selecting modifiable exercises for participants with medical conditions who have been cleared for exercise by a physician or appropriate medical personnel.

2. Skill in selecting modifiable exercises for special populations: pregnant and post-

partum women, children, and older adults.

3. Skill in selecting modifiable exercises for participants desiring increased exercise intensity.

TASK 5:

To select the appropriate music for group exercise classes by correctly evaluating music in order to plan a safe and effective exercise class.

Knowledge:

1. Knowledge of music and basic musical terms: beat, upbeat, downbeat, accent, meter, measure, phrasing, rhythm, tempo, syncopation, and dynamics.

Skills:

1. Skill in selecting appropriate music to motivate class participants and encourage adherence to exercise.

2. Skill in selecting music with appropriate tempo for safe and effective exercise participation.

TASK 6:

To accommodate the particular needs of special populations by selecting, modifying, and adapting activities in order to plan a safe and effective exercise class.

Knowledge:

1. Knowledge of the American College of Obstetricians and Gynecologists (ACOG) guidelines for pregnant and postpartum exercisers.

2. Knowledge of the common musculoskeletal conditions typically associated with older adults.

3. Knowledge of the appropriate modifications for special populations and individuals with medical conditions who have been cleared for exercise by a physician or appropriate medical personnel.

Skill:

1. Skill in the integration of safe and effective exercises for participants with medical conditions and for special populations who have been cleared for exercise by physicians or appropriate medical personnel.

TASK 7:

To demonstrate competence in the design of an exercise class by selecting appropriate equipment in order to provide a safe and effective exercise class.

Knowledge:

1. Knowledge of commonly used exercise equipment and their applications: hand-held weights, resistance bands (e.g. elastic tubing, rubber bands), and step/bench.

Skill:

1. Skill in integrating safe and effective exercises for commonly used exercise equipment and their applications: hand-held weights, resistance bands (e.g. elastic tubing, rubber bands), and step/bench.

TASK 8:

To establish a safe exercise setting by assessing and appropriately modifying the exercise environment in order to promote comfort and safety for all participants.

Knowledge:

1. Knowledge of specific environmental factors as they relate to the safety of the participants in a group exercise class (e.g. air temperature, humidity, exercise surface and area, sound, and altitude).

Skill:

1. Skill in selecting and/or adapting a safe and effective environment in order to maximize safety for class participants.

TASK 9:

To demonstrate competence in the design of the exercise class by using appropriate choreographic techniques to plan safe and effective exercise.

Knowledge:

1. Knowledge of the basic elements of

movement variation: spatial (e.g. planes, lines, direction, and floor pattern) and temporal (e.g. rhythmic, tempo, and phrasing) factors.

2. Knowledge of choreography with respect to: variation, repetition, and transition.

Skills:

1. Skill in choreographing movement for the exercise class.

2. Skill in simplifying/breaking down movements in all modes and components of a class.

3. Skill in combining movements in all modes and components of a class.

Instructional Technique

TASK 1:

To demonstrate various methods for monitoring exercise intensity by applying appropriate techniques in class in order to ensure safe and effective participation in exercise.

Knowledge:

1. Knowledge of the methods, precautions, and limitations for monitoring exercise intensity: heart rate, talk test, Borg's rating of perceived exertion (RPE), dyspnea scale, and metabolic equivalents (METS).

2. Knowledge of the techniques, precautions, and limitations for monitoring heart rate of the radial, carotid, temporal, and apical sites.

3. Knowledge of the applications, precautions, and limitations in the calculations of target heart range: percent of maximum heart rate method, age-predicted maximum heart rate, measured maximum heart rate.

4. Knowledge of heart rate responses to exercise: adequate warm-up, aerobic exercise phase, recovery, abnormal responses, and the effects of medications.

Skills:

1. Skill in palpating heart rate at the radial, carotid, temporal, and apical sites.

2. Skill in demonstrating correct technique for palpating heart rate at the radial, carotid, temporal, and apical sites.

3. Skill in explaining the talk test, RPE, and dyspnea scale as methods for monitoring exercise intensity.

4. Skill in evaluating intensity monitoring methods and making appropriate adaptations.

5. Skill in modifying group or individual exercise intensity.

6. Skill in identifying signs and symptoms of excessive effort and in making appropriate modifications.

7. Skill in selecting an appropriate intensity monitoring method in order to accommodate the effects of medications on heart rate response.

TASK 2:

To demonstrate competence in the modification of incorrect movements by applying appropriate teaching strategies in order to ensure safe and effective exercise.

Knowledge:

1. Knowledge of the three types of statements used when giving knowledge of results (KR): corrective, value, and neutral.

2. Knowledge of the appropriate uses of the three statements used when giving KR: corrective, value, and neutral.

3. Knowledge of basic exercise science principles as related to movement: cadence, muscular strength conditioning principles, body mechanics, postural assessment, and intensity precautions.

4. Knowledge of psychological factors related to feedback and KR.

5. Knowledge of psychological factors affecting participants with respect to feed-

back and KR.

Skills:

1. Skill in recognizing incorrect posture and improper execution.

2. Skill in identifying and using KR and feedback statements.

3. Skill in applying basic kinesiology to the correction of movement.

4. Skill in applying appropriate feedback and KR with respect to the participant.

5. Skill in assessing the effects of muscular imbalances when correcting individual execution.

6. Skill in analyzing posture when correcting individual execution.

7. Skill in analyzing body mechanics when correcting individual execution.

8. Skill in recognizing improper execution.

9. Skill in applying effective instructional techniques for error corrections.

10. Skill in understanding the psychological implications in communicating correction and applying appropriate response.

TASK 3:

To select appropriate techniques for modifying and adapting group and individual performance by the application of correct principles of exercise science in order to ensure safe and effective participation.

Knowledge:

1. Knowledge of the contraindications and resulting adaptations to exercise with respect to musculoskeletal, cardiorespiratory, and metabolic factors affecting exercise for participants who have been cleared by a physician or appropriate medical personnel.

2. Knowledge of the implications and modifications of exercise for older adults, pre- and post-natal women, and children.

3. Knowledge of the risk factors for coronary artery disease.

4. Knowledge of the methods used to accommodate various fitness levels and populations within a class.

Skills:

1. Skill in incorporating appropriate adaptations for musculoskeletal conditions associated with arthritis, back problems, and osteoporosis.

2. Skill in incorporating adaptations for cardiovascular conditions, including high risk participants, with respect to isometric muscle contractions, arm positions, resistance training, and exercise intensity and duration.

3. Skill in incorporating adaptations for respiratory conditions associated with chronic obstructive pulmonary disease (COPD), including asthma, bronchitis, and emphysema.

4. Skill in incorporating appropriate adaptations for metabolic concerns associated with hypoglycemia, diabetes, and obesity.

5. Skill in modifying exercises for older adults, children, and pregnant and postpartum participants.

6. Skill in adapting an exercise class to accommodate various fitness levels and populations.

7. Skill in incorporating various fitness levels and populations in the same class.

8. Skill in identifying and assigning intensity modifications for older adults, pregnant and postpartum women, children, and people with medical concerns.

TASK 4:

To demonstrate competence in instructional techniques by using correct cuing in order to ensure safe and effective exercise participation.

Knowledge:

1. Knowledge of the various types and appropriate uses of cues.

2. Knowledge of voice projection and

vocal control.

3. Knowledge of the principles of rhythm necessary for timing cues to ensure safe and effective instruction.

4. Knowledge of the principles of skill analysis necessary to sequence cues to ensure safe and effective instruction.

5. Knowledge of the principles of vocal projection and control necessary for safe and effective verbal cueing.

Skills:

1. Skill in selecting and using cues.

2. Skill in timing cues appropriately in order to ensure safe and effective exercise instruction.

3. Skill in projecting the voice safely and effectively.

4. Skill in applying basic principles of nonverbal cueing for hearing-impaired participants or participants who do not speak the language of the instructor.

5. Skill in selecting sequence of cues in order to ensure safe and effective exercise instruction.

6. Skill in using the voice safely and effectively when cueing.

TASK 5:

To demonstrate the ability to respond appropriately to the music during group exercise by applying knowledge of music and proper use of sound equipment in order to ensure safe and effective exercise participation.

Knowledge:

1. Knowledge of musical terms: beat, upbeat, downbeat, accent, meter, measure, phrasing, tempo, syncopation, and dynamics.

2. Knowledge of the methods used for appropriately counting music.

3. Knowledge of the features and operation of sound equipment.

4. Knowledge of the appropriate volume levels and sound quality needed to ensure safe and effective instruction.

Skills:

1. Skill in moving rhythmically to the music (e.g. to the beat, synchronization with musical phrases).

2. Skill in applying methods for counting music (e.g. organizing beats into metered groups, tracking measures and phrases).

3. Skill in effective operation of the various features of sound equipment.

4. Skill in determining appropriate volume levels during different phases of class and sound quality.

TASK 6:

To demonstrate competence in instructional techniques by applying appropriate teaching methodologies in order to ensure safe and effective exercise participation.

Knowledge:

1. Knowledge of the principles of exercise instruction.

2. Knowledge of the principles of evaluating performance.

3. Knowledge of the styles of instruction appropriate to the group exercise setting.

4. Knowledge of the nature of the learning process.

5. Knowledge of the domains of learning.

6. Knowledge of the stages of motor learning.

7. Knowledge of the strategies for teaching movement.

8. Knowledge of the strategies for motivating participants.

9. Knowledge of the factors affecting exercise adherence.

Skills:

1. Skill in designing an exercise class (e.g. goal setting, lesson planning).

2. Skill in selecting appropriate instructional techniques in evaluating performance in the group exercise setting.

3. Skill in using different styles of in-

struction, such as command, practice, reciprocal, and self-check.

4. Skill in selecting instructional strategies that use the cognitive, affective, and psychomotor domains of learning.

5. Skill in selecting instructional strategies appropriate to the learning level of the participant.

6. Skill in selecting the appropriate instructional strategy for teaching particular exercises.

7. Skill in selecting appropriate instructional strategies to motivate participants to excel.

8. Skill in selecting motivational strategies that affect exercise adherence.

TASK 7:

To demonstrate competence in injury prevention by applying the principles of exercise science in order to ensure safe and effective exercise participation.

Knowledge:

1. Knowledge of common chronic and acute exercise injuries.

2. Knowledge of the exercise science principles affecting safe and effective exercise.

3. Knowledge of appropriate exercise selection affecting safe and effective exercise.

4. Knowledge of high risk exercises.

5. Knowledge of health concerns that may affect safe exercise performance.

6. Knowledge of teaching techniques and their effects on safe exercise.

7. Knowledge of modifications indicated as necessary, based on health history and/or fitness assessments.

8. Knowledge of music volume control as indicated by a decibel meter.

Skills:

1. Skill in applying exercise science principles for safe and effective exercise (e.g. anatomy, applied kinesiology, body mechanics, effects of muscular imbalances, muscle physiology, and neuromuscular conditioning).

2. Skill in selecting alternatives to contraindicated exercises.

3. Skill in selecting appropriate exercises for safe and effective exercise.

4. Skill in effectively modifying or substituting exercises for participants with health concerns.

5. Skill in applying teaching techniques and their effects on safe exercise (e.g. monitoring exercise intensity, corrective techniques, modifying and adapting, cueing, music considerations, and teaching methodologies).

6. Skill in applying modifications based on health history and/or fitness assessments.

7. Skill in determining appropriate music volume levels in order to avoid hearing damage.

TASK 8:

To demonstrate competence in emergency procedures by correct implementation of first aid, cardiopulmonary resuscitation (CPR), and evacuation plans in order to ensure a safe and effective exercise environment.

Knowledge:

1. Knowledge of when to perform CPR.

2. Knowledge of how and when to activate the EMS.

3. Knowledge of the signs and symptoms of heat stress syndromes (e.g. heat cramps, heat exhaustion, heatstroke).

4. Knowledge of emergency procedures and protocol.

Skill:

1. Skill in initiating the appropriate first-aid procedure.

TASK 9:

To apply principles of fitness assessment by administering basic field tests and interpreting the results in order to ensure safe and effective exercise participation.

Knowledge:

1. Knowledge of basic field tests for evaluating cardiorespiratory endurance, body composition, muscular strength, muscular endurance, and flexibility.

2. Knowledge of the purpose and methods for administering fitness assessments in the group exercise setting.

Skills:

1. Skill in selecting appropriate field test protocols for the group exercise setting.

2. Skill in administering basic fitness assessments.

3. Skill in interpreting the results of basic fitness assessments.

Professional Responsibility

TASK 1:

To demonstrate an understanding of the various legal issues by applying current legal principles in order to avoid litigation and ensure safe and effective exercise.

Knowledge:

1. Knowledge of the assumption of risk, including waiver, warning, and informed consent.

2. Knowledge of liability, including facilities, equipment, supervision, instruction, exercise recommendations, and health screening.

3. Knowledge of negligence, both contributory and comparative.

4. Knowledge of copyright law as it applies to music, print media, and film.

5. Knowledge of scope of practice.

6. Knowledge of standard of care.

7. Knowledge of relevant legal terminology.

8. Knowledge of the difference between an independent contractor and an employee.

Skill:

1. Skill in completing an accident/incident report.

TASK 2:

To consistently apply the American Council on Exercise Code of Ethics by exhibiting behavior that is in accordance with this code in order to uphold professional standards.

Knowledge:

1. Knowledge of the ACE Code of Ethics.

TASK 3:

To demonstrate competence in business issues by application of accepted business standards and practices in order to maintain or promote the role of the group fitness instructor.

Knowledge:

1. Knowledge of employment practices.

2. Knowledge of accurate record keeping and incident/accident reporting.

3. Knowledge of personal and professional objectives.

TASK 4:

To demonstrate competence in emergency procedures by implementing first aid, cardiopulmonary resuscitation, and evacuation procedures in order to ensure the safety of participants and minimize complications in the event of an emergency.

Knowledge:

1. Knowledge of CPR procedures.

2. Knowledge of EMS system activation.

3. Knowledge of the rest, ice, compression, and elevation (RICE) principle.

4. Knowledge of contraindications to exercise.

5. Knowledge of the components of a health-screening instrument.

TASK 5:

To demonstrate an understanding of insurance as it relates to group exercise instruction by identifying insurance needs in order to minimize financial risk.

Knowledge:

1. Knowledge of professional liability insurance.

2. Knowledge of general liability insurance.

3. Knowledge of worker's compensation insurance.

4. Knowledge of health and disability insurance.

5. Knowledge of business interruption insurance.

6. Knowledge of property insurance.

TASK 6:

To demonstrate professional growth through continuing education by completion of well-rounded educational courses that are fitness-related in order to ensure safe and effective exercise and to enhance quality of service.

Knowledge:

1. Knowledge of available continuing education programs offered through individuals, conferences, colleges/universities, seminars, workshops, etc.

Note: Skill statements in this exam content outline are not evaluated on the written examination. They are provided to help candidates understand the practical application of the knowledge statements.

Appendix C
Estimated Maximal Oxygen Uptake

ESTIMATED MAXIMAL OXYGEN UPTAKE (MLO/KGBW/MIN) FOR MEN AND WOMEN, 20-69 YEARS OLD

Minute/Mile	10	11	12	13	14	15	16	17	18	19	20
Heart Rate	Men (20–29)										
120	65.0	61.7	58.4	55.2	51.9	48.6	45.4	42.1	38.9	35.6	32.3
130	63.4	60.1	56.9	53.6	50.3	47.1	43.8	40.6	37.3	34.0	30.8
140	61.8	58.6	55.3	52.0	48.8	45.5	42.2	39.0	35.7	32.5	29.2
150	60.3	57.0	53.7	50.5	47.2	43.9	40.7	37.4	34.2	30.9	27.6
160	58.7	55.4	52.2	48.9	45.6	42.4	39.1	35.9	32.6	29.3	26.1
170	57.1	53.9	50.6	47.3	44.1	40.8	37.6	34.3	31.0	27.8	24.5
180	55.6	52.3	49.0	45.8	42.5	39.3	36.0	32.7	29.5	26.2	22.9
190	54.0	50.7	47.5	44.2	41.0	37.7	34.4	31.2	27.9	24.6	21.4
200	52.4	49.2	45.9	42.7	39.4	36.1	32.9	29.6	26.3	23.1	19.8
Heart Rate	Women (20–29)										
120	62.1	58.9	55.6	52.3	49.1	45.8	42.5	39.3	36.0	32.7	29.5
130	60.6	57.3	54.0	50.8	47.5	44.2	41.0	37.7	34.4	31.2	27.9
140	59.0	55.7	52.5	49.2	45.9	42.7	39.4	36.1	32.9	29.6	26.3
150	57.4	54.2	50.9	47.6	44.4	41.1	37.8	34.6	31.3	28.0	24.8
160	55.9	52.6	49.3	46.1	42.8	39.5	36.3	33.0	29.7	26.5	23.2
170	54.3	51.0	47.8	44.5	41.2	38.0	34.7	31.4	28.2	24.9	21.6
180	52.7	49.5	46.2	42.9	39.7	36.4	33.1	29.9	26.6	23.3	20.1
190	51.2	47.9	44.6	41.4	38.1	34.8	31.6	28.3	25.0	21.8	18.5
200	49.6	46.3	43.1	39.8	36.5	33.3	30.0	26.7	23.5	20.2	16.9
Heart Rate	Men (30–39)										
120	61.1	57.8	54.6	51.3	48.0	44.8	41.5	38.2	35.0	31.7	28.4
130	59.5	56.3	53.0	49.7	46.5	43.2	39.9	36.7	33.4	30.1	26.9
140	58.0	54.7	51.4	48.2	44.9	41.6	38.4	35.1	31.8	28.6	25.3
150	56.4	53.1	49.9	46.6	43.3	40.1	36.8	33.5	30.3	27.0	23.8
160	54.8	51.6	48.3	45.0	41.8	38.5	35.2	32.0	28.7	25.5	22.2
170	53.3	50.0	46.7	43.5	40.2	36.9	33.7	30.4	27.1	23.9	20.6
180	51.7	48.4	45.2	41.9	38.6	35.4	32.1	28.8	25.6	22.3	19.1
190	50.1	46.9	43.6	40.3	37.1	33.8	30.5	27.3	24.0	20.8	17.5
Heart Rate	Women (30–39)										
120	58.2	55.0	51.7	48.4	45.2	41.9	38.7	35.4	32.1	28.9	25.6
130	56.7	53.4	50.1	46.9	43.6	40.4	37.1	33.8	30.6	27.3	24.0
140	55.1	51.8	48.6	45.3	42.1	38.8	35.5	32.3	29.0	25.7	22.5
150	53.5	50.3	47.0	43.8	40.5	37.2	34.0	30.7	27.4	24.2	20.9
160	52.0	48.7	45.4	42.2	38.9	35.7	32.4	29.1	25.9	22.6	19.3
170	50.4	47.1	43.9	40.6	37.4	34.1	30.8	27.6	24.3	21.0	17.8
180	48.8	45.6	42.3	39.1	35.8	32.5	29.3	26.0	22.7	19.5	16.2
190	47.3	44.0	40.8	37.5	34.2	31.0	27.7	24.4	21.2	17.9	14.6

ESTIMATED MAXIMAL OXYGEN UPTAKE (MLO/KGBW/MIN) FOR MEN AND WOMEN, 20-69 YEARS OLD

Minute/Mile	10	11	12	13	14	15	16	17	18	19	20
Heart Rate	**Men (40—49)**										
120	57.2	54.0	50.7	47.4	44.2	40.9	37.6	34.4	31.1	27.8	24.6
130	55.7	52.4	49.1	45.9	42.6	39.3	36.1	32.8	29.5	26.3	23.0
140	54.1	50.8	47.6	44.3	41.0	37.8	34.5	31.2	28.0	24.7	21.4
150	52.5	49.3	46.0	42.7	39.5	36.2	32.9	29.7	26.4	23.1	19.9
160	51.0	47.7	44.4	41.2	37.9	34.6	31.4	28.1	24.8	21.6	18.3
170	49.4	46.1	42.9	39.6	36.3	33.1	29.8	26.5	23.3	20.0	16.7
180	47.8	44.6	41.3	38.0	34.8	31.5	28.2	25.0	21.7	18.4	15.2
Heart Rate	**Women (40—49)**										
120	54.4	51.1	47.8	44.6	41.3	38.0	34.8	31.5	28.2	25.0	21.7
130	52.8	49.5	46.3	43.0	39.7	36.5	33.2	29.9	26.7	23.4	20.1
140	51.2	48.0	44.7	41.4	38.2	34.9	31.6	28.4	25.1	21.8	18.6
150	49.7	46.4	43.1	39.9	36.6	33.3	30.1	26.8	23.5	20.3	17.0
160	48.1	44.8	41.6	38.3	35.0	31.8	28.5	25.2	22.0	18.7	15.5
170	46.5	43.3	40.0	36.7	33.5	30.2	26.9	23.7	20.4	17.2	13.9
180	45.0	41.7	38.4	35.2	31.9	28.6	25.4	22.1	18.9	15.6	12.3
Heart Rate	**Men (50—59)**										
120	53.3	50.0	46.8	43.5	40.3	37.0	33.7	30.5	27.2	23.9	20.7
130	51.7	48.5	45.2	42.0	38.7	35.4	32.2	28.9	25.6	22.4	19.1
140	50.2	46.9	43.7	40.4	37.1	33.9	30.6	27.3	24.1	20.8	17.5
150	48.6	45.4	42.1	38.8	35.6	32.3	29.0	25.8	22.5	19.2	16.0
160	47.1	43.8	40.5	37.3	34.0	30.7	27.5	24.2	20.9	17.7	14.4
170	45.5	42.2	39.0	35.7	32.4	29.2	25.9	22.6	19.4	16.1	12.8
Heart Rate	**Women (50—59)**										
120	50.5	47.2	43.9	40.7	37.4	34.1	30.9	27.6	24.3	21.1	17.8
130	48.9	45.6	42.4	39.1	35.8	32.6	29.3	26.0	22.8	19.5	16.2
140	47.3	44.1	40.8	37.5	34.3	31.0	27.7	24.5	21.2	17.9	14.7
150	45.8	42.5	39.2	36.0	32.7	29.4	26.2	22.9	19.6	16.4	13.1
160	44.2	40.9	37.7	34.4	31.1	27.9	24.6	21.3	18.1	14.8	11.5
170	42.6	39.4	36.1	32.8	29.6	26.3	23.0	19.8	16.5	13.2	10.0

ESTIMATED MAXIMAL OXYGEN UPTAKE (MLO/KGBW/MIN) FOR MEN AND WOMEN, 20-69 YEARS OLD

Minute/Mile	10	11	12	13	14	15	16	17	18	19	20
Heart Rate	Men (60—69)										
120	49.4	46.2	42.9	39.6	36.4	33.1	29.8	26.6	23.3	20.0	16.8
130	47.9	44.6	41.3	38.1	34.8	31.5	28.3	25.0	21.7	18.5	15.2
140	46.3	43.0	39.8	36.5	33.2	30.0	26.7	23.4	20.2	16.9	13.6
150	44.7	41.5	38.2	34.9	31.7	28.4	25.1	21.9	18.6	15.3	12.1
160	43.2	39.9	36.6	33.4	30.1	26.8	23.6	20.3	17.0	13.8	10.5
Heart Rate	Women (60—69)										
120	46.6	43.3	40.0	36.8	33.5	30.2	27.0	23.7	20.5	17.2	13.9
130	45.0	41.7	38.5	35.2	31.9	28.7	25.4	22.2	18.9	15.6	12.4
140	43.4	40.2	36.9	33.6	30.4	27.1	23.8	20.6	17.3	14.1	10.8
150	41.9	38.6	35.3	32.1	28.8	25.5	22.3	19.0	15.8	12.5	9.2
160	40.3	37.0	33.8	30.5	27.2	24.0	20.7	17.5	14.2	10.9	7.7

Note: Calculations assume 170lb for men and 125lb for women. For each 15lb beyond these values, subtract 1 ml. Adapted from Kline et al. (1987).

Source: Howley, E.T. & B.D. Franks (1992). Health Fitness Instructor's Handbook, 2nd ed. Champaign: Human Kinetics Publishers.

Appendix D
Adult Basic
Life Support

Basic life support (BLS) is the phase of emergency cardiac care (ECC) that (1) prevents respiratory or circulatory arrest or insufficiency through prompt recognition and intervention or (2) supports the ventilation of a victim of respiratory arrest with rescue breathing or the ventilation and circulation of a victim of cardiac arrest with cardiopulmonary resuscitation (CPR). The major objective of performing rescue breathing or CPR is to provide oxygen to the brain and heart until appropriate, definitive medical treatment (advanced cardiac life support (ACLS) can restore normal heart and ventilation action. The prompt administration of BLS is the key to success. In respiratory arrest, the survival rate may be very high if airway control and rescue breathing are started promptly. For cardiac arrest the highest hospital discharge rate has been achieved in patients in whom CPR was initiated within 4 minutes of arrest and ACLS within 8 minutes. Early bystander rescue breathing or CPR intervention and fast emergency medical services (EMS) response are therefore essential in improving survival rates and good neurological recovery rates.

INDICATIONS FOR BLS

Respiratory Arrest

When primary respiratory arrest occurs, the heart and lungs can continue to oxygenate the blood for several minutes, and oxygen will continue to circulate to the brain and other vital organs. Such patients commonly have a pulse. Respiratory arrest can result from a number of causes, including drowning, stroke, foreign-body airway obstruction, smoke inhalation, epiglottitis, drug overdose, electrocution, suffocation, injuries, myocardial infarction, lightning strike, and coma of any cause. Establishing a patent airway and delivering only rescue breathing when respirations have stopped

or are inadequate can save many lives in such patients who still have a pulse. In addition, early intervention for victims in whom respirations have stopped or the airway is obstructed may prevent cardiac arrest.

Cardiac Arrest

In primary cardiac arrest, circulation ceases and vital organs are deprived of oxygen. Ineffective "gasping" ventilatory efforts ("agonal" respirations) may occur early in cardiac arrest and should not be confused with spontaneous respirations. Cardiac arrest can be accompanied by the following electrical phenomena: ventricular fibrillation, ventricular tachycardia, asystole, or pulseless electrical activity (incorporating electromechanical dissociation).

THE SEQUENCE OF BLS: ASSESSMENT, EMS ACTIVATION, AND THE ABCs OF CPR

The assessment phases of BLS are crucial. No victim should undergo the more intrusive procedures of CPR (positioning, opening the airway, rescue breathing, or chest compression) until the need has been established by the appropriate assessment. Assessment also involves a more subtle, constant process of observing and interacting with the victim. The importance of the assessment phase should be stressed in teaching CPR.

Each of the ABCs of CPR—airway, breathing, and circulation—begins with an assessment phase: determine unresponsiveness, determine breathlessness, and determine pulselessness, respectively. After responsiveness has been assessed, the EMS system should be immediately activated.

Activate EMS

Assessment: Determine Unresponsiveness. The rescuer arriving at the side of the collapsed victim must quickly assess any injury

Appendix D
Adult Basic Life
Support

and determine whether the person is unconscious (Fig. 1). The rescuer should tap or gently shake the victim and shout, "Are you OK?" If the victim has sustained trauma to the head and neck or trauma is suspected, the rescuer should move the victim only if absolutely necessary. Improper movement may cause paralysis in the victim with a neck injury.

Activate the EMS System. The EMS system is activated by calling the local emergency telephone number (911, if available; Fig. 1). This number should be widely publicized in each community. The person who calls the EMS system should be prepared to give the following information as calmly as possible: (1) the location of the emergency (with names of cross street or roads, if possible); (2) the telephone number from which the call is being made; (3) what happened—heart attack , auto accident, etc; (4) how many persons need help; (5) condition of the victim(s); (6) what aid is being given to the victim(s); and (7) any other information requested. To ensure

that EMS personnel have no more questions, the caller should hang up last.

Airway

In the unresponsive victim, the rescuer will need to determine if the victim is breathing. In many instances, however, this may not be accurately ascertained unless the airway is opened.

Position of the Victim. For resuscitative efforts and evaluation to be effective, the victim must be supine and on a firm, flat surface. If the victim is lying face down, the rescuer must roll the victim as a unit so that the head, shoulders, and torso move simultaneously without twisting (Fig. 2). The head and neck should remain in the same plane as the torso, and the body should be moved as a unit. The non-breathing patient should be supine with the arms alongside the body. The victim is now appropriately positioned for CPR.

Rescuer Position. The rescuer should be at the victim's side, positioned to easily perform both rescue breathing and chest compression.

Open Airway. In the absence of sufficient muscle tone, the tongue and epiglottis may obstruct the pharynx (Fig. 3.a). The tongue is the most common cause of airway obstruction in the unconscious victim. Since the tongue is attached to the lower jaw, moving the lower jaw forward will lift the tongue away from the back of the throat and open the airway. The tongue or the epiglottis, or both, may also create obstruction when negative pressure is created in the airway by inspiratory effort, causing a valve-type mechanism to occlude the entrance to the trachea.

If there is no evidence of head or neck trauma, the rescuer should use the head tilt—chin lift maneuver to open the airway, described below (Fig. 3.b). If foreign material or vomitus is visible in the

Figure 1

Initial steps of cardiopulmonary resuscitation. Determine unresponsiveness; activate the emergency medical services system. ☎ **Call 911!**

Are you okay?

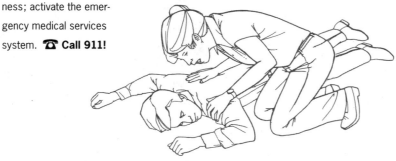

Figure 2

Positioning the victim. Victim must be supine and on a firm, flat surface.

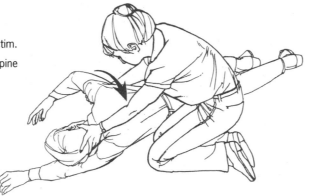

mouth, it should be removed. Excessive time must not be taken. Liquids or semi-liquids should be wiped out with the index and middle fingers covered by a piece of cloth; solid material should be extracted with a hooked index finger.

Head Tilt—Chin Life Maneuver. To accomplish the head tilt maneuver, one hand is placed on the victim's forehead and firm, backward pressure is applied with the palm to tilt the head back. To complete the head tilt—chin lift maneuver, the fingers of the other hand are placed under the bony part of the lower jaw near the chin and lifted to bring the chin forward and the teeth almost to occlusion, thus supporting the jaw and helping to tilt the head back. The fingers must not press deeply into the soft tissue under the chin, which might obstruct the airway. The thumb should not be used for lifting the chin. The mouth should not be completely closed (unless mouth-to-nose breathing is the technique of choice for that particular victim). When mouth-to-nose ventilation is indicated, the hand that is already on the chin can close the mouth by applying increased force and in this way provide effective mouth-to-nose ventilation. If the victim's dentures are loose, head tilt—chin lift makes a mouth-to-mouth seal easier. Dentures should be removed if they cannot be kept in place.

Jaw-Thrust Maneuver. This technique is recommended as an alternative for health care providers. Forward displacement of the mandible can be accomplished by grasping the angles of the victim's lower jaw and lifting with both hands, one on each side, displacing the mandible forward while tilting the head backward. The rescuer's elbows should rest on the surface on which the victim is lying. If the lips close, the lower lip can be retracted with the thumb. If the mouth-to-mouth breathing is necessary,

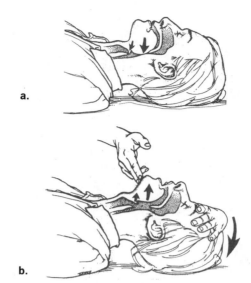

a.

b.

Figure 3

Opening the airway.
a. Airway obstruction produced by tongue and epiglottis.
b. Relief by head tilt-chin lift.

the nostrils can be closed by placing the rescuer's cheek tightly against them. This technique is effective in opening the airway but is fatiguing and technically difficult.

The jaw-thrust technique without head tilt is the safest initial approach to opening the airway of the victim with suspected neck injury because it usually can be accomplished without extending the neck. The head should be carefully supported without tilting it backward or turning it from side to side. If the jaw thrust alone is unsuccessful, the head should be tilted backward slightly.

Breathing

Assessment: Determine Breathlessness. To assess the presence or absence of spontaneous breathing, the rescuer should place his or her ear over the victim's mouth and nose while maintaining an open airway (Fig. 4). Then, while observing the victim's chest, the rescuer should (1) look for the chest to rise and fall, (2) listen for air escaping during exhalation, and (3) feel for the flow of air. If the chest does not rise and fall and no air is exhaled, the victim is breathless. This evaluation procedure should take only 3 to 5 seconds.

It should be stressed that although the

Reproduced with permission. *Guidelines for Cardiopulmonary Resuscitation and Emergency Cardiac Care,* 1992. Copyright American Heart Association

Appendix D
Adult Basic Life
Support

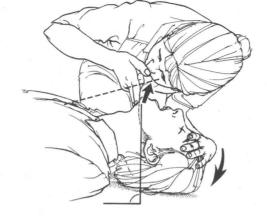

Figure 4

Determining
breathlessness.

rescuer may notice that the victim is making respiratory efforts, the airway may still be obstructed, and opening the airway may be all that is needed. In addition, reflex gasping respiratory efforts (agonal respirations) may occur early in the course of primary cardiac arrest and should not be mistaken for adequate breathing.

If a victim resumes breathing and regains a pulse during or following resuscitation, the rescuer should continue to help maintain an open airway. The rescuer should then place the victim in the recovery position (Fig. 5). To place the victim in the recovery position, the victim is rolled onto his or her side so that the head, shoulders, and torso move simultaneously without twisting. If the victim has sustained trauma or trauma is suspected, the victim should not be moved.

Performing Rescue Breathing. Rescue breathing requires that the rescuer inflate the victim's lungs adequately with each breath.

Mouth to Mouth. Rescue breathing with the mouth-to-mouth technique is a quick, effective way to provide oxygen to the vic-

tim (Fig. 6.a). The rescuer's exhaled air contains enough oxygen to supply the victim's needs. Keeping the airway open by the head tilt—chin lift maneuver, the rescuer gently pinches the nose closed with the thumb and index finger (of the hand on the forehead), thereby preventing air from escaping through the victim's nose. The rescuer takes a deep breath and seals his or her lips around the victim's mouth, creating an airtight seal. Then the rescuer gives two slow breaths, followed by 10 to 12 breaths per minute.

The rescuer should take a breath after each ventilation, and each individual ventilation should be of sufficient volume to make the chest rise. In most adults, this volume will be 800 to 1200 mL (0.8 to 1.2 L). Adequate ventilation is indicated by (1) observing the chest rise and fall and (2) hearing and feeling the air escape during exhalation. Adequate time for the two breaths (1-1/2 to 2 seconds per breath) should be allowed to provide good chest expansion and decrease the possibility of gastric distention. Too great a volume of air and too fast an inspiratory flow rate are likely to cause pharyngeal pressures that exceed esophageal opening pressures, allowing air to enter the stomach, resulting in gastric distention. When possible (eg. during two-rescuer CPR) the airway should be kept patent during exhalation to minimize gastric distention.

If initial (or subsequent) attempts to ventilate the victim are unsuccessful, the victim's head should be repositioned and rescue breathing reattempted. Improper chin and head positioning is the most common cause of difficulty with ventilation and should be carefully assessed. If the victim cannot be ventilated after repositioning the head, the rescuer should proceed with foreign-body airway maneuvers.

Figure 5

Placing the victim in
the recovery position.

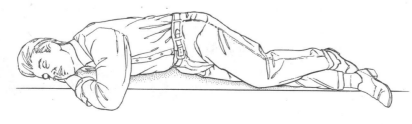

Mouth to Nose. This technique is more effective in some patients than the mouth-to-mouth technique (Fig. 6). The mouth-to-nose technique is recommended when it is impossible to ventilate through the victim's mouth, the mouth cannot be opened (trismus), the mouth is seriously injured, or a tight mouth-to-mouth seal is difficult to achieve. The rescuer keeps the victim's head tilted back with one hand on the forehead and uses the other hand to lift the victim's lower jaw (as in head tilt—chin lift) and close the mouth. The rescuer then takes a deep breath, seals his or her lips around the victim's nose, and breathes out into the patient's nose. The rescuer then removes his or her lips from the patient, allowing the victim to exhale passively. It may be necessary to open the victim's mouth intermittently or separate the lips with the thumb to allow air to be exhaled since nasal obstruction may be present.

Mouth to Stoma. Persons who have undergone a laryngectomy (surgical removal of the larynx) have a permanent opening that connects the trachea directly to the front base of the neck. When such a person requires rescue breathing, direct mouth-to-stoma ventilation should be performed (Fig. 6.c) by making an airtight seal around the stoma and blowing until the chest rises. In such patients, exhalation occurs passively when the rescuer stops breathing into the stoma.

Other persons may have a temporary tracheostomy tube in the trachea. To ventilate such persons, the victim's mouth and nose usually must be sealed by the rescuer's hand or by a tightly fitting face mask to prevent leakage of air when the rescuer blows into the tracheostomy tube. This problem is alleviated when the tracheostomy tube has an inflated cuff.

Mouth to Barrier Device. Some rescuers may prefer to use a barrier device during mouth-to-mouth ventilation. Many devices have been introduced, but few have been adequately studied. Two broad categories of devices are available, mask devices and face shields. Most mask devices have a one-way valve so that exhaled air does not enter the rescuer's mouth. Many face shields have no exhalation valve, and air often leaks around the shield. Mouth-to-barrier device breathing should ideally have low

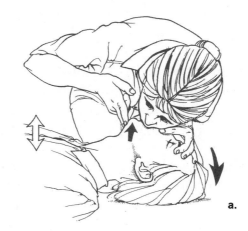
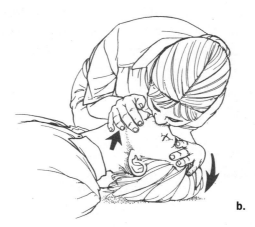
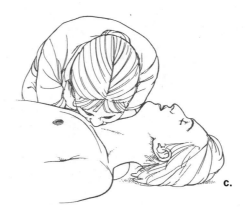

Figure 6

Rescue breathing.

a. Mouth to mouth.

b. Mouth to nose.

c. Mouth to stoma.

Reproduced with permission. *Guidelines for Cardiopulmonary Resuscitation and Emergency Cardiac Care,* 1992. Copyright American Heart Association

resistance to gas flow, or the user may tire from excessive respiratory effort. If rescuer breathing is deemed necessary, the barrier device (face mask or face shield) is positioned over the victim's mouth and nose, ensuring an adequate air seal. Mouth-to-barrier device breathing is then initiated using slow inspiratory breaths (1-1/2 to 2 seconds) as described above. Further evaluation of the effectiveness of these devices is warranted.

Recommendations for Rescue Breathing. Two initial breaths delivered over 1-1/2 to 2 seconds each should be given. Giving ventilations with a slow inspiratory flow rate and allowing complete exhalation between breaths diminishes the likelihood of exceeding the esophageal opening pressure. This technique should result in less gastric distention, regurgitation, and aspiration. For both one-rescuer and two-rescuer CPR, 10 to 12 breaths should be delivered per minute. In one-rescuer CPR, a pause for ventilation should be taken after every 15th chest compression, whereas in two-rescuer CPR, the pause for ventilation should be

taken after every five chest compressions. In such cases the 1-1/2 to 2-second pause for ventilation is devoted primarily to delivering slow inspiratory breaths. Exhalation is a passive phenomenon and occurs primarily during chest compressions.

Circulation

Assessment: Determine Pulselessness. The victim's condition must be properly assessed since performing chest compressions on a patient who has a pulse may result in serious medical complications. If a pulse is present but there is no breathing, rescue breathing should be initiated as describes above. Cardiac arrest is recognized by pulselessness in the large arteries of the unconscious victim. The pulse should be checked at the carotid artery. This should take no more than 5 to 10 seconds. The carotid artery is the most accessible, reliable, and easily learned location for checking the pulse in adults and children. This artery lies in a groove created by the trachea and the large strap muscles of the neck. While maintaining head tilt with one hand on the forehead, the rescuer locates the victim's larynx with two or three fingers of the other hand (Fig. 7.a). The rescuer then slides these fingers into the groove between the trachea and the muscles at the side of the neck, where the carotid pulse can be felt (Fig. 7.b). The pulse area must be pressed gently to avoid compressing the artery. This technique is easily performed on the side nearer the rescuer.

The pulse in the carotid artery may persist even when more peripheral pulses (eg. radial) are no longer palpable. Determining pulselessness using the femoral artery pulse is also acceptable for health care professionals; however, this pulse is difficult to locate in a fully clothed patient.

Chest Compressions. The chest compression technique consists of serial, rhythmic

Figure 7

Determining pulselessness.

a. Locate the larynx while maintaining the head-tilt position.

b. Slide the fingers into the groove between the trachea and muscles at the side of the neck where the carotid pulse can be felt.

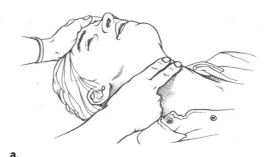

a.

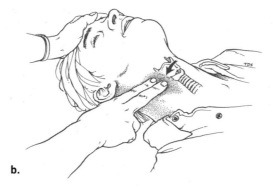

b.

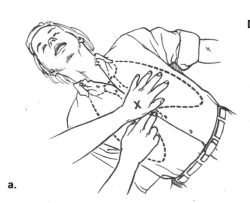

a.

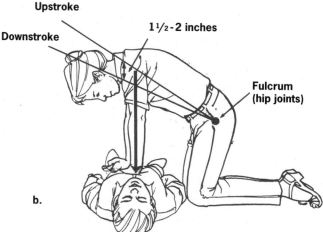

Upstroke

Downstroke

1½-2 inches

Fulcrum
(hip joints)

b.

applications of pressure over the lower half of the sternum (Fig. 8). These compressions provide circulation as a result of a generalized increase in intrathoracic pressure and/or direct compression of the heart. Blood circulated to the lungs by chest compressions will likely receive enough oxygen to maintain life when the compressions are accompanied by properly performed rescue breathing.

The patient must be in the horizontal, supine position during chest compressions. This is because even with properly performed compressions, blood flow to the brain is reduced. When the head is elevated above the heart, blood flow to the brain is further reduced or eliminated. If the victim is in bed, a board, preferably full width of the bed, should be placed under the patient's back to avoid diminished effectiveness of chest compression.

Proper Hand Position. Proper hand placement is established by identifying the lower half of the sternum. The guidelines below may be used, or the rescuer may choose alternative techniques to identify the lower sternum.

1. The rescuer's hand locates the lower margin of the victim's rib cage on the side next to the rescuer.

2. The fingers are then moved up the rib cage to the notch where the ribs meet the lower sternum in the center of the lower part of the chest.

3. The heel of one hand is placed on the lower half of the sternum, and the other hand is placed on top of the hand on the sternum so that the hands are parallel (Fig. 8.a). The long axis of the heel of the rescuer's hand should be placed on the long axis of the sternum. This will keep the main force of compression on the sternum and decrease the chance of rib fracture.

4. The fingers may be either extended or interlaced but should be kept off the chest.

5. Because of the varying sizes and shapes of hands, an acceptable alternative hand position is to grasp the wrist of the hand on the chest with the hand that has been locating the lower end of the sternum. This technique is helpful for rescuers with arthritic hands and wrists.

Proper Compression Techniques. Effective compression is accomplished by attention to the following guidelines (Fig. 8.b):

1. The elbows are locked into position, the arms are straightened, and the rescuer's shoulders are positioned directly over the hands so that the thrust for each chest compression is straight down on the sternum. If the thrust is not in a straight downward direction, the torso has a tendency to roll; part of the force is lost, and the chest compression may be less effective.

Figure 8

External chest compression.

a. Locating the correct hand position on the lower half of the sternum.

b. Proper position of the rescuer, with shoulders directly over the victims sternum and elbows locked.

2. The sternum should be depressed approximately 1-1/2 to 2 inches for the normal-sized adult. Rarely, in very slight persons lesser degrees of compression may be enough to generate a palpable carotid or femoral pulse. In some persons 1-1/2 to 2 inches of sternal compression may be inadequate and a slightly greater degree of chest compression may be needed to generate a carotid or femoral pulse. Optimal sternal compression is best gauged by using the compression force that generates a palpable carotid or femoral pulse. However, this can be implemented only by two rescuers. The single rescuer should follow the sternal compression guideline of 1-1/2 to 2 inches.

3. Chest compression pressure is released to allow blood to flow into the chest and heart. The pressure must be released completely and the chest allowed to return to its normal position after each compression. Arterial pressure during chest compression is maximal when the duration of compression is 50% of the compression-release cycle. Hence, rescuers should be encouraged to maintain prolonged chest compression. Fortunately this is more easily achieved at faster chest compression rates (80 to 100 per minute) than at rates of 60 per minute.

4. The hands should not be lifted from the chest or the position changed in any way, lest correct hand position be lost.

Rescue breathing and chest compression must be combined for effective resuscitation of the victim of cardiopulmonary arrest.

CPR PERFORMED BY ONE RESCUER AND BY TWO RESCUERS

CPR Performed by One Rescuer

Laypersons should be taught only one-rescuer CPR since the two-rescuer technique is infrequently used by laypersons in rescue situations. One-rescuer CPR should be performed as follows:

1. Activate EMS. Assessment: determine unresponsiveness (tap or gently shake the victim and shout) and activate the EMS system.

2. Airway. Position the victim and open the airway by the head tilt-chin lift maneuver.

3. Breathing. Assessment: determine breathlessness. If the victim is unresponsive but obviously breathing and if there is no trauma, the victim is placed in the recovery position and an open airway maintained. If the adult victim is unresponsive and not breathing, rescue breathing is performed by giving two initial breaths. If unable to give two breaths, (1) the head is repositioned and ventilation reattempted and (2) if still unsuccessful, the foreign-body airway obstruction sequence is performed. If the victim has a pulse but is unresponsive and not breathing, ventilation should be performed once every 5 to 6 seconds without chest compression. If respirations are restored, are adequate, and a pulse is present, the rescuer should continue to help maintain an open airway by placing the patient in the recovery position.

4. Circulation. Assessment: determine pulselessness. If pulse is present and the victim is unresponsive, continue rescue breathing at 10 to 12 times per minute if needed. Otherwise, if ventilations are also adequate, the patient should be placed in the recovery position. If a pulse is absent, begin chest compression:

• Locate proper hand position.

• Perform 15 external chest compressions at a rate of 80 to 100 per minute. Count "one and, two and, three and, four and, five and, six and, seven and, eight and, nine and, ten and, eleven and, twelve and, thirteen and, fourteen and, fifteen." (Any mnemonic that accomplishes the same compression rate is acceptable.)

• Open the airway and deliver two slow rescue breaths (1-1/2 to 2-seconds each).

• Find the proper hand position and begin 15 more compressions at a rate of 80 to 100 per minute.

• Perform four complete cycles of 15 compressions and two ventilations.

5. Reassessment. After four cycles of compressions and ventilations (15:2 ratio), the rescuer should reevaluate the patient, checking for return of the carotid pulse (3 to 5 seconds). If absent, CPR with chest compressions is resumed. If a pulse is present, the rescuer should check for breathing. If present, breathing and pulse should be closely monitored. If absent, rescue breathing should be performed at 10 to 12 times per minute and the pulse monitored closely.

If CPR is continued, the rescuer should stop and check for return of pulse and spontaneous breathing every few minutes. The rescuer should not interrupt CPR except in special circumstances.

Entrance of a Second Rescuer to Replace the First Rescuer

When another rescuer is available at the scene, the second rescuer should activate the EMS system (if not done previously) and perform one-rescuer CPR when the first rescuer, who initiated CPR, becomes fatigued. This should be done with as little interruption as possible. When the second rescuer arrives, breathing and pulse should be reassessed before CPR is resumed.

CPR Performed by Two Rescuers

All professional rescuers (EMTs and other health care professionals) should learn both the one-rescuer technique and the two-rescuer technique. When possible,

airway adjunct methods such as mouth-to-mask should to used.

In two-rescuer CPR, one person is positioned at the victim's side and performs chest compressions. The other rescuer remains at the victim's head, maintains an open airway, monitors the carotid pulse for adequacy of chest compressions, and provides rescue breathing. The compression rate for two-rescuer CPR is 80 to 100 per minute. The compressions-ventilation ratio is 5:1, with a pause for ventilation (inspiration) of 1-1/2 to 2 seconds. Exhalation occurs during chest compressions. When the compressor becomes fatigued, the rescuers should exchange positions with as minimal a delay as possible.

Monitoring the Victim

The victim's condition must be monitored to assess the effectiveness of the rescue effort. The person ventilating the patient assumes the responsibility for monitoring the pulse and breathing, which serves to (1) evaluate the effectiveness of compressions and (2) determine if the victim resumes spontaneous circulation and breathing.

To assess the effectiveness of the partner's chest compressions, the rescuer should check the pulse during the compressions. To determine if the victim has resumed spontaneous breathing and circulation, chest compressions must be stopped for 5 seconds at about the end of the first minute and every few minutes thereafter.

Disease Transmission During Actual Performance of CPR

The vast majority of CPR performed in the United States is done by health care and public safety personnel, many of whom assist in ventilation of respiratory and cardiac arrest victims about whom they

Indications and sequence of BLS/ CPR performed by one or two rescuers

Reproduced with permission. *Guidelines for Cardiopulmonary Resuscitation and Emergency Cardiac Care*, 1992. Copyright American Heart Association

have little or no medical information. A layperson is far less likely to perform CPR than health care providers. The layperson who performs CPR, whether on an adult or pediatric victim, is most likely to do so in the home, where 70% to 80% of respiratory and cardiac arrests occur.

The layperson who responds to an emergency in an unknown victim should be guided by the moral and ethical values of preserving life and assisting those in distress balanced against the risk that may exist in the various rescue situations. The presence of documentation or another reliable reason to believe that CPR is not indicated or wanted or in the patient's best interest should factor into the rescuer's decision to initiate or withhold resuscitation. It is safest for the rescuer to assume that any emergency situation that involves exposure to certain body fluids has the potential for disease transmission for both the rescuer and victim. In such situations measures recommended below should be used during CPR to minimize transmission of disease.

The greatest concern over the risk of disease transmission should be directed to persons who perform CPR frequently, such as health care providers, both in the hospital and in the prehospital environment. Providers of prehospital emergency health care include paramedics, EMTs, law enforcement personnel, fire fighters, lifeguards, and others whose job-defined duties require them to perform first-rescuer medical care. The risk of disease transmission from infected persons to providers of prehospital emergency health care should be no higher than that for those providing emergency care in the hospital if appropriate precautions are taken to prevent exposure to blood or other body fluids.

The probability that a rescuer (lay or professional) will become infected with HBV or HIV as a result of performing CPR is minimal. Although transmission of HBV and HIV between health care workers and patients has been documented as a result of blood exchange or penetration of the skin by blood-contaminated instruments, transmission of HBV and HIV infection during mouth-to-mouth resuscitation has not been documented.

Direct mouth-to-mouth resuscitation will likely result in exchange of saliva between the victim and rescuer. However, HBV-positive saliva has not been shown to be infectious even to oral mucous membranes, through contamination of shared musical instruments, or through HBV carriers. In addition, saliva has not been implicated in the transmission of HIV after bites, percutaneous inoculation, or contamination of cuts and open wounds with saliva from HIV-infected patients.

The theoretical risk of infection is greater for salivary or aerosol transmission of herpes simplex, Neisseria meningitidis, and airborne diseases such as tuberculosis and other respiratory infections. Rare instances of herpes transmission during CPR have been reported.

The emergence of multidrug-resistant tuberculosis and the risk of tuberculosis to emergency workers is a cause for concern. Rescuers with impaired immune systems may be particularly at risk. In most instances, transmission of tuberculosis requires prolonged close exposure as is likely to occur in households, but transmission to emergency workers can occur during resuscitative efforts by either the airborne route or direct contact. The magnitude of the risk is uncertain but probably low. After performing mouth-to-mouth resuscitation on a person suspected of having tuberculosis, the caregiver should be evaluated for tuberculosis using standard approaches based on the caregiver's baseline skin tests. Caregivers with negative baseline skin tests should be retested 12 weeks later. Preventive therapy should be considered for all persons with positive tests and should be started on all converters. In areas where multidrug-resistant tuberculosis is common or after exposure to known multidrug-resistant tuberculosis, the choice of preventive therapeutic agent is uncertain, but some authorities suggest two or more agents.

Performance of mouth-to-mouth resuscitation or invasive procedures can result in the exchange of blood between the victim and rescuer. This is especially true in cases of trauma or if either victim or rescuer has breaks in the skin on or around the lips or soft tissues of the oral cavity mucosa. Thus, a theoretical risk of HBV and HIV transmission during mouth-to-mouth resuscitation exists.

Because of the concern about disease transmission between victim and rescuer, rescuers with a duty to provide CPR should follow the precautions and guidelines established by the Centers for Disease Control and the Occupational Safety and Health Administration. These guidelines include the use of barriers, such as latex gloves, and mechanical ventilation equipment, such as a bag-valve mask and other resuscitation masks with valves capable of diverting expired air from the rescuer. Rescuers who have an infection that may be transmitted by blood or saliva should not perform mouth-to-mouth resuscitation if circumstances allow other immediate or effective methods of ventilation.

The perceived risk of disease transmission during CPR has reduced the willingness of some laypersons to initiate mouth-to-mouth ventilation in unknown victims of cardiac arrest. Public education is vital to alleviate this fear. In addition, if such concern is identified, rescuers should be encouraged to learn mouth-to-barrier device (face mask or face shield) ventilation. If a lone rescuer refuses to initiate mouth-to-mouth ventilation, he or she should at least access the EMS system, open the airway, and perform chest compressions until a rescuer arrives who is willing to provide ventilation or until ventilation can be initiated by skilled rescuers (arriving EMTs or paramedics) with the necessary barrier devices.

Although the efficacy of barrier devices has not been documented conclusively, those with a duty to respond should be instructed during CPR training in the use of masks with one-way valves. Plastic mouth and nose covers with filtered openings are also available and may provide a degree of protection. Masks without one-way valves (including those with S-shaped devices) offer little, if any, protection and should not be considered for routine use. Since intubation obviates the need for mouth-to-mouth resuscitation and is more effective than the use of masks alone, early intubation is encouraged when equipment and trained professionals are available. Resuscitation equipment known or suspected to be contaminated with blood or other body fluids should be discarded or thoroughly cleaned and disinfected after each use. Following these precautions and guidelines should further reduce the risk of disease transmission when providing CPR.

CPR performed by one or two rescuers

ACKNOWLEDGEMENT

Reproduced with permission. *Guidelines for Cardiopulmonary Resuscitation and Emergency Cardiac Care*, 1992. Copyright American Heart Association.

Glossary

Abduction Movement of a body part away from the body's midline.

Abrasion A scraping injury to the skin's surface.

Accent Emphasis on a given beat.

Acclimatization The process in which the body physiologically adapts to an unfamiliar environment, such as a high altitude or a hot climate.

Achilles tendinitis A chronic overuse injury characterized by inflammation of the Achilles tendon resulting from small tears in its fibers.

Acidosis A condition characterized by an above normal increase of blood acidity.

Actin One of the contractile protein filaments in muscles.

Acute Bronchitis A bout of bronchitis can develop following a cold or exposure to some irritant, such as dust or air pollution. Acute bronchitis generally lasts several days to a week.

Acute injury An injury having a sudden onset, characterized by specific pain and swelling and the inability to use the injured area normally.

Addiction To devote or surrender oneself to something habitually or obsessively.

Adduction Movement of a body part toward the body's midline.

Adenosine diphosphate (ADP) One of the chemical by-products of the breakdown of ATP during muscle contraction.

Adenosine triphosphate (ATP) The high-energy phosphate molecule that provides energy for cellular function. One of the phosphagens.

Adherence The amount of programmed exercise a client engages in during a specified time period compared to the amount of exercise recommended for that time period.

Adipose tissue A conglomeration of adipocytes (fat cells) forming the major depot of body fat.

ADP See Adenosine diphosphate.

Adult-onset diabetes See diabetes mellitus (Type II diabetes).

Aerobic Requires the presence of oxygen.

Aerobic cool-down The period at the end of the aerobics segment of an exercise session in which intensity is reduced to begin lowering the heart rate.

Aerobic dance-exercise A method of exercising to music that conditions the cardiovascular system by using movements that create an increased demand for oxygen over an extended time.

Aerobic fitness See cardiorespiratory fitness.

Aerobic glycolysis The metabolic pathway that, in the presence of oxygen, uses glucose for energy production (ATP).

Affective domain One of the three domains of learning, which involves the learning of emotional behaviors.

Afferent neurons Receptors that transmit impulses to the spinal cord and brain.

Age-predicted maximal heart rate The maximal heart rate predicted from subtracting a given subject's age from 220.

Agonist A muscle that is directly responsible for the joint movement observed. Also referred to as a prime mover.

Alkalosis A condition characterized by a decrease in acidity or hydrogen ion concentration of the blood and extracellular fluids.

Alveoli The small membranous air sacs located at the terminal ends of bronchioles. At the site of the alveoli, oxygen and carbon dioxide are exchanged between the blood and air in the lungs.

Amenorrheic The absence of menstruation.

Americans with Disabilities Act (ADA) Civil rights legislation designed to improve access to jobs, work places and commercial spaces for people with disabilities.

Amino acids Nitrogen-containing compounds that are the building blocks of protein.

Amphiarthroses A slightly movable joint.

Anacrusis The upbeat which concludes the preceding measure of music.

Anaerobic Without the presence of oxygen. Not requiring oxygen.

Anaerobic glycolysis The metabolic pathway that uses glucose for energy production (ATP) without requiring the presence of oxygen. This pathway produces lactic acid as a by-product.

Anatomical position Standing erect with the feet and palms facing forward.

Anemia A disorder caused by a low hemoglobin content in the blood, which reduces the amount of oxygen available to the body's tissues. Symptoms include fatigue, breathlessness after exercise, giddiness and loss of appetite.

Angina pectoris Chest pain caused by inadequate blood flow, and thus oxygen supply, to the heart. Often aggravated or induced by exercise or stress.

Anorexia nervosa An eating disorder characterized by an intense fear of becoming obese, a distorted body image, and extreme weight loss. A form of self starvation. Metabolic abnormalities are commonly associated with this disorder and can sometimes be fatal.

Antagonist A muscle that acts in opposition to the action produced by an agonist muscle.

Anterior The front side or to the front side of the body.

Anthropometric measurements The measurement of the human body and it's parts most commonly measured using skinfolds, girth and body weight.

Antihypertensives Medications that treat hypertension, including beta-adrenergic blocking agents and calcium-channel blockers.

Aorta The main artery exiting the left ventricle of the heart.

Apical pulse A pulse point located at the apex of the heart.

Appendicular skeleton The bones of the upper and lower extremities of the body.

Applied force An external force acting on a system (body or body segment).

Arrhythmia Abnormal Heart rhythm or beat.

Arteries Vessels that carry oxygenated blood from the heart to vital organs and the extremities.

Arterioles Smaller divisions of arteries.

Arthritis Inflammatory condition involving a joint. See also Osteoarthritis and Rheumatoid arthritis.

Articulations The joints of the body where bones come together and where all movement of the skeletal system takes place.

ASCAP The American Society of Composers, Authors and Publishers. One of two performing rights societies in the United States that represents music publishers in negotiating and collecting fees for the nondramatic performance of music.

Associative stage The second stage of learning a motor skill in which performers, having learned the basic fundamentals or mechanics of the skill, can now concentrate on refining skills.

Assumption of risk A defense used to show that a person has voluntarily accepted known dangers by participating in a specific activity.

Asthma A form of obstructive pulmonary disease. It is caused by the constriction of the smooth muscle around the small airways in the lungs. Asthma is characterized by shortness of breath and a wheezing sound during breathing. It can be induced by an allergic reaction, exercise or breathing other foreign substances.

Atherosclerosis A progressive, degenerative arterial disease that leads to occlusion of affected vessels, thereby reducing blood flow through them. Characterized by the accumulation of fatty material on the inner walls of the arteries. When blood clots form at the occluded sites in the coronary arteries (the arteries supplying the heart), a myocardial infarction (heart attack) results.

ATP See Adenosine triphosphate.

Atrium One of the two (left or right). upper chambers of the heart.

Atrophy A reduction in muscle size resulting from inactivity or immobilization.

Autonomous stage The third stage of learning a motor skill in which the skill has become automatic or habitual to performers.

Avulsion A wound involving forcible separation or tearing of tissue from the body.

Axial skeleton The bones of the head, neck and trunk.

Ballistic stretching A high force, short duration stretch using rapid bouncing movements.

Basal metabolic rate The minimum energy required to maintain life processes in the resting state.

Basic locomotor steps Steps that use the feet as the base of support and only include walking (or stepping), running (or leaping), hopping and jumping.

Beats Regular pulsations that have an even rhythm and occur in a continuous pattern of strong and weak pulsations.

Beta blockers (beta-adrenergic blocking agents) Medications, used for cardiovascular and other medical conditions, that "block" or limit sympathetic nervous system stimulation.

Biarticulate A muscle that causes motion at two articulations (joints).

Bioelectric impedance analysis (BIA) A non-invasive means of assessing body composition via an electrical current through the body. Electric flow through the body is directly related to hydrated lean body mass; hence, impedance is directly related to the level of body fat.

Blanket license A certificate or document which gives permission that may fluctuate or vary and applies to a number of situations.

Blood pressure The pressure exerted by the blood on the walls of the arteries. Measured in millimeters of mercury with a sphygmomanometer.

BMI Broadcast Music, Inc. One of two performing rights societies in the United States that represents music publishers in negotiating and collecting fees for the nondramatic performance of music.

Body composition assessment A procedure (e.g., skinfolds or hydrostatic weighing) where body density is determined which is directly related to fat mass and lean body mass, both, of which, are expressed as a relative percentage of total body weight.

Body mass index (BMI) A relative measure of body height to body weight for determining degree of obesity.

Body composition The makeup of the body in terms of the percentage of lean body mass and body fat.

Body fat That component of the body that excludes the lean body mass made up of Adipose tissues.

Bone spur A sharp or pointy outgrowth of bone.

Broad ligament The ligament which extends from the lateral side of the uterus to the pelvic wall. This ligament keeps the uterus centrally placed while providing stability within the pelvic cavity.

Bronchioles The smallest tubes that supply air to the alveoli in the lungs.

Bronchitis A form of obstructive pulmonary disease. It is caused by an inflammation of the mucus membranes and the bronchial tubes in the lungs. Bronchitis is characterized by coughing, wheezing and sputum production.

Bulimia An eating disorder characterized by episodes of binge eating followed by fasting, self-induced vomiting, or the use of diuretics or laxatives.

Burnout A state of emotional exhaustion caused by stress from work or responsibilities.

Bursa Padlike fluid filled sac located at

friction sites throughout the body.

Bursitis Irritation of a bursa, which is a padlike fluid-filled sac located at friction sites throughout the body. Bursitis occurs most often in the knees, hips, shoulders and elbows.

Caffeine A bitter, crystalline alkaloid found in coffee, tea, etc., which has a stimulating effect on the heart and central nervous system.

Calcium The most abundant mineral in the body. Involved in the conduction of nerve impulses, heart function, muscle contraction and the operation of certain enzymes. An inadequate supply of calcium contributes to osteoporosis.

Calcium-channel blockers (calcium-channel blocking agents or antagonists) Medications, used primarily for treating high blood pressure, that reduce movement of calcium ions across cell membranes.

Calisthenics Exercises to increase muscular strength and endurance which use the weight of the body or body parts for resistance.

Caloric deficit The reducing of caloric intake usually done to lose weight (a deficit of 3,500 kcal's is required to lose one pound of stored fat).

Caloric-density The concentration of calories in nutrients.

Calorie The amount of heat necessary to raise the temperature of one gram of water one degree Celsius. Often used incorrectly in place of kilocalorie. (1 kilocalorie = 1000 calories).

Cancer A malignant tumor.

Capacity The total amount of energy produced.

Capillaries The smallest blood vessels that supply oxygenated blood to the tissues.

Carbohydrates A primary foodstuff used for energy. Dietary sources include sugars (simple) and grains, rice, potatoes and beans (complex). Carbohydrate is stored as glycogen in the muscles and liver and is transported in the blood as glucose. Definition for Complex and simple carbohydrates.

Cardiac arrest The cessation of cardiac output and effective circulation.

Cardiac output The amount of blood pumped by the heart per minute. Usually expressed in liters of blood per minute.

Cardiopulmonary resuscitation (CPR) A technique that artificially produces blood flow and air exchange in a pulseless, nonbreathing victim, by mouth-to-mouth respiration and rhythmical compression on the chest.

Cardiorespiratory endurance See Cardiorespiratory Fitness.

Cardiorespiratory fitness (CRF) The ability to perform large muscle movement over a sustained period. Related to the capacity of the heart-lung system to deliver oxygen for sustained energy production. Also called cardiorespiratory endurance or aerobic fitness.

Cardiovascular endurance See Cardiorespiratory fitness.

Cardiovascular disease (CVD) General term for any disease of the heart (cardio) and blood vessels (vascular).

Carotid pulse A pulse point located on the carotid artery in the neck about 1 inch below the jaw line, next to the esophagus.

Carpal tunnel syndrome Aching pain in wrist with weakness in hand and fingers caused by compressed nerves in carpal tunnel area of wrist.

Cartilage A smooth, semi-opaque material that absorbs shock and reduces friction between the bones of a joint.

Cellulite A nonmedical term often used to describe subcutaneous fat, commonly found in the thighs and buttocks, that appears dimpled like an orange peel. Nutritional authorities agree that all forms of subcutaneous fat are the same and that cellulite is not a special form of fat.

Center of Gravity The center of a body's

mass; the actual geometric center in a rigid, symmetrical object of uniform density; in the human body, it is the point about which all parts are in balance with each other; it depends on the body's current position in space, anatomical structure, gender, habitual standing posture, and whether external weights are being held.

Central nervous system (CNS) The brain and spinal cord.

Cerebrovascular accident (CVA) A loss in function resulting from impaired blood supply to part of the brain. More commonly known as a stroke.

Cervical vertebrae The seven vertebral bones of the neck.

CHD See Coronary Heart Disease

Cholesterol A fatty substance found in the blood and body tissues and in certain foods. Its accumulation in the arteries leads to narrowing of the vessels (atherosclerosis).

Chondromalacia A gradual softening and degeneration of the articular cartilage, usually involving the back surface of the patella (kneecap). This condition may produce pain and swelling, or a grinding sound or sensation when the knee is flexed and extended.

Chronic Bronchitis Characterized by increase mucus secretion and a productive cough lasting several months to several years.

Chronic Obstructive Pulmonary Diseases (COPD) COPD includes a spectrum of airway disorders ranging from asthma and acute bronchitis to chronic bronchitis and emphysema.

Circumduction Movement of a joint in a circular pattern; combination of flexion, abduction, extension, and adduction movements.

Coccyx The four small vertebral bones making up the "tailbone."

Cognitive stage The first stage of learning a motor skill in which performers make many gross errors and have highly variable performances.

Cognitive domain One of the three domains of learning, which describes intellectual activities and involves the learning of knowledge.

Collagen The main constituent of connective tissue, such as ligaments, tendons, and muscles.

Combinations Defined as two or more movement patterns combined and repeated in sequence several times in a row.

Command style A teaching style in which the instructor makes all decisions about posture, rhythm and duration, while participants follow the instructor's directions and movements.

Compilation law An original, and hence copyrightable, sequence or program of dance steps or exercise routines that may or may not be copyrightable in themselves.

Complex Carbohydrates The starches or long chains of sugars in whole grain breads and cereals, vegetables, fruits, and dried peas and beans.

Compulsive overeating and/or overexercising A compelling urge to overeat or overexercise, which is emotionally destructive, physically draining and may progress to anorexia nervosa and bulimia.

Concentric contraction See Concentric muscle action.

Concentric muscle action Contraction of a muscle in which the muscle shortens, or the proximal and distal attachments of the muscle come closer together.

Connective tissue The tissue that binds together and supports various structures of the body. Ligaments and tendons are connective tissues.

Contractile proteins The protein myofilaments that are essential for muscle contraction.

Contracts An agreement or promise between two or more parties which creates a legal obligation to do or not to do something.

Contraindication Any condition that renders some particular movement, activity or treatment improper or undesirable.

Contusion Slight bleeding into soft tissue as a result of a blow. More commonly known as a bruise.

Copyright The exclusive right, for a certain number of years, to perform, make, and distribute copies and otherwise use an artistic, musical or literary work.

Coronary artery disease (CAD) CAD is also referred to as coronary heart disease (CHD). Cardiovascular diseases include coronary artery disease, hypertension, stroke, congestive heart failure, peripheral vascular disease and valvular heart disease. CAD is almost always caused by atherosclerosis.

Coronary heart disease (CHD) The major form of cardiovascular disease; almost always the result of atherosclerosis.

Corrective statement Used when a response is incorrect, the statement identifies the error and tells the learner how to correct it.

Coupled Reactions The linking or bonding of two substances undergoing chemical change.

Creatine phosphate (CP) A high-energy phosphate molecule that is stored in cells and can be used to resynthesize ATP immediately. One of the phosphagens.

Cross bridges The tiny projections which extend from the myosin myofilaments toward the actin myofilaments.

Cueing A visual or verbal technique, using hand signals or only a few words, to inform exercise participants of upcoming movements.

Deductible The amount the insured must pay in the event of an insurance loss.

Defendant The party in a lawsuit who is being sued or accused.

Dehydration The condition resulting from excessive loss of body fluids.

Delayed onset muscle soreness (DOMS) Muscle soreness or aching that occurs with contraction approximately 24 to 48 hours after strenuous exercise.

Dependence The condition of being influenced or controlled by something else.

Depression The action of lowering a muscle or bone.

Diabetes mellitus A disease of carbohydrate metabolism, in which an absolute or relative deficiency of insulin results in an inability to normally metabolize carbohydrates.

Diabetic coma A state of deep unconsciousness resulting from of uncontrolled diabetes.

Diarthroses A type of articulation (joint) that is freely moveable (as opposed to immovable or slightly movable).

Diastasis recti The separation of the recti abdominal muscles along the midline of the body.

Dietary Fat See Triglycerides.

Directional cueing A visual or verbal technique that tells participants in which direction to move.

Disability insurance Insurance which provides income protection in the event of an injury to the instructor.

Distal Farthest from the midline of the body, or from the point of attachment of a body part.

Diuretics Medications that produce an increase in urine volume and sodium (salt) excretion.

Dorsal Referring to the top or upper surface, as in the top of the foot.

Dorsiflexion Movement of the foot up toward the shin.

Downbeat The beat or beats receding the metrical accent.

Duration The total time of each exercise session.

Dynamic stretching See also ballistic stretching.

Dyspnea "Air hunger" resulting in difficult

or labored breathing.

Dyspnea scale A scale used to monitor exercise intensity as determined by respiration effort.

Eccentric contraction See Eccentric muscle action.

Eccentric muscle action A muscle action in which the muscle lengthens against a resistance while producing force.

Electrocardiogram (EKG or ECG) A recording of the electrical activity of the heart.

Elevation The action of raising a muscle or bone.

Emergency Medical System (EMS) A system found in many areas to provide fast, easy contact with police, fire and emergency rescue teams.

Emphysema A serious form of obstructive pulmonary disease. It is characterized by the gradual destruction of lung alveoli and the connective tissue surrounding them, in addition to airway inflammation. Most emphysema patients are long time smokers. The loss of lung tissues leads to a reduction in the ability to inhale and exhale, making breathing extremely difficult.

Energy balance The principle that body weight will stay the same when caloric intake equals caloric expenditure, and that a positive or negative balance will cause a weight gain or weight loss.

Energy imbalances The result of being overweight, underweight or obese caused by overeating or undereating, overexercising or underexercising and/or medical conditions.

Energy The potential to do work and activity: measured in calories derived from carbohydrates, fat or protein.

Epicondylitis See "tennis elbow".

Ergogenic An energy enhancer.

Essential Body Fat One of two major types of body fat, reflects that amount of body fat that is required for normal physiological functioning. This body fat is found in bone, muscle e, nerve, and major organs of the body, and also includes sex-specific fat found in women.

Essential fat Fat that cannot be produced by the body and must be supplied by the diet. The only essential fat is linoleic acid.

Estrogen The hormones produced by the ovary.

Eversion Rotation of the foot to direct the plantar surface outward.

Exercise intensity The specific level of physical activity at which a person exercises that can be quantified (e.g., heart rate, work, RPE) and is usually reflected as a percentage of one's maximal capacity to do work.

Exercise Induced Asthma (EIA) Over 80% of all asthmatics experience asthma during exercise. EIA is probably caused by the cooling and then drying of the respiratory tract that accompanies the inspiration of large volumes of dry air during exercise.

Exercise physiology The study of how the body functions during physical activity and exercise.

Exercise Specificity See Specificity Principle

Extension Movement that increases the angle between two bones of a joint, such as straightening the elbow.

External Opposed to medial or internal, exterior.

Fast twitch (FT) fiber Type of muscle fiber characterized by its fast speed of contraction and a high capacity for anaerobic glycolysis.

Fat mass The total amount of body fat stores that exist as storage fat and essential body fat. Usually, this term is expressed as either an absolute amount of weight or a relative percentage of body weight.

Fatty acid The building block of dietary fat. An important nutrient for the production of energy during low-intensity exercise.

Fatty acid oxidation The aerobic (oxygen-requiring) breakdown of fatty acids for the production of ATP.

Feedback An internal response within a

learner. During information processing, it is the correctness or incorrectness of a response that is stored in memory to be used for future reference.

Fetus   The developed embryo and growing human in the uterus, from usually three months after conception to birth.

Field tests   Fitness tests that can be used in mass testing situations.

FITT principle   Using the criteria of frequency (F), intensity (I), time (T) and type of activity (T) to individualize an exercise program.

Flexibility   The range of motion possible about a joint.

Flexion   The movement that decreases the angle between two bones of a joint.

Footwork cueing   A visual or verbal technique that tells exercisers which foot to move.

Force arm   The lever arm (the perpendicular distance from the axis to the line of the force) length of the motive force.

Force   A push or a pull, which causes or tends to cause a change in a body's motion or shape

Fracture   Any break in the continuity of a bone, ranging from a simple crack to severe shatter of the bone with multiple fracture fragments.

Freestyle method   A way of designing the aerobics segment of a class that uses movements randomly chosen by the instructor.

Frequency   Refers to the number of exercise sessions per week resulting in a training effect.

Frontal plane   A plane that divides the body into front (anterior) and back (posterior) halves.

General liability insurance   Insurance for bodily injury or property damage resulting from general negligence such as wet flooring, an icy walkway or poorly maintained equipment.

Glucose   A simple sugar; the simplest form in which all carbohydrates are used by the body for the production of energy (ATP).

Glycogen   The storage form of glucose found in the liver and muscles.

Glycolysis   The metabolic process whereby glucose is chemically broken down to produce energy (ATP). Glycolysis occurs with or without the presence of oxygen (aerobic or anaerobic).

Golgi tendon organs   A sensory organ within a tendon that, when stimulated, causes an inhibition of the entire muscle group to protect against too much force.

HDL-C-total cholesterol ratio   The ration between high-density lipoprotein cholesterol and the total of all forms of cholesterol in the body. See also High-density lipoprotein cholesterol and total cholesterol.

Heart rate   The number of beats of the heart per minute.

Heart-rate reserve   The result of subtracting the resting heart rate from the maximal heart rate. It represents the working heart-rate range between rest and maximal heart rate within which all activity occurs.

Heat cramp   A muscle spasm induced by physical work in intense heat, or at the onset of warm weather before acclimatization takes place.

Heat exhaustion   A reaction to heat marked by weakness and collapse as a result of water or salt depletion.

Heat stroke   The final stage in heat exhaustion. An extremely dangerous condition, normally manifested by cessation of sweating and dangerously high body temperature.

Hemoconcentration   An increase in the number of red blood cells as a result of a decrease in the volume of plasma.

Hemoglobin (Hb)   Protein molecule in red blood cells specifically adapted to carry (bond) oxygen molecules.

High-density lipoprotein cholesterol (HDL-C)   A plasma complex of lipids and proteins that contains relatively more protein and less cholesterol and triglycerides. High levels of HDL-C are associated with a low risk of coronary heart disease.

Homeostasis State of dynamic equilibrium or stability of physiological function.

Hydration The chemical combination of a substance with water.

Hydrostatic weighing An underwater test used to measure the percentage of lean body weight and body fat, based on the principle that fat floats and muscle and bone sinks.

Hyperextension Extension of an articulation beyond anatomical position.

Hyperglycemia An abnormally high content of sugar in the blood.

Hyperhydration The state obtained by consuming several cups of water 2-3 hours before exercising in the heat, and again shortly before exercising.

Hyperlipidemia/hypercholesterolemia Excessive amounts of cholesterol or fats in the blood.

Hypertension High blood pressure, or the elevation of blood pressure above 140/90 mmHg.

Hyperthermia A life threatening increase in body core temperature.

Hypertrophy An increase in muscle size resulting from an increase in contractile proteins.

Hyperventilation A condition resulting from a higher-than-normal volume of breathing, resulting in an abnormal loss of carbon dioxide from the blood. Dizziness may occur.

Hypocapnia The abnormal loss of carbon dioxide from the body.

Hypoglycemia A deficiency of sugar in the blood commonly caused by too much insulin, too little glucose, or too much exercise in the insulin dependent diabetic. Characterized by such symptoms as dizziness, confusion, headache and anxiety.

Hypoventilation Inability to move enough air through the lung tissues. Usually occurs as a result of either low rate or low depth of breathing.

Hypoxia The decrease in the amount of oxygen in inspired air which usually occurs at high altitudes.

Iliotibial Band Syndrome Characterized by an area of tenderness on the lateral side of the knee where the band crosses the knee. Local swelling may be present.

Incision A cut into body tissue caused by a sharp object or edge.

Inclusion style This teaching style enables multiple levels of performance to be taught within the same activity.

Incontinence The loss of sphincter control which results in the inability to retain urine, semen or feces.

Independent contractors People who conduct business on their own on a contract basis and are not employees of an organization.

Individualized medical insurance Insurance which provides hospitalization and major medical coverage.

Inferior Below.

Informed consent A written statement that is signed by each client prior to testing that informs the client of the testing purpose(s) and its processes, along with all potential risks (e.g., muscular soreness to death) and discomforts of the testing procedures.

Inguinal ligament The ligament that extends from the anterior, superior, iliac spine to the pubic tubercle.

Insulin A hormone, secreted into the bloodstream by the pancreas, that helps regulate carbohydrate metabolism.

Insulin shock The condition produced when an excessive amount of insulin is present in the bloodstream. Characterized by pale, moist skin; a full, rapid pulse; dizziness or headache; disorientation; and fainting with possible unconsciousness.

Insulin-dependent diabetes See diabetes mellitus.

Intensity The physiological stress on the body during exercise. Indicates how hard the body should be working to achieve a training effect. Heart rate is generally a reliable way to access exercise intensity.

Internal　Within or on the inside, opposed to external.

Internal fat　Fat stored deep inside the body.

Inversion　Rotation of the foot to direct the plantar surface inward.

Iron-deficiency anemia　See Anemia.

Isokinetic muscle action　A muscle contraction through a range of motion at a constant muscle tension and velocity.

Isokinetic muscle contraction　See Isokinetic muscle action

Isometric muscle action　A muscular contraction in which there is no change in the angle of the involved joint(s) and little or no change in the length of the contracting muscle.

Isometric muscle contraction　See Isometric muscle action.

Isotonic muscle action　A muscular contraction in which a constant load (resistance) is moved through a range of motion of the involved joint(s). Also referred to as a dynamic contraction.

Isotonic muscle contraction　See Isotonic muscle action.

Karvonen formula　The mathematical formula that uses heart-rate reserve (maximal heart rate minis resting heart rate) to determine target heart rate.

Kegel exercises　Exercises designed to gain control of and tone the pelvic floor muscles by controlled isometric contraction and relaxation of the muscles surrounding the vagina.

Kilocalorie (kcal)　The amount of heat needed to increase the temperature of 1 kilogram of water 1°C. One kcal equals 1,000 calories. Kcal is the appropriate term to express energy intake and energy expenditure in nutrition and exercise.

Kinesiology　The study of the principles of mechanics and anatomy in relation to human movement.

Kinesthesis　(see Kinesthetic Awareness).

Kinesthetic Awareness (Kinethesis)　The perception of body position and movement in space.

Knowledge of results (KR)　Feedback from external sources such as the instructor.

Kyphosis　Exaggerated posterior curvature of the thoracic (upper) spine.

Laceration　A wound in the soft tissue that has rough edges from tearing or cutting.

Lactic acid (LA)　A by-product of anaerobic glycolysis known to cause localized muscle fatigue.

Lateral rotation　Rotation of a body part away from the midline of the body.

Lateral flexion　Bending of the vertebral column to the side.

Lateral　Away from the midline of the body, or the outside.

Law of Acceleration　The force F acting on a body in a given direction is equal to the body's mass m multiplied by the body's acceleration a in that direction: $F = ma$, or $a = F/m$.

Law of Inertia　The tendency of all objects and matter to stay still if still, or, if moving, to continue moving in the same direction with the same velocity unless acted upon by an outside force; dependent on a body's mass.

Lean body mass　The metabolically active part of the body. The muscles, bones, nerves, skin or organs of the body. That component of the body excluding fatty tissue.

Learning　Internal changes in a person inferred from an external improvement in performance as a result of practice.

Lecithin　One of the phospholipids which is a compound of glycerol attached to fatty acids and a choline molecule. The lecithin you need for building cell membranes and for other functions is made from scratch by the liver.

Lever　A rigid bar that rotates around a

fixed support (fulcrum) in response to an applied force

Liability Legal responsibility.

Ligament Strong, fibrous tissue that connects one bone to another.

Linear Motion Movement in a straight (recti-) or curved (curvi-) line by an object which is not fixed at any point.

Linear progression Consists of one movement that transitions into another without cycling sequences.

Lipid Fat.

Lipoprotein lipase An enzyme that stimulates fat storage.

Lipoproteins A complex of lipid and protein molecules, which transport cholesterol and other lipids throughout the body. Includes high-density lipoproteins (HDLs), low-density lipoproteins (LDLs) and very low-density lipoproteins (VLDLs).

Lordosis An exaggerated anterior curvature of the lumbar spine. Often referred to as swayback.

Low back pain (LBP) A general term to describe a multitude of back conditions, including muscular and ligament strains, sprains and injuries. The cause of LBP is often elusive, most LBP is probably caused by muscle weakness and imbalances.

Low-density lipoprotein cholesterol (LDL-C) A plasma complex of lipids and proteins that contains relatively more cholesterol and triglycerides and less protein. High levels of LDL-C are associated with an increased risk of coronary heart disease.

Lumbar vertebrae The five vertebrae in the low back, just below the thoracic vertebrae and just above the sacrum.

Mass The quantity of matter anything contains; the property of a physical body that gives it inertia (its resistance to change in its state of motion). Mass is a constant and is independent of gravity.

Maximal exercise test A test that continues until a person has reached a maximal level

(VO$_2$ max) or voluntary exhaustion. The most accurate way to evaluate cardiovascular fitness.

Maximal oxygen uptake The point at which oxygen consumption reaches a period of little or no change with an additional workload.

Maximal heart rate The highest heart rate a person can attain.

Maximal heart rate formula A formula for determining target heart rate based on a percentage of the maximal heart rate.

Measure One group of beats in a musical composition marked by the regular occurrence of the heavy accent.

Medial Toward the midline of the body, or the inside.

Medial rotation Rotation of a body part toward the midline.

Medical clearance Indication by a physician that a person can safely participate in a specific exercise program.

Meniscus tears An acute injury characterized by tears in either the medial or lateral meniscus, a gristly substance (cartilage) lining the top surface of the tibia (lower leg bone).

Metabolism The chemical and physical processes in the body that provide energy for the maintenance of life.

Metatarsalgia A general term describing pain in the ball of the foot, usually under the second and third metatarsal heads caused by bruising the metatarsal joints of the foot.

Meter The organization of beats into musical patterns or measures.

Minerals Inorganic compounds that serve a variety of important functions in the body.

Mitochondria Structures located within muscle cells that contain the enzymes responsible for the generation of adenosine triphosphate by aerobic mechanisms.

Mobility The degree to which an articulation is allowed to move before being restricted by surrounding tissues.

Monounsaturated fats A type of unsaturated fat (liquid at room temperature) that has one spot on the fatty acid for the addition of a hydrogen atom. Examples: oleic acid in olive oil.

Motivation To urge or rouse excitement.

Motive force The force that starts or causes a movement.

Motor domain One of the three domains of learning, which involves the learning of motor skills.

Motor unit A motor neuron and all of the muscle fibers in innervates.

Motor end plate The synaptic connection between a motor neuron and a skeletal muscle cell.

Motor skill Physical performance or attributes including or related to agility, balance, and coordination.

Motor neuron A neuron that sends electrochemical impulses from the spinal cord to the muscle fibers causing muscular contraction.

Multiarticulate A muscle that crosses more than two articulations, causing motion at each joint. (Note: The biceps brachi is the only "multiarticulate" muscle in the body.)

Muscle spindle The sensory organ within a muscle that is sensitive to stretch and thus protects the muscle against too much stretch.

Muscular endurance The capacity of a muscle to exert force repeatedly, or to hold a fixed or static contraction over time.

Muscular strength The maximum force that can be exerted by a muscle or muscle group.

Myocardial ischemia Deficiency of blood supply to the heart muscle.

Myocardial infarction Death of a portion of the heart muscle from interruption of the blood supply. Commonly called heart attack.

Myofibril Element of muscle which contains the contractile actin and myosin proteins.

Myosin Contractile protein in a myofibril.

Negligence Failure of a person to perform as a reasonable and prudent professional would perform under similar circumstances.

Nerve Cell A neuron consisting of a cell body and an axon and one or more dendrites.

Neuron A nerve cell, consisting of a cell body, axon and dendrites.

Neutral posture To maintain the natural curves of the back without flexion, extension, rotation, or excessive anterior pelvic tilt.

Neutral statement Feedback to the student that acknowledges performance but does not judge or correct the performance.

Neutral spinal alignment See Neutral Posture.

Nitroglycerin A drug that dilates the blood vessels; used to treat angina pectoris.

Non-insulin dependent diabetes (NIDDM) See diabetes mellitus.

Nondramatic performing rights The right to play a song on its own or with other songs, but not to accompany the song with dialogue, scenery or costumes, and not to use the song to tell a story.

Numerical cueing A visual or verbal technique used by instructors to count the rhythm of the exercise, such as "1 and 2, 3, 4."

Nutrients Components of food needed by the body. There are six classes of nutrients: water, minerals, vitamins, protein, carbohydrates and fats.

Nutrition The study of nutrients in foods and of their digestion, absorption, metabolism, interaction, storage and excretion.

Obese A term to describe excess accumulation of body fat and is commonly defined when body fat for men exceeds 25 percent and 30 percent for women.

Obesity The accumulation and storage of excess body fat. Usually defined as at least 20% above ideal weight or more than 30% body fat for women and more than 23% body fat for men.

Osteoarthritis A degenerative disease caused by wearing away of cartilage, leaving two surfaces of bone in contact with each other. It is characterized by decreased mobility and pain during movement and is primarily found in older adults.

Osteoporosis A disorder, primarily affecting women past menopause, in which bone mass decreases and susceptibility to fracture increases.

Overload principle The principle that a physiological system or organ subjected to a greater-than-normal load (stress) will respond by increasing in strength or function.

Overweight A term to describe an excessive amount of weight for a given height, using height-to-weight indices.

Oxidative enzymes Protein substances needed in very small quantities to activate oxidative or aerobic metabolic processes.

Oxidative glycolysis See aerobic glycolysis.

Oxygen consumption (VO2) The process in which oxygen is used to produce energy for cellular work. Also called oxygen uptake.

Oxygen carrying capacity Refers to the quantity of oxygen that can be carried (bonded) by the blood protein, hemoglobin.

Oxygen uptake See oxygen consumption.

Oxygen debt The oxygen uptake during recovery from exercise in excess of the oxygen uptake normally observed during a rest period of similar duration. Represents the oxygen uptake that "pans back" the oxygen deficit.

Oxygen deficit The difference between the total oxygen requirement of a physical activity and the oxygen actually used during the activity. Represents the anaerobic contribution to a movement.

Palpate To examine by touch, as in determining the heart rate by feeling the pulse at the radial or carotid arteries.

Palpation Use of the finger tips to detect anatomical structures or pulse rate.

Part approach Teaching a skill part by part instead of all at once.

Partial Pressure The pressure of each gas in a multiple gas system, such as air, which is composed of nitrogen, oxygen and Co2.

Pelvic floor The muscles and tissues that act as a support or reinforcement to the lower border of the pelvis.

Performing rights society An organization to which the copyright or publisher assigns the nondramatic performing rights in the musical composition. The two performing rights societies in the United States are ASCAP and BMI.

Perfusion Pumping of a fluid through an organ or tissue.

Perineal The fibromuscular tissue located between the lower part of the vagina and the anal canal.

Phosphagen System An anaerobic pathway consisting of the ATP-CP system.

Phosphagens Adenosine triphosphate (ATP) and creatine phosphate (CP), two high-energy phosphate molecules that can be broken down for immediate use by the cells.

Phospholipid A fatty substance that has a fat-soluble end and a water-soluble end. It is an essential part of cell membranes and does not supply calories.

Phrase Composed of at least two measures of music.

Physical fitness The physical components of well-being that enable a person to function at an optimal level.

Placenta The vascular organ in mammals that unites the fetus to the maternal uterus and mediates its metabolic exchanges.

Plaintiff A party who brings a suit against another party in a court of law.

Plantar fascitis Inflammation of the plantar fascia, a broad band of connective tissue running along the sole of the foot. This inflammation is caused by stretching or tearing the tissue, usually near the attachment at the heel.

Plantar flexion Movement of the foot toward the sole of the foot.

Plaque A deposit of fatty or fibrous material

in side arterial walls, causing the arteries to narrow and lose their elasticity.

Plasma The liquid portion of the blood.

Polyunsaturated fats A type of unsaturated fat (liquid at room temperature) that has two or more spots on the fatty acid available for hydrogen. Examples: corn, safflower, soybean oils.

Posterior Toward the back or dorsal side.

Postmenopausal The period of time after menopause.

Postpartum The period of time after childbirth.

Practice style A teaching style that provides opportunities for individualization and includes practice time and private instructor feedback for each participant.

Primary bronchi The two main branches of the trachea or windpipe.

Primary risk factor A characteristic or behavior that, by itself, is significantly associated with a major health problem.

Prime mover A muscle responsible for a specific movement.

Professional liability insurance Insurance to protect against professional negligence or failure of an instructor to perform as a competent and prudent professional would under similar circumstances.

Progesterone A hormone produced by the corpus luteum, adrenal cortex and placenta whose function is to facilitate growth of the embryo.

Pronation Rotating the palm downward; a combination of ankle dorsiflexion, subtalar eversion and foot abduction.

Prone Facing downward.

Proprioceptive Neuromuscular Facilitation (PNF) A method of promoting the response of neuromuscular mechanisms through the stimulation of proprioceptors in an attempt to gain more stretch in a muscle. Often referred to as a contract/relax method of stretching.

Proprioceptors Specialized nerve endings in muscles, tendons and joints that are sensitive to changes in tension during activity, giving a body part a sense of where it is in space.

Protein A compound composed of amino acids that is the major structural component of all body tissue. A **complete protein** is a protein containing all nine amino acids essential to health.

Proximal Nearest to the midline of the body or point of attachment of a body part.

Public performance Playing a recording of a copyrighted musical composition at a place where a substantial number of persons outside of a normal circle of a family and its social acquaintances are gathered.

Publisher The entity to which the owner of a copyrighted artistic, musical or literary work assigns such copyright for licensing and income collection purposes.

Pulmonary function The functional capacity of the lungs, including lung volume, breathing rate and vital capacity.

Pulse rate The wave of pressure in the arteries that occurs each time the heart beats.

Puncture A penetrating wound caused by a pointed object.

Quality of life Overall positive feeling and enthusiasm for life, without fatigue from routine activities.

Radial pulse A pulse point located on the thumb side of the wrist.

Range of motion (ROM) The number of degrees that an articulation will allow one of its segments to move.

Rating of perceived exertion (RPE) A scale that correlates the participants perception of exercise effort with the actual intensity level.

Receptor Nerve tissue that is sensitive to changes in its environment.

Reciprocal style A teaching style that involves using an observer or partner to provide feedback to the performer.

Recommended Dietary Allowance (RDA) The daily amount of a nutrient recommended for practically all healthy persons to obtain optimal health.

Recovery heart rate The number of heartbeats per minute following the cessation of vigorous physical activity. As cardiorespiratory fitness improves, the heart rate returns to resting levels more quickly.

Regional fat distribution The location of fat storage on the body (hips, thighs, abdomen). May be as important a variable for health risk as the degree of overweight.

Rehearsal effect A learning principle. Rehearsing motor patterns in the warm-up enhances performance when the same patterns are used later in the class.

Relative humidity The amount of moisture in the air compared to the maximum amount that the air could contain at the same temperature, amount is expressed as a percentage.

Relaxin A hormone of pregnancy that softens connective tissue.

Repetition reduction Involves reducing the number of repetitions that make up a movement sequence.

Repetitions The number of successive contractions performed during each weight-training exercise.

Residual lung volume The amount of air remaining in the lungs following a maximal exhalation.

Resistive force A force that resists another force.

Respiration The exchange of oxygen and carbon dioxide between the cells and the atmosphere.

Respiratory ventilation The movement of air into and out of the lungs.

Resting heart rate The number of heartbeats per minute when the body is at complete rest; usually counted first thing in the morning before any physical activity.

Reversibility principle The principle in which training adaptations will gradually decline if the altered system or organ is not suffi-

ciently stressed on a regular basis.

Rheumatoid arthritis A chronic disease caused by an immune reaction that results in the inflammation of the membrane surrounding joints. It is characterized by pain and swelling in one or more joints.

Rhythm A regular pattern of movement or sound that can be felt, seen or heard.

Rhythmic cueing A visual or verbal technique that indicates the correct rhythm of an exercise or step pattern, such as slow (2 counts) or quick (1 count).

Rhythmic variation Allows participants to learn complex movement at a slower pace.

RICE An immediate treatment for injury: rest, ice, compression and elevation.

Risk factors A characteristic, inherited trait, or behavior related to the presence or development of a condition or disease.

Risk management Minimizing the risks of potential legal liability.

Rotary Motion Movement by an object around a fixed point or axis.

Rotation Movement of a body part around its longitudinal axis.

Round ligament The ligaments which are found on the side of the uterus near the fallopian tube insertion to help the broad ligament keep the uterus in place.

Sagittal plane A plane that divides the body into right and left halves.

Sarcomere A repeating unit of muscle fiber; sarcomeres shorten when muscles contract.

Saturated fats Fatty acids carrying the maximum number of hydrogen atoms. These fats are solid at room temperature and are usually of animal origin.

Sciatica Severe pain in the leg running from the back of the thigh down the inside of the leg as a result of the compression of, or trauma to the sciatic nerve.

Scoliosis A lateral curvature of the vertebrae column, usually in the thoracic area.

Scope of practice The range and limit of

responsibilities normally associated with a specific job or position.

Secondary risk factor A characteristic symptom, behavior, or condition that, by itself, has a weak association with a disease, but increases the risk when other risk factors are present.

Seizure An attack, such as a convulsion.

Self-check style A teaching style that relies on individual performers to provide their own feedback.

Sensory neuron A neuron that sends electrochemical impulses from a sensory organ to the spinal cord. Responsible for sensation.

Serum ferritin A storage iron which is measured, in conjunction with hemoglobin, to determined if an iron deficiency is present.

Shin splints A general term for any pain or discomfort on the front or side of the lower leg, in the region of the shin bone (tibia). A common, chronic aerobics injury with several causes.

Shock A circulatory disturbance produced by severe injury or illness, in which there is inadequate perfusion of blood through the body tissues.

Simple carbohydrates The refined sugars, such as table sugar, honey, brown sugar, corn syrup and the naturally occurring sugars in milk and fruit.

Skinfold assessment The most widely used method to ascertain body fat, which is determined by specific anatomical location and measurement of subcutaneous fatfolds.

Skinfold caliper An instrument used to measure the thickness of skinfolds at various sites on the body. The measurements are used to estimate the percent of body fat.

Sliding filament theory A generally accepted theory explaining the interaction between actine and myosine proteins and ATP to cause muscle contraction.

Slow twitch (ST) fiber A type of muscle fiber characterized by its slow speed of contraction and a high capacity for aerobic glycolysis.

Specificity Principle A specific exercise demand made on the body will result in a specific response by the body.

Sphincter A circular muscle whose function is constricting an opening.

Sphygmomanometer Blood pressure cuff.

Spot reducing The effort to reduce fat at specific sites by exercising the muscles at those sites. A popular but false concept.

Sprain Overstretching or tearing of a ligament and/or joint capsule, resulting in discoloration, swelling and pain.

Stabilizer muscles Muscles that stabilize one joint, so a desired movement can be performed in another joint.

Standard of care Appropriateness of an exercise professional's actions, in light of current professional standards and based on the age, condition and knowledge of the participant.

Static Stretching A low force, long duration stretch that holds the desired muscle at their greatest possible length for 15 to 30 seconds.

Statute of Limitations A formal regulation limiting the period within which a specific legal action may be taken.

Step cueing A visual or verbal technique that refers to the name of the step in an aerobics routine, such as "step, ball, change".

Step test (submaximal) A test for cardiovascular fitness which requires the subject to step up and down from a bench at a prescribed rate for a given period. There are several different step test protocols.

Storage fat The fat (adipose tissue) that surrounds internal body organs for protection and at least 50% of storage fat is found just under the skin (subcutaneous fat).

Strain Overstretching or tearing of a muscle or tendon.

Strength See Muscular strength

Stress fracture An incomplete fracture caused by excessive stress (overuse) to a bone. Most common in the foot (metatarsal bones) and lower leg (tibia).

Stretch Reflex An involuntary muscle contraction initiated by stimulation of a muscle spindle within that muscle.

Stroke volume The volume of blood pumped from the left ventricle in one cycle of a heart beat.

Structured method A way of designing the aerobics segment of a class that uses formally arranged step patterns, repeated in a predetermined order.

Subcutaneous fat One site of storage fat that is located beneath the skin and is directly related to the amount of total body fat.

Submaximal exercise test A test to evaluate cardiorespiratory fitness, performed at less than maximal effort and terminated before exhaustion.

Substrate A fuel source for energy metabolism.

Superior Located above.

Supination A combination of ankle plantar flexion, subtalar inversion and foot adduction.

Supine hypotension An abnormal reduction in blood pressure related to position (lying on the back).

Supine Face up.

Sympathetic Related to the sympathetic nervous system, which is a division of the autonomic nervous system that activates the body to cope with some stressor, (i.e. fight or flight).

Symphysis pubis The fibrocartilaginous joint between the pelvic bones in the midline of the body.

Synarthroses A type of articulation that is immovable.

Syncopation A rhythmic device which temporarily shifts the normal pattern of stresses to unstressed beats or parts of beats.

Synergist A muscle that aids another muscle in its action.

Systolic blood pressure The pressure exerted by the blood on the vessel walls during ventricular contraction.

Talk test A method for measuring exercise intensity using observation of respiration effort and the ability to talk while exercising.

Target heart rate The number of heartbeats per minute that indicate appropriate exercise intensity levels for each person. Also called training heart rate.

Target heart-rate range The exercise intensity that represents the minimum and maximum intensity for safe and effective exercise. Also referred to as training zone.

Task complexity The number of parts or components within a task and the level of information processing required to complete the task.

Task organization The extent to which the parts of a task are interrelated. In a task that is high in organization, the parts that constitute the task are closely related to one another. In a task low in organization, the parts are independent.

Tempo The rate of speed at which a musical composition is played.

Temporal pulse Pulse point located on either temple.

Tendinitis An inflammatory response to microtrauma from overuse of a tendon.

Tendon Strong, fibrous connective tissue that attaches a muscle to a bone.

Tennis elbow Pain on the outside of the elbow at the attachment of the forearm muscles.

Teratogenic Nongenetic factors that can cause birth defects in the fetus.

Thoracic vertebrae The twelve vertebrae to which the ribs are attached.

Tidal volume The amount of air that passes in and out of the lungs in an ordinary breath.

Torque A force causing rotation about a fixed point; the act or process of turning around a center or axis.

Transient osteoporosis The temporary increase in the porosity of the bone as a result of dietary calcium deficiency.

Transverse plane A plane that divides the

body into upper (superior) and lower (inferior) parts.

Triglycerides　The storage form of fat consisting of three free fatty acids and glycerol.

Type I Diabetes　A result of destruction of the insulin producing beta cells in the pancreas. Type I diabetics produce little or no insulin and are thus required to inject insulin on a daily basis.

Type II Diabetes　The most common form of diabetes. It results from an inability to use the insulin produced by the pancreas because of reduced sensitivity of the insulin target cells. Type II diabetics produce insulin, but are not able to use the insulin they produce. Type II diabetes is often corrected by diet, exercise and oral medication.

Underweight　Condition in which lack of body fat and/or lean muscle tissue puts the individual in health risk or at a disadvantage for certain competitive sports.

Unsaturated fats　Fatty acids that contain double bonds between carbon atoms and thus are capable of absorbing more hydrogen. These fats are liquid at room temperature and usually of vegetable origin.

Upbeat　The beat or beats not receding the metrical accent.

Uteroplacental insufficiency　The inability of the uterus and the placenta to transfer nutrients and oxygen to the fetus due to constriction of the umbilical cord.

Valsalva maneuver　Increased pressure in the thoracic cavity caused by forced exhalation with the breath held.

Value statement　Feedback that projects a feeling about a performance, using such words as "good," "well done," or "poor job."

Vascular disturbances　A disruption of circulation.

Vascularity　The amount of blood vessels in a muscle.

Vasoconstriction　Narrowing of the opening (lumen) of blood vessels caused by contraction of the smooth muscle cells in the

walls of the vessels.

Vasodilation　Widening of the opening (lumen) of blood vessels caused by a relaxation of the smooth muscle cells in the walls of the vessels.

Vein　A blood vessel that carries blood to the heart.

Ventricle　One of the two (left or right) lower chambers of the heart.

Venules　Small blood vessels that carry deoxygenated blood back toward the heart, after converging into veins.

Vertebrae　The bones that form the spinal column.

Vital signs　Measurable bodily functions, including pulse rate, respiratory rate, blood pressure, skin color and temperature.

Vitamins　Organic compounds that function as metabolic regulators in the body. Classified as water soluble or fat soluble.

VO2 max　See Maximal oxygen uptake.

Waiver　Voluntary abandonment of a right to file suit.

Warm-up　The preparatory portion of a workout or exercise session designed to ready the body for vigorous motion. A warm-up period consists of stretching, walking and general exercises designed to stimulate the muscles, heart and lungs.

Water　The most important nutrient in the body responsible for all energy production, temperature control (especially during vigorous exercise), transportation of all nutrients and waster products in and out of the body and lubrication of joints and other structures. A few days without water may result in death.

Wet bulb temperature　A temperature that combines the temperature of the air and the humidity into one reading. When humidity is low, the wet bulb temperature is below air temperature. When humidity is high, the wet bulb temperature is similar to air temperature.

Whole approach　Teaching an entire skill all

at once, instead of part by part.

Yo-yo dieting   A pattern of periodic weight reduction followed by often rapid weight gain. Associated with progressive difficulty with weight maintenance.

Index

Index

Index

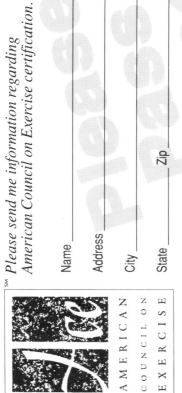

*SM Please send me information regarding
American Council on Exercise certification.*

Name _____

Address _____

City _____

State _____ Zip _____

Home Phone ( ) _____

Work Phone ( ) _____

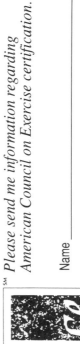
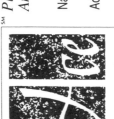

---

*SM Please send me information regarding
American Council on Exercise certification.*

Name _____

Address _____

City _____

State _____ Zip _____

Home Phone ( ) _____

Work Phone ( ) _____

AMERICAN
COUNCIL ON
EXERCISE

---

*SM Please send me information regarding
American Council on Exercise certification.*

Name _____

Address _____

City _____

State _____ Zip _____

Home Phone ( ) _____

Work Phone ( ) _____

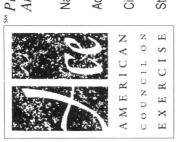

AMERICAN
COUNCIL ON
EXERCISE

---

*SM Please send me information regarding
American Council on Exercise certification.*

Name _____

Address _____

City _____

State _____ Zip _____

Home Phone ( ) _____

Work Phone ( ) _____

AMERICAN
COUNCIL ON
EXERCISE

BUSINESS REPLY MAIL
FIRST CLASS MAIL   PERMIT NO. 202113   SAN DIEGO, CA

POSTAGE WILL BE PAID BY ADDRESSEE

American Council on Exercise
P.O. Box 910449
San Diego, CA 92191-9966

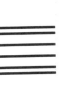

NO POSTAGE
NECESSARY
IF MAILED
IN THE
UNITED STATES

BUSINESS REPLY MAIL
FIRST CLASS MAIL   PERMIT NO. 202113   SAN DIEGO, CA

POSTAGE WILL BE PAID BY ADDRESSEE

American Council on Exercise
P.O. Box 910449
San Diego, CA 92191-9966

NO POSTAGE
NECESSARY
IF MAILED
IN THE
UNITED STATES

BUSINESS REPLY MAIL
FIRST CLASS MAIL   PERMIT NO. 202113   SAN DIEGO, CA

POSTAGE WILL BE PAID BY ADDRESSEE

American Council on Exercise
P.O. Box 910449
San Diego, CA 92191-9966

NO POSTAGE
NECESSARY
IF MAILED
IN THE
UNITED STATES

BUSINESS REPLY MAIL
FIRST CLASS MAIL   PERMIT NO. 202113   SAN DIEGO, CA

POSTAGE WILL BE PAID BY ADDRESSEE

American Council on Exercise
P.O. Box 910449
San Diego, CA 92191-9966

NO POSTAGE
NECESSARY
IF MAILED
IN THE
UNITED STATES